Nutrition and Clinical Dietetics

Herbard Hon

NUTRITION AND CLINICAL DIETETICS

BY

HERBERT S. CARTER, M.A., M.D.

ASSISTANT PROFESSOR OF MEDICINE, COLUMBIA UNIVERSITY; ASSOCIATE ATTEND-
ING PHYSICIAN TO THE PRESBYTERIAN HOSPITAL; CONSULTING
PHYSICIAN TO THE LINCOLN HOSPITAL, NEW YORK

PAUL E. HOWE, M.A., PH.D.

ASSOCIATE IN ANIMAL PATHOLOGY, ROCKEFELLER INSTITUTE FOR MEDICAL
RESEARCH; FORMERLY ASSISTANT PROFESSOR OF BIOLOGICAL CHEMISTRY,
COLUMBIA UNIVERSITY, N. Y.; NUTRITION OFFICER, CAMP KEARNY,
CALIFORNIA; OFFICER IN CHARGE OF LABORATORY OF NUTRITION
ARMY MEDICAL SCHOOL, WASHINGTON, D. C.

HOWARD H. MASON, A.B., M.D.

INSTRUCTOR IN DISEASES OF CHILDREN, COLUMBIA UNIVERSITY, NEW YORK;
ASSOCIATE ATTENDING PHYSICIAN TO THE PRESBYTERIAN HOSPITAL;
ATTENDING PHYSICIAN TO THE RUPTURED AND CRIPPLED
HOSPITAL, NEW YORK

SECOND EDITION, THOROUGHLY REVISED

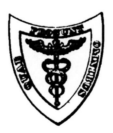

LEA & FEBIGER
PHILADELPHIA AND NEW YORK
1921

PREFACE TO THE SECOND EDITION

The Authors present the second edition of Nutrition and Clinical Dietetics with the hope that it may be found increasingly useful to the general student body as well as to the practitioner.

In Parts I and II there has been made an adequate revision of the chapters on Energy, Metabolism and Digestion, particularly with regard to the physiology of digestion; also an *entire* revision of the chapter on Vitamines, and as well a new chapter on Metabolism in Pregnancy and Lactation together with the Feeding of Children over Two Years O'd.

In Part III there has been a general overhauling of the material in the light of the more recent literature. To Part IV there have been added some fifty odd pages of new material gathered from a careful review of the subject of Dietetics in Disease as found in the publications of the past three years. These additions have been chiefly in the form of the amplification of already existing chapters. In all parts of the book obsolete matter has been eliminated.

H. S. C.
P. E. H.
H. H. M.

CONTENTS

PART I.

FOODS AND NORMAL NUTRITION.

CHAPTER I.

DIGESTION, ABSORPTION AND EXCRETION.

CHAPTER II.

ENERGY REQUIREMENT.

CHAPTER III.

PROTEIN REQUIREMENT.

CHAPTER IV.

INORGANIC SALTS AND WATER.

CHAPTER V.

FOOD REQUIREMENTS IN PREGNANCY AND LACTATION. FOOD REQUIREMENTS AND FEEDING OF CHILDREN. FASTING.

CHAPTER VI.

NORMAL FEEDING AND FOOD ECONOMICS.

PART II.

FOODS.

CHAPTER VII.

INTRODUCTION—MILK.

CHAPTER VIII.

Protein Foods.

CHAPTER IX.

Meat or Flesh Food.

CHAPTER X.

Fish and Shell Fish—Poultry and Game.

CHAPTER XI.

Eggs and Cheese.

CHAPTER XII.

Protein-rich Vegetable Foods.

CHAPTER XIII.

CARBOHYDRATE-RICH FOODS.

CHAPTER XIV.

FAT-RICH FOODS.

CHAPTER XV.

FOODS VALUABLE FOR THEIR SALTS, WATER, AND BULK.

PART III.

FEEDING IN INFANCY AND CHILDHOOD.
CHAPTER XVI.
BREAST FEEDING—FEEDING NORMAL AND ABNORMAL CHILDREN.

CHAPTER XVII.
ARTIFICIAL FEEDING.

CHAPTER XVIII.
FEEDING OF THE PREMATURE INFANT. FEEDING AFTER THE FIRST YEAR. FEEDING DURING ACUTE ILLNESS AND IN NUTRITIONAL DISTURBANCES.

PART IV.

FEEDING IN DISEASE.

CHAPTER XIX.

DIET IN DISEASES OF THE CIRCULATORY ORGANS.

CHAPTER XX.

DIET IN DISEASES OF THE LUNGS.

CHAPTER XXI.

DIET IN DISEASES OF THE STOMACH.

CHAPTER XXII.

DIET IN DISEASES OF THE INTESTINES.

CHAPTER XXIII.

DIET IN DISEASES OF THE ACCESSORY DIGESTIVE GLANDS.

CHAPTER XXIV.

DIET IN DISEASES OF THE SKIN.

CHAPTER XXV.

DIET IN DISEASES OF THE GENITO-URINARY SYSTEM.

CHAPTER XXVI.

DIET IN DISEASES OF PATHOLOGICAL STATES DUE TO DISTURBANCES OF NORMAL METABOLISM.

CHAPTER XXVII.
Diet in Blood Diseases.

CHAPTER XXVIII.

DIET IN DEFICIENCY DISEASES.

CHAPTER XXIX.

DIET IN DISEASES OF THE NERVOUS SYSTEM.

CHAPTER XXX.

DIET IN ACUTE AND CHRONIC INFECTIONS.

CHAPTER XXXI.

DIET IN RELATION TO SURGICAL OPERATIONS.

CHAPTER XXXII.

DIET IN DISEASES OF THE DUCTLESS GLANDS.

CHAPTER XXXIII.

DIET IN MISCELLANEOUS CONDITIONS.

CHAPTER XXXIV.

FOOD PROTECTION.   ACCESSORY FOOD.   BEVERAGES.

CHAPPTE XXXV.

TABLES OF FOOD VALUES AND WEIGHTS AND MEASURES.

NUTRITION AND CLINICAL DIETETICS

INTRODUCTION

THE term food may be applied to any material with the aid of which the body is able to maintain its characteristic functions: temperature regulation, the performance of work, the repair of wasted tissues, the production of new tissues, and those countless factors—connoted by digestion, absorption, circulation, etc.—involved in the preparation and transportation of the ingested food to the seat of action of the prime factor of organization, the cell.

In the various kinds of cells of a complicated organism such as the human body, transformations are in progress which are qualitatively similar but which vary quantitatively according to their specific functions: thus we have the cells of the muscular system, whose chief function appears to be the performance of work and the liberation of energy for the maintenance of body temperature, or the cells of the glandular organs which form substances to be secreted into or from the body, and of the nervous system which are concerned in the conveyance of impulses. Whatever may be the specialized function of any cell, it is imbued with the fundamental characteristic activities of all cells. The sum total of the activities of the individual cell or of the body as a whole are grouped under the term metabolism, by which we mean "all chemical and physical changes which occur in living matter and which constitute the basis of the material phenomena of life." When such changes involve the transformation of simple into more complex substances, they are usually associated with an increase in the energy content of the compounds formed, and are designated as *anabolic processes*. Changes which are concerned with the disintegration of complex material with the formation of simpler products are designated as *catabolic processes* and are ordinarily associated with the liberation of energy. By means of anabolic processes the products of digestion are built up

2

into the active structural compounds of protoplasm, into secretions, or into complexes suitable for storage and future use. Such processes predominate in growth and in those organs or tissues associated with the elaboration of secretions. The catabolic processes involve a disruption of food-stuffs, of cell components, or of reserves, and the liberation of energy in the form of heat or mechanical work, the end-products of this activity being finally eliminated from the body. The cellular activities associated with muscular contraction and the regulation of body temperature are pre-eminently catabolic. In normal individual cells and in the body in general there is a nice balance between the anabolic and catabolic processes. Any disturbance of this equilibrium may result in a pathological condition. Considerations of diet in disease are concerned almost entirely with alterations in the balance between anabolic and catabolic activities.

Five important classes of food-stuffs are required to satisfy the needs of the body; the lack of any one of these would result in grave metabolic disturbances. They are: proteins, carbohydrates, fats and lipins, salts and water. To this list of general classes may be added a sixth, the accessory food substances designated as vitamines.

The collective expression, food, is applied to naturally occurring combinations of the food-stuffs enumerated or to products from these. Since most foods are themselves conglomerates of materials which have been associated with life, they contain in different proportions some of all the elements required by the human organism. Thus we have such foods as meat, eggs, etc., in which protein predominates, but which contain also fat, carbohydrates, water, and salts; or certain vegetable foods whose solid material is largely carbohydrate and salts, with a very small proportion of protein and fat.

The functions of the food-stuffs are varied; proteins, carbohydrates, and fats may be utilized by the body as a source of energy, the greater proportion of the energy requirement of the body is supplied, however, by the carbohydrates and fats. Protein serves not only as a source of energy but as the source of amino-acids and radicles necessary for the formation of body protein, secretions, etc. Salts and water, while not the source of energy, are essential factors in the constitution and activity of all parts of the body.

Proteins are, as we have just indicated, important as the chief source of nitrogen-containing substances necessary for life, being colloidal in nature and capable of combining with both acids and bases, and absorbing or entering into loose chemical combinations with salts and water, they share in a most varied activity in the body processes.

In the cycle of life protein is synthetized in the vegetable kingdom, and this protein is utilized in the construction of animal protein. Animals appear to be unable to synthetize the greater number of amino-acids present in the protein molecule, particularly those containing cyclic nuclei. Plants, however, can form the amino-acids and conjugate them into protein. The animal organism is, then, dependent upon the plant for the basal units of its protein molecule. Before plant protein can be used it must be broken down into amino-acids or simple combinations of these, which are then built up into the type of protein characteristic of the particular tissue concerned. The object of feeding is to supply not only protein to the individual, but protein which will furnish the proper kinds and amounts of amino-acids.

The second class of food-stuffs, carbohydrates, are used by the body as a source of energy in the performance of its many internal activities as well as of external work. They are, apparently, more readily accessible for such purposes than protein or fat; in all cases in which a sudden expenditure of energy is involved or in states in which the body is forced to draw upon its reserve supplies the depots of carbohydrate (glycogen) are the first to become depleted, after which the fats and proteins furnish the required nutritive materials. The absence of carbohydrates from the diet often results in pronounced metabolic disturbances, *e. g.*, acidosis.

Chemically, carbohydrates consist of carbon, hydrogen, and oxygen; the hydrogen and oxygen being often present in the proportions in which they occur in water. This last fact was responsible for the name. From the structural point of view we find carbohydrates to be oxidation products of polyhydric alcohols (ketone- or aldehyde-alcohols). Human food usually contains molecules consisting of chains of five or six carbon atoms or multiples of these. Starch, in which form the greater proportion of ingested carbohydrate food exists, is a polymer of the six carbon sugar—glucose.

Fats and lipins serve in a varied capacity in the body. The terms include a number of different types of substances which may be roughly divided into two groups: *fats*, which are combinations of fatty acids and glycerol or other alcohols, and *lipins*, which resemble the fats in certain properties but which differ in chemical constitution. Lipins are substances of a fat-like nature yielding fatty acids or derivatives of fatty acids and some other radicle containing nitrogen or nitrogen and phosphorus. Of the latter group lecithin has been studied extensively; the other groups, such as complexes containing other lipins, protein, carbohydrate, various organic and inorganic compounds, have received little attention and our knowledge of their functions is limited. Recent investigation has indicated that the lipins are important factors in the transportation of fat by the blood stream to the tissues and particularly to the mammary gland. The "fat" of food is a mixture of fats and lipins.

Fats are used almost exclusively in the production of energy or in the regulation of temperature. In temperature regulation it functions in a two-fold manner: it yields energy in the form of heat as the result of oxidation, and it serves as an insulating medium in the form of deposited subcutaneous fat. Chemically considered, fats are combinations of carbon, hydrogen and oxygen. As contrasted with the carbohydrates, fat molecules contain little oxygen, and consequently yield a greater amount of energy upon oxidation. A gram of fat will yield more than twice as much energy in the form of heat as will a gram of carbohydrate. The body appears to prefer carbohydrates, however, for the production of heat, at least for short intervals of time. It stores its energy yielding material as fat; the quantity of carbohydrate stored in the body is comparatively small, not sufficient to last a man more than a day or two even when some fat and protein are consumed at the same time, as in fasting.

Water and salts are concerned not only in the structure of the cells but in the maintenance of normal physical and chemical relations between the parts of the cells—intracellular water and salts—and between the groups of cells which constitute the tissues and organs of the body—extracellular water and salts. Water gives to the blood its fluidity, and this enables it to permeate the cellular structures of the body, carrying with it the dissolved gases and substances used in the activities of the cell. Suspended in the water (colloidal solution) are proteins and organized bodies, the blood cells. The salts which are dissolved in the water assist not only in maintaining normal osmotic conditions between all parts of the body, but also a uniform reaction by combining with acids and bases and transporting them to the lungs and kidneys for excretion.

Recent work has demonstrated the presence of other substances in food which are essential to the normal functioning of the body. The absence of these materials results in pathological changes, and the ingestion of very small amounts is accompanied by rapid recovery. The name "vitamines" has been applied to these substances by Funk. There appear to be at least three types: a substance soluble in fat, designated fat-soluble A, protective against xeropthalmia; a substance soluble in water, designated water-soluble B, protective against beriberi, and another water-soluble substance protective against scurvy. We know little of the chemical nature of these substances but their importance in the diet is, on the other hand, unquestioned.

These, then, are the facts which underlie dietetics, and while they are indisputably exact, much of the success of feeding in disease still must rest on clinical experience; for given hard-and-fast scientific facts the personal equation always enters into the picture and it will always be true that certain individuals will not react to food stimuli in the logical way, idiosyncrasy playing a not inconsiderable role. Since this is true in health, how much greater must be the variation in disease when one considers that all people differ in their habits, environment, age, activity of the glands of secretion, and susceptibility to certain food elements, etc.?

It is undoubtedly true that in health some people eat too much, this being the larger error than that they eat too little; on the other hand, in disease many if not most people eat too little and add an element of starvation to an organism already handicapped by functional disturbances, infections or what not. The crux of the matter lies in selecting a diet suited to the individual conditions under varying circumstances, not alone in quantity but in quality as well. Recent advances in our knowledge of the specific dynamic action of food-stuffs have made it easier to say what food should theoretically suit a certain set of circumstances and on this basis one can, to a certain extent, choose suitable feedings, provided the personal equation is not too insistent.

In certain diseases the indications for diet are clear cut and are largely a matter of rule, adherence to which will usually bring about the result desired, *e. g.*, in obesity, while in others there is no counting on the results, for the foods which suit conditions in one individual will fail to produce the desired result in another, so that while the principles remain the same the individual requirements may be quite different and opportunity is afforded for the practise of nice judgment. In such a disease as typhoid fever this is particularly true, and the best feeding results will be obtained by the medical attendant who gives the most attention to details and uses the best judgment in the selection of foods, both quantitatively and qualitatively. In such conditions it is possible only to indicate the principles to be used in ordering foods, leaving the rest to the individual attendant's discretion. So it is throughout the entire range of disease—there must be a knowledge of the facts in the biochemistry of foods, combined with clinical experience and good judgment if one wishes the best results.

PART I.

FOODS AND NORMAL NUTRITION

CHAPTER I.

DIGESTION, ABSORPTION AND EXCRETION.

DIGESTION

Enzyme Action.—Food, when ingested, is, with but few exceptions, potential nourishment. Before it can be used in the body it must be reduced to simpler forms or liberated from structures unavailable for absorption into the blood. Until food is in a condition readily to pass through the walls of the alimentary tract, it is not available as a factor in metabolism. Such transformations are accomplished in the processes of digestion. As the result of these, solid masses of food are disintegrated, insoluble carbohydrates, fat, and protein complexes are transformed into compounds which are soluble or of such size (ultramicroscopic) that they may readily traverse the walls of the alimentary tract and finally reach the blood and be carried to the various cellular structures of the body. This conversion of heterogenous food masses into a pabulum of comparatively simple and uniform consistency is accomplished with the aid of enzymes (ferments),[1] whose activities are furthered by the mechanical movements of the alimentary tract.

Enzyme action is catalytic in nature. In the presence of enzymes the rate of digestive activity increases. In the presence of water or dilute solutions of alkalis or acids, the conversion of starch into maltose proceeds slowly. The addition of the salivary amylase, ptyalin, to a starch mixture under suitable conditions of alkalinity and temperature, increases the rate of the process; instead of requiring a period of days and weeks for the completion of the digestion of a

[1] While we will confine our discussion largely to the enzymes of the digestive tract, it must be remembered that enzymes are present in all tissues and fluids of the body.

given mass of material, a few minutes or hours suffice. These changes are produced, furthermore, at the comparatively low temperature of the body.

Enzyme action is specific; for each kind of substance to be changed a special enzyme is elaborated. If many intermediate products are formed, more than one enzyme may be required to reduce a food material to its simplest state. Ptyalin, the salivary amylase, can carry the digestion of starch only as far as the maltose stage. Another enzyme, maltase, is required for the cleavage of maltose in the formation of glucose. This enzyme is restricted in its action to maltose and glucose; it cannot change sucrose or lactose or any other carbohydrate. To complete the digestion of food, then, many different enzymes are necessary.

Enzymes are classified according to the types of chemical reactions they affect. They are named by adding the suffix "ase" to the type of reaction, or to the substrate, the substance upon which they act. Practically all the enzymes of the digestive tract are members of the group designated as hydrolases. Their function is to aid in the disintegration of complex food molecules, changes which involve cleavages of the molecule with the addition of the elements of water. The more important digestive enzymes will be discussed in connection with the digestive processes.

The activities of any particular kind of enzyme are influenced by its environment. Such factors as (*a*) reaction, (*b*) temperature, (*c*) concentration of the enzyme, (*d*) concentration of the products of reaction, (*e*) presence of electrolytes —salts, alter the degree and intensity of enzymatic transformations.

For each kind of enzyme there is a degree of acidity (excess of hydrogen ion) or alkalinity (excess of hydroxl ion) at which it will produce its maximum effect. If this optimum concentration of hydrogen (or hydroxl) ion is not reached or is exceeded, the action will be retarded because of the absence of sufficient ions to promote the activity of the enzyme or of an excess of ions which would result in an inhibition or destruction of the enzyme. Most enzymes act best at a temperature between 35° and 45° C., approximately body temperature; they are destroyed at higher temperatures (70° to 100° C.), and inhibited at lower temperatures. Although a small quantity of enzyme is capable of effecting the conversion of a large amount of food, with a greater concentration of enzyme the same result may be produced in a much shorter time, the increase in rate being in most cases approximately proportional to the concentration. An accumulation of the products of digestion tends to retard the speed with which the reaction proceeds.[1] This is in accord with the usual course of chemical reactions in which the products are not removed. They proceed in one direction until an equilibrium is reached between the reacting substances and the end-products, or until all of the reacting substances are consumed, when demonstrable reaction ceases; a change in the concentration of any of the factors results in a reaction which tends to restore the equilibrium, or cause it to go to completion. Certain enzymes have been shown to possess the power of reversibility such that they can cause a reaction to proceed in a direction opposite to that normally followed. Electrolyte facilitates or retards enzyme activity according to the kind and concentration; small quantities of certain electrolytes are apparently essential.

Some enzymes when secreted from the cell are in an inactive form which requires the action or presence of another substance or enzyme before they become active. Such enzymes are called zymogens, or mother substances, and the activation is caused by a zymo-exciter or kinase. For example, the activation of the zymogen, pepsinogen, is caused by the zymo-exciter hydrochloric acid and that of the zymogen, trypsinogen, by the kinase, enterokinase.

Oral Digestion.—In the mouth the physical activities of the alimentary tract predominate over the chemical. Here, through mastication, the food is finely divided and thoroughly mixed with the salivary secretion. Three results are accomplished. By fine division the food is prepared for the subsequent action of the digestive juices. By the admixture of water and mucus dry and hard food masses are moistened and softened and swallowing is facilitated. The salivary amylase, ptyalin, is brought into intimate contact with the food and thus amylolytic digestion is promoted. Food remains for so short a time in the mouth that relatively very little digestion occurs there. Thorough mastication of food affects the digestion and consumption of food, aside from the chemical activities of salivary digestion. An increased flow of appetite juice results from the prolonged stimulation of the taste organs of the mouth. A decreased food consumption results in part from a developing sense of satiety and in part from fatigue of the muscles of mastication. Thorough chewing also prepares the food for complete digestion in the stomach and intestines—including salivary[1] digestion in the

---

[1] In the ordinary course of digestion, particularly in the intestines, the end-products are removed by absorption so that hydrolysis is facilitated rather than retarded,

stomach. The function of saliva has been held by certain investigators to be primarily that of a lubricant in swallowing. The fact that the saliva of certain animals, particularly carnivora, contains no amylase or other enzymes and that in aquatic mammals there is apparently no salivary secretion of importance, are cited as proof of that inference. We shall see, however, that for man the digestive function of saliva is desirable although probably not essential.

The quantity and quality of saliva secreted has been shown to vary with the nature of food ingested; coarse (dry), granular, or acid food elicits the production of a thin, watery flow of saliva, while moist foods stimulate the flow of a more viscid secretion. The amount of saliva secreted is affected by the sight or smell of food, it is stimulated by appetizing food and inhibited by non-appetizing food. The total daily excretion is estimated at 1500 cubic centimeters, 50 ounces.

The chemical constituents of saliva are principally water, mucin, inorganic salts—phosphates, chlorides, sulphates and carbonates and traces of thiocyanates, nitrites—and enzymes. Saliva is slightly alkaline to almost neutral in reaction, hydrogen-ion concentration $2-4 \times 10^{-8}$, approximately that of blood. The reaction fluctuates slightly with changes in the acid-base equilibrium of the blood. A slightly acid saliva, 2×10^{-7} gram molecules of hydrogen-ion, has been observed to flow from the salivary glands, particularly in association with acidosis. An acid, mixed saliva is obtained from the mouths of some individuals. In the latter case the acidity is often the result of fermentation (bacterial) of food debris on and between the teeth.

Salivary digestion is confined almost entirely to the transformation of starch and dextrins; cellulose is not attacked by it. Salivary amylase, or ptyalin, is the principal enzyme in the saliva of man. Through its action insoluble or colloidal starch is converted into soluble and diffusible maltose and this, through the action of maltase present in the saliva and also in the intestines, is changed to glucose. The reaction best suited for the activity of salivary amylase is neutral to slightly acid, a hydrogen-ion concentration of 2×10^{-7}, has been found to be the optimum reaction; the presence of even a slight excess of acid inhibits its action. Protein combines with acid and the resulting compound is not sufficiently acid to prevent the action of salivary amylase.

Starch digestion continues for some time after the food has reached the stomach—half an hour or longer, according to the quantity and nature of the food ingested. This is particularly true in the case of solid food because of the thorough mixing of food and saliva in the mouth and the collection of food in the fundus of the stomach. Furthermore, when protein is ingested with starch it combines with the acid of the stomach and for a time a reaction is maintained in the food mass which is suitable for the activity of salivary amylase. That amylolytic digestion in the stomach is desirable is indicated by the fact that protein food mixed with starch when subjected to the action of saliva has been shown to digest more rapidly with gastric juice than when not so mixed. This increased digestibility has been found to be due to physical changes in the starch. Boiled colloidal starch absorbs pepsin and thus inhibits its action. If, however, the starch be changed to its soluble form through the action of salivary amylase, the activity of pepsin is unaffected. Thus salivary digestion of starch is an important aid to active gastric digestion.

Gastric Digestion.—The stomach serves as a reservoir in which the food masses accumulate, are thoroughly mixed, acidified, partially digested, and passed on in small quantities to the intestines for further digestion and absorption. Milk is coagulated in the stomach at the beginning of its digestion. Very little absorption of food material takes place in the stomach.

The resting empty stomach is practically collapsed. The fundus or cardiac portion of the stomach is in a sense a reservoir which accommodates itself to the size of the entering material. As additional masses of food are passed into the stomach, the preëxisting material is forced forward and to one side in such a way that the last portions of swallowed food are, in general, received within the mass already present in the stomach. Gastric juice is then secreted upon the surface of the solid contents of the stomach and, in the fundus, digestion proceeds from the surface toward the center. The partially liquefied products are forced to the pyloric portion of the stomach by the tonic contractions of the stomach walls for acidification, further digestion and passage to the intestine. The tonic contraction of the stomach is not a steadily increased tension, but appears as tonus waves of from one to three minutes duration. As the stomach gradually empties, and when the stomach is empty, these waves pass into the hunger contractions of the empty organ. This arrangement and sequence of events permit of rather extensive salivary digestion in the center of the solid food masses in the stomach. The processes described above apply particularly to the more solid foods. Liquid or semisolid foods do not necessarily follow such a course.

The walls of the fundus of the stomach are in a continual state of contraction and force the food forward by steady pressure. The pyloric portion of the stomach, in contrast with the fundus, is in active motion; contraction waves pass from the fundus toward the pylorus carrying some of the food mixture before them and against the closed pylorus. While the pylorus remains closed the material is not only carried forward by these waves but is also returned through the advancing rings of contracted muscles.

Through the mixing of the food and the digestive action the heterogeneous food mass is converted into the liquid or finely divided semiliquid chyme. The addition of gastric juice increases the acidity of the mass. According to Cannon the pylorus is caused to open primarily by the acidity (true or hydrogen-ion concentration) of the chyme forced against it. Hence when the acidity is sufficiently great, the pylorus opens and a portion of the acidified food is forced into the small intestine. The presence of acid in the intestine causes the pylorus to close and remain so until the acid forced into it is neutralized and the chyme in the stomach is again acid enough to cause the pylorus to open. Carlson's recent work on man has led him to question the acid control of the pylorus, especially from the stomach side. He found that in normal man and animals there is a correlation between the opening of the pylorus and the tonus rythmn of the fundus of the stomach in such a way that the pylorus opens at the height or near the end of each tonus wave. This co-ordination is relatively independent of the chemical reaction of the stomach. In a normal person a certain degree of acidity or of alkalinity or complete neutrality on the stomach side of the pylorus is compatible with normal pyloric rhythm. Under all conditions acid acting on the duodenal side of the pylorus never fails to introduce reflex contractions of the pyloric sphincter, even after the resection of all extrinsic nerves to the pylorus. Hard particles of food may temporarily prevent the opening of the pylorus, and as we shall see later, certain material, particularly some of the liquid foods, may pass the pylorus without being acidified. Later in the process of digestion the pylorus permits even comparatively large masses of undigested food and indigestible material to pass into the intestines.

For liquids the processes just described do not always occur. When water is taken, even on a full stomach, it passes through into the intestines in a comparatively short time and without becoming acid in reaction. Examination of men and animals with the radiograph, and studies of the structure of the stomach and of the arrangement of its contents, have shown that water, in passing through the stomach, follows the lesser curvature of the stomach. Raw white of egg also passes through the stomach without becoming acidified.

Milk is usually coagulated as soon as it enters the stomach; it has been shown, however, that during the early days of infancy, milk may pass directly into the intestines without becoming acidified or coagulated. Experiments with semi-solid foods and with milk have shown that when such foods do not pass directly into the intestines, the greater portion of the water and dissolved matter pass on and the more solid foods remain behind for digestion. Thus two portions of food containing the same amount of solid material, but one having a greater proportion of water than the other, will require practically the same time for digestion and passage out of the stomach.

Aside from effecting mechanical mixture, the gastric processes are essentially proteolytic in effect. A milk-coagulating enzyme, rennin, and a lipase are also present, both of which are important under special conditions—rennin when milk is taken and lipase when finely divided, emulsified, fats are ingested. Carbohydrates are undoubtedly hydrolyzed by hydrochloric acid, the extent depending upon the concentration of the acid and the time it has to act. Such action is, however, under ordinary conditions, very slight. An excessive concentration of acid in the stomach, whether it be unneutralized appetite juice, ingested acid or the presence of fat, is usually accompanied by a regurgitation of material from the duodenum. This regurgitated material tends, by neutralization, to reduce the acidity of the gastric contents. It has been suggested that such regurgitation is a normal mechanism by means of which the reaction of the gastric contents is maintained at the optimum reaction for the activity of the gastric enzymes. In the regurgitated material are the enzymes of the pancreatic and intestinal juices and also bile. The extent of the activity of these substances in gastric digestion is not known. The most important chemical factors in gastric digestion are, then, the enzymes —pepsin, rennin and lipase—and hydrochloric acid. The salts present are important aids to digestive activity.

Pepsin (gastric protease) is secreted as pepsinogen from all parts of the gastric mucosa. The hydrochloric acid in gastric juice changes pepsinogen into pepsin and produces an acidity favorable for the accelerating action of pepsin. Carlson has found that the average normal person secretes from

600 to 700 c.c. of gastric juice on the average palatable meal, or about 1,500 c.c. per day. This secretion corresponds to 240 to 250 milligrams of pepsin per dinner; capable of digesting 630 to 750 grams of protein in three hours. The total pepsin secreted in twenty-four hours is capable of digesting one and one-half kilograms of coagulated egg white in three hours. These amounts are far in excess of the needs of digestion, which may explain the clinical findings of a great reduction in pepsin content without evidence of impaired gastric digestion.

Hydrochloric acid is secreted chiefly in the fundus of the stomach; its concentration when freshly secreted is from 0.45 to 0.55 per cent., expressed clinically, 120 to 130. The acidity of the gastric juice is dependent upon the rate of secretion. With rapid secretion the maximum acidity is obtained, while juice secreted at a slow rate has a lower acidity. The low acidity sometimes ascribed to gastric juice 0.2 per cent., or 40 to 50 expressed clinically, is the acidity of the contents of the empty stomach and represents the continuous secretion plus swallowed saliva and the occasional admixture of intestinal contents. According to Carlson, there is no type of deviation from the normal in which the gastric glands are capable of secreting juice greater than normal acidity. There may be hyposecretion but no physiological hypersecretion. Deviations of acidity from the normal may occur but they are always in the direction of hypoacidity down to anacidity. The clinical hyperacidity is, then, apparently a symptom and not a cause of this syndrome. The optimum acidity for peptic action is about 0.2 to 0.5 per cent. of hydrochloric acid or in terms of hydrogen-ion concentration, between 1×10^{-4} to 4×10^{-4} gram molecules of hydrogen-ion. The acidity of the gastric contents varies during the course of digestion, normally increasing gradually to a maximum and then decreasing somewhat. Hawk has found the variations of the acidity of the gastric contents following a test meal when determined from hour to hour to be characteristic of certain diseases. Fluctuations occur in the acidity with variations in the relative amount of associated substances, particularly proteins, that combine with acid.

Through the action of hydrochloric acid and pepsin some solid protein materials are first swollen. This swollen protein, together with the remaining protein material, is then broken down into simpler protein complexes, the proteoses and peptones. If the action be sufficiently prolonged artificially, pepsin may hydrolyze protein to the simplest protein products, amino-acids, but in the body in the time during which protein ordinarily remains in the stomach, digestion proceeds to the proteose and peptone stages. Pepsin facilitates the digestion of all proteins with the exception of keratin. While peptic digestion may not be complete in the chemical sense, it prepares the protein material for further digestion in the intestine. This is particularly true of collagen in connective tissue which permeates all animal parts. Collagen is swollen and partially hydrated in the stomach, an essential process for its subsequent digestion by the proteolytic enzyme of the pancreatic juice, trypsin. As the result of peptic digestion, then, solid protein masses of food are disintegrated into smaller particles, and "peptonized," wholly or in part, forming a thin soupy mass which is readily passed on to the intestines.

Fatty material is warmed by the stomach and, with the exception of the very solid fats, melted, the connective membranes of the fatty tissue are digested and the fat liberated, and thus it is prepared for digestion in the intestines. Finely emulsified fats, *e. g.*, cream, egg yolk, etc., are acted upon by gastric lipase and hydrolyzed into fatty acids and glycerol; such action is, however, of little practical importance.

Since salivary digestion is stopped by the presence of "free" hydrochloric acid, carbohydrate digestion ceases as soon as the stomach contents become distinctly acid.

The caseinogen of milk is transformed by rennin into insoluble casein, which forms a clot. In the formation of the clot fat and other substances present in milk are entangled and held in the stomach with the casein. It has been shown that the watery portion of milk, whey, passes on quite rapidly into the intestines and that the solids (casein clot) are retained for digestion. This coagulative process permits the ingestion of a highly nutritious liquid without burdening the intestine with large quantities of complex undigested protein material. For a further discussion of rennin, see Milk, p. 150.

Appetite.—Appetite is an important factor in digestion; that this is true is particularly evident in the case of gastric secretion and digestion, and the subsequent digestive processes. True gastric juice is secreted continuously even in the absence of food or obvious nervous excitatory factors, in quantities varying from a few cubic centimeters to 150 c. c. per hour, average 30 to 60 c. c. per hour. This secretion is usually lower in acid than the appetite secretion. It is not markedly increased in prolonged starvation and is decreased and may be entirely absent in fevers and various types of gastritis. Two particular types of stimuli increase the rate of secretion of gastric juice, psychical and chemical. The sight, thought, smell, or taste of food, or familiar sounds associated with food or its preparation will produce a flow of gastric juice.[1] This juice is highly acid in character and has a strong digestive power. It is designated "appetite juice" and is the result of nervous stimulation of the gastric glands. The flow of appetite juice appears upon the mastication of food and begins to decline at the end of a meal when the taste of food has disappeared from the mouth. The rate of secretion is from 1.5 to 12 c. c. per minute, average about 3.5 c. c. per minute. This secretion is absent in normal infants. It is gradually diminished or absent in gastritis or any inflamatory condition of the gastric mucosa, in fevers and in strong emotions of anger or pain. Stomachics or bitters have little or no effect in stimulating the flow of appetite juice. A flow of appetite juice is important but not essential. Adequate digestion of food has been observed in the absence of appetite juice in (a) normal infants and (b) under experimental conditions in animals and man when food is introduced directly into the stomach and (c) the complete digestion of unpalatable food by both man and animals. Under such conditions a flow of gastric gastric juice is stimulated through chemical means. The composition of "appetite juice" has been shown by Povlov to be approximately the same in quality regardless of the nature of the diet ingested; it varies in amount according to the extent and nature of the appetite stimulus.

Secretion of gastric juice under the influence of chemical stimulation is varied: bread produces a copious flow of juice with a greater digestive capacity than meat; fats and alkalis in low concentration inhibit the flow of gastric juice; alkali in higher concentration may cause an increased flow of gastric juice. The apparent specific effects of foods are probably the result of variation in the degree of stimulation resulting from the extractives and digestive products contained in the food or produced by digestion. This stimulation is probably excited through liberation of a gastric hormone. The importance of a secretion of appetite juice is, then, evident, for, in the case of food substances, which are not in themselves "chemical" stimulants, products of digestion obtained under the influence of the psychical stimulation become the chemical stimulants of the gastric

---

[1] Similar and readily recognizable phenomena occur in the secretion of saliva the "mouth waters" at the thought, sight, or smell of appetizing food, while unpalatable food does not have this effect.

secretion which carries on the digestive process after that induced by nervous stimulation has ceased.

Appetite has a secondary effect upon the flow of pancreatic juice, for this is in large measure related to the flow of gastric juice. Acid from the gastric mixture in the duodenum produces the hormone, or "chemical messenger" called secretin from an inactive mother substance: prosecretin.[1] Secretin is carried in the blood and lymph to the pancreas and intestinal glands where it stimulates the flow of the pancreatic and intestinal juices, and to the liver where it stimulates a flow of bile. The flow of pancreatic juice is also affected by nervous stimuli. The indirect effect of lack of appetite is a slowing of all digestive processes. A good appetite becomes, then, a most important factor in digestion. After suitable preparation food is more readily digested.

Appetite is not to be confused with hunger—it is an entirely pleasant state of consciousness associated with our memories of food, particularly the taste, sight and smell of food, hunger is a sensation of pain. Appetite may exist without hunger and is apparently a matter of individual experience which may be modified by experience. It is not a certain guide to the wholesomeness or nutritive value of food—particularly when food is modified by modern processes of manufacture in which certain important food factors may be removed, as in milling, purification, etc. There has been some recent evidence to the effect that animals allowed to choose their food from a number of foods will choose the diet best suited to their needs—but this is not entirely a proven fact. For man, particularly, this does not necessarily hold for his tastes are more often affected by the method of cooking and the manner of serving.

The appetite is stimulated or depressed by the manner in which food is prepared, the way in which it is served and by the mental state of the individual concerned. Food properly cooked, well seasoned and attractively served tends to stimulate the appetite, whereas undercooked or overcooked food served in a careless manner does not stimulate the appetite and may even create a dislike for the food. The determination of what constitutes a well-cooked and attractively served meal rests to a large degree with the taste and

[1] A hormone is a specific chemical substance produced, under a definite stimulus, in one organ which passes in the circulating blood and lymph to another organ in which it excites a secretion or change characteristic of that organ. The quantity of secretion or action produced is related directly to the quantity of hormone formed; a distinction from enzymes. Hormones are comparatively simple chemical substances, diffusible, heat stable, and readily oxidized.

habits of the one who is to eat it. Food which is properly cooked for one person may be unfit to eat in the estimation of another. Likewise, attractive service is purely a relative term. An illustration of the varied tastes of individuals and even peoples is evident from a consideration of the diets of different countries and even in the same country. The mental state of the individual as affected by pleasure, worry, excitement, pain or disappointment, also tends to stimulate or depress the appetite. Appetite is not, however, an absolute necessity for complete and ready digestion of food, for it has been shown that food which was actually distasteful to the person eating it was just as completely digested and utilized as food which was eaten with a relish.

Hunger.[1]—The sensations of hunger have been held to originate through various sources, among them the lack of food substances in the blood or tissues, to the stimulation of the nerves of the stomach by an accumulation of gastric juice in the secreting cells and to a stimulation of the nerves of the mucous membrane of the stomach. Cannon has shown, and Carlson has further confirmed the fact, that the sensation of hunger is in its most important components, due to a type of contractions of the empty or nearly empty stomach, which are not directly related to the immediate needs of the body for nutrient material.

The term empty stomach is a relative one for there is usually some gastric juice, saliva or duodenal contents present (25 to 50 c.c.). The empty stomach in healthy individuals, is never completely at rest but, in general, exhibits a greater degree of tonus than the full stomach. At the height of digestion the contractions of the stomach begin in the lower portion of the stomach and involve only the antrum, as the stomach empties these digestion contractions start further and further up the body of the stomach until they finally begin at or near the cardiac end when the stomach is nearly or completely empty of food. The chief difference between digestion contractions and hunger contractions is, then, in the greater vigor of the empty stomach, the involvement of the entire stomach and the effect of the contractions upon the consciousness. The contractions of the empty stomach come in periods varying from fifteen minutes to an hour—sometimes longer—characterized by a gradual increase in tonus and on these tonus waves are superimposed a series of rapid contractions each lasting from eighteen to thirty sec-

[1] Much of this discussion of hunger is based on a lecture given by Lt.-Col. A. J. Carlson to the Section of Food and Nutrition, Surgeon General's Office, U. S. Army.

onds and increasing in intensity until at the end an incomplete tetanus may result lasting from two minutes up to fifteen minutes. This latter condition is followed by a period of relative quiescence for from a half hour to several hours.

The contractions of the stomach just described give rise, in the normal person at least, to the varied degrees of pressure, pain and emptiness which we associate with or call hunger. The sensations associated with hunger such as nervousness, headache, and feeling of weakness and dizziness and even fainting, are largely of reflex origin involving stimulation of nerves in the muscular coats of the stomach by the strong hunger contractions. In sick individuals or a person suffering from neurosis, or in prolonged starvation the effect of the contractions upon the consciousness may give rise to other effects such as the feeling of sick stomach, nausea, or of general epigastric distress. It is the gastric contractions which give rise to the sensation of hunger and not the central consciousness of hunger which induce the contractions. Hunger is a type of muscle sense for the sensations are due to the stimulations of the nerve-endings in the muscular coats of the stomach. In general, the presence or absence of hunger contractions parallel the call for or refusal of food.

Hunger contractions decrease with age; they are at their maximum in early life. They persist or even increase in prolonged starvation, although in the later stages of starvation mental depression and other central changes may lead to alteration in the conscious effects, such as nausea or epigastric distress. In disease the hunger contractions are increased in diabetes and decreased in most fevers, including thermic or heat prostration.

The control of hunger, therefore, lies in the control of the emptying of the stomach and of the contractions of the empty or nearly empty stomach. Disturbances of gastric motility, in vagi conductions or in parts of the nervous system concerned with the elaboration of the conscious sensation of hunger will interfere with the mechanism. There does not appear to be any certain way to increase hunger except through physical work or external cold—with the accompanying increase in body metabolism. The various stomachics or bitters, long in use to improve hunger, have no effect when given in therapeutic doses into the stomach (fistula). When given by mouth such substances inhibit or depress the hunger mechanism in proportion to the bitter taste or strong stimulation of the nerve endings of the mouth.

Intestinal Digestion.— The digestion of food which has been started in the mouth and stomach is completed in the small intestine. The pancreatic and intestinal juices con‑tain enzymes which accelerate the transformation of all three of the principal food-stuffs into soluble and diffusible products. The action of these enzymes is facilitated by bile.

Carbohydrates are changed into monosaccharides. Starch is hydrolyzed into maltose by the pancreatic amylase or amylopsin, and into glucose by the enzyme maltase. The sugars, maltose, sucrose, and lactose, are broken down into fructose and glucose, and galactose and glucose respectively by maltase, sucrase and lactase. Unaltered protein with the exception of unhydrated collagen and keratin, and the pro‑ducts of peptic digestion are transformed into amino-acids by the trypsin present in the pancreatic juice and erepsin contained in the intestinal juice.

Erepsin, the protease of the intestinal juice, secreted from glands in the intestinal mucosa, acts chiefly upon peptone and peptides, transforming them into amino-acids, thus completing the digestion of protein which has been started by pepsin and trypsin. Erepsin does not digest natural complex proteins, with the exception of caseinogen, his‑tones and protamines. Enterokinase, another intestinal enzyme, is an activating enzyme which is capable of chang‑ing trypsinogen into trypsin.

Nucleoproteins are only partially digested by pepsin and trypsin; their digestion is completed by special enzymes contained in the intestinal juice and in the walls of the intes‑tines. Fats are emulsified in the intestines in the presence of soaps and hydrolyzed into fatty acids and glycerol by the pancreatic lipase, steapsin. Bile also aids in the digestion of fat by increasing the solubility of the soaps and fatty acids; and by accelerating the action of the lipase. Bile contains no enzymes of importance.

The most favorable condition for intestinal digestion is in a neutral to slightly alkaline medium. The pancreatic juice is alkaline in reaction equivalent to approximately 0.5 per cent. Na_2CO_3. It has a hydrogen-ion concentration of about 2×10^{-8} gram molecules per liter.

The structure and movements of the intestines facilitate digestion and absorption but do not enable them to hold large quantities of food. Small quantities of chyme are received from the stomach as often as conditions in the stomach and intestines are suitable for its transference; in general, when the acid chyme passed into the intestine be‑comes practically neutral. The reciprocal action between the two organs prevents overloading of the intestines with large quantities of acid material.

The movements of the intestines have been described by Cannon after examination, with röntgen rays, of the intestines of a cat fed with food mixed with bismuth subnitrate. He found that food masses passed from the stomach were collected together in the duodenum, mixed with pancreatic and intestinal juices and bile, and moved along the intestines in a continuous column. After the food mass had been carried for a short distance, the forward movement stopped and the solid column was broken up into short segments by a number of constrictions in the intestinal wall. These segments were again divided, the halves of two adjacent segments forming a new one. In this way the food masses were repeatedly divided without a forward movement of the total mass. After a time the material was moved along as a continuous column, as before, to another portion of the intestine where segmentation again took place. By this means the intestinal juices are thoroughly mixed with the chyme, the enzymes have the maximum opportunity to act and the food is brought into intimate contact with the walls, of the intestines, thus facilitating digestion and absorption.

Sensibility of the Alimentary Canal.— The sensations associated with the alimentary canal which influence consciousness in normal persons are (*a*) hunger, (*b*) appetite, (*c*) satiety, (*d*) fullness, (*e*) defecation urge, and (*f*) peculiar sensations of heat that may follow strong chemical stimulation of the gastro-intestinal mucosa. In persons with gastro-intestinal disorders we may have (*a*) nausea, (*b*) anorexia, (*c*) bulimia, (*d*) pains of peptic ulcer, (*e*) pains of gastralis, (*f*) pains of gastro-intestinal colic or cramp, gas pains, and (*g*) ill defined and not definitely localized general discomfort or tension referred to the viscera frequently experienced in mild gastritis, enteritis, and constipation. In addition to these recognized sensations there are undoubtedly other sensory components which affect only the reflex or subconscious processes. There does not appear to be any tactile sensibility of the mucosa of the alimentary tract. Temperature sensibility exists in the esophageal, gastric, and anal mucosa and possibly to a less extent in the intestinal mucosa for both heat and cold but which is much less delicate than that of the skin. The gastro-intestinal mucosa appears to be entirely devoid of pain nerve endings.

The sensation of warmth or heat experienced when taking strong acids or concentrated alcohol into the stomach may be due to stimulation of heat nerve-endings in the mucosa. Weaker chemical stimuli such as cold water or very weak alcohol produce an effect on the consciousness similar to, if not identical with, the sensation of appetite.   It is evident, therefore, that moderate chemical stimulation contributes to the element of appetite.   Such sensations may originate from various substances in the food.   This gastric component of appetite is not ordinarily recognized when food is eaten in the ordinary way because of the more powerful stimuli produced by tasting, seeing or smelling palatable food.

ABSORPTION

Absorption of the products of digestion takes place largely in the intestines.   The mucous membrane of the mouth exhibits absorptive powers, but the short time food remains in the mouth precludes any extensive absorption.   In the stomach soluble food and the products of digestion are undoubtedly absorbed to a certain extent, but again absorption is so slight as compared with intestinal absorption as to have no practical value.   A considerable degree of gastric absorption has been demonstrated, however, for water, salts, and alcohol.   Absorption is stimulated by condiments.

The maximum absorption of digestive products takes place in the small intestine: in the duodenum and the jejunum.   Normally the absorption of food products in the small intestine is fairly complete and consequently in the large intestine there is relatively little absorption; and this is limited chiefly to water.   Under certain conditions, as in rectal feeding, the large intestine appears to be capable of a considerable absorption of food products.

Attempts to correlate intestinal absorption with the known laws of diffusion and osmosis have failed to account entirely for the apparently selective absorptive powers of the mucous membranes.   Since a dead membrane does follow these laws it has been suggested that certain "vital" forces are concerned.   When we are fully conversant with the physicochemic structures of the cell, it may be found that these apparently "vital" phenomena are due to special adaptations of simple laws of solutions and diffusion modified by the colloidal state of the substances present.

The manner and form of absorption of protein or its products are subjects of considerable controversy.   Protein may be broken down in the processes of digestion into aminoacids and simple complexes of these, polypeptides.   It was formerly supposed that protein material was absorbed either unchanged or as a proteoses or peptone, and converted into blood protein or destroyed. This view was based largely upon the fact that it was impossible to detect the presence of amino-acids in digestive mixtures or in the blood. Refinement of the methods of analysis and more careful investigation have shown conclusively, however, that digestion of protein proceeds beyond the peptone stage and that protein is probably transformed almost entirely into amino-acids. This is in many ways the more logical conclusion, since there are a number of cell and tissue proteins which contain different proportions of amino-acids than do the food proteins, and these are undoubtedly arranged after their absorption in a different manner in the various protein molecules in the cells and tissues. The absorption of amino-acids and their simple complexes through the intestinal wall is more readily understood than that of colloidal protein structures, because the amino-acids are diffusible.

Two views with regard to the way in which these simple products of protein hydrolysis are carried in the blood have received the most consideration: (*a*) that the amino-acids in their passage through the intestinal wall are resynthetized into protein material, principally serum albumin or serum globulin, and are carried in this form by the blood to the cells for use in the processes of repair and growth or deaminized; (*b*) that the absorbed amino-acids are carried by the blood to the various cells in the body and used directly by the cells or destroyed either there or in the liver. The first conception is probably incorrect; it was based, in part, upon the fact that the products of protein digestion had not been found in the portal blood, and on the presence of large quantities of ammonia in blood coming from the region of the intestines. According to this theory at least a partial disintegration of the nutrient serum proteins into simpler forms was necessary before they could be of use in the structure of the qualitatively different muscle and organ proteins. The excess of simpler forms, *e. g.*, amino-acids, remaining after the formation of such more or less specific protein structures from the heterogeneous mass of structural forms presented were supposed to be deaminized in the intestinal wall or possibly in the blood. The carbon moiety, or mass of amino-acid material minus the animo radicle, was either oxidized as are the fats and carbohydrates, or synthetized to carbohydrates or possibly fats. The nitrogen appeared as ammonium salts which were transformed by the liver into urea.

The second theory is based upon recent investigations which have demonstrated quite conclusively that considerable quantities of amino-acids are present in the blood of the portal vein and in the blood and tissues in general, and that the ammonia of the portal blood is not chiefly the result of deaminization in the small intestine but originates in the large intestine as the result of putrefactive processes. In the light of these investigations opinion with respect to the fate of the absorbed amino-acids and simple peptides has changed. Instead of being either synthetized into protein material during their passage through the intestinal wall or destroyed, a part, if not all, of the amino-acids is now believed to be absorbed into the blood stream without change. These simple digestive products are carried in the blood and lymph and taken up by the tissues for use in the general processes of repair and growth. The excess is deaminized, the amino radicle is transformed into urea, chiefly in the liver, partially in the muscles, while the carbon moiety is oxidized or used in the formation of carbohydrates or fat.

Carbohydrates are normally absorbed as simple sugars, monosaccharides. Of these glucose predominates, since it is the end-product of the digestion of starch and maltose, and constitutes half of the yield from the molecule of sucrose and lactose. Fructose and galatose are converted either in the intestinal wall or in the liver into glucose, the carbohydrate characteristic of the body. These carbohydrates pass in the portal blood stream to the liver. This organ acts as a storehouse and regulator of the supply of carbohydrate used in the body. The normal glucose content of the blood is approximately 0.1 per cent. The blood from the intestines during digestion, however, contains more than this amount. Under ordinary circumstances the liver removes this excess of glucose and transforms and stores it as glycogen. When the glucose content of the blood entering the liver falls below the normal amount, it receives sufficient glucose to keep this value constant.

When readily absorbable carbohydrates, such as sucrose, maltose, or lactose, are ingested in excess, they may be absorbed unchanged. But the blood apparently does not contain an enzyme capable of hydrolyzing or utilizing sucrose or lactose, for they are treated as foreign substances in the blood and are removed by the kidneys. Maltose, however, may be utilized by the tissues to a certain extent; excess quantities are excreted. When glucose appears in the blood in amounts greater than normal or which exceed the threshold value of the kidney it appears in the urine. Such conditions exist in certain diseases such as diabetes and may also result from the rapid absorption of glucose from the intestines in quantities so great that the liver cannot take care of it.

The appearance of sugars in the urine following too rapid absorption from the intestine is called "alimentary glycosuria," The quantity of any sugar which can be ingested without causing alimentary glycosuria is termed the assimilation limit, and is more or less specific for each sugar. Taylor holds that there is apparently no limit, beyond the capacity of the individual to retain it, to the quantity of glucose which may be ingested and absorbed. Some of his subjects took as much as 500 grams of glucose at one time without eliminating sugar in the urine; the limit of others was lower than this. Since starch requires a longer time for digestion the absorption of the resultant glucose extends over a longer period of time. With such a gradual absorption glucose does not normally appear in the blood in concentrations which will result in an alimentary glycosuria.

Glucose is used in the body, particularly in the muscles, for the production of energy. One of the intermediate products appears to be lactic acid, which, upon further oxidation, gives carbon dioxide and water, which are excreted. Carbohydrates ingested in amounts more than sufficient to maintain the stores of glycogen in the liver and muscles and for the ordinary oxidative processes may be transformed into fat. Careful experiments have been conducted to prove this, for in spite of the general evidence obtained from feeding herbivorous animals, the formation of fat from carbohydrates has been questioned. By determining that a greater amount of fat was deposited in the body or excreted in milk than was contained in the food fed or could have been formed from the protein, it has been demonstrated quite conclusively that carbohydrates are used by the body in the formation of fat; careful respiration experiments have also shown this.

Ingested fat is transformed in the intestines into fatty acids, soaps, and glycerol and absorbed in these forms. In their passage through the intestinal mucosa these products are resynthetized into neutral fats. Instead of passing directly into the blood through the capillaries of the intestines, as do the carbohydrates and the greater part of the protein digestion products, fat is taken up by the lymph ducts and poured into the blood stream with the thoracic lymph. It has been shown that fat-like substances such as petroleum (hydrocarbon) and esters saponified with difficulty (not fat) are not absorbed from the intestines. The use of petroleum oil to relieve constipation depends upon this fact.

Studies of fat absorption have shown that fat which appears in the blood, or which is deposited in the tissues, or which is excreted in milk, may retain certain of the characteristics of the food fat, such as the iodine number, etc. Fats are, however, changed in the process of absorption for, following the ingestion of a food fat with a high melting-point the blood fat shows a lowered melting-point while the reverse is true when fat with a low melting-point is ingested.

The fat content of the blood increases during feeding, for the absorbed fat is poured into the blood stream above the liver. Studies of the fat content of the blood have shown that fat begins to be absorbed about two hours after ingestion and reaches a maximum of absorption in about six hours. Bloor has suggested that lecithin takes part in fat absorption and that it is the first stage through which fat passes in the processes of utilization. In dogs, and by analogy probably in man, the fat content of the blood is fairly constant, except at times of active absorption from the intestines, showing a regulation somewhat similar to that observed in the case of glucose. When large quantities of fat are being utilized, as in fasting or diabetes, there is often an increase in the blood fat.

BACTERIAL ACTION AND FECES

Intestinal Bacteria.—Food is disintegrated through the action of bacteria as well as by the digestive processes which take place in the intestines as the result of the action of the digestive enzymes. Such digestion takes place normally and to a greater extent in the large intestine in the case of poor digestion and absorption in the small intestine. The bacteria active in the intestines may be grouped into two general classes: first, those which act primarily upon carbohydrate material and which produce alcohol and organic acids, such as lactic, acetic, butyric, benzoic, succinic, valerianic acids, accompanied by the evolution of carbon dioxide and methane. These are ordinarily classed as fermentative bacteria. Their action is not restricted to soluble carbohydrates; certain kinds are capable of digesting cellulose. Bacteria which act upon cellulose are of practical importance to the herbivora which obtain a portion of their carbohydrate material through such action. Fermentative bacteria require in general a neutral to slightly acid medium for their growth and activities.

To the second class of bacteria of importance in the digestive tract belong those whose action is confined primarily to protein material, often classed as putrefactive bacteria, and which are chiefly anaërobic.

The relative number of bacteria excreted per day in the feces has been placed at between 33 to 128 x 10^{12}. A large proportion of these are dead. One estimate has placed the relative proportion of dead bacteria in feces at 99 per cent.; this value is difficult to determine because of the varying conditions in the intestines. The actual weight of dry bacteria excreted per day has been found to be between 5 to 8 grams.

Among the products of putrefaction are the proteoses, peptones, and amino-acids obtained in the usual digestive processes. In addition to these, however, are a number of products more or less characteristic of bacterial action, such as the nitrogenous substances of the aromatic series—indol and skatol, phenol, cresol, phenyl-propionic acid, certain of the amines, accompanied often by the development of gas; hydrogen, sulphide, carbon dioxide, methane, hydrogen, and ammonia. Certain of these products are toxic, particularly those of the aromatic series and the amines.

It has been demonstrated that indol, phenol, skatol, etc., are detoxified, conjugated, with sulphuric acid, by the liver to form compounds of the type of indican (indoxyl potassium sulphate) in which form they are excreted in the urine. During or after excessive putrefaction these products may not be entirely conjugated when various abnormal effects, among them nervous disturbances, occur which are ordinarily included in the meaning of the term auto-intoxication. The quantity of indican in the urine during a given period has been generally accepted as a good index of the extent of intestinal putrefaction.

An alkaline reaction is particularly favorable for the growth of putrefactive bacteria. The large intestine is the only portion of the intestinal tract in which such a condition normally prevails. Some bacteria particularly of the B. coli type may be both fermentative and putrefactive in effect. They tend, however, to antagonize the putrefactive anaerobes.

In the stomach the action of bacteria ingested with the food is retarded if not completely destroyed. The hydrochloric acid of the gastric juice is sufficiently concentrated to destroy certain types of bacteria; only the active bacteria of other types are destroyed while the spores are resistant to its action. Bacterial action, then, in the normal stomach is practically negative. It is quite probable that pathogenic bacteria, which are ordinarily destroyed by the hydrochloric acid of the gastric juice may enter the intestine with undigested food particles and oil globules or in water that passes through the stomach without becoming acidified to any extent. In the presence of large quantities of protein, which combines with the hydrochloric acid of the gastric juice and tends to lower the acidity of the gastric contents or following the ingestion of alkaline drinks or doses of alkaline salts, bacteria may develop or escape destruction. In certain abnormalities, hyperchlorhydria, atony of the stomach, etc., or conditions in which the concentration of the hydrochloric acid is lowered through any cause, fermentative bacteria often develop, and produce organic acids, alcohol and carbon dioxide. The excessive ingestion of carbohydrate, particularly sucrose (cane sugar) and glucose, often leads to such fermentation. Yeasts grow even in acid solutions. Their development in the stomach is accompanied by the production of organic acids, *e. g.*, lactic and butyric acids, particularly following the ingestion of sugars, in cases in which there is a slow emptying of the stomach.

The reaction of the small intestine is favorable for the growth of fermentative bacteria. This is true particularly in the lower parts of the small intestine, for the contents of the upper portion of the duodenum are slightly alkaline. Here the acid contents of the stomach are wholly or partly neutralized by the relatively large volumes of pancreatic and intestinal juices and the bile, which, while only slightly alkaline in reaction, are capable of neutralizing considerable acid. In the lower portions of the small intestine, particularly the jejunum and ileum, the intestinal contents are nearly neutral to slightly acid as the result of the partial neutralization of the intestinal and pancreatic secretions by the hydrochloric acid, and of the organic acids—produced during the digestion of fat and probably also by bacterial action. These portions of the intestine are, then, favorable to the growth of fermentative bacteria. Examination of intestinal contents has demonstrated a pronounced growth of such bacteria. The effect of bacterial action in this region is not particularly harmful, for the products of fermentation are not, in general, toxic. The evolution of considerable quantities of carbon dioxide often leads to flatulence. Herter has suggested that the presence of an excess of fatty acids causes intestinal irritation, and diarrhea.

Putrefaction and Feces.— Putrefactive processes predominate over fermentative in the large intestine. The protein material which comes from the small intestine is here acted upon by the putrefactive bacteria of which, *B. coli*, *B. lactis aerogenes*, *Bact. welchi*, *B. bifidus* and certain cocci predominate. The character of the bacteria present depends to a certain extent upon the nature of the food ingested. In a favorable medium certain types of bacteria will grow rapidly and in so doing form products which inhibit the growth of other types. The predominance of *B. bifidus* in the intestinal tract of the infant has been explained as due, in part at least, to the continual presence of lactose in the diet and to the slight acid reaction of the feces, a condition which results from the activities of *B. bifidus*. Acidity of the feces is sufficient to inhibit the growth of practically all putrefactive bacteria. The gradual change in the diet of the infant, even a change from the breast milk with its relatively high lactose and low protein content, to cow's milk with its lower lactose and higher protein content, tends to make *B. bifidus* disappear and other types, particularly *B. coli*, to predominate. A large proportion of the bacteria cultivable on artificial media present in adult feces are *B. coli*. This organism is not entirely dependent upon carbohydrate; it can grow either in a carbohydrate-protein medium or in one in which available carbohydrate is entirely absent.

Material which is passed from the small into the large intestine throught the ileocecal valve is of practically the same consistence as that ejected from the stomach into the small intestine; a semiliquid mass. This is true because the active absorptive processes of the small intestine, which remove both water and solids, are compensated by subsequent excretion of water through the intestinal walls. The total mass of the material is, however, greatly reduced. The large intestine in man is essentially a concentrating, absorptive, organ; its secretion, which is rich in mucus and alkaline in reaction,has not been shown to exert material digestive action. Digestion continues, however, as a result of enzymes from the small intestine and other transformations result from the action of bacteria. The latter processes are of particular importance in certain of the lower animals in which the cecum is larger than in other animals.

In the upper portion of the large intestine the semiliquid mass from the small intestine is concentrated; water in particular is absorbed. This thickened mass is then passed to the transverse and descending portions of the colon, and finally out of the body. Observations of the passage of food through the large intestine by means of the *x*-rays have lead to the conclusion that, in general, two hours are required for transit through each of the three parts of the colon, *i. e.*, ascending, transverse, and descending. Sleep appears to retard, while the ingestion of meals accelerates the movement of material in the large intestine.

The time required for the passage of food through the alimentary tract varies with the nature of the food ingested and with the condition of the individual. According to the observations just noted the time is usually from eight to twelve hours. Under conditions of regular routine and uniform mixed diet, the residue from food ingested on a given day may be eliminated on the following morning. Even under such circumstances characteristic particles of food in a certain meal may appear in the feces days after the ingestion of that particular food. With the ingestion of a diet which is almost completely absorbed, or in fasting, defecation may take place only once in two or three days. On the other hand, foods which irritate the intestinal mucosa pass out promptly.

The material passed from the large intestine varies with the nature of the food ingested. It consists chiefly of undigested and unabsorbed food, bacteria and bacterial products, cast-off cells, the residues of intestinal secretions and salts. Fecal material is formed even in fasting, such feces consist of the residue from intestinal secretions, cellular material, bacteria, and bacterial products.

In the course of digestion relatively large quantities of secretions are poured into the alimentary tract and a considerable quantity of epithelial cells is mechanically removed. A large proportion of this material is reabsorbed, a certain quantity is, however, eliminated in the feces.

When considering the absorption of foods from the intestine, it is necessary to make a distinction between the material remaining undigested and unabsorbed and that secreted into the intestines in the process of digestion, designated as "metabolic products." The quantity of such material eliminated has been studied particulary with regard to the utilization of nitrogenous foods in which case the "metabolic nitrogen" is involved. A determination of the fecal nitrogen excreted in fasting would seem a most logical manner of estimating approximately the "metabolic nitrogen" in this relation. Studies of the influence of indigestible non-nitrogenous materials in their passage through the intestine upon the excretion of nitrogen indicate an increase in the fecal nitrogen in their presence over that excreted in their absence; for a large mass of inert material, in addition to holding a certain amount of the secretion by absorption, tends to increase the rate of peristalsis. To determine the "metabolic nitrogen," then, it is essential that a mass of non-nitrogenous material[1] be ingested which will yield a fecal residue of approximately the same size as that of the diet under consideration. Estimates of the metabolic nitrogen of man indicate the amount to be approximately 1 gram of nitrogen per day. Recent experiments in which agar agar was used as the inert material have placed this value at 0.5 gram of nitrogen per day.

The degree of indigestibility of the food-stuffs affects the quantity of feces formed. Foods which contain a large proportion of indigestible material result in a greater fecal mass than those which are readily digested and absorbed. Foods rich in cellulose yield large watery stools containing considerable undigested protein and fat which have been protected from the action of the digestive enzymes by the indigestible cellulose. The relative composition of the feces from easily digestible and completely absorbed food is approximately the same irrespective of the nature of the diet. This has been demonstrated by feeding diets of meat and of rice alternately, in which it was found that the figures for percentage composition of the undigested residues were quite similar, *i. e.*, the quantity of nitrogen and fat excreted in the feces was roughly the same. In these cases the fecal material consisted largely of the metabolic products. An increase in the quantity of food does not result in an equivalent increase in the fecal output. An increase of 80 per cent. in the quantity of food ingested (bread) has been found to cause an increase of only 15 per cent. in the quantity of feces. With meat the effect is less—because of its greater digestibility. Milk has a different effect; an increase in the quantity of milk ingested results in a proportional increase in the fecal output, because of the unabsorbed inorganic constituents of the milk, calcium, and phosphorus, and, to a less extent, of the nitrogenous material.

We conclude, then, that for easily digestible diets, such as meat, eggs, milk, rice, cheese, starches, etc., the fecal material consists essentially of the residues from the intestinal secretions, cellular material, inorganic salts, bacteria, and bacterial products. Diets containing relatively indigestible material, such as vegetables, or those which have not been properly digested because of insufficient mastication or deficient peristalsis, will yield stools containing food residues and probably a greater quantity of non-reabsorbed metabolic products than easily and properly digested diets.

[1] Agar agar has been suggested for this purpose.

The reaction of the feces is normally neutral to slightly alkaline to litmus. Feces from a highly nitrogenous diet exhibit an alkaline reaction due to the production of ammonia in the process of putrefaction. When fermentation predominates, the reaction of the stool will probably be slightly acid because of the presence of organic acids produced.

The large intestine is capable of absorbing considerable nutriment when it is presented to it as in rectal feeding, particularly the products of protein digestion, proteoses, peptones, amino-acids and the diffusible carbohydrates. This is of practical importance in the feeding of the sick, which will be discussed later. Cannon has observed the action of the large intestine after rectal injection of enemata. He studied the effect in cats, of large and small amounts of thin fluid masses, and of thick, mushy masses, and found that the food was largely in the upper part of the large intestine, to which it was carried by antiperistaltic waves. After abundant injections the food passed the ileocecal valve and into the small intestine. Nitrogen equilibrium has been maintained for fifteen days in a boy with a stricture of the esophagus when fed per rectum, with a mixture of protein (meat) digestion products obtained by digestion *in vitro* with trypsin and erepsin.

EXCRETION.

The excretion of the products of general metabolic activity takes place through the lungs, kidneys, large intestine and skin. Of the products of carbon metabolism, carbon dioxide and water, the former is excreted almost entirely through the lungs; water is excreted through all excretory channels. The nitrogenous end-products of protein metabolism, salts, and, to a certain extent, the carbon end-products are excreted through the kidneys. The feces contain metabolic end-products that are excreted through the liver and the walls of the intestines, and in addition undigested food material and epithelial cells from the intestinal tract, bacteria and their products. The extent to which excretion takes place, or may take place through the intestine is not well understood. Certain mineral salts, such as calcium, magnesium, together with the phosphate radicle, iron, and salts of silicon, are excreted into the lumen of the intestine. Intestinal excretion of inorganic salts depends to a large extent upon the nature of the food ingested, *i. e.*, whether or not it yields an excess of acidic or basic radicles as the result of metabolic processes. Because of the appearance of the salts of calcium, phosphate and iron in the feces it was formerly supposed that these salts taken in the inorganic form were absorbed with difficulty, and hence they must be supplied in organic combinations. It has been shown, however, that they are actively excreted through the bile and walls of the intestine. A larger proportion of calcium and magnesium appears in the urine following an acid diet than occurs from an alkaline diet. Certain substances are excreted through the bile—cholesterol, lecithin, and bile pigments. Salts of the heavy metals which are toxic when ingested appear largely in the bile, and subsequently in the feces.

Epidermal excretion consists chiefly of water with small amounts of nitrogenous waste products, lipins and salts.

In the course of protein metabolism, the amino-acids, and possibly more complex molecules are absorbed from the intestinal tract, and are taken up in part by the tissues and synthetized into protein molecules. Amino-acids not used in the processes of synthesis are deaminized, and the resultant ammonia is converted into urea and excreted; a small proportion of the absorbed amino-acids may be stored for a time. Such processes take place throughout the body, but they occur to a greater extent in the liver and the intestines. The carbon-containing fragments of the molecules of amino-acids may be oxidized or synthetized into carbohydrate or fat. In the tissues protein molecules are broken down entirely or in part into amino-acids or simple complexes of these which meet a fate similar to those ingested.

Among the constituents of food and tissues are nitrogenous compounds other than simple amino-acids, such as nucleo-proteins and products of their hydrolysis, purin and pyrimidin bases, uric acid, creatine, creatinine, heterocyclic ring compounds, urea, and ammonium salts. Some of these are not available for body functions and are excreted unchanged; others may take part in cellular activities, although our knowledge on this point is not definite.

Nitrogen is excreted chiefly as urea, ammonia, uric acid, creatinine, creatine, and purine. The following table[1] gives the composition of urine obtained after the ingestion of two types of diet: high and low protein content.

[1] Folin: Am. Jour. Physiol., 1905, xiii, 118.

COMPOSITION OF NORMAL URINE EXCRETED FOLLOWING THE INGESTION OF A
HIGH PROTEIN AND A LOW PROTEIN DIET.

	High protein diet.	Per cent. of total nitrogen.	Low protein diet.	Per cent. of total nitrogen.
Volume of urine . .	1170 c.c.	..	385 c.c.	
Total nitrogen . .	16.80 gm.	..	3.60 gm.	
Urea nitrogen . .	14.70 "	87.5	2.20 "	61.7
Ammonia nitrogen .	0.49 "	3.0	0.42 "	11.3
Uric acid nitrogen .	0.18 "	1.1	0.09 "	2.5
Creatinine nitrogen .	0.58 "	3.6	0.60 "	17.2
Undetermined nitrogen	0.85 "	4.9	0.27 "	7.3

		Per cent. of total SO_3.		Per cent. of total SO_3.
Total SO_3 . . .	3.64 "	..	0.76 "	
Inorganic SO_3 . .	3.27 "	90.0	0.46 "	60.5
Ethereal SO_3 . . .	0.19 "	5.2	0.10 "	13.2
Neutral SO_3 . . .	0.18 "	4.8	0.20 "	26.2

The greater proportion of the urinary nitrogen is excreted as urea. The daily excretion of urea is approximately 30 grams, equivalent to about 80 to 90 per cent. of the total nitrogen in the urine. These values vary with the nature of the diet, its protein content, the activity and rate of metabolism and the degree of retention of nitrogen-containing substances. An excessive ingestion of protein or increased body activity is accompanied by an increased urea output, both absolute and relative; a decreased protein ingestion or retention of nitrogen is accompanied by a lowered urea excretion. Since urea represents a large proportion of the urinary nitrogen determinations of this factor are sometimes taken as an indication of the extent and nature of protein metabolism.

The amounts of urea and ammonia which appear in the urine are closely related. Urea is formed from ammonium carbonates and carbamates. Any factor which prevents the transformation of ammonia into urea, such as the formation of ammonium salts of highly dissociated acids or the production of excessive quantities of organic acids which are neutralized by ammonia, induce decreased urea excretion accompanied by increased ammonia excretion. When there is an excess of acidic over basic radicles in the body, the acidity is reduced by two processes in particular: excretion of the acid radicle as a salt of a strong base and of the hydrogen in combination with a phosphate radicle, or excretion in combination with ammonia. Thus a diet whose ash yields an excess of acidic over basic radicles will be accompanied by a relatively high ammonia excretion. Or, the presence of an excessive quantity of organic acids in the body as the result of a failure to oxidize them is followed by an increased excretion of ammonia.

Creatinine appears in the urine of normal adults in amounts comparatively constant from day to day—1 or 2 grams— but with slight fluctuations throughout the day. Diet has little effect upon the excretion of creatinine. According to Folin the excretion of creatinine is a measure of endogenous metabolism. It has been suggested that there is a relation between the mass and activity of the muscular system and the quantity of creatinine excreted in the urine. This relationship may be expressed in terms of body weight; it varies with different individuals but is fairly constant for each. The normal value for the average person has been found to be from 7 to 11 milligrams of creatinine per kilogram body weight.

Creatine, which is closely related to creatinine, appears in the urine of women at cyclic intervals of menstruation and following childbirth and is a normal constituent of the urine of children. It also appears during fasting and in diseases involving carbohydrate metabolism. There seems to be a certain relation between carbohydrate metabolism and the excretion of creatine such that in the absence of carbohydrates or in disturbed carbohydrate metabolism creatine appears in the urine. The ingestion of creatinine is followed by an increased creatinine elimination. Creatine, when ingested, is accompanied by an increased creatine excretion, but has little effect upon the excretion of creatinine. Our knowledge of the importance and significance of creatine and creatinine is very limited.

Uric acid is, in man, an end-product of the metabolism of nucleins either of the food or of the tissues, or both. It is derived chiefly from the oxidation of purine bases. The average excretion for man is about 0.6 gram per day; it varies from 0.3 to 1.2 gram per day. The ingestion of purine-containing foods, or accelerated nuclear metabolism, is accompanied by an increased uric acid excretion. Uric acid is practically insoluble in water; its solubility is decreased in acid solutions and increased in alkaline solutions. By varying the nature of the diet, and consequently the reaction of the urine, it has been found that the quantity of uric acid which the urine is capable of dissolving (or holding in solution) is increased by a diet yielding an alkaline ash and decreased by one yielding an acid ash.

DIGESTIBILITY OF FOOD

The food value to the body, of any particular food, depends upon the quantity of assimilable matter it yields as the result of digestion. The relative digestibility of foods is, then, an important factor in determining the diet from either a clinical or an economic point of view. In feeding the sick or delicate persons the *ease, rapidity* and *completeness* with which the ingested food is digested, absorbed and assimilated are essential factors. The economist is particularly concerned with the completeness or extent of digestion, while the physician must know something of the ease with which food is digested and assimilated. These attributes of metabolic availability are subject to considerable variation. Digestion is influenced by many modifying factors; such as psychical influences which accelerate or inhibit the motor as well as the secretory activities of the alimentary tract; the kind of food; the mode of preparation; the degree of comminution, including mastication, and (considering individual food stuffs) the nature of material with which it is associated. Psychical stimuli accompanying contentment, pleasurable surroundings, well-served and appetizing food tend to facilitate digestion, while those which originate from fear, anger, worry, keen anticipation, and even high degree of happiness inhibit the activities of the alimentary tract and thus delay digestion; fortunately the unfavorable emotions are usually accompanied by a loss of appetite which prevents the ingestion of food.

The quantitative measure of digestibility of a particular food-stuff is the ratio between the quantity absorbed and that ingested. The degree of absorption is determined by subtracting the amount of undigested food-stuff from that ingested. In estimating the quantity of undigested material in the feces, allowance must be made for the constituents which have been secreted or excreted into the intestine during digestion, such as those in the digestive juices, epithelial cells, fats, etc., and which, originating in the body, arise ultimately from food that has been absorbed. This form of excretion, so far as it is related to nitrogenous constituents, has been called "metabolic nitrogen." Under abnormal conditions, such as excessive or retarded peristalsis the digestibility of food varies. With excessive peristalsis, the digestive juices do not have sufficient time to act, and there is a consequent lower utilization. Such a condition may be associated normally with a very bulky diet, such as with a predominantly vegetable regimen.

Studies of the comparative digestibility of protein, fat, and carbohydrate of various types of foods, when ingested by man as a mixed diet, have been made by Atwater. A summary of his results is as follows:

COEFFICIENTS OF DIGESTIBILITY OF FOOD-STUFFS IN DIFFERENT GROUPS OF FOOD MATERIALS. (ATWATER.)

	Protein.	Fat.	Carbohydrate.
Protein-rich food:			
Animal food—meat, eggs, dairy products	97	95	98
Vegetable food—legumes, dried	78	90	97
Carbohydrate-rich foods:			
Cereals	85	90	98
Sugars and starches	..	..	98
Cellulose-rich foods:			
Green vegetables	83	90	95
Total food:			
Mixed diet	92	95	97

These values are for ordinary mixed diets. Special methods of preparation will modify them to a certain extent, *e. g.*, when finely divided vegetable proteins were fed with starch and fat the utilization of these substances, in the dog, is approximately that of meat, whereas according to Atwater's tables they are much less digestible. Degree of absorption does not, however, necessarily determine availibility to the body, for a food which is completely absorbed may not be of the proper composition for its most economical utilization by the body (assimilation).

When considering foods for the purpose of regulating a diet, we are usually concerned with the *ease* or *rapidity* with which they are digested. A food may be completely digested and still be "indigestible" in the sense in which this word is used with reference to the facility with which it is digested. Our measure of "facility" is rather indefinite. It is ordinarily taken as the time required for a particular food to leave the stomach, because until comparatively recently we have been unable to study the processes which go on in the intestine from a time-relation point of view. The rapidity with which food is absorbed from the alimentary tract may also be accepted as an indication of the ease or difficulty with which a food is digested. The rate at which nitrogenous or carbonaceous end-products are excreted has been used as an index of the rate of digestion and particularly of absorption.

The rate of passage of food from the stomach has been systematically studied by Cannon, who showed that the three important food-stuffs, carbohydrate, protein and fat, in equal masses and of approximately the same consistency, when fed alone, leave the stomach at different though characteristic rates. Carbohydrate-rich foods passed out rather rapidly and appeared in the intestines in relatively large quantities. Protein did not begin to pass out of the stomach for some time. Once it began to appear in the intestines it came at a fairly uniform rate for a period of two or three hours. Fat also passed slowly from the stomach, more so than protein. Mixtures of foods were ejected from the stomach at rates which were intermediate between those characteristic of the types of foods concerned. The closing of the pylorus is dependent largely upon the appearance of acid in the duodenum. A food which combines with acid, as protein, or which retards the secretion of the gastric juice, as fat, passes more slowly from the stomach than carbohydrate, a food which does not neutralize the acid. The order in which foods are ingested also affects the length of time required for the stomach to empty itself. A starchy food taken after protein food is retarded in its passage out of the stomach. Acid foods, those which do not absorb (neutralize) much acid, or those which stimulate the secretion of large quantities of gastric juice, pass out more rapidly than foods which absorb considerable acid, are alkaline, or inhibit the secretion of gastric juice. Hence the rate of movement from the stomach is dependent upon the presence of free acid in the gastric juice. Exceptions to this general fact occur in disease—such as achylia in which the stomach empties rapidly.

The consistency of the food likewise affects the rapidity with which it passes from the stomach: hard particles retard evacuation of the stomach; protein-food in lumps remains longer in the stomach than hashed protein, but is more completely liquefied than the latter. Dilution of the food masses, on the other hand, does not retard their passage from the stomach. Practically no difference has been observed in the rate with which equal volumes of thick and watery mixtures of starchy foods are passed from the stomach; watery protein mixtures pass out more quickly than thick mixtures because of the smaller amount of protein present.

London, using equal masses of solid food, found that the quantity of food remaining in the stomach after a definite period was the same whether a watery or partially desiccated food was fed, but that the degree of digestion was greater in the latter case. The water, apparently, tends to pass out of the stomach first. Groebbels found, however, that for dogs water ingested after bread doubles the time required for the food to leave the stomach, and that bread and water taken simultaneously remained even longer. The absolute amount of food taken determines, however, the length of time required for the complete evacuation of the stomach.

Selection of the time required for a particular kind of food to disappear from the stomach, as a criterion of the ease or rapidity of its digestion is, as we have seen above, of doubtful value. To overload the intestine is undoubtedly as harmful as to overload the stomach. This is a more difficult matter, for the interrelation between the conditions in the intestine and the opening and closing of the pylorus are very intimate. Our knowledge of the factors affecting the rate of passage of foods from the stomach permits us, however, to select diets which are suited to the needs of the particular case under consideration. Thus a food, highly digestible from the quantitative point of view, when fed in fairly large masses, would remain for a longer time in the stomach than when finely divided as in thick soup, and consequently the protein and perhaps the carbohydrate would be more completely digested before it passed into the intestines; this increased digestion in the stomach should tend to reduce the digestion required in the small intestine. The relative digestibility of particular foods will be discussed when they are taken up.

CHAPTER II.

ENERGY REQUIREMENT

The energy utilized by man in the performance of work and in the maintenance of body temperature is derived from the oxidation of the various food-stuffs in the body, particularly carbohydrates and fats. Extensive studies of animal and human metabolism have demonstrated that the law of conservation of energy holds for the living organism just as it does in the inanimate world. The performance of a definite amount of work or the maintenance of a definite temperature involves the transformation of amounts of potential energy into kinetic energy equivalent to the work performed or the heat produced. Life is accompanied by the continual performance of work in one form or another. A knowledge of energy changes in the various conditions and states of life is fundamental to a satisfactory understanding and control of the diet.

CALORIC VALUE OF FOOD-STUFFS.

Oxidation, or combustion, of food-stuffs is accompanied by the liberation of energy in the form of heat. When this process takes place under properly controlled conditions, it is found that for each unit of material oxidized a definite quantity of heat is liberated. The measure of heat is the calorie; the heat required to raise the temperature of 1 gram of pure water 1 degree at 15°C. Since this is a relatively small unit, for convenience the kilo calorie or Calorie is used, *i. e.*, the quantity of heat required to cause the same change of temperature in one liter (kilogram) of water.[1] Typical food-stuffs measured by this standard yield definite though different amounts of energy.

[1] Determinations of the calorific value of foods are conducted with the bomb calorimeter. Dried food is placed in a closed metal bomb, lined with a virtually unoxidizable metal, such as platinum or gold, charged with oxygen under great pressure. The bomb is then immersed in a known weight of water contained in receptacle of insulating material to prevent the rapid loss of heat. The food is ignited with a small piece of iron wire heated by an electric current. In the presence of the large excess of oxygen combustion proceeds rapidly to completion and the heat developed increases the temperature of the surrounding water. The amount of increase is determined by means of an accurate and sensitive thermometer. The caloric value of the food is then calculated from the observed change, with proper corrections for radiation, etc.

Investigation of the body processes has shown that the production of body heat and of work is accomplished at the expense of energy obtained by reactions entirely similar to those observed in the calorimeter. The quantity of heat liberated and the end-products of the *complete oxidation* of carbohydrate or fat are entirely analgous to those obtained by experimentation outside the body. But since the end-products of *complete utilization* of protein in the body—urea, creatinine, uric acid, etc.—are themselves capable of being burned with the liberation of energy, the energy derived by the body from protein is less than that obtained in the calorimeter.

In calculating the amount of energy derived from the food by the body we must consider that food as eaten is not entirely digested nor is the absorption from the intestinal tract complete. If allowance is made for that portion of the food-stuff which is not assimilated (approximate values: carbohydrate 2 per cent., fat 5 per cent., protein 8 per cent.), and for variations in degree of utilization, we may assume the physiological fuel values as 4.1 Calories per gram for carbohydrate, 9.3 Calories per gram for fat, and 4.1 Calories per gram for protein. Knowing the relative proportions of these primary food-stuffs in any food, we can calculate, with the above values, the approximate quantity of heat energy, which the body may derive from it. Most of the fuel values of foods presented in the various tables in this book are computed in this manner.

In the calculation of diets the fuel value of food is usually expressed in two forms: (*a*) the number of calories available from a given weight of food, as the pound or gram, and (*b*) the weight of food (grams, ounces, or pounds) which will yield a certain number of calories, 100 Calories (kilo-calories) or 1000 Calories (kilo-calories). The first method of recording unit values is most useful in calculating the caloric value of a diet which has been consumed as in statistical investigations of diet, or where the food is taken *ad libitum*. When it is desired to prepare a diet having a given caloric value from a diet list composed of dishes of known weight and composition, the second procedure is particularly satisfactory.

One Hundred Calorie Portion.— The 100 Calorie portion, or the weight of food which will supply 100 large calories, has been suggested by Fisher as a unit for comparisons. This unit is useful in comparing not only the relative nutritive value of various foods but also their cost. The use of this unit facilitates the preparation of diets in which foods of the same types may be substituted one for another to avoid monotony. The proportions of protein, carbohydrate, and fat which furnish energy are expressed in terms of percentages, an arrangement which permits rapid calculations in the selection of a properly balanced diet.

The 100 Calorie portion can be used advantageously in the preparation of diets only when slight variations are not important, since the results are expressed in terms of portions or individual pieces; variations will occur in the interpretation of a portion, composition of food, etc. When the portions are weighed out exactly the accuracy is increased, but then the usefulness of the method is not realized, for it is designed as a ready measure of the caloric value of the diet. Books[1] containing data for the composition of various prepared dishes and their equivalent caloric yields and protein contents, the percentage of calories in the form of fat and carbohydrates and of protein are now obtainable. With such data a fairly accurate diet may be prepared by serving definite proportions of the total recipe after it has been prepared.[2]

Combustion of food-stuffs *in the calorimeter* in the presence of an excess of oxygen, is initiated by means of a red-hot wire and continued rapidly in the presence of heat developed as the result of the primary oxidation. Had we been able to observe the reaction, we should have noted an intense momentary production of heat. Combustion of food *in the body*, on the other hand, involves smaller masses of food, molecular in size, and the total quantity of energy liberated in one place and at any moment is neither as great nor as intense as in the calorimeter. The oxidation proceeds in stages: thus a molecule of glucose is oxidized gradually, passing through a number of different and successively simpler compounds before it is finally converted into carbon dioxide and water. Enzymes (oxidases) facilitate these processes; the extent and rapidity of which are controlled by a close interrelation of numberless enzymic and physical factors. The result is the gradual liberation of heat under the most favorable conditions for bodily activity.

Proteins, carbohydrates, and fats all yield energy when utilized by the body.

---

[1] Jurgenson, Kochlehrbuch und praktisches Kochlehre, 1910. Cooper, The New Cookery, Battle Creek, Michigan, 1916. Rose, Feeding the Family, New York, 1916.

[2] The use of the data obtained by Gephart and Lusk (Analysis and Cost of Ready to Serve Foods, Jour. Am. Med. Assn., 1915), in conjunction with the purchase of food at the particular restaurants concerned will serve to increase the knowledge of a patient with regard to the relative food values of various prepared dishes.

Determination of Energy Requirement. Calorimeter.— Heat liberated by an organism in the course of its activities can be estimated in two ways: directly by measurement with a calorimeter (direct calorimetry) and indirectly, through the measurement of the oxygen consumed and the carbon dioxide excreted (indirect calorimetry); by means of a respiration apparatus. A combination of the two procedures is often pursued. In the first case the subject is placed in a room constructed on the same general principle as a bomb calorimeter; the calorimeter most used in this country (Atwater, Rosa, Benedict) is of the adiabatic type, *i. e.*, the temperature of the walls is kept practically constant and the heat given off by the subject is absorbed by water circulating through metal coils *within* the chamber. The volume of water passed through the pipes and the increase in temperature are noted and from this data the heat evolved is calculated, with suitable corrections. To this result must be added the heat carried by vaporized water, calculated from the water absorbed from the air which has circulated through the chamber. This type of apparatus differs from the bomb calorimeter, in which the heat evolved is absorbed by water *surrounding* the chamber.

Respiration Apparatus.— The respiration apparatus is a closed, air-tight chamber in which the subject is placed and through which is circulated a current of air. The products of oxidation, carbon dioxide and water, are removed from the air by absorption, by soda lime and sulphuric acid respectively, as they pass from the chamber. These determinations are made either on the total volume of air or from an aliquot portion. Knowing the composition of the entering air and the amount of carbon dioxide and water produced during the experiment, the extent of oxidation can be calculated. In the Atwater-Rosa-Benedict apparatus the respiration apparatus and calorimeter apparatus are combined. In this case the air passed through the apparatus is circuated through a closed system. Oxygen is added to the air just before it enters the chamber, and carbon dioxide and water are removed after it has passed out of the room. By this method not only the carbon dioxide and water given off can be determined but also the absolute amount of oxygen used by the subject can be measured. Comparison of the results of direct calorimetry with the calculated values from CO_2 excreted and oxygen consumed has shown them to be comparable and for short periods—two or three hours—the latter method yields results which are perhaps more accurate.

A less elaborate type of respiration apparatus is also in use, in which the subject breathes through a closed system of the same general nature as that described above without being confined in a specially constructed room.

Respiratory Quotient. — The oxidation of different types of food-stuffs involves combination with various quantities of oxygen and the liberation of variable proportions of carbon dioxide. According to Avogadro's law equal volumes of gases under the same conditions of temperature and pressure contain equal numbers of molecules; hence, when in the oxidation of an atom of carbon a molecule of oxygen (O_2) is used and a molecule of carbon dioxide (CO_2) is produced, no change occurs in the volume of the reacting gases provided the system is returned to the original temperature and pressure. Since carbohydrates contain sufficient oxygen to form water with the hydrogen present in the molecule, combustion therefore involves only the oxidation of the carbon present, consequently the ratio of carbon dioxide produced to oxygen consumed $\frac{CO_2}{O_2}$ is 1. Fats, on the other hand, do not contain sufficient oxygen to combine with their hydrogen to form water, and oxygen is utilized for this purpose in addition to that used in the oxidation of carbon. The ratio of $\frac{CO_2}{O_2}$ is therefore less than 1, in this case approximately 0.7. Protein is intermediate between fats and carbohydrates in its state of oxidation. Its $\frac{CO_2}{O_2}$ ratio is, therefore, less than one, approximately 0.8.

From data obtained with the respiration apparatus the ratio of carbon dioxide formed to oxygen consumed can be calculated; this ratio is designated the respiratory quotient. A high respiratory quotient (above 0.8) is taken as evidence of the utilization of considerable quantities of carbohydrates, a low quotient (near 0.7) as evidence of the extensive utilization of fat by the body. When carbohydrate is transformed into fat, oxygen is derived from the carbohydrate and the respiratory quotient may be greater than 1, whereas in the case of diabetes, protein is converted into carbohydrate and excreted in the urine, less oxygen is excreted as CO_2 than would normally be the case, and the respiratory quotient may be less than 0.7. Results obtained through the calculation of such quotients have been of great value in indicating the differential utilization of food-stuffs in the body.

Basal Metabolism. — Two methods of attack have been employed in determining the total quantity of energy required and the relative proportions of the food-stuffs most suitable for individuals under varying conditions. One, the statistical method, consists in estimating, from observations of a large number of individuals the average quantity and composition of the food eaten by normal individuals during comparatively long periods of time. Such experiments have been carried out in many countries and upon groups of individuals employed in different occupations. These data form a very substantial basis for our deductions regarding the food requirements of man.

The second and more exact method is to determine by means of a calorimeter, or respiration apparatus, the energy exchange of the body under different conditions of activity and states of nutrition. A combined study of the energy exchanged and of the excreta, including the carbon dioxide and water expelled by the lungs (universal respiration apparatus) enables us to estimate the relative amounts of the various food-stuffs utilized by the body. Studies of this sort yield very definite results. The accuracy of these experiments tends to counter-balance the deficiencies arising from the smallness of the number, and the shortness of the periods of observation in this mode of investigation. Atwater, and later his collaborator, Benedict, have collected a large amount of data by both methods of investigation upon the dietetic habits of the American people. It is largely upon their results that our ideas of food requirements are based.[1]

For the estimation of the energy requirements of different individuals and as a basis of comparison between them in experimental work it is essential to have some standard by which they may be measured.

Such a standard in metabolism or basal energy requirement is taken as equivalent to the heat liberated by a fasting man (post-absorptive condition twelve to fifteen hours after the last meal) when lying down, asleep and comparatively relaxed. It may be expressed in terms of the total daily energy requirement, or in smaller units, such as the energy liberated per-kilogram of body weight or square meter of body surface in an hour. Values based on the unit of body weight are suitable only when comparing individuals of approximately the same size, shape and weight; since, in general, a greater amount of energy is produced per unit of weight by a small than a large organism. For the comparison of different individuals, as a man and a child, or of two men of different sizes, expressions of the energy metabolism,

[1] Benedict, Lusk, DuBois, Howland and Murlin have recently contributed a large amount of work bearing upon the fundamental basis of energy exchange, basal metabolism, in the normal adult and child in disease.

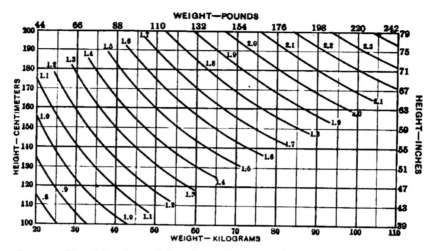

Fig. 1.—Chart[1] for determining the surface area of man in square meters from weight in kilograms (Wt.) and height in centimeters (Ht.) or their equivalents in pounds and inches, according to the formula:

$$\text{Area (sq. cm.)} = \text{Wt.}^{0.425} \times \text{Ht.}^{0.725} \times 71.84.$$

STANDARDS OF NORMAL METABOLISM. AVERAGE CALORIES PER HOUR PER SQUARE METER OF BODY SURFACE.[2]

Subject, age in years.	According to Meeh's formula.	According to linear and height-weight formulas.
Boys, twelve to thirteen	45.7	49.9
Men, twenty to fifty	34.7	39.7
Women, twenty to fifty	32.3	36.9
Men, fifty to sixty	30.8	35.2
Women, fifty to sixty	28.7	32.7

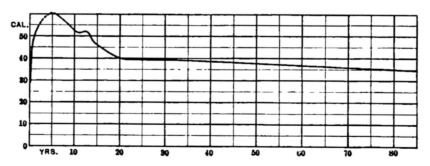

Fig. 2.—Variation of basal metabolism with age: Calories per square meter of body surface per hour. Only the results of male subjects were used in making this curve; the metabolism of female subjects is slightly lower. (Russel Sage Institute of Pathology.)

[1]DuBois and DuBois; Arch, Intern. Med., 1916, xxvii, p. 863.
[2]Gephart and DuBois: Arch, Int. Med., xvii, 913.

PERCENTAGE INCREASE OR DECREASE IN THE HOURLY BASAL METABOLISM FOR VARIOUS FACTORS AFFECTING THE EXTENT OF ENERGY METABOLISM. (ADAPTED FROM THE WORK OF LUSK AND DUBOIS.)

	Increase or decrease, per cent.	Additional Calories per hour for average man.
Average man, 154 pounds (70 kg.), at complete rest, 70 Calories per hour:	Increase.	
Ingestion of food	5 to 10	4 to 7
Lying in a chair, supported	0	0
Sitting up in chair	8	6
Moderate activity in chair	29	20
Very restless in bed	20 to 100	14 to 70
Exercise:		
Walking on level, 2.7 miles per hour	230	160
Climbing, 2.7 miles per hour	580	407
Hard labor, bicycle riding	756	529
Thin but healthy	0	0
Fat but healthy	0	0
Disease:		
Most patients not seriously ill	+10 to —10	+7 to —7
Obesity	+10 to —10	+7 to —7
Diabetes with severe acidosis	0 to 15	0 to 10
Severe pernicious anemia	0 to 20	0 to 14
Acromegaly	0 to 30	0 to 21
Cancer, severe heart and kidney disease and high fever	20 to 40	14 to 28
Leukemia	30 to 60	21 to 42
Typhoid fever	40 to 50	28 to 35
Convalescence	10 to 20	7 to 14
Exophthalmic goiter:		
Mild	25 to 50	18 to 35
Severe	75 to 100	53 to 70
	Decrease.	
Prolonged undernutrition	—10 to —30	—7 to —21
Diabetes, emaciated	—10 to —35	—7 to —25
Cretinism and myxedema	—25 to —50	—18 to —35

EXAMPLE: Man, aged fifty to sixty years; height, 67 inches (170 cm.); weight, 154 pounds (70 kg.); office work most of day (fourteen hours); walks two hours; bed, eight hours.

Calories per hour.

(a) Area, from chart, 1.8 square meters.

(b) Basal metabolism per square meter of body surface (Table, p. 62, man 50–60) 35.2

(c) Basal metabolism of 1.8 × 35.2 . . . . 63.4 (drop 0.4)

(d) Increase for food, 10 per cent. (used in all calculations), 63 × 0.1 6

(e) Increase for bed, resting basal metabolism plus food (c + d), or 63 + 6 69

(f) Increase for office work, moderate activity in chair, 29 per cent.; 63 × 0.29 18

(g) Increase for walking (on level), 230 per cent.; 63 × 2.3 145

Then for the day: Calories per day.

Bed: Eight hours = (c + d) × 8 or (63 + 6) × 8 . 552

Office work: Fourteen hours = (c + d + f) × 14 or (63 + 6 + 18) × 14 1218

Walking: Two hours = (c + d + g) × 2 or (63 + 6 + 145) × 2 428

Total for day 2198

in terms of unit surface, are more accurate and comparable; the number of Calories per square meter per hour is usually selected as the unit of reference. Benedict has recently proposed that basal metabolism be expressed in calories per day or hour determined from equations which involve weight, height and age as factors.

The relative value of body weight and body surface as the basis of comparison between different individuals has recently been studied by Benedict and by DuBois and their co-workers. DuBois has studied the relation of body surface and basal metabolism, and as a result, advocates the use of body surface as the basis of comparison between different individuals. His conclusions are based upon data obtained from the measurements of the energy exchange and of body surface; the latter was determined by a new and more accurate method than any hitherto described. With the aid of this data DuBois has shown that Meeh's formula[1] for calculation of body surface which has been in general use, does not give accurate results for any but a selected (average) group of individuals. DuBois and DuBois[2] have derived a formula (linear formula) in which only linear measurements are concerned; determinations of length and circumference. This formula necessitates a number of careful observations and calculations. For any but the most exact work the following simple formula may be used. It involves but two factors, height and weight (height-weight formula): $A = W^{0.425} \times H^{0.725} \times 71.84$, where A is the area in square centimeters; H, height in centimeters, and W, weight in kilograms. With this formula, or more conveniently with the chart on page 62, the extent of body surface can be readily calculated.

The errors in the linear formula and the height-weight formula have been estimated at a maximum of ±5 per cent., average ±1.5 per cent. while Meeh's formula gives a variation of ±30 per cent., average 15 per cent. The maximum deviations obtained with DuBois' formula apply particularly to those of unusual shape.

While the basal metabolism of various individuals is nearly the same per square meter of body surface, such a comparison is not exact in all cases. Benedict and more recently Harris and Benedict have considered the factors which modify basal or standard metabolism. From an analysis of data obtained in a series of investigations conduc-

[1]Meeh's formula: $S = C\sqrt{W^2}$ where S is surface; W, weight and C a constant dependent upon the shape of the solid; for man C is 12.3.
[2]Arch, Int. Med., 1916, xvii, 855.

ted under similar conditions, in the post-absorptive condition, Benedict called attention to various factors which modify the basal metabolism of different individuals, such as height, weight, activity, age and sex. Harris and Benedict[1] have made a statistical study of the determinations of the basal metabolism of 136 men, 103 women, and 93 infants. A correlation was found between body weight and heat production and between stature and heat production which was higher in the first case than in the second. These factors, weight and height, appear to have independent significance for the prediction of basal metabolism. The degree of correlation is higher for men than for women, but apparently not greater for male infants than for female infants. With increasing age throughout adult life, there is a decrease in heat production which is less for women than for men. This decrease in total daily heat production is essentially uniform from year to year; the daily metabolism is reduced 7.15 Calories for men and 2.29 Calories for women each year. Women are, in general, smaller than men, if then, the metabolism of the two sexes to be compared on the basis of unit of body weight or unit of body surface it is found that there is a much smaller difference than that given above. The difference between men and women is less when compared on the basis of body weight than of body surface. In any case the metabolism of women is found to be less than that of men. When the effect of body weight, stature and age are taken into consideration women show a metabolism approximately 6.4 per cent. less than that of men.

The value of the unit of body weight and of body surface in predicting the basal metabolism of different individuals has been questioned by Harris and Benedict. These authors show that the "body surface law," which assumes that the heat production of an organism is proportional to its superficial area, is open to question. Such a law presupposes the constancy of heat production in the same individual at different times and also a constancy of heat production per square meter of body surface in different individuals. These conditions are not fulfilled in the case of fasting men or men subjected to under-feeding in which the changes in metabolism are not commensurate with the changes in body surface. The influence of sex, age, and activity are also deviations from the body surface law.

[1] Harris and Benedict: Carnegie Publications, 1919, 279; Proc. Natl. Acad Sciences, 1918, 370.

5

Heat production was found to be highly and apparently equally correlated with body weight and body surface. Predictions of basal metabolism on the basis of body surface, using DuBois height weight chart, have apparently a slight superiority over the use of body surface when these two methods are compared upon a statistical basis. The apparent greater accuracy of body surface as a unit of comparison is held to be due to the fact that body surface takes into account both weight and height.

An equation for calculation of a standard of basal metabolism for adults in the range covered by Harris and Benedict has been developed. This equation takes into consideration the factors found to be most evidently related to the quantity of heat produced in human adults; height, weight and age. These equations for the total *daily basal metabolism* are:

For men, $h = 66.4730 + 13.7516\ w + 5.0033\ s - 6.7550\ a$. For women, $h = 655.0955 + 9.5634\ w + 1.8496\ s - 4.6756\ a$. Where h=total heat production per 24 hours, w=weight in kilograms, s=stature in centimeters and a=age in years.[1] These equations predict the total daily basal metabolism of various individuals more accurately than the DuBois formula. Calculations of the total daily metabolism must take into account the daily activities of the individual under consideration. The hourly basal metabolism calculated from these equations can be used with the percentage variations in activity indicated on page 63 if desired.

Basal metabolism varies with activity, age, size, sex, training and disease. In considering the average energy requirement the effect of these factors must be recognized even though we do not have at present all the necessary data to correct them in our estimations. Sufficient data have been collected with regard to age to indicate the trend of the variation and to permit the use of such data in calculating energy requirements during certain periods of life. Benedict holds that "the basal metabolism is a function of both the total mass of active protoplasmic tissue and of the stimulus to cellular activity existing at the time the measurement of metabolism is made." Body composition *i. e.*, proportion of active protoplasmic tissue to the inert body fat, has an effect upon the basal metabolism, thus the

---

[1] Tables have been prepared by Benedict and Harris in their publication to facilitate calculation, which involve only the addition of two figures. These tables are too extensive for publication here. If the above equations be abbreviated such that all figures below unity except the first be eliminated these equations will be found to be easily handled and accurate for practical purposes.

tendency of athletes toward a higher metabolism when compared with non-athletes is to be ascribed to their greater muscular development; the lower metabolism of women than of men, is apparently associated with their greater proportion of inert body fat (lower muscular development) and in part to an inherent characteristic of sex; tall persons have a greater metabolism than short individuals since they have proportionately greater amounts of muscular tissue. Another factor that modifies the basal metabolism, stimulation of cellular activity is influenced by a number of factors: age, sleep, character of preceding diet and after-effects of severe muscular work; there are also variations in the diurnal as well as day-to-day metabolism.

The effect of age has been more extensively studied than the other factors which affect the basal mtabolism. The active youth has a higher rate of metabolism than a person in middle life, while an old man has a still lower metabolism. The metabolism of an infant is low during the first month, after which it becomes much higher. In childhood the basal metabolism is above that of the adult, with increasing age the rate of metabolism decreases until it reaches that of the adult at about twenty years of age; there is a slight rise at about puberty. During adult life the rate of decrease of basal metabolism is fairly uniform and rather gradual; it is greater for men than for women. The chart on page 62 indicates the variations in basal metabolism with age. In calculating the metabolism of persons of different ages, no correction need be made when the Harris-Benedict formula is used (for adults); with the DuBois chart page 62 the standards of normal metabolism proposed by Gephart and DuBois may be used.

Daily habits and the nutritional condition affect the energy changes. A fasting subject lying perfectly still immediately after waking in the morning has been shown to have an average metabolism which was 13 per cent. higher than when asleep. Later in the day under similar conditions the metabolism increased to 22 per cent. above the resting state. Prolonged fasting results in a lower metabolism than before fasting. Severe muscular work is accompanied by a continued higher rate of metabolism some time after the cessation of work. These variations have been ascribed by Benedict, as indicated above, to an alteration in the stimulus to cellular activity. The effect of a decrease in body weight in the same individual is a lowered rate of metabolism. A 12 per cent. loss of weight was found to be accompanied by an energy requirement which was approximately one-third less, and the heat output per kilogram of body weight or per square meter of body surface was 18 per cent. less than that required at the original weight (Benedict).

In addition to the factors which modify the basal metabolism there are others which have a direct effect upon the total daily metabolism: food, activity, temperature and disease. The ingestion of food causes an increase in the rate of metabolism. Experiments upon fasting men and animals have established the fact that after the removal of the effect of the previous diet, which affects metabolism during the first part of a fast, the energy production is low and practically constant. If to such an organism food be given, there will be an increase in the basal energy metabolism which will vary with the kind and quantity of food ingested. Protein exerts a greater stimulation than carbohydrate or fat. Small quantities of food will increase the basal energy metabolism from 5 to 10 per cent. While following the ingestion of large quantities of food, the increase may be as high as 40 per cent. This increase begins in the case of proteins and carbohydrates, in from a half-hour to an hour after the ingestion of food, while following the ingestion of fat there is little increase until five or six hours afterward. The increase in the basal metabolism following the ingestion of food is designated as the *specific dynamic effect* of food. The effect of protein has been shown by Lusk to be due to a stimulation of the metabolism of the cells by certain of the amino-acids. The effect of carbohydrate and fat, on the other hand, is due to the mass action of these food-stuffs in the circulation—as the result of plethora. Benedict has also suggested that this increased metabolism is the result of stimulation of cellular activity.

Muscular activity has a direct effect upon the energy requirement of an individual. In studying the basal energy metabolism of a fasting man, as indicated above, it was found that the metabolism was increased 13 per cent. above that of the sleeping metabolism merely as the result of being awake, and that continued mental activity and prolonged muscular activity resulted in a further increase of 9 per cent. in the basal metabolism measured under conditions of complete repose later in the day. As the intensity increases there is a proportionate increase in the energy exchange. Energy-yielding food must be supplied to meet this increase.

Training in the performance of work has a tendency to reduce the energy requirement for a given piece of work. The beginner makes a greater effort to perform his work, for many false motions are made; the result is an increased metabolism. Experience and routine gradually reduce the number of unnecessary movements with a corresponding reduction in the energy exchange.

Studies of the relative efficiency of the human body—the proportion of energy contained in food which is transformed into work—shows the body to be a very efficient machine. Experiments in which a man rode a specially constructed bicycle, by means of which the work performed in riding could be measured, showed that 35 per cent. of the total energy transformed during muscular work was used in the accomplishment of the work. In general, however, the efficiency of the body in converting the potential energy in the food into work is found to be approximately 20 per cent.

The energy required to accomplish a given[1] amount of work was found to be the same irrespective of whether the body was in the best of nutritive condition or had lost weight as the result of fasting. The effect of loss of weight is to result in an economy in the basal metabolsim and a lower energy requirement for the performance of work because of the smaller weight, but for similar amounts of work the energy expended was the same. Work performed following the ingestion of carbohydrate, glucose, did not result in an increased energy output above that for the same amount of work without carbohydrates, *i. e.*, there was not a summation of the energy required for work and extra heat produced following the ingestion of carbohydrate. Meat and alanine, however, exerted their specific dynamic effect upon the metabolism with the production of energy which was not utilizable for the production of work. In this case the energy production for a given amount of work was equal to that required for the work performed without food plus the extra heat resulting from the effect of the protein or its products.

To meet the increased energy requirement which accompanies muscular activity the body must be supplied with greater quantities of energy-yielding food. Protein metabolism, as we will show later, is not increased to any extent during work provided sufficient fat and carbohydrate are present. Fat is capable of yielding a greater quantity of heat per gram than carbohydrate. Carbohydrate, on the other hand, is apparently more readily oxidized in the body. Studies of the respiratory quotient during work has demonstrated an increased utilization of carbohydrate at such times. These observations indicate that the stores of carbo-

[1] Anderson and Lusk: Jour. Biol. Chem. 1917, xxxii, 421.

hydrate are being utilized for the performance of work in preference to the fats. The use of carbohydrate as a prime source of energy is emphasized by the fact that following the cessation of work the body appears to be subsisting in the presence of a depleted store of carbohydrates (Benedict). Other experiments show, however, that fat is capable of supplying the energy requirement of the body, particularly in the presence of small quantities of carbohydrate. In a sudden burst of activity, then, carbohydrates are more satisfactory than fats. In long-continued activity the fats which are apparently oxidized with difficulty are extensively utilized. Where there is an excessive prolonged energy requirement such as in continuous severe labor and in cold climates, an increase in the more concentrated fats in the diet is desirable; for, were the heat derived entirely from carbohydrates it would entail an excessive ingestion of vegetable food.

Age, with its variation in the processes of metabolism—in the young the predominance of anabolic over catabolic functions (formation of new tissues) continuous activity and greater rate of metabolism as contrasted with the slower movements, lowered rate of metabolism and muscular tone accompanied usually by decreasing weight with age—exhibits a variation from the requirements of the average adult in the prime of life.

Disease affects the basal metabolism; it may be increased as in exophthalmic goiter (Grave's disease) 75 to 100 per cent.; in typhoid fever, 40 to 50 per cent.; in anemia, cancer, severe cases of heart and kidney disease and high fevers, 20 to 40 per cent.; it may be decreased as in cretinism and myxedema 20 to 50 per cent.; or it may approximate the normal rate as in diabetes. Considerations of the energy requirement in various diseases will be found in discussions relating to them. It is an interesting fact that in typhoid fever when the basal metabolism is markedly increased, the ingestion of food is not accompanied by a marked increased heat production or specific dynamic effect. This fact is of impotance, for it permits, on a scientific basis, the feeding of fever patients with the large quantities of food necessary to meet the requirements of their increased metabolism without fear of materially augmenting the metabolism because of the inherent stimulating effect of the food itself.

To summarize our discussion: The energy metabolism of various individuals of different sizes may be quite accurately compared on the basis of the extent of their body surface The intensity of metabolism varies with the mass of active protoplasmic tissue and the stimulation to cellular activity as represented, for example, by sex and age. Food-stuffs have their specific effects upon the rate of heat production. The varied activities of life aside from those included in the basal metabolism are associated with an extra expenditure of energy. Evaluations of the daily average metabolism include allowances for all such variations in activity and they must be used accordingly.

When it is desired to know the energy requirements of an individual with a fair degree of accuracy the value should be calculated with the use of the height weight formula of DuBois or the equation of Benedict, see p. 62 to 66, making suitable corrections for activity and disease if present. When a rough approximation is all that is desired the data in the tables given below are sufficient.

	Calories per hour.
Man sleeping	65
Man sitting at rest	100
Man at light muscular exercise	170
Man at active muscular exercise	290
Man at severe muscular exercise	450
Man at very severe muscular exercise	600

In estimating the daily energy requirement of a man the day is considered as being made up of a number of periods of various types of activity whose hourly energy transformations are approximately known. The total requirement is, then, a summation of these hourly transformations. Such calculation of the heat exchange has been made for an average man at light muscular work, taking into consideration the variation in activity.

	Calories per hour.	Heat output.
At rest, sleeping eight hours	65	520
At rest, awake, sitting up six hours	100	600
Light muscular exercise ten hours	170	1700
Total output of heat for twenty-four hours		2820

The daily energy requirement of man under various conditions has been given by Lusk as follows:

	Calories per day.
In bed twenty-four hours; absolute rest without food	1,680
In bed twenty-four hours; absolute rest with food	1,840
In bed eight hours; work in which sitting in a chair, sixteen hours; with food	2,170
In bed eight hours; in a chair fourteen hours, moderate exercise, two hours	2,500
In bed eight hours; in a chair fourteen hours, vigorous exercise two hours; with food	3,000
Farmer, active exercise	3,500
Lumberman	5,000
Rider in a six-day bicycle race	10,000

The following table gives the extra calories attributable to occupation and the total daily metabolism for average men and women at various occupations:

Occupations of men.	Extra calories per hour	Total daily metabolism. Average man 5 ft. 8 inches and 155 lbs.
Basal		1770
Hospital ward		1900
Tailor	44	2240
Bookbinder	81	2530
Shoemaker	90	2600
Metal worker, filing and hammering	141	3000
Painter of furniture	145	3050
Carpenter making table	164	3200
Stonemason chiseling tombstone	300	4300
Man sawing wood	378	4900

Occupations of women.		Average woman 5 ft. 4½ inches and 134 lbs.
Basal		1480
Hospital ward		1580
Seamstress, needlework	6	1630
Typist, 50 words per minute	24	1770
Bookbinder	57	2030
Seamstress using sewing machine	63	2080
Housemaid, moderate work	81	2220
Laundress, moderate work	124	2560
Housemaid, hard work	157	2830
Laundress, hard work	214	3490

The following daily energy requirements for infants and children have been suggested.

ENERGY REQUIREMENTS FOR CHILDREN.

	Total Calories per day.
1 to 2	900 to 1200
2 to 5	1200 to 1500
6 to 9	1400 to 2000
10 to 13	1800 to 2200
14 to 17 girls	2200 to 2600
boys	2500 to 3000[2]

Atwater has given comparative values for the metabolism of the different members of a family. On the basis of the father having a rate of 1, the energy requirements of the rest of the family would be:

Father	1.0
Mother	0.8
Sons: 14 to 17	0.8 to 1.5
Daughters: 14 to 17	0.7 to 1.0
Children: 10 to 13	0.6 to 1.0
6 to 9	0.5
2 to 5	0.4
Under 2	0.3

[1] Jour. Am. Med. Assoc., 1918 lxx 821.
[2] Lusk and Gephart have found from a study of the food eaten by boys in a fashionable boarding school that an active boy may consume food equivalent to 4000 to 5000 calories per day.

CHAPTER III

PROTEIN REQUIREMENT.

In our previous discussions, as well as in our subsequent discussions relating to protein-rich foods, we have taken up the composition of protein material in general, its digestion, absorption, and the change which it undergoes in the process of assimilation. At present we are concerened with the quantitative relation of protein in the diet and the factors which influence this.

Protein as we have already found, is an essential constituent of our daily dietary. Energy may be derived from portein, fat or carbohydrate but only protein or its products of hydrolysis can furnish the amino-acids necessary to replace the loss of nitrogenous material in the tissues resulting from the general bodily functions or for the constructive processes of growth.

The necessity for the presence of protein in the dietary was early recognized. It was, in fact, a more difficult task to demonstrate that this food constituent was concerned more particularly in the structural changes of the body than primarily as a source of energy for muscular work. We no longer say, as did Liebig, that protein is the source of muscular energy, but recognize that this function belongs to the carbohydrates and fats, and consider protein as the chief source of material for the repair of the wear and tear in the muscles and other parts of the body.

Admitting that the necessity for protein is so well established that it is practically self-evident, we may take up the question of the quantity of protein necessary for the body, how it may be supplied, and the relative efficiency of protein for the needs of the body.

Methods employed for the study of these problems are in general the two considered in our discussion of the energy requirements of the body: the purely experimental and the statistical. In the experimental studies use is made of the nitrogen balance or of the rate of growth of young animals, such as rats, when compared with the normal rate of growth. For the determination of the nitrogen balance the nitrogen content of the food—representing the protein material—

feces, urine, and in some cases the hair, scurf and excretions from the skin, are analyzed for definite periods of time. The quantity of nitrogen found in all of the excretions is then subtracted from that in the food. If the result is a positive figure, that is, if there is less nitrogen in the excretions than in the food, then the subject is said to have a positive nitrogen balance, for he has retained in his body a certain amount of nitrogen-containing material. If the result be a negative value, *i. e.*, more nitrogen in the excretions than was contained in the food, the subject has supplied nitrogenous material from his tissues and is said to have a negative nitrogen balance. A normal adult is usually in an approximate nitrogen equilibrium. During growth and regeneration—youth, pregnancy and convalescence—the organism normally shows a positive balance. In conditions of emaciation, fever or wasting diseases a negative balance is obtained.

The average daily protein metabolism or plane of nitrogen equilibrium varies in the same individual, according to the quantity of protein ingested. A sudden change from a low to a high protein diet, or *vice versa*, is not accompanied by an equally abrupt variation in the daily excretion of nitrogen. Instead there is a gradual increase or decrease in the quantity of nitrogen eliminated until the new plane of metabolism is finally attained and the subject is once more in nitrogen equilibrium, approximately three days. When protein food is completely removed from the diet the total nitrogenous excretion is an index of the internal, or endogenous, metabolism of the individual.

An exact determination of the endogenous protein metabolism of man is the ideal basis for the study of the needs of the body. This is a difficult procedure, for many contributing factors modify the quantity of nitrogen excreted—our measure of the rate of the protein metabolism. When all of the food elements are removed as in fasting, we might expect to obtain a measure of the endogenous protein. metabolism. Experiments upon men and animals have shown, however, that this is not the case, for a number of modifying factors, such as the previous diet and the quantity of fat and carbohydrate (glycogen) present in the body, will modify the course of the cellular activities and the protein metabolism.

The plane of protein metabolism in the early stages of fasting is affected by the previous dietary regimen. When this diet has been rich in protein, a larger quantity of nitrogen is excreted in the urine than would have been obtained had the diet been poor in protein—just as with a normal diet, if the protein quota be decreased, the nitrogenous excretion changes gradually and not abruptly from one level to another. It is evident, therefore, that it would not be accurate to accept the quantity of nitrogen excreted in the early part of a fast as a measure of the endogenous protein metabolism. Neither can we accept the nitrogen excreted after the effects of the previous nitrogenous diet have passed, for during this period of readjustment other factors have been developing an abnormal influence. The normal man is accustomed to derive the greater portion of his energy from the oxidation of carbohydrates and fats. A fast is commenced with a small reserve of carbohydrate, glycogen, and a somewhat larger reserve of fat. During the first few days, while the effects of the previous diet have been disappearing, practically all of the glycogen reserve has been utilized and after this the body subsists upon a diet, so to speak, of fat and protein. The removal of carbohydrate material from the diet of a man who is accustomed to this food element in his diet results in a disturbance of his metabolism, particularly a change in the fat metabolism. Under such conditions the body seems to be unable completely to oxidize fats. Partially oxidized fatty acids are passed into the blood stream and these cause a disturbance of the equilibrium between the acidic and basic radicles which has its effect upon the respiratory and salt metabolism and ultimately, if not directly, upon the protein metabolism. We have evidence of the incomplete oxidation in the beta-hydroxybutyric and aceto-acetic acids, in the urine, and of a disturbed equilibrium in the increased ammonia and acidity of the urine. Such disturbances are experienced not only in fasting man but in diabetes, in which there is a failure to oxidize glucose, and they have been demonstrated experimentally by feeding a carbohydrate-free diet to men and to animals accustomed to a carbohydrate-rich diet. Acidosis increases the rate of protein metabolism. In fasting a further increase of protein metabolism results when the fat supply is reduced and the organism is forced to utilize protein material as a source of energy. A measure of endogenous metabolism cannot therefore be obtained by means of fasting experiments.

A study of the metabolic changes on a protein-free diet containing carbohydrates, fats and salts in the proper proportions is perhaps a better index of the endogenous protein metabolism. This procedure is also open to question for under these conditions the body is supplying from its own tissues the protein material needed for repair.

Studies of the endogenous protein metabolism show that the average man metabolizes from 0.04 to 0.03 gram of nitrogen per kilogram of body weight—2.1 to 3.8 grams of nitrogen for a 70-kilogram (154 lb.) man—in the form of protein in the processes associated with the general wear and tear of the body.

In constitution the protein molecule varies in both the quantity and the kind of amino-acids according to its source. If we compare the quantities of amino-acids in certain proteins we see that were a man to eat the vegetable protein gliadin alone he would have considerable more glutamic acid than was absolutely necessary and to obtain sufficient lysine to form a protein of the approximate composition of, say, beef protein he would have to ingest a much larger quantity of gliadin than beef or other animal proteins.

Protein.	Glutamic acid.	Lysine.
Gliadin	43.7	0.15
Zein	26.2	0
Legumin	13.0	3.03
Casein	15.6	6.00
Gelatin	16.8	6.00
Beef protein	15.5	7.60
Fish protein	10.1	7.50

The chemical structure of the protein ingested must therefore be considered in determining the protein requirement. If the ingested protein contains a proportion of any essential amino-acid that is less than the quantity needed by the body or lacks the acid entirely, it becomes necessary for the body to synthetize the required amino-acid from other available acids or products, or to supply the amino-acid either by an increased ingestion of the protein itself, if the failure be due only to a lowered content, or by the ingestion of other proteins, or of the amino-acid itself if it be entirely absent. Conversely, if the protein contain a greater proportion of certain amino-acids than the body can utilize they will not be used but deaminized, oxidized and the products excreted.

Our knowledge of the synthesis of amino-acids in the body is very limited. Glycocoll is apparently synthetized and, under experimental conditions, perfusion of the liver, the formation of alanine, phenylalanine, and tyrosine have been demonstrated. The extensive synthesis of amino-acids in the body has not, however, been shown. Studies of such problems are complicated by the possibility that apparent synthesis may be due to the formation of the amino-acid by bacteria in the intestines and its subsequent utilization by the body. Synthesis of amino-acids with cyclic nuclei appears to be particularly difficult. The body cannot, then, be depended upon to supply the missing amino-acids; they must be added to the diet as such or in the form of protein containing them.

The fact that gelatin cannot of itself satisfy the total protein requirement is due to its lack of the amino-acids, tryptophan, tyrosine, and cystine. The addition of tyrosine and cystine and trytophan has been found to improve its value and make it satisfactory, for short periods at least. Experments with growing rats have likewise served to demonstrate the effect of various quantities of amino-acids in the diet. A protein of corn, zein, which is deficient in the amino-acids, lysine and tryptophan, is found to be unable to support growth or even to maintain the rats without loss of weight. With the substitution of equivalent quantities of other complete proteins the rats grow normally. The addition of tryptophan to the zein diet serves to maintain the rats without growth; while the addition of both tryptophan and lysine makes the diet sufficient for both growth and maintainance. The importance of lysine for growth has been shown in experiments in which gliadin, a vegetable protein containing no lysine but tryptophan, was fed. The rats maintained their body weight but did not grow: the addition of lysine made the diet satisfactory. In one of Osborne and Mendel's experiments with gliadin a rat which failed to grow gave birth to a litter of young which grew at the normal rate on their mother's milk. Later these rats were fed different diets. Those which received complete proteins grew at the normal rate while one which received the diet fed to the mother failed to grow. From experiments of this nature carried out by Willcocks and Hopkins, Osborne and Mendel, and Hart and McCollum, it has become evident that, other necessary factors being present, the absence or a slight deficiency in the protein fed of an amino-acid essential in cellular metabolism, determines the extent of tissue construction, or rate of growth. With the absence of such units the other amino-acids which would have been used in the formation of a protein molecule cannot be utilized; they may be used in some processes in the formation of tissue or secretions not involving the missing radicle or are deaminized and oxidized. McCollum has suggested that the processes of repair do not necessarily involve the decomposition and synthesis of an entire protein molecule.

The quantity of protein needed also depends upon other factors in the diet. McCollum in studying the presence of toxic substances in natural foods (wheat) and their effect upon growth found that protein tends to neutralize the effect of such substances. He explained his findings as follows: "A single factor (protein) in a ration may appear to admit the maximum performance of the animal with respect to growth, without itself representing the optimum amount or character. When this circumstance prevails it may entirely escape notice, yet if in another ration exactly like it, except that a second factor tends to injure the animal, nutritive failure may result. In such a case as the latter the improvement of the protein factor by the addition of more protein or by the substitution of a better protein, the plane of protein intake remaining unchanged, the animal may make the maximum performance notwithstanding the unfavorable character of the injurious factor of the ration." This finding is an argument, in general, for a high rather than a low protein diet whenever the protein is not carefully selected.

The addition of protein nitrogen in amounts equivalent to the basal nitrogen requirement, to a diet containing a sufficient quantity of fat and carbohydrate may not necessarily serve to prevent a loss of protein from the body. This may be due to the nature of the protein as already discussed, or to the number of portions into which the daily quota is subdivided and ingested, in other words, the number of meals per day. Ingested protein is rapidly metabolized and there is little storage of protein or amino-acids in comparison to the reserves of fat and carbohydrate in the body. If the protein required for one day be ingested at one time a large proportion of it will be utilized or deaminized in from six to nine hours; and to satisfy the needs of the actively functioning tissues the body will draw upon its own protein reserves. By taking the protein in smaller quantities a number of times a day the body will be more continuously supplied with the necessary amino-acids derived from its digestion. A similar effect can be produced in part by mixing the protein with more or less indigestible material which apparently delays the digestion and absorption of protein. Nitrogen equilibrium has been maintained upon a diet low in protein when ingested in six equal portions which was not sufficient when ingested in three portions.

The following studies by Thomas of the relative efficiency of protein in the maintenance of nitrogen equilibrium illustrate the variable usefulness of different proteins. The basis of valuation of the food proteins is such that 100 represents protein which satisfies the basal requirement determined on a protein-free diet when fed in equivalent quantities—with ample quantities of carbohydrate and fat.

BIOLOGICAL VALUE OF PROTEINS.

Meat	104.7
Milk	99.7
Fish	94.5
Rice	88.3
Potato	78.9
Bean	55.7
Flour (wheat)	39.6
Corn	29.5

The high efficiency of meat protein has been ascribed by Thomas as due to the effect of extractives which may be concerned in the maintenance of nitrogen equilibrium. This is only one possibility for we know little of the relative structures and combination of proteins in different foods or of associated factors, all of which might be effective. It is certainly true that animal proteins in general are more efficient in the human economy than vegetable proteins.

Our discussion has confined itself more or less to particular proteins. In the average diet a mixture of proteins is ingested so that the sum total is entirely sufficient for the needs of the body. In meat inefficient gelatin (collagen) occurs with the eminently satisfactory muscle protein, and likewise in corn the incomplete zein is associated with other proteins which contain the requisite amino-acids. Studies of the value of particular types of protein rich foods have indicated that a diet restricted to a single kind of seed (pea or bean), or grain, supplies protein of low biological value. Mixtures of protein from different vegetable products are better than the single food but no combination is superior to the milk proteins in supplying adequate protein (McCollum).

The protein requirement is influenced by the quantity of fat and carbohydrate, energy-yielding foods, present in the diet. The effect of these food-stuffs is to lower or raise the plane of protein metabolism when added or subtracted from a nitrogenous diet; fat is, however, less effective than carbohydrate. If the carbohydrates of a mixed diet, upon which nitrogen equilibrium is being maintained, be replaced by an isodynamic quantity of fat, a negative nitrogen balance will result; that is, the body will use some of its protein reserve. The replacement of fat by carbohydrate is accompanied by a lowered protein utilization. This is particularly true when the protein ingestion is low. When carbohydrates are fed to a fasting man or dog, or to one who is receiving a carbohydrate-free diet, either with or without protein, the rate of nitrogen excretion is lowered. Fat also is capable of reducing the plane of nitrogen metabolism of a fasting organism, particularly when the subject is poor in fat. Variations of fat and carbohydrates within certain limits when both appear in the diet at the same time do not result in marked variations in the protein metabolism. It may be that the failure of fat to maintain nitrogen equilibrium when it replaces carbohydrates is due to the fact that the body requires a certain amount of carbohydrate for its normal functioning and, that since fat apparently does not yield carbohydrate, and the amino-acids of the protein molecule may do so, the body breaks down an additional quantity of protein to furnish the necessary carbohydrate. Thomas has suggested that the beneficial effect of carbohydrate is concerned with the synthesis of amino-acid in the body.

Lusk has suggested that 10 to 15 per cent. of the total energy requirement be in the form of protein. This applies approximately to people of all ages. For the average protein requirement of man see the following discussion of standard dietaries.

STANDARD DIETARIES—AVERAGE PROTEIN REQUIREMENT

Practically all the standard dietaries which have been proposed have been determined by the statistical method. Observations have been made of the quantity and kind of food ingested by a large number of persons under different circumstances; the composition of various kinds of food has been determined; on the assumption that the results of these analyses approximate the composition of the food eaten in the dietary investigated, the amounts of protein, fat, and carbohydrate in the diet have been determined. Voit's standard was the first to attract widespread attention and it has been the nucleus of controversy concerning the optimum protein requirement for man. Voit proposed for a man at moderate work:

Protein	118 grams.
Fat	56 "
Carbohydrate	500 "
Total calories	3055 "

Investigations of the dietary habits of groups of people in various countries and conditions have been the basis of other dietary standards. The following table contains some of the standards which have been suggested:

STANDARD DIETARIES.

Author and conditions.	Protein. gm.	Fat, gm.	Carbohydrate, gm.	Fuel value, Calories.
Atwater (man):				
Hard work	150	..	..	4150
Moderate work . . .	125	..	..	3400
Sedentary life	100	..	..	2700
Rest (or woman at light				
work)	90	..	..	2450
Voit (Germany):				
Average diet	118	56	500	3053
Hard work	145	100	450	3300
Playfair (England) . .	119	51	531	3060
Gautier (France) . . .	107	65	407	2630
Chittenden	60	..		2800

From this table we see that the quantity of food in the form of protein, fat and carbohydrate varies with the kind and degree of work performed; the amount of food required varies also with age, and with the sex of the individual.

The influence of work upon the energy and protein requirements has been discussed in general. A greater consumption of energy-yielding material is required to satisfy the needs of a man at work than is required by a person at rest. This fact has been established by careful experiments in confirmation of the results obtained by dietary studies.

External temperature also modifies energy requirements. A man exposed to the cold requires a greater quantity of energy-yielding food than the one who does the same work at a moderate temperature. For this reason studies of the daily habits of people of different climates show the ingestion of diets of different energy contents. Differences in the size and age of individuals involve diets of different energy content. The infant has a higher energy metabolism than an adult in the prime of life; and an old man, a smaller requirement. Two adults of the same size and weight, performing the same work, require approximately the same amount of energy. But where there is a difference in size, as in the case of a lean man and a fat man of the same weight, and approximately the same body surface, the energy requirement of the thin man is much higher because of the greater mass of functioning tissue.

To these physiological factors, which influence the energy requirement of man, the physical and economic factors must be added. Such considerations as taste, habit and custom, the kind of food available, and the ability to purchase, modify the quantity and kind of food eaten by any given group of individuals. Hence the standards based upon the study of the food consumption of various classes and races of people reveal not only the *actual needs but also the habits and propensities* of the people.

6

When considering the basal protein requirement of man we found that muscular activity had practically no effect upon the protein metabolism. An examination of the table containing the proposed standard diets of various investigators shows an increase in the quantity of protein where the fat and carbohydrate have been increased to meet the changed energy requirements. The studies on which these standards are based apply to men of different physique and muscular development, which difference is in itself reason for different amounts of protein in the diets. When it is considered, however, that the protein consumption of a man at moderate labor is already greatly in excess of his basal requirements, it is difficult to understand the reason for for large increases in the protein portion of the diet of individuals at hard labor whose muscular development probably is not greatly increased.

The increased production of heat (specific dynamic action) following the ingestion of protein, with the accompanying feeling of warmth is a partial explanation of the desirability of an increased protein ingestion by those exposed to cold; and, conversely, of the undesirability of a high protein diet in the tropical climates. The heat derived from such action of protein has been shown to be available for the maintenance of body temperature, but not for work.

The optimum protein requirement of man has been a subject of considerable controversy. The discussion concerns chiefly the standards which we have already discussed—approximately 100 to 150 grams of protein per day—and an amount considerably less than this, 50 to 75 grams of protein per day. On the one hand there is evidence of the amount of protein which various peoples have been in the habit of eating and apparently crave. On the other hand there is a physiological basis for a low protein diet in that the minimal requirements of the average man are much lower than 100 grams of protein per day, that the body can satisfy its energy requirements with fats and carbohydrate and that the protein material taken in excess of the body needs is decomposed, and the nitrogen portion is excreted in the kidneys chiefly in the form of urea, while the carbon moiety is utilized for the production of energy. Chittenden has been the chief advocate of the low protein diet. Hindhede, from his work on the use of the potato as the chief article in the diet, has recently advocated an even lower diet than that of Chittenden.

Various arguments have been advanced for and against a low protein diet. Those who believe that such a diet is advisable base their opinion, in addition to the facts indicated above, on observations which indicate that such a diet results in greater strength and endurance, is more economical and is accompanied by a lowered intestinal putrefaction. Against a low protein diet arguments have been presented to the effect that men do not eat a low protein diet from choice, that there is the danger of the selection of a diet with a low total caloric value, that the "minimum is not necessarily the optimum," and that low planes of mental, moral and physical development exist in countries in which the population subsist on a low protein plane. One of the most telling arguments in favor of a high protein diet where the nature of the protein and the qualitative nature of the diet is not known, is the finding of McCullom that an increase of the protein portion of a diet will in certain cases overcome the effect of toxic substances present in food.

The values for the *average protein requirement* given in the table on page 81 have been determined chiefly by statistical means. The protein requirement is apparently not affected by as many variables as the energy requirement. Muscular work does not materially affect the protein metabolism provided the increased energy requirements are met with sufficient quantities of non-nitrogenous food-stuffs: fat and carbohydrates. When the body is already meeting a part of its energy requirements with protein material, such as might exist in underfeeding or in fasting, increased activity is associated with an increased protein destruction. There might in the course of time be an indirect increase in the protein metabolism following work as a result of an increase in the quantity of muscular tissue with its greater "wear and tear."

The protein requirement varies with the age of the individual considered. An infant, which is forming new protein as well as repairing the wear and tear of its body, requires proportionately more protein than does an adult who needs only to supply the protein for repair. An old man, with relatively diminished muscular development and tone, requires less protein material than the adult who is in the prime of his life. Muscular development undoubtedly affects the amount of nitrogenous material required; while the protein needs of the pregnant woman or nursing mother are increased because of the storage of nitrogenous material in pregnancy, and the drain upon the stored protein experienced during lactation. Although the average diet contains sufficient protein material to cover any variations in the requirements due to size, age, and sex, these factors must be considered when an insufficient or a restricted diet is prescribed.

CHAPTER IV.

INORGANIC SALTS, WATER AND VITAMINES

THE importance of inorganic salts has not been emphasized in dietetics so much as the energy and protein parts of the diet. That this is so has been due in part to the fact that the average mixed diet contains a sufficient amount of the various inorganic constituents for all general purposes. Studies of pathological conditions, however, have repeatedly demonstrated that a diet may be entirely satisfactory from the stand-point of protein and energy and still be lacking in some inorganic constituent, or group of constituents, which, when supplied, rectified the trouble. Recent studies of the biological value of various foods and in the use of diets composed of purified food-stuffs in the study of the presence or absence of the vitamines have emphasized the importance of the necessity for the proper kinds and proportions of inorganic salts in the diet. In such work it has been found that an improper salt mixture may be as detrimental to growth as one which lacks other food factors, such as inadequate protein or the vitamines.

A consideration of the role played by inorganic substances in nutrition will serve to bring out their importance in the dietary. Whereas fat, protein, and carbohydrate serve to furnish energy to the body, inorganic salts are not concerned directly with this. In their capacity, however, of regulating the body functions they contribute toward the oxidation of these various food substances. Iron in particular appears to be concerned in oxidation. We find this element in the red blood corpuscles as an important and apparently active constituent of the hemoglobin. Certain investigators have attempted to show that the action of oxidases is due to the inorganic elements or salts which are contained in them.

The fluids and tissues of the body are maintained in osmotic equilibrium by the contained salts. The accumulation of water in one portion of the body or the desiccation in another is prevented by the diffusibility of salts or the attraction for water when separated from the surrounding medium by a semipermeable membrane. When there is a perversion of this property by a change in the physical structures or the chemical properties we find pathogenic states to exist, such, for instance as the condition of edema.

The inorganic elements occur in the body in two general forms: (*a*) Combined with organic material as such, as radicles or held in an insoluble form such as the iron of hemoglobin, the phosphorus of nucleoprotein, the iodine of the thyroid gland, and the constituents of the structural tissue and of all actively functioning tissues, *e. g.*, the calcium and magnesium and phosphorus of the bone; (*b*) in solution as ionizable salts where they are active in maintaining osmotic equilibrium, and the constant reaction of the body fluids, assisting in the transportation of the oxygen and carbon dioxide in the blood, concerned in the permeability of the cell walls, and affecting the irritability of muscle and nerve.

The mere enumeration of a few of the important uses of the inorganic element brings out strikingly their significance. The multiplicity of their function has likewise rendered the study of these substances difficult, for with one element having a varied function, its removal from the diet may be responsible for many secondary reactions which will mask the direct result.

Experiments designed to show the effect of the complete removal of salts have demonstrated that an ash-free diet is detrimental to the organism. It was early shown that a diet containing the requisite amount of carbohydrate, fat, and proteid but which did not contain the ash constituents resulted in an early death. Von Bunge suggested that these harmful effects were due largely to an excess of acidic radicles present in the body caused by the sulphuric acid formed in the process of metabolism from the sulphur present in the protein molecule. Ordinarily this acid would be neutralized by the fixed bases present in the diet. In the absence of these, however, they derive a certain portion of their required base from the alkali radicles in the tissues. He suggested the addition of carbonates to combat this acidity.

Studies of the effect of an ash-free diet upon man have been made. In one case symptoms were experienced which were analgous to that associated with acidosis, including muscular weakness and the presence of acetone on the breath. Other investigators failed to obtain any symptoms of acidosis. In both experiments there was a loss of weight as the result of the ingestion of an ash-free diet. It is apparent that individual differences must be considered in the interpretation of such data. With rats it has been found (Osborne and Mendel) that a fair amount of growth is attained in the absence of all but very minute amounts of the elements, magnesium, sodium, potassium or chlorine but not in the absence of calcium or phosphorus. Sodium and potassium cannot both be absent from the diet at the same time.

The analyses of various foods for the inorganic elements they contain, and a consideration of the latter on the basis of whether they yield ash which is predominantly acidic or basic in nature, have shown that some foods, upon oxidation in the body yield an excess of acidic over the basic elements, while of others the opposite is true. An excess of inorganic acid radicles in the blood, whether they occur as the result of the ingestion of the acids themselves or are produced in the processes of metabolism from neutral compounds, is neutralized in one of two ways—by combination (*a*) with ammonia or (*b*) with some of the fixed alkalies of the body. Since there is at all times an equilibrium, both changes occur. Such changes produce an excess of salts in the blood which is excreted in the urine. The fixed bases which accomplish this neutralization may come from the alkaline carbonates of the blood, perhaps from the calcium or magnesium of the bones. The ultimate result, if the diet be continued, is the reduction of the body's store of basic elements. Such a condition we have already considered in our discussion of the effect of a salt-free diet. The effect of an excess of basic elements in the body is not so serious, for they may be neutralized by the carbonic acid formed in the process of oxidation. The urine excreted after the ingestion of a diet which contains an excess of potential basic ash constituents will tend to be alkaline, while that obtained after a potentially acid diet will be acid.

Sherman and Gettler have recently considered some of the more important foods on the basis of their acid- or base-yielding properties, and have called attention to the desirability of balancing potentially acid foods in the diet with predominantly base-yielding foods. The table on page 87 gives the result of their work, grouped according to predominating acid- or base-yielding power (extremes in each case).

It will be seen in general that, with the exception of milk, animal products yield an excess of acid radicles whereas plant foods with the exception of cereals and some nuts yield an alkaline ash. Vegetables and fruits are chiefly base-yielding foods. That foods which are rich in the salts of organic acids should yield an excess of base is due to the fact that the acid portion of the molecule is oxidized in the body yielding carbonates which are potentially basic.

Calcium, phosphorus, potassium, sulphur, sodium, lithium, chlorine, magnesium, manganese, iron, boron, iodine, fluor-

EXCESS ACID OR BASE IN REPRESENTATIVE FOODS IN TERMS OF NORMAL SOLUTIONS.[1]

Article of food.	Potential acid.		Potential base.	
	Per 100 gm.	Per 100 calories.	Per 100 gm.	Per 100 calories.
Succulent vegetables:				
Asparagus	..	..	0.8	3.6
Potatoes	..	..	7.2	8.6
Carrots (or beets)	..	..	10.8	23.7
Fruit:				
Cranberries	..	..	1.8	3.8
Pineapple	..	..	6.8	15.7
Nuts:				
Almonds	..	..	12.0	1.8
Walnuts	..	1.1	..	..
Legumes	..	..	23.9	6.9
Cereal:				
Oatmeal (or wheat)	12.9	3.2	..	..
Rice	7.8	2.5	..	..
Lean meat	12.0	10.4	..	..
Fish	7.8	..	..	..
Milk	..	..	1.8	2.6
Cheese	..	1.2	..	..
Eggs	11.1	7.5	..	..

ine and silicon are the more important "mineral" elements found in the body. The bases are combined chiefly as phosphates, sulphates, chlorides, and carbonates. Of the chlorides in the body the sodium salt predominates. It is the most abundant inorganic constituent of the diet and also of the urine. The fluids of the body are particularly rich in sodium salts and, consequently, in sodium chloride; while the potassium salts predominate in the tissues, chiefly as the phosphates. The quantity of chlorides in the urine is directly related to that ingested, for the body tends to maintain itself in chlorine equilibrium.

CHLORINE REQUIREMENT OF MAN

The sodium chloride requirement of the body is difficult to determine. Studies of the minimum chloride requirement in which there is a complete removal of salt, as in fasting or an ash-free diet or sodium chloride-poor diet, fail to determine the optimum requirement; they always show the lowest excretion under conditions in which the body has lost its reserve and is tending to conserve that amount which is left. Such studies on man indicate a loss of approximately 10 to 12 grams of sodium chloride, calculated as chlorine, in the course of ten days. The daily excretion decreases gradually until it reaches a low level when between 0.1 and 0.2 gram of chlorine are excreted per day. That, in such

[1]Compiled from Sherman: Food Products 1915. Sherman and Gettler: Jour. Biol. Chem. 1912, xi, 363.

INORGANIC SALTS, WATER, VITAMINES

CHLORINE CONTENT OF FOODS.

	Per cent. of edible portion.	Chlorine in 100-Calorie portion, gm.	Weight of 100-Calorie portion, gm.
Protein-rich foods:			
Cheese	1.0	0.2	23
Chicken	0.6	0.02	45–93
Beef and veal	0.5	0.05	35–50
Cheese, cottage	0.5	..	31
Fish:			
Salmon	0.28	0.13	70
Cod, haddock	0.24	0.33	216
Egg white	0.15	0.28	196
Milk, whole	0.12	0.17	145
Milk, butter	0.10	0.275	280
Egg, whole	0.10	0.06	68
Egg, yolk	0.10	0.03	28
Lentils	0.08	0.02	29
Peanuts	0.04	0.007	18
Peas, dried	0.04	0.01	28
Beans, dried	0.03	0.008	29
Walnuts	0.01	0.001	14
Carbohydrate-rich foods:			
Potatoes	0.12	0.10	81
Flour, wheat	0.07	0.02	28
Cornmeal	0.06	0.02	28
Rice	0.05	0.01	29
Oatmeal	0.035	0.009	25
Potato, white	0.03	0.04	120
Barley, pearled	0.02	0.005	28
Rye	0.02	0.005	28
Honey	0.01	0.01	31
Sugar	..	..	..
Water- and salt-rich foods:			
Celery	0.17	0.9	540
Lettuce	0.06	0.3	524
Cauliflower	0.05	0.16	328
Radish	0.05	0.17	341
Beets	0.04	0.08	217
Carrots	0.036	0.078	221
Rhubarb	0.035	0.15	433
Cabbage	0.03	0.09	317
Tomatoes	0.03	0.09	439
Spinach	0.02	0.08	418
Corn, green	0.014	0.014	99
Cherries	0.01	0.01	128
Grapefruit	0.01	..	..
Grapes	0.01	0.01	104
Lemons	0.01	0.02	226
Oranges	0.01	0.02	195
Peaches	0.01	0.02	242
Peas, green	0.01	0.01	100
Squash	0.01	0.02	217
Beans, green	0.009	0.007	82
Apples	0.004	0.006	159

Fat-rich foods:
Butter; lard; olive oil; salt pork; bacon; salt content, high and varies.

6

case, chlorides have been lost beyond the reserve that is related to the quantity of chlorine ingested (which results in part from a lag in its excretion) is evidenced by the marked retention of chloride during the first days of feeding after a fast or after the ingestion of a salt-free diet.

The sodium chloride requirement is affected by the nature of the diet. This is brought out most strikingly by a consideration of the quantity of sodium chloride taken by the herbivora as contrasted with the carnivora. Von Bunge was the first to call attention to the fact that the carnivora do not exhibit the marked craving for salt that is evidenced by the herbivora. He ascribed this difference to the greater quantity of potassium salts ingested with a vegetable diet, which caused an increased excretion of potassium chloride, with the consequent depletion in chlorine. That potassium salts do cause an increased chlorine excretion has been shown by direct experimentation. From these considerations it is evident that the estimation of the quantity of sodium chloride required per day is a difficult matter. The quantity of chlorine necessary to protect the body against loss of chlorine has been placed at 3 or 4 grams per day. The average consumption has been estimated at from 15 to 20 grams of sodium chloride per day.

Ingestion of large quantities of sodium chloride increases the excretion of nitrogen. The explanation of this is not clear; it seems probable that it is due to the accompanying diuresis.

The table on page 88 gives the average chlorine content of various foods arranged (1) according to whether they are particularly valuable as sources of protein, carbohydrate, or for the salts and water which they contain and (2) in each group in the order of their decreasing chlorine content.

PHOSPHORUS REQUIREMENT OF MAN.

Phosphorus[1] occurs abundantly in the body almost exclusively in the oxidized form as the phosphoric acid radicle. As such, however, it appears in a variety of combinations. Thus it occurs in the body or in the combined form with the protein molecule as nucleoprotein of the cell nuclei and as the phosphoproteins casein and vitellin; combined with fatty acids as lecithoprotein, the lecithins, and the phosphatides of the nervous tissue; in simple organic combination in the

[1]For a review of the metabolism of phosphorus the reader is referred to the excellent and complete review of the literature on this subject by Forbes and Keith: Ohio Agric. Exp. Sta., Tech. Bull., 1914, No. 5.

plant as phytin, and finally in the inorganic state combined with the various bases in the skeleton, particularly with calcium and magnesium and in the body in general as the sodium and potassium salts.

As a constituent of the nuclei the phosphoric acid takes part in one of the most vital processes of the body, the formation of new cells. Combined with calcium and magnesium it becomes the constituent which gives permanence and hardness to the bones, while as a soluble salt dissolved in the fluids of the body in conjunction with the carbonates and proteins it serves to maintain the neutrality of the tissues.

The question of the ability of organic and inorganic phosphorus to supply the body needs has been one which has received a great deal of attention. This problem is particularly important in connection with the artificial feeding of infants and the treatment of disease. The weight of the evidence shows that only a small amount of organically combined phosphorus is necessary in the diet provided a sufficient amount of inorganic phosphorus is present. Forbes has recently summed up the evidence with regard to the availability of organic and inorganic phosphorus. In his review of the factors which might affect the correct interpretation of the data considered—in which he calls attention to the fact, the importance of which has become daily more evident, that it is necessary to consider the presence or absence from the experimental diet of such substances as the "vitamines" or lipoids (see p. 102) before we shall be able to demonstrate conclusively the greater advantage of one form of phosphate over the others or their equality, Forbes concludes with the following statement:

"It therefore seems not at all unlikely that the many demonstrations of the superior nutritive value of organic phosphorus compounds have been influenced by other beneficial substances occurring in association with them in natural foods, and contained as impurities in these organic phosphorus compounds as isloated and used in nutrition investigations. As to the relative importance of this factor and others we are as yet unprepared to make positive assertions; but these recent studies at least raise the question as to whether the apparent superiority of organic to inorganic phosphorus compounds is due to these organic compounds by themselves, or whether their superiority is dependent upon minute quantities of certain associated compounds. However this question may be settled the studies, certainly suggest that, if the natural organic phosphorus compounds are not of superior usefulness, or are not essential to the

PHOSPHORUS (P_2O_5) CONTENT OF FOODS (AVERAGE DAILY REQUIREMENT 3.3 GRAMS).

	Per cent. of edible portion.	P_2O_5 in 100-Calorie portion, gm.	Weight of 100-Calorie portion, gm.
Protein-rich foods:			
Cheese, hard	1.45	0.39	23
Beans, dried	1.14	0.326	29
Egg, yolk	1.0	0.27	28
Peas, dried	0.91	0.24	28
Peanuts	0.90	0.16	18
Almonds	0.87	0.132	15
Beans, lima, dried	0.77	0.22	29
Walnuts	0.77	0.11	14
Lentils	0.66	0.29	29
Cheese, cottage	0.50	0.40	31
Meat and chicken	0.50 (fat)	0.15–0.18	45–93
	(lean)	0.24–0.30	..
Fish	0.40	0.60	50
Egg, whole	0.37	0.24	68
Milk, whole	0.22	0.303	145
Milk, skimmed	0.22	0.60	273
Egg, white	0.03	0.05	196
Carbohydrate-rich foods:			
Oatmeal, dry	0.827	0.216	25
Barley, pearled	0.46	0.127	28
Bread, whole wheat	0.40	0.16	39
Cornmeal	0.30	0.08	28
Potato, white	0.14	0.166	81
Rice	0.203	0.057	29
Bread, white	0.20	0.075	39
Wheat flour	0.20	0.05	28
Potato, sweet	0.09	0.08	101
Water- and salt-rich foods:			
Wheat bran	3.0		
Beans, green	0.27	0.22	82
Peas, green	0.26	0.24	100
Corn, green	0.22	0.21	99
Cauliflower	0.14	0.45	328
Spinach	0.13	0.54	418
Beans, string	0.12	0.28	241
Carrots	0.10	0.22	221
Celery	0.10	0.54	540
Lettuce	0.09	0.47	524
Asparagus	0.09	0.39	450
Cabbage	0.09	0.28	317
Beets	0.09	0.19	217
Squash	0.08	0.08	217
Cherries	0.07	0.09	128
Tomatoes	0.059	0.257	439
Oranges	0.05	0.09	195
Peaches	0.047	0.11	242
Apples	0.03	0.05	159
Lemons	0.01	0.04	226
Fat-rich foods:			
Cocoa	1.1	0.22	20
Chocolate	0.90	0.14	16
Cream	0.18	0.10	51
Butter	0.03	0.004	13

maintenance of growth in animals, then other nutrients associated with them in the natural foods *are* essential, and the result is to put a new emphasis on the value of the natural organic food-stuffs as compared with inorganic or artificially synthetized nutrients and certain manufactured foods.''

The phosphorus requirement of man has not been determined with any certainty. The procedure is difficult because, unlike many of the products of metabolism, a large proportion of the phosphorus may be excreted in the feces. The daily requirement of the adult man has been placed at 1.44 grams of phosphorus (P) or 3.3 grams of P_2O_5. Under special conditions the requirement may be as low as 0.9 gram P or 2 grams of P_2O_5.

The quantity of food phosphorus that may be retained depends upon the nature of the diet. Since a large proportion is deposited in the bones, the presence of a sufficient amount of the bases, calcium and magnesium, associated with it in such structures is essential. When these are not present the phosphoric acid radicle is excreted in combination with the more soluble bases and thus fails to satisfy the requirements. The ingestion or formation of acids or acid-yielding substances results in an increased excretion of phosphorus.

The phosphorus of the food, obtained as it is from both the animal and vegetable kingdom occurs in a variety of organic compounds, the particular advantage of any one of which has not been determined. Feeding experiments in which one type of phosphorus is fed to the exclusion of all others do not necessarily demonstrate the true availability of the compound. In selecting diets, then, for their phosphorus content we cannot lay stress on any given food as presenting the constituents in a more available form than another. In considering data with regard to the P_2O_5 content of foods and particularly the vegetables, it is to be remembered that in their preparation a certain proportion of the phosphorus is removed. This is particularly true in the removal of the outer coating of cereals.

The table on page 91 gives the relative quantity of P_2O_5 in some of the more common foods.

CALCIUM REQUIREMENT OF MAN.

Calcium salts play a varied role in the body economy. Calcium occurs in the bones chiefly as phosphate. Dissolved in the body fluids calcium is an important factor in the coagulation of the blood and in the contraction of the muscles. Underhill has suggested that calcium salts play an important role in the regulation of the blood-sugar content.

During the period of growth the importance of calcium salts is most easily demonstrated, for at this time the body is utilizing relatively large quantities of calcium, the removal of which from the diet at this time results in arrested or poor development of the bones. It is for this reason that consideration of the calcium requirement of the growing child is very important. The disease most commonly associated with calcium metabolism, rickets, may not be entirely the result of a lack of calcium in the diet but of a failure to assimilate it. In the adult the temporary removal of calcium is not followed by such marked effects as those observed in growth, for the body can call upon its reserve for a considerable time without showing any undesirable effect. Calcium, like phosphorus, is excreted largely through the intestine, and its excretion is continued in fasting.

The importance of calcium and the fact that it is impossible to consider each salt by itself is well illustrated in the use of such solutions as Ringer solution and the antagonistic action of salts. Physiological salt solution is sufficient to maintain the osmotic properties of muscle. In such a solution, however, muscle will not exhibit its properties of irritability and contractibility for any length of time. If, to the physiological salt solution, calcium and potassium chloride be added in the proper proportions, it will exhibit these properties for a much longer period; an isolated heart when supplied with oxygen will continue to beat spontaneously for a long time in Ringer solution which contains these salts. An excess of calcium may produce a condition of tonic contraction called "calcium rigor." Loeb has recently shown that the ions antagonize each other in their their effect upon body processes; particularly the permeability of cell membranes. Membranes such as those surrounding sea-urchin eggs are permeable to certain concentrations of sodium chloride and dilute acids. If to such solutions a bivalent ion, such as calcium or magnesium, be added the permeability is greatly reduced. Clowes has been able to produce results analogous to these in purely physical systems. Thus we see that the role of salts in the body, aside from their structural value is very complex.

In discussing the cathartic action of salts, Meltzer calls attention to the fact that the salts of magnesium are essentially inhibitors of intestinal movement and suggests that the purgative effect produced by such salts is the result of the combined action of sodium salts which stimulate contraction and of magnesium salts which cause a relaxation. This inhibitory effect of magnesium, which extends to other parts of the body, may be counteracted by subsequent injections of calcium salts. Anesthesia has been produced by the injection of magnesium sulphate.

The calcium requirement of man varies with the period of life. The growing child requires a greater proportionate quantity of calcium per day than an adult in middle life; while an old man requires much less. During pregnancy and lactation there is a necessity for an increased consumption of calcium. Dietary studies show that an ingestion of approximately 0.7 gram of calcium (calculated as oxide) per day is the smallest amount which will maintain the average normal adult in calcium equilibrium on an ordinary diet. Since absorption is not always complete, a somewhat larger quantity is desirable, 1 to 1.5 grams per day.

Whether or not the average mixed diet satisfies the calcium requirement without special selection of food is a matter which is open to question. When the food consists chiefly of meat and cereals, foods low in calcium, it is probable that the calcium ingestion is not sufficient. If the diet contains milk, eggs (yolk), legumes, and fruits the diet will probably contain a sufficient quantity of calcium. It has been found that, apparently, the calcium in vegetables is not as well utilized as that of milk or soluble calcium salts. In the absence of milk in the diet it would be best to augment the diet of children with soluble calcium salts rather than to rely entirely upon vegetables for this element (Mendel).

The diet of pregnant and nursing mothers and of children requires special consideration. During pregnancy and lactation the mother is nourishing the young through her own system. At this time, too, there is an especial necessity for calcium and the other constituents which are concerned in the structural tissues of the body—magnesium, iron, and phosphorus. Forbes has recently shown that the cow when producing milk apparently draws upon her own calcium reserve, even though there be ample supplies of calcium in the diet. It is essential, then, that the mother have a plentiful supply of those foods which furnish these inorganic elements. Decay of teeth during pregnancy, has been ascribed to the drain upon the calcium reserves caused by the secretion of milk.

The nature of the diet of a child is also important after it has ceased to depend upon its mother for food. Particular attention should be given to the calcium content of the food,

CALCIUM (CaO) CONTENT OF FOODS (AVERAGE DAILY REQUIREMENT
1.0 GRAM).

	Per cent. of edible portion.	CaO in 100-Calorie portion, gm.	Weight of 100-Calorie portion, gm.
Protein-rich foods:			
Cheese:			
Hard	1.1	0.25	23
Cottage	0.3	0.30	31
Almonds	0.30	0.046	15
Beans, dried	0.22	0.063	29
Egg, yolk	0.20	0.05	28
Milk, whole	0.168	0.24	145
Milk, skimmed	..	0.465	273
Buttermilk	0.15	0.415	280
Peanuts	0.14	0.04	18
Lentils	0.12	0.04	29
Walnuts	0.11	..	14
Beans, lima, dried	0.10	0.028	29
Egg, whole	0.093	0.06	68
Egg, white	0.015	0.028	196
Fish	0.015–0.08	0.033	50
Meat	0.01–0.03	0.005–0.01	45–93
Carbohydrate-rich foods:			
Oatmeal	0.13	0.03	25
Wheat	0.06	0.01	27
Bread, whole wheat	0.04	0.016	39
Bread, white	0.03	0.011	39
Barley, pearl	0.025	0.007	28
Potato, sweet	0.025	0.02	101
Wheat flour	0.025	0.007	28
Potato, white	0.016	0.019	81
Cornmeal	0.015	0.004	28
Rice	0.012	0.003	29
Honey	0.005	0.001	..
Sugar	..	..	..
Starch	..	..	..
Water- and salt-rich foods:			
Cauliflower	0.17	0.55	328
Olives	0.17	0.06	40
Celery	0.10	0.54	540
Dates	0.10	0.03	29
Spinach	0.09	0.37	418
Beans, string	0.075	0.177	241
Carrots	0.077	0.168	221
Oranges	0.06	0.11	195
Rhubarb	0.06	0.26	433
Lemons	0.05	0.12	226
Lettuce	0.05	0.26	524
Radish	0.05	0.17	341
Asparagus	0.04	0.17	450
Beans, lima	0.04	0.033	82
Peas, green	0.04	0.032	100
Beets	0.03	0.06	217
Cherries	0.03	0.04	128
Squash	0.02	0.054	217
Tomato	0.02	0.087	439
Prunes (dried)	0.02	..	33
Apples	0.014	0.022	159
Fat-rich foods:			
Cocoa	0.14	0.027	20
Chocolate	0.14	0.052	16

for here the diet changes from one consisting of milk, which is richest in calcium, to a mixed diet which, unless properly chosen, may be poor in calcium. A calcium deficit for a growing child results in soft bones with the resulting abnormalities of structure.

The table on page 95 contains the more common foods arranged according to calcium content in each type group.

IRON REQUIREMENT OF MAN.

Iron occurs as a constituent of the blood pigment. We find it also in the chromatin of cells in which it is in part concerned, with the processes of oxidation, not only as a carrier of oxygen but as a catalyzer of enzyme action. The total quantity of iron in the body has been estimated at from 3 to 4 grams.

The iron requirement of man has been estimated at from 0.01 to 0.012 gram of iron per day. Until a more careful determination of the actual requirements has been established a slightly higher value of 0.015 gram per day has been suggested (Sherman). Women require much more iron than men. During the periods of pregnancy, lactation and menstruation of women there is a considerable loss of iron which must be replenished and in the growth period of children there is a greater demand for iron than in the adult. Observation has shown that the body is proportionately richer in iron at the time of birth than at any other time in its development. Analyses of milk and of the newborn and young have shown that during gestation the fetus accumulates a store of iron. During the suckling period the quantity of iron is almost constant and milk is comparatively poor in iron. The conclusion from these facts is, then, that the child derives from its mother, before birth, a store of iron sufficient for its needs throughout the period when it is nursing, and that the mother supplies, in the milk, approximately enough iron to replace the iron lost in the processes of metabolism. After the child stops nursing it is important that the iron content of the diet be given careful consideration, for both the small daily losses made good by the milk and the iron needed for the processes of growth must be furnished.

The degrees of availability of iron, in the organic and inorganic forms has been, as in the case of phosphorus, a matter of great controversy. Experiments have shown that both forms of iron are absorbed from the small intestines. That inorganic iron may be used in the production of hemoglobin

IRON (FE) CONTENT OF FOODS (AVERAGE DAILY REQUIREMENT 0.015 GRAM).

	Per cent. of edible portion.	Fe in 100-Calorie portion, gm.	Weight of 100-Calorie portion, gm.
Protein-rich foods:			
Lentils	0.0086	0.0024	29
Egg, yolk	0.0085	0.0023	28
Beans, dried	0.007	0.002	29
Beans, lima, dried	0.007	0.002	29
Peas, dried	0.0056	0.0015	28
Fish	0.004	0.0009	80–100
Meat	0.0038	0.0008–0.003	35–50
Egg, whole	0.003	0.0019	68
Walnuts	0.0021	0.00029	14
Almonds	0.002	0.0003	15
Chicken	0.002	0.0013	45–93
Peanuts	0.002	0.0035	18
Milk, skimmed	..	0.00066	273
Milk, whole	0.00024	0.00034	145
Egg, white	0.0001	0.0002	196
Carbohydrate-rich foods:			
Wheat	0.0053	0.0014	28
Oatmeal, dry	0.0036	0.0009	25
Bread, whole wheat	0.0015	0.0006	41
Wheat, flour	0.0015	0.0004	28
Barley, pearled	0.0013	0.00036	28
Potato, white	0.0013	0.0015	120
Cornmeal	0.0011	0.0003	28
Honey	0.001	0.0003	31
Bread, white	0.0009	0.0003	38
Rice	0.0009	0.0003	29
Potato, sweet	0.0005	0.0004	81
Water- and salt-rich foods:			
Dandelion greens	0.027	0.0044	164
Spinach	0.0032	0.0133	418
Dates	0.003	0.001	29
Olives	0.0029	0.0009	33
Beans, lima	0.0025	0.002	82
Beans, string	0.0016	0.0038	241
Peas, green	0.0016	0.0016	100
Cabbage	0.0011	0.0035	317
Asparagus	0.001	0.0043	450
Lettuce	0.001	0.005	524
Carrots	0.0008	0.0016	221
Corn, green	0.0008	0.00075	99
Squash	0.0008	0.0017	217
Beets	0.0006	0.0013	217
Lemon	0.0006	0.0013	226
Radish	0.0006	0.002	341
Celery	0.0005	0.0027	540
Cherries	0.0005	..	128
Turnips	0.0005	0.0013	254
Tomato	0.0004	0.0017	439
Apples	0.0003	0.0005	159
Oranges	0.0003	0.0006	195
Peaches	0.0003	0.0007	242
Onions	..	0.0011	205
Fat-rich foods:			
Butter			
Cream	..	0.0001	51
Cocoa	..	0.0005	20

has not been proven, it does increase the production of hemoglobin, in which case it apparently acts as a stimulant to the cellular activities. Iron in simple organic combination, lactate, has been used successfully as the source of iron for growing rats. There is ample evidence that iron was found in organic combination is assimilated and used in the processes of growth and in the formation of hemoglobin. Although inorganic iron appears to be as effective as organic iron it has been recommended by some that at least a part of the iron ingested being the "organic" form. Iron is eliminated chiefly in the feces. The table on page 97 contains the iron content of some of the more important foods.

In using the table it is essential to remember that fat meat contains a smaller proportion of iron than does a lean piece, for fat contains practically no iron. The preparation of cereals for the market (milling) results in the removal of a considerable portion of the iron contained in the whole grain. The advantage of foods, such as vegetables and fruits, which are not particularly valuable to the body for protein or a source of energy, is shown when it becomes desirable to increase the inorganic salt content of the diet.

IODINE REQUIREMENT OF MAN.

Iodine is present in its greatest amount in the thyroid gland. The function of iodine in the thyroid is not known. The quantity of iodine in the gland is variable. Ingestion of iodine or the application of iodine to the skin is accompanied by an increased iodine content of the thyroid. It appears to be in combination with protein material. The name thyroglobulin has been given to an iodine-rich protein isolated from the thyroid gland. Regions in which the iodine content of the water is low have been shown to be, in many cases, those in which goiter is prevalent. If, as general observation seems to indicate, there is a relation between the lack of iodine and the prevalence of goiter, it is important to know the foods which contain iodine.

Iodine is contained in the water of various districts; it also occurs in sea water and in foods grown near the sea. Recent analyses of foods have shown that iodine is not a constant constituent of foods; that when present it is usually found in exceedingly minute proportions, and that in general, at least, it must be regarded as an accidental constituent in the sense of standing in no vital relation to the growth of food products. The presence of iodine in most vegetable food products clearly depends upon the fact of its presence in the soil and the lack of a selective capacity in the feeding of plants.[1] Of the plants examined, Irish moss, from which blanc mange is prepared, and agar agar are the best sources of iodine. Garden vegetables, some kinds of legumes, or seeds, beans, and peas, are shown to be fair sources of iodine, although the presence or absence of iodine and the quantity contained are uncertain. Studies of foods from different sections of the country, particularly from localities in which goiter is prevalent, failed to show any uniformity in the presence of iodine over districts which were comparatively free from goiter.

WATER REQUIREMENT OF MAN.

Water as an essential constituent of the diet receives very little attention in the usual consideration of the foods. That this is so is but natural, for it is one of the most readily obtainable and generally used food-stuffs. The lack of water is, however, sooner and more keenly felt than the absence of protein, carbohydrate, or fat. An animal receiving neither food nor water will die sooner than one which is given only water; while an earlier death will result from dry food and no water.

The relative importance of water from a quantitative point of view is indicated by the water content of the body tissues. The fat-free organs show a comparatively constant water content, being about 80 per cent. The presence of fat affects the percentage of water content of the tissues as a whole, but being inert so far as holding water is concerned, it does not appear to influence extensively the composition of the tissues which hold it. The secretions are particularly rich in water (86 to 99 per cent.). while the skeletal tissues, such as bone and connective tissue, have a much lower water content (10 to 50 per cent.). The tissues of young animals, of regenerating and probably of recuperating tissues are richer in water than those of an adult organism.

The functions of water are numerous: it is a constituent of all protoplasm; as a solvent it aids in carrying to the cell the food material produced by digestion in the removal of the waste products; it maintains the osmotic equilibrium between the various organs and tissues; by reason of its high specific heat its evaporation assists in the maintenance of a constant body temperature; and it is the vehicle for the transportation of the blood elements throughout the body.

[1] Cameron: Jour. Biol. Chem., 1914, xviii, 335. Forbes and Beegle: Jour. Med. Research, 1916, xxxiv, 445.

The water present in the body is not necessarily to be considered as *free* water in the sense that after its complete removal from the cellular structures they will not cease their activities or that its return will initiate them anew. A certain amount of water is probably held in loose chemical combination or by physical attraction with the various molecular structures, such as the protein. It is known that much of the organic material in the body exists in swollen colloidal masses and that the removal of water from them affects their physical and perhaps their chemical properties. Our knowledge on this point is rather meagre. We do know, however, that the complete removal of water results in the disappearance of the phenomenon known as life. Since the water content of various tissues is relatively constant a decided diminution in the water content is fatal. Certain organisms, such as the frog, insects, etc., can lose a considerable proportion of their water under favorable conditions and still remain alive, although usually dormant; seeds exhibit similar phenomena. Water is never entirely absent under such conditions; there is a minimum which if passed, results in the disappearance of life.

Water is ingested either as such or associated with food. Most water contains a considerable quantity of salt.[1] The quantity of water ingested with the food may be considerable; many foods are roughly three-fourths water. A certain amount of water is liberated in the tissues as the result of oxidation.

The quantity and manner in which water is excreted is affected chiefly by the temperature and humidity of the surrounding air, the activity of the individual and the quantity and nature of the food and water ingested. Under normal conditions the equivalent of the water ingested in a day is excreted in a similar time chiefly through the lungs and skin, and in the urine and feces. A considerable proportion of the water ingested under average conditions of temperature and humidity appears in the urine within a comparatively short time after its ingestion. After large volumes of water have been taken as much as three-fourths of the amount appears in the urine within an hour after its ingestion. Higher temperatures outside the body, or excessive muscular activity increase the loss of water through the lungs and skin; while with low temperatures and relative quiet the

[1] The specific effects of certain mineral waters is due to their salt content. It may be, however, that the increased water ingestion, under such circumstances which usually accompanies the use of such waters, may also contribute to the beneficial effects of water cures.

amount of water which appears in the urine is increased. Twenty-five per cent. of the heat lost from the body in a day has been found to be through the evaporation of water—at approximately the rate of 29 grams per hour or 700 cc. per day. With an increase in the quantity of water ingested, other conditions being the same, a greater proportion of the ingested water appears in the urine. The body may suffer a loss of water as the result of excessive perspiration, the action of diuretics or of cathartics. Under such circumstances the ingestion of water results in a restoration of the amount lost, for the tissues tend to maintain the concentration of water at a constant level.

With the loss of water there is usually a loss of salt from the body either in the urine or through the skin. One investigator has studied this loss with regard to increased perspiration and the processes attending the restoration of water. He suggests that thirst resulting from excessive perspiration is quenched most readily by water containing salts, or taken with food, than with distilled water; for unless salt is present the water ingested will not be retained but will be rapidly excreted. In the process of recuperation following emaciation there is a very rapid restoration of the lost water. Thus the tissues of fasting animals, which show an increased water content, upon the ingestion of food and water, even though large quantities of water have been ingested throughout the fast, show a marked water retention. Because of the varied activities of man the quantity of water which is necessary for the normal functioning of the body is a difficult matter to determine. It has been placed at from 2 to 5 liters (or quarts) per day.

The effect of water on metabolism has been studied from many angles. Ingested water passes rapidly through the stomach and is readily absorbed in the intestines. In spite of this it has been shown that it affects the rate and extent of digestion. Water taken into the stomach in large quantities increases the secretion of gastric juice; small amounts have no effect. When water is taken with food the flow of gastric juice has been shown to be not only greater in amount but to contain more acid. The secretion of bile and pancreatic juice is also stimulated by water, probably because of the interrelation between the acid reaction in the stomach and the flow of these secretions. The passage of food from the stomach has been held to be accelerated as the result of the ingestion of water. This is not entirely correct, for it has been shown that there is a slight retardation of the passage of bread from the stomach when water is taken after bread. Experiments with fistulous animals and anatomical and *x*-ray studies have shown, however, that water, when ingested alone, does not mix to any extent with the food mass in the stomach in its passage to the pylorus. A sort of trough is formed along the lesser curvature of the stomach through which the water flows from the esophagus to the pylorus. Practically neutral water has been observed to pass the pylorus when the stomach is full of food and the digestive processes are at their height.

A large ingestion of water serves to increase the excretion of nitrogen in the urine. This effect is the result apparently of stimulated cellular activity and in part to a flushing out of the soluble nitrogenous end-products of metabolism.

Mattill and Hawk have studied the influence of copious water drinking with meals and found a more complete utilization of food, protein, carbohydrates, and fat and decreased putrefaction and bacterial development in the feces. From the results of such work we may conclude that for the normal individual the ingestion of water with meals is not harmful.

VITAMINES OR ACCESSORY FOOD-STUFFS

Investigations of the dietary factors concerned in growth and of certain diseases, such as beri-beri and scurvy, have shown that for normal growth and maintenance of health and of weight at least two substances are necessary in a diet in addition to (*a*) an adequate protein or mixture of proteins, (*b*) a proper combination of inorganic salts and (*c*) energy (obtained from carbohydrate, protein or fat) in amounts sufficient to meet the needs of the body. The quantities of these substances required for normal nutrition are exceedingly small. Their identification is not on the basis of their chemical composition—they are apparently not protein, fat or carbohydrate in nature—but through their effects upon the growth and health of animals or individuals when known to be absent or when added to a deficient diet. Various names have been applied to these unidentified dietary essentials such as, vitamines, accessory factors, food hormones, growth determinants, growth stimulants, body regulators, etc. The term vitamine has become rather generally used as a class name for these substances both in the scientific and popular literature and this term will be so used in our discussions.

Vitamines occur in both plants and animals but appear to be present in greater concentration in some foods than in others. While these substances are present in animal tissues animals are unable to synthetize them and are, therefore, dependent upon plants or other animals as their source of vitamines. Two types of unidentified substances or vitamines have been detected and a third appears probable. The first vitamine, designated fat-soluble A, is soluble in fats and accompanies them when isolated from food-stuffs. It is associated with fats particularly those obtained from the tissues and organs of both plants and animals rich in cellular material, such as butter fat (milk), egg yolk, kidney fat, cod liver oil, etc., from animals and the leaves of plants— alfalfa, spinach, celery tops, chard, dandelions, beet tops, lettuce, cabbage, etc. Extracts of spinach leaves have been found to be exceedingly rich in this substance. Those portions of plant and animal life which serve as places for the storage of reserve food material such as the fatty tissue and muscle tissue of animals and the fleshy portion of oily fruits and the seeds of plants—olives, peanuts, cotton seeds—or the carbohydrate rich (starchy) portions of plants and seeds,—tubers, roots, stalks, endosperm of seeds, etc.,—are comparatively poor in fat-soluble A. The products obtained from these portions of the plants and starch, sugars, wheat flour, degerminated corn meal, polished rice, olive oil, cotton- seed oil, peanut oil, etc., are practically lacking in this sub- stance. Fat-soluble A is relatively thermo-stable although purified products rich in it appear to lose their activity as the result of keeping or heating for long periods.

The second unidentified food factor, water-soluble B is, as the name implies, soluble in water; it is also soluble in alcohol. This substance is widely distributed in both plant and animal foods, milk, eggs, meat and vegetables—leaves and entire seeds, grains, roots and tubers. It is not associa- ted with the fats or oils extracted from foods. As in the case of fat-soluble A this substance is most abundant in cellular rich structures of plants and animals. Thus the outer coat- ing and germ of seeds and grains, yeast, glandular organs, etc., are rich in water-soluble B. Products obtained from the storage portions of grain by milling, lack, or are very poor in this second factor—white flour, polished rice, degerminated and bolted corn meal. Water-soluble B is not completely destroyed under ordinary conditions of heating, as in cooking and preserving, provided the solution or material is not made alkaline, such as by the addition of soda. The origi- nal vitamine of Funk, the anti-neuritic vitamine is the same as water-soluble B of McCollum.

The third vitamine, the anti-scorbutic vitamine, has only recently been established as an entity. Fresh foods, particularly fruits and vegetables, and meat and milk are capable of curing scurvy. Drying or cooking for long periods at comparatively high temperatures diminishes or destroys the curative property.

A full recognition of the existence of such accessory substances has come through two channels in particular, the study of deficiency diseases, such as beri beri and scurvy, and qualitative studies of the diet, in which the rate of growth and increase in body weight are taken as the criteria of its sufficiency or insufficiency. As an example of the first class of work we may take beri beri. In considering the diet of individuals susceptible to beri beri it was noted that those living largely upon polished rice were more susceptible than those ingesting a diet of unpolished rice. It has been shown further that when chickens or pigeons are fed on polished rice they develop polyneuritis, a disease similar to beri beri, while those fed unpolished rice do not do so. They have, therefore, been used extensively in the study of substances capable of curing beri beri. Analysis of rice polishings has shown them to be richer in phosphorus than other parts of the grain. Yet attempts to associate beri beri with phosphorus metabolism have had little success beyond showing that the accessory substances occur in those parts of grains rich in phosphorus. The injection of an alcoholic or water extract of rice polishings, of certain plants or of animal organs into birds affected with polyneuritis will bring about rapid recovery. Funk has made attempts to isolate the substance which is the active factor in such cures. He has obtained from rice polishings and autolyzed yeast a crystalline product possessing the property of curing polyneuritis even when given in as small quantities as a few milligrams. The exact nature of the material is unknown. Funk proposed the name vitamine for substances capable of curing "deficiency" diseases and suggests that it contains nitrogen of the amine type and that it is related to the pyrimidine nucleus. The substance prepared by Funk is soluble in water and alcohol, insoluble in ether, chloroform, benzene, and acetone; is destroyed by alkalies, but is more stable in the presence of acids; heat, that is by boiling for some time, destroys it. It is readily absorbed by silicious earth, fuller's earth, or Lloyd's reagent, and extracts prepared by this method have been found to be quite effective.

Williams[1] has studied the effect of certain hydroxypyridine derivatives upon birds afflicted with polyneuritis gallinarum in an attempt to determine the nature of the vitamine of

[1] Jour. Biol. Chem., 1916, xxv, 437.

Funk. He found partial curative effects less satisfactory than the natural "vitamine" preparation with one of the isomeric forms of hydroxypyridine, while another isomer was entirely ineffective. From this and other considerations Williams came to the conclusion that isomeric changes are at least partially responsible for the instability of "vitamines" in food-stuffs and that anti-neuritic properties may be related to certain types of isomerism. This work is suggestive but has not been fully substantiated.

The second source of our knowledge of accessory substances, studies in which the rate of growth has been taken as a criterion of the sufficiency or insufficiency of a given diet, has perhaps been more fruitful than the study of diseases in extending our conception of their relation to nutrition in general. Such studies were initiated originally to learn the effect upon nutrition of variations in the amounts and kinds of amino-acids in the diet. It was in the selection of a suitable diet consisting of simple purified food substances which would form the basis for subsequent variations in the diet that the importance of accessory substances for growth became evident.

It has been shown (Hopkins and Wilcox; McCollum and Davis; Osborne and Mendel) that when rats are fed on a practically fat-free diet, composed of protein (such as casein or edestin), starch, and a suitable salt mixture which was entirely sufficient with regard to its energy, protein, and salt content, they did not grow normally, nor did they maintain their weight. The addition of lard to this diet yielded slightly better but still unsatisfactory results. When, however, milk was added to the mixture containing lard, growth would continue. In studying the constituents of milk which were responsible for this correction in the diet it was found that butter would accomplish the same result.

To determine which constituent of the butter carried the accessory substance, the butter fat was separated from the other constituents, protein, salts, and water, by centrifugalizing warm butter. When this purified butter oil, a substance practically free from nitrogen and phosphorus, was fed the results were just as satisfactory as those obtained from ordinary butter, indicating that the active agent was contained in butter fat. This substance (or substances) is resistant to heat and a certain amount of chemical action for butter which has been heated with live steam or subjected to the process of saponification does not lose its efficiency. When kept for long periods of time products rich in fat-soluble A tend to decrease in potency. The fats closely associated with metabolic activity are more effective in maintaining growth than "storage" fats, lard, beef fat, etc., which are in general ineffective or less satisfactory. The substance contained in butter fat remains efficient for over a year; while "butter oil," in which it is more concentrated, begins to lose its efficiency in half a year and becomes entirely inefficient in a year, even when kept at o° C. and in the dark. Egg yolk fat, cod-liver oil, kidney fat, the ether extract of ripe cod testicle and forage plants also supply the substances necessary for growth. The liquid portion of beef fat obtained by fractional crystallization from alcohol will accomplish similar results. Certain fats, such as lard, olive oil, cold pressed almond oil, the more solid portions of beef fat obtained in the preparation of beef oil, as indicated above do not contain this substance or substances. The deficiency is not due to a lack of the lipoids, lecithin and cholesterol, for phosphorus-containing substances are practically absent from butter oil, and lard contains a greater amount of cholesterol than butter. This active material bears certain quantitative relations to the diet, for there is a minimum value which must be present to produce results.

The presence of a water-soluble accessory factor was demonstrated (McCollum) through the case of diets in which lactose was substituted for dextrin in an otherwise complete food mixture. With such a substitution the diet was not effective in promoting growth. The addition of the water extract of egg yolk or the alcoholic extract of wheat germ to such a defective diet was sufficient to correct it. This led them to believe that lactose carried a water-soluble factor and that there were two factors necessary for growth in addition to the customary food-stuffs. Investigations of various lactose preparations served to confirm the suspicion with regard to the presence of the water-soluble factor and it has since been demonstrated in a number of foods.

Further studies have brought out with renewed emphasis the variety of factors which must be considered and controlled in the regulation of the diet and the possibility and the danger of neglecting modifying factors in our zeal to correct the most apparent defects. "A moderate shortage of one or another of the chemically unidentified dietary factors" is not to be regarded "as of greater gravity than faulty character in any other dietary factor." (McCollum.)

A toxic factor may influence the dietary value of a food. The relative biological values of foods has recently been emphasized by McCollum. Foods are divided into two classes (*a*) those particularly rich in vitamines, adequate protein and salts, *protective foods*, which include milk, egg yolk and the leaves of vegetables (*b*) foods deficient in one or more particular, which include all other foods such as the endosperm of seeds and grains, meat, roots and tubers. The protective foods are those which are particularly rich in cellular material whereas the other foods represent the portions of plants and animals which serve as storage tissues. It has been found that in the case of rats, a diet containing a proper supply of protein, energy, salts, and "fat-soluble A" and "water-soluble B" may be apparently satisfactory for growth and reproduction, while a diet composed of naturally occurring food-stuffs may be inadequate because of the presence of a substance or substances which exert a toxic influence upon the body, but if to such a diet a substance containing a toxic substance be added, a failure to continue to grow may result. If, however, the protein portion of the diet be increased or a better, more complete protein be substituted, the animal may continue to grow at a normal rate. The disturbances in metabolism accompanying a diet containing a large proportion of the wheat germ is apparently, in part, deficient because of the presence of a toxic substance.

Scurvy.— Scurvy has been recognized for many years as a disease associated with diet. It has been found to occur under conditions in which there was an absence of fresh fruit, vegetables and meat. Scurvy has occurred in the early days when sea-going vessels were required to remain out for long periods of time, in sieges, following crop failures and in arctic expeditions, *i. e.*, under conditions in which the diet was restricted to preserved foods or very limited quantities of fresh foods. The addition of fresh foods or fruit juices served to cure or prevent the disease. It has occurred recently in the war in Europe among troops subsisting largely upon a limited dietary. Scurvy in infants is sometimes recognized as a separate disease from that occurring in adults. Since infantile scurvy is referable to the same dietary defects which cause scurvy in adults and the symptoms are in general the same it is probably similar.

The subject of scurvy has received considerable attention recently in its relation to the vitamines and, as the result of the war and limited food supplies, with regard to the antiscorbutic properties of various foods and the effect of heat and preservation on these properties. Scurvy has been held to result from (*a*) a limited consumption of potassium, particularly the "acid vegetable potassium," (*b*) infection following a deficient diet, (*c*) acidosis following the ingestion of a preponderance of acid yielding foods, (*d*) the absence of some dietary factor which leads to the development of substances in the intestines and these in turn are the cause of the symptoms (autointoxication), (*e*) stasis in the large intestine as a result of the physical character of the diet and the production of toxic putrefactive products and (*f*) the absence of a specific vitamine. Recent controversy has involved particularly the last three factors.

Following the demonstration of a vitamine in connection with beri beri, Holst and Frölich and also Funk came to the conclusion that scurvy was a deficiency disease in the same sense in which beri beri is a deficiency disease, *i. e.*, there was a substance involved in the etiology of the disease of the nature of a vitamine. The deductions were based upon the similarity in the way beri beri and scurvy are produced by the ingestion of one-sided diets, particularly those derived from milled products in contrast with whole grains and seeds or fresh foods, and their cure by the addition of such foods. Furthermore, grains which would produce scurvy in guinea pigs would when sprouted prevent the occurrence of the disease. The guinea pig was used to study the anti-scorbutic value of foods. The findings confirmed the observations on men in that fresh, raw, or boiled succulent vegetables are anti-scorbutics. Fresh raw milk was an anti-scorbutic but heated milk was not. Boiling of vegetables diminished the anti-scorbutic value. Extracts of vegetables would cure scurvy and if acidulated with citric acid did not lose their anti-scorbutic value when heated as readily as the natural extracts. Extracts of acid fruits and vegetables were more resistant to heat with regard to their ability to cure scurvy than the non-acid foods.

The work of Holst and Frölich, then, tended to indicate the presence of a substance of the nature of a vitamine. Subsequent data seemed, however, to discountenance such a conclusion. Jackson found that guinea pigs would develop experimental scurvy in various degrees on diets of pastuerized, raw, boiled, skimmed and condensed milk, as well as after the ingestion of grains. The presence of bacterial infection was demonstrated in the swollen joints which she held to be specific for the disease. Soon after this McCollum and his co-workers maintained that while scurvy in guinea pigs was due to a faulty diet the effects were not due to the absence of a specific substance but to constipation associated with the physical character of the diet which resulted in the accumulation of toxic fecal products. They based their conclusions upon a series of observations; (*a*) that the oat kernel contained all the food factors necessary for the growth of rats when corrected with purified foods for its deficiency in certain inorganic salts, fat-soluble A, and the character of the protein; (b) in the course of their autopsies the ceca of guinea pigs fed on oats or milk and oats were impacted with putrifying feces; (c) the addition of inert liquid petrolatum to the diet of oats and milk would check the disease in certain animals in which it was well developed and phenolphthlein, another laxative, would prevent the occurence of the disease over long periods; (d) an artificial orange juice, composed of citric acid, cane-sugar and inorganic salts, exerted a decided protective action when added to the oat-milk diet. These workers were not ready entirely to accept the bacterial infection theory of Jackson and proposed an alternative hypothesis in which they held that bacterial infection was probably secondary to the injury of the intestinal walls through the formation of bacterial toxins as the result of putrefaction in the impacted cecum.

These conclusions of McCollum were radical and yet attractive in their simplicity. Evidence was soon presented from many sources, Chick and Hume, Harden and Zilva, Mendel, Hess, Givens, Emmett and others tending to discredit the interpretation of certain of McCollum's findings. It was found that in studies of experimental scurvy the quantities of foods ingested must be taken into consideration. Raw milk, which serves as an anti-scorbutic for infants and which did not serve as such for guinea pigs on the oat-milk diet, was found to be capable of preventing scurvy if fed in sufficient quantities. Instead of lacking the anti-scorbutic factor it was merely low in its anti-scorbutic value. Substances which will prevent impaction of the feces in the guinea pig did not prevent scurvy when added to diets which produced scurvy in their absence. Artificial orange juice, similar to McCollum's preparation was found to be inefficient nor did the removal of citric acid and other acids from lemon juice render it inactive. Fuller's earth which absorbs the water-soluble B vitamine does not absorb the anti-scorbutic factor. Water-soluble B can be removed from a mixture which contains both vitamines.

McCollum has recently repeated much of the work of the investigators mentioned above and his own work in which he has also measured the quantities of food consumed and has modified his views[1] so as to recognize a protective substance against scurvy. His observations on the curative

[1] Private Communication, June, 1919.

effect of petroleum oil and phenolphthlein were doubtless due, as Harden and Zilva stated, to the fact that the appetite of the animals, which were furnished a diet of milk and oats, fell off because of infection of the cecum, and when the intestinal canal was cleaned out by the laxatives they took sufficient milk to have a curative effect.

The evidence is, then, that there is a protective substance or vitamine active against scurvy as well as one for beri beri and for xerophthalmia.

The anti-scorbutic vitamine has been found in green leaves, fresh fruit juices, onions, root vegetables (swedes and potatoes), fresh milk, meat and sprouted seeds. The different foods show variations in their content of the vitamine. Orange juice or a water extract of orange pulp, 2:1, lemon and lime juice, have been found to be particularly active. Hess found that a slightly alkalinized solution of orange juice, if injected soon after preparation, is an effective anti-scorbutic. In general, however, alkaline extracts deteriorate rapidly. Tomato juice, fresh or canned, and potato water have been found to be good anti-scorbutics for children. Hess noted a case of scurvy which did not react to orange juice but did to potato.

Foods which have been found to be low in their anti-scorbutic value or lack the vitamine are: yeast and its extracts, wheat embryo, egg yolk, prunes, beets, cod liver oil, olive oil, "malt soup," (unless prepared from fresh raw milk) and dried foods or foods cooked for a long time. Desiccation tends to reduce the content of the anti-scorbutic vitamine in foods, least apparently in acid foods. There is some evidence that the method of drying and the age of the fresh food has a relation to the degree of destruction of the vitamine. Cooking, heating, or boiling, to 100° C. tends to destroy the anti-scorbutic vitamine; cooking vegetables for a short time at a high temperature is not as destructive as subjection to a low temperature for a long period.

Milk has already been referred to as an anti-scorbutic. In comparison with oranges, however, it is relatively poor in the vitamine. The effect of heat upon milk is to lower or to destroy the anti-scorbutic property. According to Hess the aging of milk with the subsequent development of an abnormal flora is an important factor in the destruction of the anti-scorbutic factor, more so perhaps than heating. Milk heated to 145° F. or boiled milk is less apt to produce scurvy in infants than milk which has been heated to 165° F. The explanation is that boiling tends to destroy all bacteria and heating to 145° F. does not destroy all of the lactic acid producing organisms, which are in a sense protective against

the growth of putrefactive organisms. Milk heated to 145°
F. will not sour unless reinoculated with the lactic acid
bacillus. Raw milk kept for some time tends to lose its
anti-scorbutic value. Dried milks and evaporated milks
lack the anti-scorbutic vitamine. There is some evidence
that dried milks made from *fresh* raw milk exposed to relatively high temperatures for a short time may retain a
part at least of their anti-scorbutic value.

Pellagra.— Pellagra is held to be a disease resulting from
a lack of a specific substance of the nature of vitamines in
the diet, arising from an improper selection of foods or loss
of the vitamine in cooking. It still appears possible that
the effect of diet is only secondary in that the deficient diet
may be a predisposing factor to infection due to decreased
resistance.[1] According to Goldberger[2] pellagra is due directly to a faulty diet as the result of one or a combination
of the following factors, (*a*) a physiologically defective protein supply, (*b*) a low or inadequate supply of fat soluble
vitamine or of water-soluble vitamine, (*c*) a defective mineral
supply. McCollum after analyzing various supposed pellagra producing diets finds them generally deficient in the
character of the protein, fat-soluble A, calcium, sodium and
chlorine.

Rickets.—The status of rickets as a deficiency disease has
not been established. The evidence of Hess in which cod-
liver oil was found to prevent the occurrence of rickets
among negro children and the experiments of Mellanby who
was able to prevent experimental rickets in pups with meat,
water extract of meat free from protein, malt extract, commercial yeast extract, large quantities of milk, butter, margarine or cod-liver oil, whereas the protein of meat, casein,
linseed oil, or yeast would not do so, tend to indicate the
necessity for the presence of some particular dietary factor.

[1] MacNeal; Jour. Am. Med. Assn., 1916, xvil, 975; Jobling and Peterson:
Jour. Infect. Dis. 1916, xviii, 501.
[2] Jour. Am. Med. Assn. 1918, lxxi, 944.

CHAPTER V.

FOOD REQUIREMENTS IN PREGNANCY AND LAC-
TATION. FOOD REQUIREMENTS AND FEED-
ING OF CHILDREN. FASTING.

FOOD REQUIREMENTS IN PREGNANCY AND LACTATION

During pregnancy food is required for the development and maintenance of the fetus, and associated tissues, growth of the uterine musculature, body musculature and of the breasts as well as for the maintenance of the maternal organism itself. In certain stages of gestation additional food is required to meet the extra calls upon the mother. In the early stages of pregnancy food beyond that normally required by the mother, is not needed since the food required for the growth and maintenance of the embryo is comparatively small. Later, however, from about the middle of the period of gestation, the embryo and associated tissues begin to make considerable demands upon the mother and provision must be made in her diet for these purposes. Following parturition the additional demands upon the maternal organism continue but the method of nourishing the young is transferred from the continuous nourishment through the blood stream to intermittant feeding through the breasts. The mother must still maintain herself but the quantity of tissue to be maintained is lowered to the extent of the special tissues elaborated in the body for the proper growth of the embryo; a difference which is not great.

Energy.—In the early stages of gestation there is little increase in the energy requirement of the mother plus the fetus. During the last stages of pregnancy an extra metabolism has been determined equivalent to approximately four per cent. of that of the mother in sexual rest. This extra metabolism represents the additional energy necessary to maintain the child and the associated tissues. Studies of the respiratory quotient of the fetus indicate that heat is produced largely from carbohydrate. Following parturition the total metabolism of the mother and infant is almost exactly that which existed before parturition. In other

[1]Murlin, Amer. Jour. of Obstetr., 1917, lxxv, 913, has discussed the data with regard to the metabolism of mother and offspring.

words, the extra metabolism of the child required to maintain itself outside its mother's body is approximately that of the additional tissues associated with the fetus *in utero*. The demands made upon the mother soon after parturition are no greater than those just beforehand. As the child grows and requires more food, the added energy requirements must be met to compensate for the milk produced. The heat production of puerperal women was found to be 11 per cent. higher than the average for non-pregnant women and seven per cent. higher than that of the same subjects just before delivery. This difference in the rate of metabolism has been ascribed in part to the increased activity of the mammary glands and in part to the stimulating effects of the products of involution.

The energy metabolism of the infant soon after birth is slightly lower, per unit of body surface, than that of the mother. This is due possibly to the undeveloped heat regulating mechanism. From the time of birth the rate of metabolism increases until a maximum is reached between one and two years; during the time of most rapid growth and maximum milk consumption. Following this the rate of metabolism decreases rapidly at first and then more gradually (adult) until old age with a slight rise at the time of puberty. The basal metabolism of an infant at birth is 48 Calories per kilogram of body weight. Between six and twelve months the basal metabolism is 60 calories per kilogram. Severe crying increases the metabolism 40 per cent. per hour. Fifteen per cent. of the calories ingested are retained for growth. The energy intake for infants to cover the basal metabolism and increase for activity and growth has been placed at from 80 to 90 Calories per kilogram of body weight.

Protein Requirement.—Data with regard to nitrogen metabolism in pregnancy indicate a negative nitrogen balance during the early stages of gestation. Such a loss takes place in animals no matter what the nature of the diet may be, indicating that this loss is not essentially a matter of the quantity of food. The limited data with regard to human metabolism does not demonstrate a negative balance but does show a lower positive balance at the corresponding stage of gestation than at any other time. This tendency toward a negative balance occurs at about the third month of gestation; the time of placental formation and morning sickness. With the completion of the placenta this increased catabolism gives place to predominant anabolic activity. From this time on we find a retention of nitrogen for the

8

growth of the fetus and development of the maternal tissues. Retention of nitrogen from the seventeenth week
to the end of the period of gestation is greater than the requirement of the fetus, associated tissues and the mammary
glands. The increased retention of nitrogen has been suggested as being in anticipation of the demands of labor and
the period of lactation. The quantity of nitrogen retained
by the fetus has been estimated by Michel:

COMPOSITION OF THE FETUS. (MICHEL, AFTER MURLIN.)

Age, weeks.	N. grams.	P. grams.	Ca. grams.	Mg. grams.
16	2.94	0.66	0.42	0.02
20	6.05	1.45	2.21	0.08
24	11.05	2.44	4.08	0.13
28	16.01	3.53	5.88	0.19
40	72.70	18.67	33.26	0.82

The data indicate very clearly, the fact that the greatest
quantitative growth takes place in the last fourth of pregnancy. During this period particularly it is necessary that
the diet of the mother be adequate with regard to inorganic
salts as well as other foods; milk is one of the best single
foods for this purpose.

Immediately following the birth of the child the mother
exhibits a negative nitrogen balance arising chiefly from the
involuting uterus. When these processes are practically
completed the positive balance present in the later stages
of gestation is again found.

The character of the protein ingested is of importance in
pregnancy and lactation. The maternal system cannot
synthetize amino-acids to any extent, hence it is necessary
to provide adequate protein to meet the increased draft
imposed by the growing infant. A deficient diet reacts
more upon the mother than upon the child. During gestation the fetus draws upon the resources of the mother for
the food factors necessary for growth. Under-feeding has
been found to have little effect upon the young. This
applies particularly to under-feeding following the normal
full development of the mother before becoming pregnant.
Long continued under-nutrition during the period of growth
of the mother and subsequent pregnancy has been found to
interfere with the normal processes of gestation or to result
in inferior young. The same conditions apply to lactation;
the *tendency* is to continue to produce a normal milk in
spite of under-nutrition. If, however, the period of under-
feeding is sufficiently prolonged the quantity of milk appears
to diminish rather than the proportions of the constituents
present. In any case the mother is the first to suffer and

afterward, when her tissues fail, the young. As McCollum has expressed it—the mother is the factor of safety in the nourishment of the young.

The extra demands upon the maternal body for inorganic salts during pregnancy and lactation are confined chiefly to calcium and phosphorus, *i. e.*, the mother ordinarily takes with her food sufficient of the other inorganic salts, sodium, chlorine, iron, magnesium, etc., to meet her own needs and those of her child. The quantities of calcium and phosphorus needed for the production of the fetus and later of milk are rather large. The data of Michel indicates a large retention of calcium in the last quarter of the period of gestation. At the beginning of lactation in such high milk producing animals as the cow there is a loss of calcium (Forbes) from the body of the mother which cannot be offset, at the time, by an increased consumption of calcium. In the later stages of lactation and after milk production has ceased the loss of calcium from the body is probably replaced.

Diet and Lactation.—The relation of the diet to the quantity and quality of milk produced is of considerable importance. The original stimulus to the milk flow originates in the placenta or associated tissues. Later (Eckles), this stimulus loses its force and is replaced by a nervous stimulus. The flow of milk is maintained and apparently may be increased to a maximum for the individual through the constant stimulus of nursing or the removal of the milk. The extent to which milk flow can be increased by nursing is not known. Observations have been made in which it was increased in wet nurses from the quantity necessary for one child to that sufficient for three children.

Diet has little effect upon the composition of milk during the early stages of lactation.[1] Over-feeding has practically no effect. If the stimulus to produce milk is not present feeding will not increase the quantity of milk. The consumption of large quantities of nitrogenous food will not affect, appreciably, the percentage composition of milk. Under-nutrition does not affect the quantity of milk produced for some time; the percentage of fat tends to decrease. In this case the milk is produced at the expense of the mother. Later in the period of lactation the effect of under-nutrition is to reduce the quantity of milk and to cause some modification in the percentage of fat (increase) and protein and lactose (decrease). If under-nutrition is sufficiently pro-

[1] The composition of milk varies slightly according to the stage of lactation.

longed the character of the milk is undoubtedly affected. Recent work on the distribution and occurrence of the vitamines has shown that the animal organism apparently cannot synthetize these food factors but must obtain them, ultimately, from plant sources. Where the store of vitamines in the mother is low her milk will tend . to be deficient in these substances. Women with beri beri have been found to produce a deficient milk such that normal infants allowed to nurse develop beri beri. Experiments with rats indicate that the milk is deficient in vitamines when the diet of the mother lacks these substances. There is some indication that the quantity of vitamine in cow's milk is related to the nature of the diet.

The quantity and quality of the diet necessary for human milk production has been studied by Hoobler. For women performing light work diets containing 2600 to 2900 calories per day maintained a better milk flow without affecting the maternal tissues than those consuming a diet of from 3400 to 3700 calories. Where the mother is engaged in more active work a slightly higher diet would be indicated. Over feeding did not result in an increased milk flow. The best results were obtained with a ratio of protein calories to fat (calculated as carbohydrate) and carbohydrate calories of 1:6. This is rather a high protein diet. Animal protein was found to be better than vegetable protein for the production of milk. A combination of nut protein and vegetables gave very satisfactory results. Milk as a source of protein is the best for the production of milk and the protection of the maternal tissues.

FOOD REQUIREMENTS AND FEEDING OF CHILDREN.

Children differ from adults in that they are in the process of growing; they are daily increasing the size of their muscles, bones and organs and are also very active. The food of a growing child must meet not only the daily wear and tear and furnish energy for the daily activities but it must supply additional quantities of all types of food-stuffs for use in the formation of the increasing mass of tissue. The rate of increase in weight for boys and girls is given in the table[1] on page 117.

The rate of increase in weight is not uniform but proceeds in cycles. Robertson[2] has shown from an analysis of the rate of growth that the increase in weight is periodic, in the

[1] Manny, from data obtained by Holt, Burke and Boas, Pub. 115. New York Association for Improving the Condition of the Poor.
[2] Amer. Jour. Physiol, 1915, xxxvii, 37.

form of S-shaped curves. For man there is, (*a*) probably a short cycle preceding the implantation of the ovum, (*b*) a second cycle beginning with the development of the embryo and extending nearly to the end of the first year of extra-uterine life with a maximum velocity at 1.66 months in the male and 2.47 months in the female, (*c*) a third cycle starting during or near the completion of the first year of extra-uterine life and practically fusing with the preceding cycle with the maximum rate at about 5.5 years for both sexes. (*d*) a fourth cycle which attains its maximum velocity at 14.5 years for females and 16.5 years for males and ending with the attainment of adult weight.

AVERAGE WEIGHT, AND INCREASE IN WEIGHT PER YEAR FOR BOYS AND GIRLS.

Age	Boys		Girls	
	Weight lbs.	Increase per year lbs.	Weight lbs.	Increase per year lbs.
Birth	7.55		7.16	
6 months	16.00	16.90	15.50	16.68
1 year	20.50	9.00	19.80	8.60
2 years	26.50	6.00	25.50	5.70
3 "	31.20	4.70	30.00	4.50
4 "	35.00	3.80	34.00	4.00
5 yrs. 6 mos.	41.20	4.14	39.80	3.87
6 " "	45.20	4.00	43.40	3.60
7 " "	49.50	4.30	47.70	4.30
8 " "	54.50	5.00	52.50	4.80
9 " "	59.60	5.10	57.40	4.90
10 " "	65.40	5.80	62.90	5.50
11 " "	70.70	5.30	69.50	6.60
12 " "	76.90	6.20	78.70	9.20
13 " "	84.80	7.90	88.70	10.00
14 " "	95.20	10.40	98.30	9.60
15 " "	107.40	12.20	106.70	8.40
16 " "	121.00	13.60	112.30	5.60

When the food supply is restricted in amount growth is retarded particularly with regard to weight. In experimental animals it has been noted that when restricted to diets adequate in the nature of the constituents but inadequate in amount such that they maintain a fairly constant weight that they grow in length and height but become emaciated. If after such a period of feeding an adequate diet is given the animal will gain in weight and in circumference and will return approximately to normal provided the restriction has not been too prolonged. Such recovery has been noted in children.

Energy Requirements of Children.—The basal metabolism of children is higher than that of adults. The variation in the basal metabolism with age for male subjects is given in Fig. 2, p. 62. From the chart it is evident that from birth to approximately five years of age the rate of metabolism is increasing. From five years on until maturity the rate of metabolism falls with a slight rise at about the thirteenth to fourteenth year, puberty, after which it continues to decrease. Following the attainment of maturity the basal metabolism shows a gradual and regular decrease until death. The data are not complete for female subjects but the general trend of the curve is the same except that the values are slightly lower. In addition to the increased rate of metabolism of children over that of adults we find an increased rate of energy consumption as the result of marked activity. It is evident, therefore, that children require food out of proportion to their size when compared with adults. Girls are both smaller and less active than boys and they require less food. The following table gives the difference in total calories for boys and girls in given age-groups and the calories per pound for boys and girls from three types of study of the metabolic requirements of children.[1]

DIFFERENCE IN TOTAL CALORIES CONSUMED BY BOYS AND GIRLS AT DIFFERENT AGES.

	2-5 years.	6-9 years.	10-13 years.	14-17 years.
Boys and girls	1308	1718	2190	2525
Boys	1309	1797	2337	2534
Girls	1245	1575	2015	2253
Boys and girls, protein, grams	47	57	68	90

CALORIES PER POUND FOR BOYS AND GIRLS FROM EACH OF THREE TYPES OF METABOLIC DATA.

Age group Years	Boys			Girls		
	Dietary Expts.	Metabolism Expts.	Respiration Expts.	Dietary Expts.	Metabolism Expts.	Respiration Expts.
2-5	38.7	44.1	61.9	35.0	42.8	....
6-9	32.8	36.9	49.6	32.8	34.1	49.6
10-13	30.9	27.8	38.7	25.0	27.3	33.2
14-17	28.2	29.1	26.9	20.5	20.0	26.9

From a consideration of the data available with regard to the energy requirement of children Miss Gillett has prepared the table on page 119 giving the caloric intake required by children of different ages. In this table allowance is made for individual variation. Boys have been found to ingest food equivalent to 4000 to 5000 calories per day.

Protein Requirement.—Less is known with regard to the protein requirement of children than that of adults. It appears that protein calories to the extent of 10 to 15 per cent. of the total calories is sufficient; this is the proportion found for adults. Such a proportion of protein amounts to a re-

[1] Gillett; Food Allowances for Healthy Children, Pub. 115, New York Assoc. for Improving the Condition of the Poor, 1917.

latively high protein intake per unit of body weight when it is considered that the caloric intake of children is from two to three times that of the resting adult,

FOOD ALLOWANCES FOR CHILDREN (GILLETT).

Age. Years.							Boys.	Girls.
							Calories per Day.	
Under 2	.	.	.	.	.	.	900–1200	900–1200
2– 3	.	.	.	.	.	.	1000–1300	980–1280
3– 4	.	.	.	.	.	.	1100–1400	1060–1360
4– 5	.	.	.	.	.	.	1200–1500	1140–1440
5– 6	.	.	.	.	.	.	1300–1600	1220–1520
6– 7	.	.	.	.	.	.	1400–1700	1300–1600
7– 8	.	.	.	.	.	.	1500–1800	1380–1680
8– 9	.	.	.	.	.	.	1600–1900	1460–1760
9–10	.	.	.	.	.	.	1700–2000	1550–1850
10–11	.	.	.	.	.	.	1900–2200	1650–1950
11–12	.	.	.	.	.	.	2100–2400	1750–2050
12–13	.	.	.	.	.	.	2300–2700	1850–2150
13–14	.	.	.	.	.	.	2500–2900	1950–2250
14–15	.	.	.	.	.	.	2600–3100	2050–2350
15–16	.	.	.	.	.	.	2700–3300	2150–2450
16–17	.	.	.	.	.	.	2700-3400	2250-2550

The character of the protein ingested is of as great importance in growth as the quantity of protein. The nature of protein deficiencies has been discussed on page 76. Data obtained on the biological value of proteins, complex foods and vitamines in which growth is the index of the relative value of various foods have contributed many interesting and important facts with regard to food requirements in growth. Milk protein was found by McCollum[1] to be of greater value for the purposes of growth in the pig than certain cereal proteins. The following table contains a protion of the data.

PER CENT. OF INGESTED PROTEIN RETAINED FOR GROWTH BY THE PIG.

Source of protein.	Per cent. of protein retained.
Milk	63
Oats, rolled	26
Wheat	23
Corn	20

Meat undoubtedly has a value approximating that of milk. It is to be remembered that the growth impulse of the pig is much greater than that of the human infant and the capacity to store protein in the latter case, is, therefore, less. Similar relative values have been obtained with regard to milk protein in experiments on rats. The lower value of vegetable proteins for growth and maintenance is not to be construed as meaning that they are not valuable

[1] Jour. Biol. Chem., 1914, xix, 323.

sources of protein. The work of Mendel and Osborne has repeatedly shown that the limiting factor in the inefficient protein is the low content or absence of one or more amino-acids. A combination of two proteins when either alone would be insufficient may be entirely satisfactory. This is possible since the deficiencies in amino-acids are different for different proteins and that one protein may contain an excess of an amino-acid in which another protein is deficient. All animal proteins ordinarily used for food may be considered as relatively complete proteins; gelatin is an exception. In using a large proportion of vegetable foods it is necessary to correct for the low biological value of these proteins. Milk is the best source of protein for this purpose in the diet of children, not only because of the high value of its protein but because of the associated food constituents which it contains, calcium salts and the vitamines.

Inorganic Salts.—Our knowledge of the quantities of inorganic salts required for growth is rather limited. Those salts needed in the greatest quantities are, calcium, phosphorus, iron, sodium and chlorine. With the exception of sodium and chlorine these are the elements most likely to be deficient in the diet. Ample quantities of milk and vegetables will ensure an adequate consumption of the necessary inorganic salts. Milk supplies calcium and phosphorus, but little iron, the vegetables, particularly leafy vegetables, furnish iron in addition to the other salts. The infant when subsisting entirely on milk apparently depends upon its reserve of iron in its tissues until it is past the nursing stage and can obtain iron from other foods. Insufficient inorganic salts will result in a retardation of growth. That this is not true for limited periods has been shown by Mendel and Osborne who observed normal growth in rats on diets balanced with regard to acid and base but poor in sodium, potassium, magnesium or chlorine, but not when deficient in calcium or phosphorus.

Vitamines.—The subject of vitamines has been discussed page 102. It is in the feeding of children that particular attention must be given to the question of vitamines. An ample supply of all three types of vitamine should be assured fat-soluble A, water-soluble B, and the anti-scorbutic vitamine. Water-soluble B is rather widely distributed in nature and is fairly resistant to drying and preserving. Unless the diet is restricted to highly milled or purified foods there is little danger of a failure to obtain this anti-neuritic vitamine. Fat-soluble A is less widely distributed and more consideration must be given to its presence in the diet.

This vitamine is found particularly in milk fat (butter) and organ fats, as distinct from body fats and vegetable fats, and in the leaves of vegetables. It is resistent to heat but apparently undergoes deterioration upon long standing. Particular attention must be paid to the presence of the anti-scorbutic vitamine in the feeding of small children.

Water.—Children need a plentiful supply of water. It has been found that an adult man will lose 25 per cent. of his daily heat production through the evaporation of water from the skin and lungs. Children with their marked activity and higher rate of metabolism will certainly equal if not surpass this figure. The necessity for water is, therefore, evident.

Selection of Diets for Children after the Second Year.[1]— In feeding children during the period of growth the important considerations are (a) that the diet be selected to furnish the necessary food factors, (b) that the food be wholesome and plentiful, and (c) that good food habits are established and maintained. In selecting foods, milk, eggs, cereals, vegetables and fruits, should form the basis of the diet; meat should be served only occasionally and in small amounts. Methods of cooking should be confined entirely to boiling, roasting and baking; no fried food should be served. Cereals should be thoroughly cooked, preferably the night before, and warmed for breakfast. All foods should be comparatively bland in flavor; the use of highly seasoned foods and sweets for young children is unpardonable. Rich or highly flavored foods are not necessary for a child. To permit children to eat such foods and sweets is to encourage them to eat increased quantities of food which are likely to lack necessary food factors, particularly the vitamines and calcium or lime, with a resulting deficiency in growth. The natural appetite of a child is sufficient to insure an adequate consumption of wholesome food and a healthy child will do so provided it has not been allowed to acquire improper food habits. A child does not naturally *crave* rich foods, it acquires, or is allowed to acquire, a taste for them. If it is taught to eat only wholesome bland foods it will crave only such foods. There is plenty of time later in life to learn about rich foods.[2]

[1] See page 269 for the feeding of children through the second year.
[2] This discussion is adapted in part from Diet for the School Child, Bureau of Education, U. S. Dept. of Interior and the publications of the Dietetic Bureau, Boston, Mass. A bibliography on Child welfare,—Bascom and Mendenhall, has been published by the Amer. Med. Assn., 1918; other material may be obtained from Rose, Feeding the Family; the New York Assoc. for the Improvement of the Condition of the Poor; Child Health Organization New York; and publications of the U. S. Dept. of Agriculture.

Food for Children. *Milk and Eggs.*—Milk is the most important single food in the diet of children and should be the chief source of their protein,—it is a protective food— *i. e.*, it contains adequate protein, is rich in calcium, phosphorus and has a plentiful supply of fat-soluble vitamine and a moderate amount of water-soluble B and the anti-scorbutic vitamine; it is deficient only in iron. Children between the ages of three to six should receive from 1½ to 2 pints of milk a day and above these ages at least three cups of milk a day. Warm milk is preferable to cold milk. When there is an objection to drinking milk as such it should be incorporated in other dishes—cocoa, custards, milk soups, etc. Dried or evaporated milk may be used when fresh milk cannot be obtained, but these milks must be corrected for their loss of anti-scorbutic properties. With dried skimmed milk, plenty of leafy vegetables or cream or butter should be given to supply the fat-soluble vitamine. Eggs are included among the protective foods and next to milk should be in the dietary of a child. A quart of milk and an egg a day will furnish sufficient protein, with that obtained in the other foods, for a child up to seven years. Eggs should be soft boiled, poached, scrambled or as an omelet, but not fried.

Meat.—The use of meat in the form of beef, mutton, veal, fish, etc., is not desirable for young children. The objection is not so much to the meat itself as to the fact that it is highly flavored. The result is that the child acquires a particular liking for meat and unless carefully watched will tend to eat it in place of other necessary forms of food; meat is deficient in the fat-soluble vitamine and in calcium. Meat should be used as flavoring material for cereals, rice, vegetables, soups and stews to stimulate the consumption of these foods if necessary, rather than meat as such. The allowance of meat should not be more than 60 grams (2 ounces) for a child between seven to ten years and 90 grams (3 ounces) for a child ten to fourteen years old. When meat and eggs are scarce or prohibitive cereals and pea or bean soup with spinach or other green leafy vegetables should be used with milk.

Cereals, Bread, or Other Grain Products.—Approximately one-third of the food required by a child should come from the cereals or legumes. Products containing a large proportion of the whole grain, brown rice, cracked wheat (thoroughly cooked), whole wheat, oatmeal, are preferable to the highly milled foods such as polished rice, or white flour, since in the process of milling much of the organic material, a part of the protein and most of the vitamines are removed. The relative economic value of cereals will be found on page 141. Cereals should·be thoroughly cooked, long slow cooking in a double boiler or fireless cooker are desirable. Cereals should be served with milk and only a small amount of sugar or no sugar at all. The dry partially cooked cereals may be used for variety; such foods are both expensive and bulky. The flaked products cost approximately two to three times as much as the cooked cereal and the puffed products six to seven times as much. The best cereals are oatmeal, wheatena, pettijohn, cornmeal, hominy, rice, farina or cream of wheat.

Vegetables.—Vegetables are an essential constituent of the diet of children, because of the salts and vitamines which they contain and because of the indigestible residue which tends to prevent constipation. They may be divided into two classes, (*a*) the leafy vegetables which may be considered as protective foods in that they supply the fat-soluble, water-soluble and anti-scorbutic vitamines, inorganic material and bulk to the diet and (*b*) the roots and tubers which contain relatively smaller quantities of each of the articles enumerated under (*a*) but have in addition more energy producing carbohydrates. Potatoes are a very important food and should be served practically every day, particularly when boiled or cooked in their skins, since in peeling potatoes as in milling grains much of the valuable salts and vitamines are removed in the process. Rice is another vegetable product which can be used continuously without a distaste arising from monotony. For young children vegetables should be thoroughly cooked and then macerated and eaten as such or made into thick soups. Up to the fifth year, potatoes, peas and beans, fresh or dried (in soups) spinach, onions, string beans, squash, cauliflower, asparagus, carrots, and stewed celery may be used. Above the fifth year all vegetables, except cabbage, cucumbers and corn, can be eaten. Corn should not be given until the twelfth year. In preparing vegetables the water in which they are cooked should be served with them or used in soups since a large proportion of the salts are removed in the water.

Fruit.—Fruit should be used each day. If fresh fruit is not obtainable cooked, dried or evaporated fruits may be used. Fresh fruit should be very ripe. Fruits such as oranges, stewed or fresh apples, ripe pears or peaches, stewed dried figs, dates, prunes or peaches or ripe or cooked bananas may be given.

Fats.—Fats, particularly butter fat (or cream) are important factors in the diet of children because of the fat-soluble vitamine they carry and the energy which they contain. If skimmed milk is used, butter fat should be added to the diet or plenty of the leaves of fresh vegetables given to furnish the fat-soluble vitamine. Butter substitues may be used—the oleomargarines are better than the nut butters—if the same correction is made in the diet as for skimmed milk. Children should not have cooked fat, except bacon.

Water.—Give plenty of good water—care must be taken that the food is not washed down before it is properly chewed.

Planning the Meals.[1]—*Breakfast.*—Breakfast should consist of milk and bread and butter and when possible in addition cereal, fruit and an egg.

Dinner.—The heaviest meal should be in the middle of the day except for children of school age who are compelled to hurry back to school immediately after their meal. Dinner should consist of soup, eggs or meat, vegetables, bread and butter and dessert. The soup should be made of dried peas or beans or fresh or canned vegetables, such as spinach, carrots, potato or onions. The addition of rice or barley and milk will make a most nutritious dish. If a thick vegetable soup is not made another vegetable should be added. The desserts should be plain and wholesome, such as fruit, cereal pudding, rice, oatmeal or farina with fruit, baked Indian pudding, or bread pudding, plain cookies, or cakes, and cocoa, fruit custards, junkets, ice cream or ices, sliced oranges.

Supper.—For supper dishes made of milk, eggs, strained vegetables (for young children) cereals and fruits are to be preferred to meat, whole vegetables, or sweet desserts. For example, (*a*) bread or cereal and milk, potato and fruit or eggs; (*b*) potato, bread and butter, apple sauce and ginger bread.

School Lunches.—When it is not possible for the children to come home to a hot dinner at noon and to eat without hurrying it is preferable for them to carry their lunch. Such a lunch should be both nutritious and appetizing. If possible hot cocoa or soup should be served at the school. It is essential that the child should have a convenient and attractive place in which to eat his lunch and it is desirable that a definite time be set aside for a lunch hour, otherwise he will be in a hurry to finish and go out to play. A failure to make such provision has been found to result in undernourishment even when ample food was supplied.

Food Habits of Children.—An important factor in the proper feeding of children is the establishment of good food

[1] See also page 131.

habits. They should be taught, (*a*) to eat what is given them, provided of course that only wholesome food is offered, (*b*) to eat slowly but without delay and in an orderly manner, (*c*) to be regular to their meals, and (*d*) to have clean hands and faces. Children should not be forced to eat when not hungry, not be allowed to eat between meals and particularly not to eat sweets just before meals for such a practice will invariably destroy the appetite for the wholesome and necessary foods. They should not be allowed to drink tea or coffee. The food habits of children are influenced by those of the parents. If the parents do not care for the food their children should have they must refrain from comment with regard to their own likes and dislikes. If a dislike for a certain food is expressed by the parents, they cannot expect the child to like it. It is on the whole better that the child should eat apart from the parents and preferably before the regular meal until the third or fourth year or even until the sixth year. It is better to modify the habits of the parents than to teach the children to like and to demand highly flavored foods to the exclusion, or partial exclusion at least, of the essential foods a child should have. It is to be remembered that food habits are *habits per se* and not essentially natural cravings for particular types of food. Depend upon healthy exercise and outdoor living to create an appetite rather than to stimulate it with special foods or methods of cooking.

The food habits of delicate children have been studied by Emerson.[1] It was found that the food habits of children are very uniform in that they take the proper amount too much or too little food with great regularity. Delicate children invariably take too little food. Such children (*a*) show signs of malnutrition in which weight is affected more than height, (*b*) may or may not have retarded mental development, (*c*) have an unstable nervous system. Physical causes modify the food consumption through fatigue, mental distress and body defects. To bring about proper nutrition delicate children should be treated for the physical defects, particularly nasal pharyngeal obstructions (adenoids, tonsils, deviated septum, and sinus infections) and carious teeth. These children must be kept out of doors and sleep out doors if possible. Sweet and rich foods, if the children are addicted to them, must be replaced by wholesome, simple foods, gradually if necessary, by selecting foods as near those of the likes of the child as possible and compat-

[1] New York Med. Jour. February 24, 1917.

able with the changes required. Records should be kept of the diet to be assured of the value of the changes. Weights should be taken to determine the gain or failure to gain.[1] Periods of rest in bed should be instituted, preferably before lunch and before the evening meal or better, after exercise and a bath. The meals should be cheerful. Mental distress over school work should be reduced as much as possible. If addicted to fast eating this fault must be corrected.

Malnutrition clinics[2] in connection with schools have demonstrated the possibilities of correcting the effects of malnutrition in children through careful supervision of the diet, instruction with regard to food and the arousal of interest in the individual gain by weekly weighing and plotting of the weights. Such clinics were first started by Emerson and are now carried out in connection with the work of the Bureau of Education, Department of Interior, Child Health Organization of New York, and in other cities.

FASTING.

The fasting state sometimes prevails in disease as a result of obstruction of the alimentary tract or the inability of the individual to retain ingested food. Conditions of undernutrition from similar causes are much more common than complete fasting. Short fasts are often used in the treatment of various diseases. A knowledge of the changes in the body that result from fasting is of a purely scientific as well as practical interest, for it aids in understanding and explaining the normal metabolism and certain pathological conditions.

Life is accompanied by various cellular and systemic changes which we ordinarily designate as metabolism—processes of synthesis and of decomposition; oxidation with the liberation of carbon dioxide, water, and energy; the formation and disintegration of proteins, and the coördination of these activities in all parts of the body. Even though food no longer be supplied these processes continue. Since the

[1] Emerson believes that any child seven per cent. under weight is to be considered as under-nourished. There is some difference of opinion with regard to the value of the comparison of body weights with average body weights for a given age. The element of race may introduce a factor as great as the one indicated. It is wise, however, to consider a child who deviates from the stanard weights as undernourished until he proves himself to be an exception. The taking of weights enables one to follow the rate of growth and to note a failure to grow. It is more important that a child should follow the *rate* of growth than it is that he should attain the actual weight indicated in tables of weights.

[2] A bibliography on malnutrition has been compiled by Mrs. Dorothy Reed Mendenhal for the Child's Bureau, U. S. Dept. of Labor.

losses sustained in metabolism are then no longer replenished from ingested material, the more active and essential organs make use of similar substances contained in the body. Thus we find that the heart, brain, lungs, kidneys, testicles, and liver lose a much smaller proportion of their weight during fasting than do the muscles and adipose tissue. From this we conclude that the former organs which are, in a sense, more essential for life obtain the necessary food material from the blood which in turn is replenished largely from the muscle and adipose tissue. This process of drawing upon the tissues for continued activity is not an unusual one. There are undoubtedly times between the ingestion of food, particularly late during the long interval between the evening meal and breakfast, when but little food is received from the alimentary tract and the body lives at the expense of its own stores.

Not only does the body draw upon its own tissues for the material necessary for its activity but it appears to be able to utilize these much more economically than it does ingested food. In the light of our present knowledge of protein metabolism in which, as McCollum has expressed it, the processes of repair do not involve the destruction and resynthesis of entire protein molecules, it seems quite probable that one tissue is able to utilize in part the amino-acids which have been removed from material in another tissue and that the more or less complete disintegration of protein in one part of the body serves to supply material for the repair of the losses from a number of different tissues in other portions of the body.

The activity of the kidneys, liver, and digestive tract are reduced to a minimum in fasting, for they are no longer required to take care of an excess of food-stuffs. The kidneys are concerned only with the elimination of the products of endogenous metabolism which, as we know, is small in comparison with the exogenous metabolism of the average individual. The elimination of abnormal urinary constituents, as aceto-acetic acids and β-hydroxybutyric acid or bile constituents is sometimes imposed upon the fasting kidneys.

The period of time during which an organism may fast depends upon a number of factors. The previous nutritive condition has its effect in that the quantity of fat and protein which are available determines in part the body reserves. The size of the individual affects the rate of metabolism; small persons have in general a greater metabolism for the body weight than a large person. Age is accompanied by a varied rate of metabolism; children metabolize at a greater rate than adults and therefore utilize their body stores more rapidly than an adult. The external conditions surrounding the body, such as temperature and humidity, may either increase or decrease the body activities. The ingestion of water tends to lengthen the period an organism may fast as compared with a fast without water. Finally, fasting experience in a given individual is a modifying factor; as the result of repeated fasts the body appears to acquire such a resistance that it is better able to withstand the effect of each subsequent fast. This appears to be particularly true when the organism is permitted to recover from the previous fast before being subjected to another.

Men have fasted for as long as fifty days without apparent harm. There are authentic records of a number of thirty-day fasts. Benedict[1] has recently reported the result of a most careful study of a thirty-one-day fast by a man. Animals have been known to fast for much longer periods. The longest fast of a warm-blooded animal is that observed in a dog which continued for 117 days, after which the animal was fed and restored to its original condition and fasted again for the second longest fast, 104 days. Cold-blooded animals, such as the frog, salamander, etc., have been known to fast for much longer periods of time. It is evident, therefore, that the body can obtain from itself sufficient material on which to exist for a considerable length of time. Death, as the result of fasting in the case of normal individuals, is probably due to the failure of some organ or tissue and not to the complete utilization of the body stores. Certain investigations seem to show that a definite minimum quantity of nitrogen-containing material is necessary in order that life may exist.

During a fast the general rate of metabolism is lowered. Studies of the respiratory changes show that the total quantity of carbon dioxide excreted per day is lowered, and the respiratory quotient falls to a value which indicates the oxidation, chiefly, of fat and protein. Protein metabolism is also decreased; the daily nitrogen excretion after the first few days becomes low and fairly constant. It may fall as low as 4 to 6 grams of nitrogen per day. The excretion of salts is also diminished. All phases of normal body metabolism are greatly reduced in fasting.

[1] Benedict has reported a very complete experiment on a man during a thirty-one-day fast, Carnegie Institution of Washington, 1914, Pub. No. 203. The data from this fast are published in chart form in Mathew's Physiological Chemistry, New York, 1915.

CHAPTER VI

NORMAL FEEDING AND FOOD ECONOMICS.

THE application of the principles of human nutrition to the feeding of the normal individual or to the family group is at once involved and difficult. Though the scientist may determine and the physician prescribe an ideal dietary, its adoption by the individual may be quite impractical, due to cost, inconvenience, or lack of market facilities. But since foods are interchangeable within wide ranges, a summary of the principles of nutrition which underlie the selection of food, together with typical menus and a discussion of the cost of food may aid in the interpretation and application of these principles.

Our previous discussion of the various food-stuffs and their digestibility has shown that the source of food is of no particular importance so long as it possesses all of the necessary material and is wholesome, that is, does not contain or yield products which are detrimental to the health of the normal individual. For example, disregarding for the moment the psychological factor, the stomach and intestines can digest a cheap cut of meat or fish as thoroughly as an expensive steak; American cheese as well as Roquefort cheese; cottonseed oil as well as olive oil. The psychical factor cannot, however, be completely ignored for two reasons:

1. Studies of the secretion of the digestive juices and of the rate with which food passes from the stomach indicate that appetite, which in its psychological sense is to a large extent the reflex of palatability, serves to stimulate an early flow of gastric juice and thus facilitate digestion. Once a food is digested and absorbed its value to the body is mainly a matter of its intrinsic composition.

2. A diet which contained all of the necessary food factors might still prove to be unsatisfactory because of psychical objections on the part of those who are to eat it. Such factors as habit, taste, and custom must be taken into consideration. The likes and dislikes for food are to a large degree governed by the kind and variety of food, method or preparation, etc., which have been observed in the household or community in which individuals are reared—a change of the usual dietary regimen is accepted with hesitation, which

can only be overcome by palatability or force of will. If, in the latter case, the diet prove to be unsatisfactory, its continuance is accomplished with greater difficulty or not at all. On the other hand, food well prepared is usually acceptable. It is the factor of *palatability*, based largely upon the proper selection and preparation, which determines the success or failure of diets selected because they are economical. Palatability is, as we have said before, entirely a relative factor, tempered by custom. The diet of the Eskimo, rich in fat and very high in protein, is apparently satisfactory to him. The peasant's diet of porridge and black bread is acceptable, while added white bread or meat constitute luxuries. The absence of choice meats, rich sauces or sweets from the diet of the well-to-do American is regarded as a hardship. A variation of diet outside the range of the dietary habits is a matter of acquired taste or necessity. When it is necessary or desirable to cause a marked change in a diet, careful preparation and serving will do much to accomplish that purpose.

DIETARY ESSENTIALS.—A diet which will supply the needs of the body must contain:

(*a*) Energy-yielding food sufficient in quantity to supply the basal energy requirement and to meet the increased need resulting from activity. The energy may be derived from the oxidation of protein, carbohydrate, or fat, although the requirement beyond that obtained from the protein necessary in other relations, and a minimum amount of fat, is satisfied chiefly by carbohydrates.

(*b*) Protein, containing the necessary amino-acids, or in variety which will yield them in sufficient amount.

(*c*) Carbohydrate.

(*d*) Lipins (fat), natural and unmodified.

(*e*) Mineral matter—salts in quantities and kind sufficient to maintain the skeletal structure, equilibrium between the fluid portions of the body, and to supply the specialized needs of protoplasm in general and of certain organs in particular.

(*f*) Substances of unknown chemical nature classed as accessory food-stuffs, termed vitamines, found particularly in vegetables, coverings of grains and in fatty material. Preserved or highly milled foods are less likely to contain these substances than raw or freshly prepared food.

(*g*) Bulk or indigestible material to stimulate peristalsis.

(*h*) Water.

The absolute quantities of the various food-stuffs needed vary with the size, age and activity of the individual concerned, and with the external conditions to which he is subjected.

The quantitative food requirements of man are as follows:

Energy.—Forty calories per square meter of body surface per hour plus the energy required for general activity; increased muscular work and external conditions. The daily requirement for the average individual at various ages and activities may be found on pages 71 and 72.

Protein.—Equivalent to 10 to 15 per cent. of the total calories required per day. For the adult this amounts to from 60 to 120 grams per day.

Carbohydrate and Fat.—The total quantity and the relative proportions of these food-stuffs vary with the energy requirements. It has been found that fat and carbohydrate may be used in the diet in the proportion of 7 to 2 without apparent marked disturbance in metabolism. The average diet, however, contains a preponderance of carbohydrate. The average fat intake is from 25 to 75 grams per day.

Mineral Matter.—With the exception of phosphorus, calcium and iron, little is known in regard to quantitative requirements. The quantities of inorganic constituents which are required daily by the average individual have been estimated as follows:

Phosphoric acid (P_2O_5)	3.3
Calcium oxide (CaO)	1.0
Iron (Fe)	0.015

Accessory Foods and Bulk.—The average mixed diet contains sufficient quantities of these substances. For further discussion see pp. 102 and 238.

PLANNING MEALS.—The object to be attained in planning meals is to furnish the necessary food elements in their proper proportions and in an attractive manner. To accomplish this end not only the food factors must be considered but the types of food acceptable to the individuals who are to eat which will supply these factors. The following typical menus prepared by Miss Rose as suggestions in planning the diet of a family of moderate means, including children above two years of age, may be regarded as illustrations of properly selected diets. Certain foods, as pancakes and sausages, are included to increase the variety for adults who are accustomed to a more varied diet than children.

MENU I.

Breakfast:

Wheaten grits with cream or whole milk.

For all members of the family.

Oranges.

For all members of the family except very little children, to whom orange juice may be given between meals.

Bread and butter.	For all members of the family.
Sausages.	For adults.
Pancakes.	For adults.
Coffee.	For adults.

Dinner:

Soup.	For adults and older children.
Roast mutton.	For all members of the family except children under seven years of age.
Baked potatoes.	For all members of the family.
Spinach.	For all members of the family.
Bread and butter.	For all members of the family.
Milk to drink.	Especially for children.
Apple pie.	For adults.
Apple sauce.	For children.

(An egg for children under seven years of age may be included in the above meal plan.)

Supper:

Milk toast.	For all members of the family.
Scrambled eggs.	For adults.
Bread and butter.	For all members of the family.
Peach sauce } Cookies. }	For all members of the family except very small children.

Menu II.

Breakfast:

Rolled oats with cream or whole milk.	For all members of the family.
Stewed prunes.	For all members of the family.
Bread and butter.	For all members of the family.
Milk to drink.	For all members of the family.
Eggs:	
Poached.	For children.
Fried.	For adults.
Coffee.	For adults.

Dinner:

Soup.	For adults and older children.
Pot roast.	For adults and older children.
Boiled potatoes.	For all members of the family.
Creamed onions.	For all members of the family.
Bread and butter.	For all members of the family.
Milk to drink.	Especially for children.
Custard pie.	For adults.
Baked custard.	For children.

Supper:

Scalloped rice with cheese.	For adults and older children.
Plain boiled rice with cream or whole milk.	For younger children.
Bread and butter.	For all members of the family.
Milk to drink.	Especially for children.
Fruit sauce or baked apples } Molasses cookies. }	For all members of the family.

Menu III.

Breakfast:

Cornmeal mush with cream or whole milk.	For all members of the family.
Stewed fruit.	For all members of the family except very little children; to be given to children between meals.
Bread and butter.	For all members of the family.
Milk to drink.	Especially for children.
Bacon.	Especially for adults.

Waffles.	For adults.
Coffee.	For adults.
Dinner:	
Baked Hamburger steak.	For all members of the family except children under seven years of age.
Creamed potatoes.	For all members of the family.
Mashed potatoes.	For small children.
Buttered carrots.	For all members of the family.
Bread and butter.	For all members of the family.
Milk to drink.	Especially for children.
Steamed suet pudding.	For adults.
Baked apples.	For children.
Supper:	
Cream of bean soup.	For all members of the family.
Bread and butter.	For all members of the family.
Prune sauce.	For all members of the family.
Sponge cake.	For all members of the family.

The table on page 134 suggests the fuel value or calories for the meals of a day apportioned among the various types of foods suitable for persons of different ages, under normal conditions.

In this table a distinction is made between the starch-rich vegetables which supply considerable quantities of energy in the form of carbohydrates and the green vegetables which are particularly valuable for the bulk which they give to the contents in the alimentary tract, because of the indigestible cellulose contained, and for the salts and accessory substances in which they are particularly rich. The dishes classed as meat may often be combined with another class of food such as starch-rich foods or milk, as for example meat-pie, creamed beef, or oyster stew.

It must again be emphasized that the physician who prescribes as well as the housekeeper who plans meals for a family must be sufficiently familiar with the composition of most of the common foods to be able to class them as valuable sources of protein, fat, carbohydrate, or salts. If they do not possess this knowledge one type of food may exceed its most satisfactory proportion in the diet. It is necessary, too, that correct dietary habits be established by children. Preference for a particular food must not lead to the habit of "making a meal" of it. Likes and dislikes for food are largely a matter of habit, and the importance of an early establishment of good food habits cannot be overestimated. While it is not necessary that each meal or the combined meals of one day be complete in meeting the requirements of an individual, such a balance should be approximated and satisfied at least within the course of a few days. The following menus, and the table giving the relative proportion of protein, fat and carbohydrate in them, will serve to illustrate

THE APPORTIONMENT OF CALORIES AMONG THE DIFFERENT TYPES OF FOODS FOR THE MEALS OF A DAY FOR PERSONS OF DIFFERENT AGES.[1]

Total daily requirement.	Man.		Woman.		Child.				Aged 70–80 years.
	Sedentary.	Active.	Sedentary.	Active.	3–4 years.	5–7 years.	8–12 years.	Adolescent 14–16 yrs.	
	2200–2800	3500–4000	1800–2300	2600–3000	1100–1400	1400–1700	1700–2000	1800–2300	1500–1800
MORNING MEAL.									
Fruit	100	...	100	50–100	25–50	50–100	50–100	50–100	75–100
Cerel	50–100	150–300	...	50–150	50–75	50–100	75–100	100–150	100–200
Meat or eggs	100–200	200–300	50–100	100–200	...	...	...	...	75–150
Bread, rolls or hot cakes	100–200	300–400	50–200	50–150	50–150	50–100	50–100	100–200	...
Butter or oleomargarine	100	150–300	33–100	...	...	25–50	50–75	100–200	100–200
Milk or cream (for coffee or cereal—adults)	100–250	100	100–200	250–500	150–270	150–200	...	50–100	...
Sugar	50–100	100	...	...	...	...	...	...	100–200
Milk to drink } 10.30 lunch	...	...	...	...	170	125–175	...	...	...
Bread and butter }	...	...	...	...	50–75	75–125	...	...	4 P.M. tea 75–100
MID-DAY MEAL OR DINNER. / OR LUNCHEON.									
Soup	50–75	...	25–100	25–100	150–200	50–75	50–75	...	100–150
Meat (egg for children)	100–300	150–300	150–300	200–350	60–80	50–100	75–100	200–300	100–200
Starch-rich vegetables	100–150	150	100–150	150–250	...	...	10–25	50–100	75–100
Green vegetables (including salads)	100–250	100–200	100–200	200–350	5–15	5–15	75–100	125–150	...
Bread	50–100	200–400	75–200	50–200	75–150	50–100	150–200	100–300	100–200
Dessert	200–300	250–400	200–300	200–400	100–200	100–200	75–100	150–200	100–200
Milk (and sugar for coffee or cocoa—adults)	...	200	...	...	...	50–100	150–200	...	...
Butter	...	...	50–200	...	150–200	...	50–100	...	...
Milk to drink	...	...	...	...	...	100–150	100–150	100–300	...
EVENING MEAL.									
Soup, light meat or cheese dish	100–200	200–400	150–250	250–400	...	50–100	200–300	...	100–130
Bread or rolls	100–200	200–400	100–150	100–200	...	...	50–100	100–300	75–100
Dessert	200–400	300–552[2]	100–150	200–400	25–150	100–200	100–200	150–200	100–200
Butter	...	...	...	100–200	...	...	...	...	...
Cream or milk and sugar for coffee or cocoa	100–150	200	150–175	...	...	...	...	...	...
Cereal for children, with milk	...	...	...	...	200–303[3]	150–300	...	100–150	100–200

the possibility that even in an apparently well selected diet, some one foodstuff may predominate.

Examples of one-sided diets, predominantly protein, fat, or carbohydrate and an analysis of their composition have been given by Langworthy. [1]

MENUS WITH PROTEIN PREDOMINATING.

Breakfast: Cereal cooked in milk, chicken hash with egg, popovers, butter, and milk as a beverage.
Dinner: Dried-bean puree, halibut steak, potatoes scalloped in milk, tomatoes stuffed with chopped beef, bread and butter, and frozen custard with nut cookies.
Lunch or Supper: Baked beans, nut bread and butter, old-fashioned rice pudding, and a glass of milk.

MENUS WITH A LARGE PROPORTION OF FAT

Breakfast: Oatmeal with cream, sausage, and corn bread and butter.
Dinner: Cream of tomato soup, mutton chop with creamed potatoes, greens cooked with bacon or pork, bread and suet pudding with hard sauce.
Lunch or Supper: Creamed salmon, lettuce with oil dressing, tea biscuits and butter, pumpkin pie and a cup of chocolate.

MENUS WITH CARBOHYDRATE PREDOMINATING.

Breakfast: An orange followed by corn cakes with maple syrup, and bread or toast and butter.
Dinner: Meat pie and baked potato, green peas, bread and butter, and cottage pudding with chocolate sauce.
Lunch or Supper: Rice croquettes with jelly, rye bread and butter, baked apples, and sugar cookies.

THE COMPOSITION OF THE NUTRIENTS AND THE ENERGY SUPPLIED BY THE ABOVE MENUS USED FOR ILLUSTRATION.

	Weight of edible food served, gm.	Protein, gm.	Fat, gm.	Carbo-hydrates, gm.	Fuel value, Calories.
Protein meals:					
Breakfast	471	36	50	54	810
Dinner	772	58	64	120	1288
Lunch or supper	639	33	38	105	894
Total	1882	127	152	279	2992
Fatty meals:					
Breakfast	353	24	69	58	949
Dinner	617	33	88	108	1356
Lunch or supper	621	29	83	98	1259
Total	1591	86	240	264	3564
Carbohydrate meals:					
Breakfast	509	15	32	168	1020
Dinner	529	40	33	133	989
Lunch or supper	376	14	27	127	807
Total	1414	69	92	428	2816

[1]Scientific Monthly, 1916, ii, 294.

Cost of Food.—No discussion of the question of normal nutrition is complete without a consideration of the cost of food. To those persons into whose hands falls the planning of a dietary for the normal family, the problem is not entirely one of furnishing a diet in which correct relative amounts of protein, fat, carbohydrate, mineral constituents as well as accessory substances are provided. Their problem is, in addition, to select such a diet which can be supplied at a cost not exceeding a fair proportion of the income of the family.

The following table shows the proportion of the income to be spent for food, as observed by the Bureau of Labor[1] for 92 industrial centers in the United States.

PROPORTION OF INCOME SPENT FOR FOOD.

Income per year.	Percentage for food per year.	Total for food per year.	Average number in family.	Amount per day per person.
Under $900	44	$371	4.3	$0.24
900–1200	42	456	4.5	.28
1200–1500	39	515	4.7	.30
1500–1800	37	572	5.0	.31
1800–2100	36	626	5.2	.33
2100–2500	35	711	5.7	.34
Over 2500	35	860	6.4	.33

From considerations of the energy value of the food purchased by the families represented in the accompanying data it was found that, in general, for any community a higher energy content was purchased with an increase in income. Comparisons of income groups in different communities showed that a low income group in some cases purchased for a smaller expenditure food value equal to that of a higher income group of another community. The underlying causes of such variations are rather ill-defined but are related, apparently, to the congestion and size of the city and to the geographical location as well as to the food habits. Comparisons of families having the same income but of varying size showed a decreasing food value purchased per member with an increase in the size of the family.

Fortunately there is not a direct relation between the cost of food and its nutritive value. An inexpensive diet, so far as the needs of the body are concerned, may be as satisfactory as an expensive diet. Too often, however, lack of knowledge and training in the selection and preparation adds unduly to the cost of food, especially among the poorer classes who can least afford unwise expenditures.

[1] Monthly Labor Review, 1919, ix.

The physician is particularly interested in prescribing a diet which contains the special nutrients needed by his patient at a cost within the means of the family. Too often diet lists are not flexible, although good results might be obtained by the use of other and less expensive equivalents. The work of Hess in studying the effect of extract of orange peel and potato water as a preventative of scurvy in infants has shown possibilities in this direction.

It would seem, then, incumbent upon the purchaser of the family food supply to familiarize herself with the composition of the common foods and at least roughly with the cost in relation to their total food values. The tables on page 138 show foods typically high and low in cost in proportion to their food values.[1]

It is readily seen from such tables that but few foods were obtainable at a cost of less than one-third of a cent per 100 calories and that few of the foods in the first table are perishable or difficult of transportation. Fresh fruits and vegetables, fresh meat, milk and eggs all cost one cent or more per 100 calories.

Lusk and Murlin have suggested that the labels on food containers should indicate the energy value of the contents and the percentage of protein contained. The nature of the proteins would be indicated by letters—complete proteins, such as animal proteins would be designated as proteins, of "Grade A," while incomplete proteins, such as gelatin, would be "Grade D." Mixtures of complete proteins "A" and incomplete proteins "D" are in what would be marked "Grade B," while foods containing a large proportion of incomplete protein, as corn, would belong to "Grade C." The label might read: "This can contains X calories of which Y per cent. are in protein of "Grade C.""

An illustration of the variation in the cost of a menu while maintaining the calorie content of the diet constant is found in the summary of menus on page 139 prepared by Mrs. Rose for prices in 1916. The reduction is accompanied by a reduction in protein calories.

The factors which influence the cost of various foods are, as we have noted before, in many cases independent of their food values, but depend upon quite external conditions, such as source, perishability, supply and demand, proportion of waste, etc. This is particularly true of our most expensive food-stuffs. An understanding of the relative cost of food necessitates, therefore, a knowledge of the factors which underlie the relation between food value and cost.

[1]Bevier: Planning of Meals, Univ. of Ill. Bull., 1914, xi, No. 30.

FOODS LOW IN COST IN PROPORTION TO THEIR TOTAL FOOD VALUE.[1][2]

Kind of food.	Cost per pound (Jan., 1913).	Calories per pound.	Ounces in 100 Calories.	Cost of 100 Calories.	Grams of protein in 100-Calorie portion.
Cornmeal	$0.025	1655	.96	$0.0015	2.59
Wheat flour	.03	1655	.96	.0018	3.87
Oatmeal	.45	1860	.86	.0024	4.20
Sugar, granulated	.06	1860	.86	.0032	0.00
Beef heart	.05	1320	1.21	.0037	6.40
Beans, navy dried	.062	1605	.99	.0038	6.82
Cross ribs of beef	.08	1765	.906	.0040	5.10
Lard, best leaf	.18	4220	.37	.0040	0.00
Potatoes at $1 bushel	.016	385	4.15	.0041	2.64
Peanuts, shelled	.12	2560	.62	.0046	4.69
White bread	.07	1225	1.30	.0057	3.60
Brisket of beef	.07	1165	1.37	.0060	4.90
Rice	.10	1630	.98	.0061	2.28
Oleomargarine	.22	3525	.45	.0062	0.00
Flank of mutton	.125	1900	.85	.0065	3.75
Bacon	.20	3030	.52	.0066	1.68
Dates	.10	1450	1.10	.0068	0.61
Corned beef	.14	1990	.80	.0070	5.22
Skim milk at $0.10 gal.	.0125	170	9.40	.0073	9.26
Whole milk at $0.10 qt.	.046	314	5.09	.0101	4.76
Salt mackerel	.10	1155	1.38	.0086	5.65
Butter	.36	3605	.44	.0099	4.54
Cheese, cheddar	.22	2145	.74	.0120	6.50
Walnut meats	.45	3300	.48	.0139	2.61
Round steak	.15	895	1.70	.0167	12.62

FOODS HIGH IN COST IN PROPORTION TO THEIR TOTAL FOOD VALUE.[1][2]

Kind of food.	Cost per pound (Jan., 1913).	Calories per pound.	Ounces in 100 Calories.	Cost of 100 Calories.	Grams of protein in 100-Calorie portion.
Mushrooms	$0.65	210	7.6	$0.309	$7.54
Lettuce	.15	75	21.3	.200	5.44
Lobster, fresh	.25	140	11.4	.178	19.07
Black bass	.30	205	7.8	.146	20.56
Chicken, broiler	.30	295	5.4	.101	19.6
Sweetbreads	.80	825	1.93	.095	9.05
Oysters	.20	230	6.9	.087	12.27
Cauliflower	.12	140	11.4	.085	8.16
Rhubarb	.05	65	24.6	.077	2.79
Celery	.05	70	22.8	.070	4.08
White fish	.20	325	4.9	.061	14.72
Oranges	.10	170	9.4	.058	1.6
Tenderloin of beef	.60	1330	1.2	.045	5.51
Porterhouse steak	.30	1110	1.44	.027	7.8
Sirloin steak	.25	985	1.62	.025	7.58
Roquefort cheese	.45	1700	.94	.024	6.02
Leg lamb, medium fat	.18	870	1.80	.020	8.11
Rib roast, medium fat	.20	1155	1.38	.017	5.52

[1] Based on Bulletin 28, "Composition of American Food Materials." Office of Experiment Stations, U. S. Dept. of Agriculture.

[2] The prices given apply to the year 1913, and are for comparative purposes only. Present prices of food are abnormal (1919). According to statistics published by the Bureau of Labor, Monthly Labor Review, Vol. 8, May 1919, the increase in cost of food using 1913 prices as a basis, or 100, is as follows: 1913, 100; 1914, 102; 1915, 101; 1916, 114; 1917, 146; 1918, 168; 1919, 234.

TYPICAL MENUS OF VARYING COST OF A FAMILY OF EIGHT.[1]

Requirements of family (man, woman, baby one year, boy three years, two girls six and nine years, boy twelve years, grandmother ninety years). Protein Calories, 1424-2061. Total Calories, 14,252.

Menu I.	Menu II.	Menu III.	Menu IV.
1¾-2 c. per 100 Cal.	1¼-1½ c. per 100 Cal.	¾-1 c. per 100 Cal.	-¾ c. per 100 Cal.

BREAKFAST.

Oranges.	Oranges (small).	Bananas (prune pulp for two youngest).	Stewed dried apples.
Wheatena with top milk.	Wheatena with top milk.	Wheatena with top milk.	Cornmeal mush with milk and sugar.
Puffy omelet with bacon.	. . . .	. . . .	Bread, pork fat; sausage for father and mother.
Toast, coffee, milk.	Toast, coffee, milk.	Toast, coffee, milk, cereal coffee.	Cereal coffee for older children and adults. Milk.

MID-DAY MEAL.

Creamed chicken on toast.	Creamed dried beef on toast.	Macaroni and cheese.	Baked samp, with cheese.
Baked bananas.	Baked bananas.	Stewed apricots.	Stewed raisins.
Boston brown bread.	Boston brown bread.	Boston brown bread.	Oleomargarine.
Rice pudding.	Rice pudding.	Oatmeal cookies.	Brown bread.
Tea, milk.	Tea, milk.	Tea, milk.	Oatmeal wafers.
			Tea for adults, cocoa for children.

EVENING MEAL.

Consomme.			
Baked halibut, egg sauce.	Baked halibut, white sauce.	Creamed salt cod.	Beef stew with vegetables.
Potatoes on half shell.	Potatoes on half shell.	Baked potatoes.	
String beans, buttered.	String beans, buttered.	Boiled onions.	
Bread and butter.	Bread and butter.	Bread and butter.	Bread and oleomargarine.
Tomato salad, French dressing.	Cold slaw.		
Apple snow with boiled custard.	Chocolate blanc mange cream and sugar.	Rice pudding, cream and sugar.	Date pudding with liquid sauce.
Lady fingers.	Plain cookies.		
Protein Calories, 2202.	Protein Calories, 2106.	Protein Calories, 1791.	Protein Calories, 1526.
Total Calories, 14,410.	Total Calories, 14,414.	Total Calories, 14,330.	Total Calories, 14,299.

Our food is derived from two sources, animal and vegetable. Animal foods are particularly valuable as a source of protein and fat; they contain little carbohydrate. Vegetable foods are our chief source of carbohydrate, and they are to a less extent a source of protein. Both animal and vegetable food supply inorganic salts and accessory substances; green vegetables are valuable largely because of these materials.

Food derived from animals fed with cultivated fodder is much more expensive than the vegetable foods used in its production. This is true because animal food is developed largely at the expense of vegetable food; a process the efficiency of which is comparatively low. Furthermore, animals must often be kept for a period of years for their proper development, during which time they must be carefully tended; and they are also subject to disease with the possibility of loss by death. Flesh foods obtained from wild animals, such as fish and game, might be relatively cheaper because the only factors of cost involved are those of catch-

[1] Rose: Feeding the Family, New York, 1916.

ing or killing the animals, preserving and sending them to the market. Although game may be procured cheaply, it is expensive to the average individual because of its scarcity. Similarly, fish is expensive in certain parts of the country because of the cost of transportation and storage.

The perishability of fresh animal food also tends to make it expensive. With the exception of the isolated fat products, meat decomposes rapidly at ordinary temperatures. It must be preserved therefore by processes which are comparatively expensive, such as refrigeration. Furthermore, care must be exercised in handling it to prevent contamination. In addition there is a certain loss by deterioration when such food passes through the hands of the retailer, and this loss must be made good in the price charged for the remainder.

Various methods of preservation of animal food in common use operate to lower its cost to the consumer. Cold storage or refrigeration is a comparatively expensive process of preservation and tends to increase the cost of flesh foods; in spite of this it is a means of actually reducing the cost of such foods because it permits the slaughter of animals in large quantities and their transportation to the consumer with a relatively low loss by deterioration. Refrigeration permits the storage of other perishable animal food, such as eggs, in seasons in which they are plentiful. The net result of such preservation is a gain to the consumer, for while it tends to increase the cost when the foods are in season, it brings the cost of the same food out of season below what it would be were there no refrigeration.

Other methods of preservation, such as drying (beef and fish), smoking, pickling, and canning, which do not require extensive refrigeration and which are performed where the supply is plentiful, also tend to lower the cost of animal foods. Processes which involve special manipulation of the food, such as the preparation of cheese and the extraction of fat, are also means of lowering the cost of animal foods.

Plant foods are cheaper sources of food material than animal foods. They are used directly and the only loss to the body is that which results from a failure to absorb or to utilize them completely. Their cultivation is comparatively simple, and they mature in one season. Artificial preservation is not so essential and, when practised, is comparatively cheaper than the preservation of more perishable foods in their natural state. Plant foods, such as carrots, potatoes and apples when ripe can be stored for some months with little deterioration; with a slightly increased expense for cold storage they may be kept for even longer periods. Foods which would decay at ordinary temperatures, such as oranges, can be preserved in cold storage. Many plant foods are preserved in the dry state. Some become relatively dry before they are gathered, such as the legumes—beans and peas—and the grains—corn, oats, and wheat; while other foods used extensively in the fresh state—prunes, apples, apricots—are dried under special, artificial conditions. Milling of cereals and grains helps to extend the period of preservation without deterioration; this is particularly true of fat-rich grains, such as corn. Some plant foods, such as corn, peas, and tomatoes may also be preserved in the fresh, water-rich state by canning. This is done at times when they are plentiful and in districts in which they are produced, thus furnishing a supply of these foods at reasonable prices during seasons in which they would otherwise be unobtainable.

RELATIVE ECONOMY OF FOODS.
(Dietetic Bureau, Boston, Mass.).

1. Very Economical.	*2. Economical.*	*3. Expensive.*
	CEREALS.	
Oatmeal up to 16 cts. per lb.	At any reasonable price.	Corn Flakes at any price.
Barley up to 10 cts. per lb.	At any reasonable price.	Puffed Wheat at any price.
Cornmeal up to 9 cts. per lb.	At any reasonable price.	Puffed Rice at any price.
Hominy up to 8 cts. per lb.	At any reasonable price.	Post Toasties at any price.
Rice	Up to 15 cts. per lb.	Krumbles at any price.
	Pettijohn at any reasonable price.	
	Shredded Wheat up to 15 cts. per box.	
	Cream Wheat } up to 25 cts.	
	Farina } for 1¼ lb. box.	
	FRUIT.	
Prunes up to 16 cts. per lb.	Up to 23 cts. per lb.	Fruit in column *2 above* the prices named
Raisins up to 16 cts. per lb.	Up to 23 cts. per lb.	Plums over 1 cent each.
Dates up to 17 cts. per lb.	Up to 25 cts. per lb.	Peaches over 1 cent each.
Dried apples } up to		Pears over 1 cent each.
Dried peaches } 14 cts.	Up to 20 cts. per lb.	
Dried apricots } per lb.		
Fresh apples up to 2 cts. per lb.	Up to 3 cts. per lb.	
	Bananas up to 30 cts. per doz.	
	Grapes up to 8 cts. per lb.	
	An occasional orange (once a week for the baby) at 50 cts. per dozen.	
	VEGETABLES.	
Dried beans } at any ordinary		Any of the foods *above* the price named in column 2
Dried peas } price, even 25		
} cts. per lb.		
Spinach up to 10 cts. per lb.	Up to 16 cts. per lb.	Canned peas above 15 cts. per can.
Potatoes up to 5 cts. per lb.	Up to 8 cts. per lb.	Canned corn above 17 cts. per can.
Cabbage up to 5 cts. per lb.	Up to 7 cts. per lb.	Any other canned vegetable purchased at the store.
Onions up to 4 cts. per lb.	Up to 6 cts. per lb.	
Cauliflower at 8 cts. per lb. (provided outside leaves are used in some way).	Up to 13 cts. per lb.	
Beets up to 4 cts. per lb.	Up to 6 cts. per lb.	Celery above 11 cts. per bunch (3 roots).
Carrots up to 4½ cts. per lb.	Up to 7 cts. per lb.	Asparagus above 10 cts. per lb.
Turnips up to 4 cts.	Up to 6 cts. per lb.	Lettuce above 5 cts. a head .
	String beans up to 10 cts. per lb.	
	Fresh peas and beans up to 10 cts. per lb.	
	Squash up to 3 cts. per lb.	
	Tomatoes at 5 cts. per lb.	

The table on page 141 gives the relative economy of vegetable foods. It is of value in determining the wisest expenditure of money for these articles.

Many foods which appear cheap, *i. e.*, are sold at a low cost per pound, are in reality expensive on account of the large amount of waste in skin, bone, seeds, etc.; for example, a chicken weighing 4.65 lbs., costing 40 cents per lb. alive, weighed 4.09 lbs. dressed, and yielded but 1.11 lbs. cooked meat, which brought the cost up to $1.69 per pound. Small prunes prove more expensive than larger ones costing 5 to 8 cents per lb. more, owing to the greater waste in skin and seeds of the smaller prunes.

The cost of food is also influenced by supply and demand. In the case of meat, the demand for special cuts of which there are but a few in each carcass, such as tenderloin steaks and sweetbreads, results in prices which are out of proportion to the food value of these cuts. These unnatural prices react favorably upon the less desirable cuts, for they are

COST OF MEAT REQUIRED TO FURNISH ONE POUND OF PROTEIN AND 1000 CALORIES FROM WHOLESALE CUTS AT MARKET PRICES.[1,2]

Wholesale cuts.	Retail price per pound, cents.	Boneless meat in the cut, per cent.	Cost of pound boneless meat in cut, cents.	Cost of pound protein in cut, cents.	Cost of 1000 Calories in cut, cents.
Fore shank	5	59.56	8.4	50	7
Hind shank . . .	5	48.84	10.2	63	9
Neck	6	84.31	7.1	46	5
Flank	8	99.44	8.0	85	3
Plate	8	91.23	8.7	82	4
Clod	10	95.18	10.5	63	10
Chuck	11	87.99	12.5	84	9
Rump	12	79.85	15.0	119	8
Round	15	90.39	16.6	101	15
Rib	18	85.56	21.0	171	11
Loin	22	90.23	24.4	188	14

RELATIVE FUEL VALUES OF THE BONELESS MEAT OF THE WHOLESALE CUTS.[1,2]

	Calories furnished by 100 grams of boneless meat.			Percentage distribution of Calories.		Pounds of boneless meat required to furnish 1000 Calories.
	Fat x 9.	Protein x 4.	Total.	In fat.	In protein.	
Flank . .	514.4	40.5	554.9	92.7	7.3	0.40
Plate . .	437.1	46.0	483.1	90.5	9.5	0.46
Rib . .	365.6	54.1	419.7	87.1	12.9	0.52
Rump . .	350.5	55.3	405.8	86.4	13.6	0.54
Loin . .	339.4	57.4	396.8	85.5	14.5	0.56
Chuck . .	247.9	65.8	313.7	79.0	21.0	0.70
Neck . .	235.1	67.9	303.0	77.6	22.4	0.73
Hind shank .	186.9	71.0	257.9	72.5	27.5	0.86
Fore shank .	179.8	73.9	253.7	70.9	29.1	0.87
Round . .	176.9	73.6	250.5	70.6	29.4	0.88
Clod . .	161.6	73.5	235.1	68.7	31.3	0.94

[1] Hall and Emmett: Univ. of Ill. Agri. Exp. Sta., 1912, Bull. 158.
[2] See foot-note, page 138.

sold at somewhat lower rates. Other animal foods, such as game and shad-roe, are plentiful only at certain seasons of the year. Vegetables which are difficult or expensive to cultivate, such as mushrooms, or are rare or transported long distances when out of season in a particular locality, bring high prices.

The relation between supply and demand, and the lack of correspondence between food value and cost, is well illustrated by meat. Studies of the food value of the various cuts bring out the fact that the cost of protein—and meat is most valuable because of its protein content—increases

COST OF LEAN AND OF TOTAL MEAT IN THE VARIOUS RETAIL CUTS AT MARKET PRICES.[1,2]

Retail cuts.	Diagram number, p. 176.	Retail price per pound of cut, cents.	Cost per pound of lean meat in cut, cents.	Cost per pound of lean and fat meat in cut, cents.
Steaks:				
Porterhouse, hip-bone	8	25	38.6	28.9
Porterhouse, regular	10	.25	40.2	27.2
Club steak	18	20	32.1	22.6
Sirloin, butt-end	1	20	25.3	20.6
Sirloin, round-bone	3	20	28.3	21.1
Sirloin, double-bone	5	20	28.7	22.7
Sirloin, hip-bone	7	20	32.3	24.2
Flank steak	1	16	19.3	16.0
Round, first cut	2	15	17.0	15.3
Round, middle cut	6	15	17.3	15.6
Round, last cut	14	15	19.3	16.0
Chuck, first cut	2	12	18.3	14.1
Chuck, last cut	9	12	15.7	13.1
Roasts:				
Prime ribs, first cut	1	20	40.5	22.9
Prime ribs, last cut	4	16	26.1	18.8
Chuck, 5th rib	1	15	22.8	17.3
Rump	1	12	19.4	12.8
Boiling and stewing pieces:				
Round pot roast	16	10	11.6	10.1
Shoulder clod	14	10	12.3	10.5
Shoulder pot roast	11	10	14.3	11.6
Rib ends	3	8	16.2	9.2
Brisket	1	8	15.0	8.7
Navel	2	7	12.8	7.7
Flank stew	2	7	10.9	7.1
Fore shank stew	1	7	8.5	7.0
Neck	15	6	8.5	7.0
Soup bones:				
Round, knuckle	2	5	26.3	12.5
Hind shank, middle cut	18	5	7.5	6.3
Hind shank, hock	19	5	62.5	26.6
Fore shank, knuckle	2	5	17.2	12.5
Fore shank, middle cut	4	5	12.5	9.4
Fore shank, end	6	5	28.8	20.9

[1]Hall and Emmett: Univ. of Ill. Agr. Exp. Sta., 1912, Bull. 158.
[2]See foot-note, page 138.

roughly 175 per cent. from the tougher cuts to the most expensive cuts of beef. As the result of the high price of meat during the war and the consequent demand for the "cheaper cuts" of meat the cost of such cuts has increased more in proportion than the more desirable cuts.

The *relative* costs of the protein for 1000 Calories in the various cuts of beef are indicated in the tables on pp. 142-143 which may be used in conjunction with the table and charts on pages 174-176.

The cost of lean beef is a rough index of the relative economy of steaks and roasts; in comparing boiling and stewing meats, however, the cost of both fat and lean, gross meat, should have more weight because in the utilization of these cuts the fat is usually incorporated with the lean in the form of meat loaf, hash, hashed meats (Hamburger steak), and corned beef. Since soup bones are of particular value for their flavoring material, their food value is not entirely comparable with the other portions of the carcass, as can be seen from the table. From the table we can see that the cheap cuts of meat actually furnish protein at a much lower price than the expensive cuts. It is to be remembered that in purchasing cheaper cuts of meat one often receives a larger proportion of connective tissue with its incomplete protein, gelatin, than in the case of the more expensive cuts; this lowered food value is, however, more than compensated by the decreased cost of the complete protein.

Fish may be used to vary the diet or as a source of relatively cheaper protein food; they are practically interchangeable with meat and are in general less expensive.

In considering animal and vegetable food from an economic point of view, it is necessary to know whether the food-stuffs of the same kind which they contain are of equal value to the body; otherwise the apparently cheaper food may be in the end actually more expensive. Such considerations are particularly important with regard to protein. Comparative studies of the digestibility of foods have shown that as ordinarily prepared the protein of animal food is more completely absorbed than the protein of vegetables—meat protein, 91 to 97 per cent.; vegetable proteins, 80 to 85 per cent.; bread protein, 70 per cent.; rye protein, 40 to 76 per cent.; barley protein, corn protein, 61 to 83 per cent. The lower degree of absorption of vegetable proteins is due chiefly to the cellulose layer which surrounds the protein and prevents its digestion. A larger amount of total food in general must be ingested to obtain the same amount of protein from vegetable than from animal protein. In finely ground cereals and legumes, however, the protein has been found to be as thoroughly digested as animal protein. Certain vegetable proteins are low in their content of the amino-acids necessary for growth and maintenance; but associated with these are other proteins which contain the necessary amino-acids. Consequently the natural mixture of proteins is more or less complete and unless particular isolated or concentrated deficient proteins are involved, vegetable proteins may be used as the sole source of protein. That animal proteins are more efficient in satisfying the body needs than vegetable proteins has been found in studies of the comparative utilization of animal and vegetable proteins. A comparison of proteins of different origin on the basis of their availability (biological value) to the body has shown that the different quantities of protein indicated when added to a carbohydrate diet will protect the body from protein loss after it has been reduced to a minimum on a purely carbohydrate diet:

	Grams
Meat protein	30
Milk protein	31
Rice protein	34
Potato protein	38
Bean protein	54
Bread protein	76
Indian corn protein	102

It is evident, therefore, that naturally occurring protein mixtures of vegetable origin are not as efficient as animal protein and that larger quantities must be ingested not only because of their lower digestibility but also of their lower biological value.

The economic question with regard to the use of proteins of animal and vegetable origin therefore resolves itself into which is cheaper, the ingestion of a large amount of vegetable protein or a smaller amount of animal protein. The answer must be tempered by a consideration of the increased activity of the body required to metabolize and to excrete the excessive unavailable amino-acids of vegetable origin and of the possible effect of such increased activity upon the general well-being of the body. It is impossible at present to answer the question. When our knowledge of the amino-acid content of proteins is sufficiently developed we may be able to furnish the deficient amino-acids of an economical diet with comparatively small quantities of a more expensive protein. Even now we recognize the advisability of using a certain proportion of protein of animal origin with vegetable protein, for safety; there are very

10

few diets which do not contain such protein, at least in the form of milk, eggs, or cheese. The inclusion of protein of animal origin in the diet is commendable from another point of view, for with the animal protein is purchased a certain amount of fat, a food of high caloric value. This addition of fat is desirable because it reduces the quantity of bulky carbohydrate food which must be ingested to meet the energy requirement of the body and also because it meets the need of a certain proportion of fat which would otherwise have to be purchased separately and added to the diet.

A diet consisting largely of vegetables has been objected to on the ground that it is bulky; that a large quantity of food must be eaten in order to obtain sufficient protein, or else one must live on a low protein diet, for, with the exception of legumes and nuts, vegetable foods are relatively poor in protein. Since hunger is satisfied not so much by the quality of the food as by the quantity which is ingested, the appetite is in danger of being satisfied before sufficient material has been consumed to supply the protein requirement. For this reason and because vegetable proteins are less completely absorbed and less efficient in the body economy than animal protein a strictly vegetable diet is likely to be a low protein diet.

It has been maintained by people who restrict their diet largely to vegetables, that they are able to utilize their food more efficiently and that the body activities take place at a lower level than those who eat meat. Benedict has shown, however, that the basal metabolism of vegetarians is not essentially different from that of those living upon a mixed diet. It is possible that a vegetarian may be able to live on a low protein diet more readily than a man upon a high protein meat diet, because of the retarding effect of the indigestible cellulose upon the rate of digestion and of the absorption of products of digestion of vegetable proteins. Experiments have shown that the admixture of indigestible material results in a more uniform rate of excretion of nitrogen in the urine than in the absence of such material; the inference is that the absorption from the intestine is likewise slower. On a vegetarian diet, then, instead of the rapid absorption of protein products of digestion and the disintegration of the excess characteristic of a high protein meat diet, the material is absorbed more slowly and the amino-acids are consequently more completely utilized for actual processes of repair and of growth. Proof of this fact has been presented in which a man was able to maintain nitrogen equilibrium on a lower plane of protein ingestion when food was taken in small amounts a number of times a day than when food was taken less often.

In determining the value of a diet from an economic point of view consideration must be given to the quantity, proportion and kind of inorganic salts which it contains. While the average mixed diet contains a sufficient quantity of calcium, phosphorus and iron for the needs of the normal adult, the diet of children and nursing and pregnant women requires special attention in order that the mineral constituents be present in suitable proportions. A diet to be satisfactory with regard to its content of inorganic constituents must have the salts present in quantities which will meet the needs of the body and in such a form that the ash does not predominate potentially in acidic constituents —the same applies to foods which are potentially basic but to a much less degree, for an excess of base is not as harmful as an excess of acid.

From a consideration of the kinds and quantities of inorganic elements in foods it is evident that the vegetable foods and eggs are, in general, rich in calcium, iron and phosphorus and yield an alkaline ash (oatmeal yields an acid ash), while the ash of the egg is acid; meat is rich in iron and phosphorus and poor in calcium and has an acid ash; milk and cheese are rich in calcium and phosphorus, poor in iron; milk yields an alkaline and cheese a slightly acid ash. Certain foods, particularly the prepared and purified products of both plant and animal origin, such as the fats and sugars, are very poor in salts.

A diet in which vegetables and milk or cheese are the chief source of protein will therefore be predominately basic and contain, from a quantitative point of view, the most important inorganic constituents. In such a diet the low iron content of milk or its protein products is compensated by the relatively high iron content of vegetables. A diet in which meat or eggs predominate will, on the other hand, tend to lower the alkaline reserve on the body, because of the acid ash, and meat will at the same time be deficient in calcium, while eggs will furnish this element in comparatively large amounts. Milk and cheese are therefore much more desirable not only as an economical source of animal protein but also for the salts contained in them. They can be included to advantage in a diet even when their cost is comparatively high. Eggs are next in order when the ash constituents are considered, and meat is the most expensive.

PART II.

FOODS

CHAPTER VII.

INTRODUCTION—MILK.

THE preceding chapters have dealt with the digestion, absorption and utilization of food; and the factors which determine the quantity and nature of food required for the needs of the human body. The discussion was confined almost entirely to the materials which are the *basic* ingredients of food—protein, carbohydrate, fat, salts, water, and vitamines. Oxygen is also a food; its presence is so general, however, that it is ordinarily omitted from a quantitative discussion of diet. Any food in the general sense is composed of one or more of these ingredients. One food may contain a preponderance of protein, another of fat, etc. For the discussion of the various foods, a basis of classification is necessary. A classification may be based upon the origin or composition of foods, or on the need which they supply. In the following chapters we classify foods according to their composition in terms of food-stuffs. For complex foods the particular food-stuff for which they are most valuable to the body determines the placement of them in the classification. Thus, we shall consider protein foods; fat foods; carbohydrate foods; and foods valuable for their salts, water, or vitamines, such as fruits, condiments, and beverages. A classification of this kind not only emphasizes the principal use of the food, but also aids in the search for foods that supply the elemental food factors; and it differs from the usual method of considering only the origin of foods in that there is no distinction recognized between vegetable and animal food. The dried legumes are placed with the protein-rich foods and certain animal products are placed with the fats. There is one food, however, which is difficult to classify under these circumstances but which is of sufficient importance to be considered alone, viz., milk, for it is the most complete food available.

A more recent subdivision of foods has been suggested by McCollum. Certain foods are of such a constitution that they contain some of all of the necessary food factors, and particularly those most likely to be deficient in other foods, *i. e.*, adequate protein, inorganic salts, and the vitamines. Milk and the leaves of green vegetables are of this class. Such foods have been designated *protective foods*. The grains, seeds (bean and pea), meat, roots and tubers are deficient in one or more of the food factors, although they contain considerable amounts of protein, fat or carbohydrate. The grains, seeds, roots and tubers are deficient in the character of the protein, inorganic salts and fat-soluble A. Meat is deficient in calcium and fat-soluble A.

MILK

Milk is one of the most important foods in the human diet. It contains adequate protein, calcium, phosphorus, and the fat-soluble vitamine in considerable amounts. The water soluble vitamine and the anti-scorbutic vitamine are present to a fair degree. Milk is very poor in iron. As a supplement to the dietary deficiencies of the seeds and grains milk is invaluable. Lusk has stated that a family of five should not buy meat until it has bought three quarts of milk.

Milk[1] is a complex food—a product of the activities of the mammary gland—prepared for the nourishment of the growing young. It is a whitish liquid with a characteristic odor and sweetish taste. The white color is due to the emulsified state of the fat and to the opalescence of the caseinogen solution. A slight yellowish tinge is imparted to milk, particularly when rich in fat, by certain coloring matters. This pigment apparently comes from the coloring constituents of plants (see p. 232) and consequently varies in amount with the diet. A lactochrome, which is similar to urochrome in urine, occurs in the whey of milk.

The specific gravity of milk varies between 1.027 and 1.035. Two counteracting factors influence the specific gravity of milk—the fats, which tend to lower it, and the other solid constituents, protein, carbohydrates and salts, all heavier than water, tend to increase it. The specific gravity is not necessarily a criterion of purity, for a skimmed, diluted milk may have the same specific gravity as fresh milk. Milk is an amphoteric liquid and is approximately neutral

[1] We shall confine our present discussion largely to the milk of the cow. Unless otherwise designated the term milk refers to cow's milk.

in reaction, hydrogen-ion concentration 2.6 x 10⁻⁷ gram molecules. Human milk is slightly more alkaline 0.6–1.1 x 10⁻⁷.
The freezing-point of milk is –0.55° C.

A microscopic examination of milk reveals the presence of
fine droplets of emulsified fat, leukocytes, and bacteria,
particularly streptococci. Milk that has not been carefully
handled will contain dirt, and in some cases pathogenic
bacteria. Bacteria may come from the udder itself or from
the air. Leukocytes are normal constituents of milk that
increase in number when the udder is diseased. With proper
precautions milk which will contain very few bacteria (200
to 500 per cubic centimeter) may be obtained from a healthy
cow. The number of bacteria per cubic centimeter has been
taken as a standard of purity. The following values are
those recommended by the Commission on Milk Standards
as the maximum for each grade.

NUMBER OF BACTERIA PERMITTED IN THE VARIOUS GRADES OF MILK.

Grade.	Bacteria count shall not exceed per cubic centimeters.	
	Before pasteurization.	After pasteurization at time of delivery.
A	200,000	10,000
B	1,000,000	50,000
C	+1,000,000	–50,000

Non-pathogenic bacteria have very little effect upon adults
but appear to be detrimental to infants. It is essential,
then, that infants receive a milk containing very few bacteria. For the adult a milk of low bacterial count is desirable because of the greater probability of the absence of
pathogenic organisms.

Chemical Properties.—Milk contains all of the food-
stuffs necessary for the growing organism: protein, fats,
carbohydrates, vitamines, and salts are present in amounts
best adapted to the young for which it is prepared. It is a
most satisfactory dietary constituent in the regimen of the
adult. Water is quantitatively the most important constituent of milk. It exists to the extent of from 80 to 90
per cent., the average being about 87 per cent.

Milk may readily be separated into products which are
particularly rich in one or more of its constituents. By
gravity, or more rapidly by centrifugalization, the greater
proportion of the fat may be removed as cream. Conglomeration of the fat droplets gives butter; coagulation
with rennin or precipitation with acid separates casein or

caseinogen respectively from the other proteins, salts and lactose.

The following tables give the percentage composition of milk and various milk products arranged in the order of their increasing fat content.

MILK AND ITS PRODUCTS ARRANGED ACCORDING TO THEIR INCREASING FAT CONTENT.

	Fat, per cent.	Protein, per cent.	Carbohydrate, per cent.
Centrifuged milk	0.2 }	3.8	4.4
Skim milk	0.6 }		
Buttermilk	0.6	3.8	4.4
Whole milk } . . .	3.5	3.7	4.4
Rennin coagulated milk }			
Evaporated (unsweetened) . .	8.3	7.5	9.7
Condensed (sweetened) plus cane			
sugar, 41 per cent.	9.0	8.5	13.3
Curds	10.0	11.0	3.0
Cream, usual	15.0	3.0	4.0
Cream, fat	20.0	3.0	4.0
Dried (whole)	28.5	24.3	36.8
Cream, very fat	30.0	3.0	4.0
Butter	85.0	0.5	..

MILK AND ITS PRODUCTS ARRANGED ACCORDING TO THE PROTEIN CONTENT.

	Protein, per cent.	Fat, per cent.	Carbohydrate, per cent.
Whey	0.8	0.1	5.0
Whole milk } . . .	3.7	3.5	4.4
Rennin coagulated milk }			
Evaporated (unsweetened) . .	7.5	8.3	9.7
Condensed (sweetened) plus cane			
sugar, 41.0 per cent. . . .	8.5	9.0	13.3 (54.3)
Curds (cottage cheese)	10.0	11.0	3.0
Cheese, fat	27.0	30.0	..
Cheese, medium fat	35.0	10.0	..
Cheese, skim milk	35.0	4.0	..
Dried (whole)	24.3	28.5	36.8

Protein.—The proteins of milk constitute about 3 per cent. of the total weight or 25 per cent. of the solid constituents. Of the three predominating proteins in milk, lactalbumin, lactoglobulin and caseinogen, the latter presents the most characteristic properties. Caseinogen[1] belongs to the class of conjugated proteins called phosphoproteins. It is an acid protein, insoluble in dilute acids and dissolved by alkalis. Neutral solutions of caseinogen are not coagulated by boiling but a pellicle is formed, such as is observed upon boiled milk. The flocculent precipitation observed in sour milk consists of caseinogen which

[1] There is a certain confusion in the use of the terms caseinogen, the protein existing in fresh milk, and càsein, the product of the action of rennin upon caseinogen. (Halliburton: Jour Physiol., 1900, ii, 448). Certain authors, particularly the German writers, designate the protein of fresh milk as casein and the clot as paracasein.

has become insoluble in the acid (lactic) produced by the action of bacteria upon the lactose. The changes in the protein molecule are simple and appear to involve only processes such as occur in the precipitation of inorganic substances. Precipitated casein may be dissolved by the addition of an alkali; water-soluble casein preparations are of this nature.

The phenomena of the coagulation of milk by rennin also concerns caseinogen. The transformations are more profound than those mentioned above for sour milk. In this case the caseinogen is split into two molecules of casein or perhaps into a soluble whey, albumose and casein. The calcium salts of casein are insoluble; in the presence of soluble calcium salts calcium caseinate is formed and the characteristic clot is produced. The coagulum formed holds by absorption or entanglement certain quantities of fat and lactose. A comparative study of cow's milk and human milk shows that the quantity of caseinogen is greater in cow's milk than in human milk.

Lactalbumin and lactoglobulin have not been shown to differ materially from the albumins and globulins of blood serum. The albumin forms about 0.6 per cent. of the whole milk or 15 per cent. of the proteins, while the globulin exists only in traces. Minute traces of fibrin and a protein called opalisin have been detected.

Fats.—The fat in milk is a mixture of several different fats, the more important of which are the triglycerides of palmitic, stearic, and oleic acids, and to a less extent of myristic, butyric, caproic, caprylic and capric acids. Fat is the most variable constituent of milk, the proportion may vary from 25 to 2 per cent.; the average is between 3 and 4 per cent. Further discussion of the fats of milk will be found under butter, p. 232. Milk is also rich in fats with low melting-points; factors which tend toward increased digestibility. Milk fat exists normally in the form of a fine emulsion. The degree of emulsion of fat in milk differs with the various breeds. The greater availability of the fat from the milk of the Holstein cow over that of the Jersey cow is ascribed to the finer state of division of the fat of the former. The value of condensed milk in the feeding of some infants has been ascribed to the fact that such milks are "homogenized" and consequently the fat is very finely divided.

Carbohydrates.—Lactose, or milk-sugar, the principal carbohydrate constituent of milk, is a specific product of the mammary gland. Chemically it is a disaccharide. Hydrolysis, as in digestion, yields a molecule each of galactose and glucose. Compared with cane-sugar from which it differs only in the arrangement of its atoms, lactose is not as sweet or as soluble. These properties account in part for the use of lactose as a vehicle for drugs and, the lack of sweetness particularly, for its use in diets which must have a high caloric value and still be completely assimilable. Lactose is dextrorotatory, has a strong reducing power and is not fermented ordinarily by yeast. Alcohol and lactic acid are formed from it by the action of certain bacteria, chiefly *Bacillus lactis acidi* and yeast. In these processes lactose is first hydrolyzed into its monosaccharide components and then transformed into alcohol or lactic acid, according to the organism concerned. The production of lactic acid commonly occurs in the souring of milk. Alcoholic fermentation is induced in the preparation of "koumyss" and "kefir." The quantity of lactose in cow's milk varies from 4 to 6 per cent. of the whole milk, the average being about 5 per cent., or 38 per cent. of the total solids.

Salts.—The salts, inorganic and organic, consist of combinations of calcium, magnesium, sodium, potassium, and iron with the acid radicles of hydrochloric, sulphuric, phosphoric and citric acids. In addition there are probably combinations of these substances with the proteins. The proportion and importance of the salts in milk will be considered later (p. 156).

Besides their direct food value, particularly for bone formation, the combinations of calcium and the phosphoric acid radicle, calcium phosphates are associated with the caseinogen in its natural state and are concerned in the coagulation of milk by rennin.

The modification of cow's milk for infants by dilution with water, lime water, etc., reduces the proportion of salts in the modified milk. Forbes suggests the use of whey for the dilution of milk which permits the reduction of the quantity of caseinogen without reducing the proportion of the other constituents, particularly the salts.

The iron content of milk varies with the species. Cow's milk contains a half to a fifth as much as human milk; human milk, 1.6 to 1.7 milligram of Fe_2O_3 per liter; cow's milk 0.3 to 0.7 milligram of Fe_2O_3 per liter. This marked difference indicates that children fed on cow's milk get much less iron than when fed on human milk; a difference which is increased when cow's milk is diluted with water.

Citric acid is present in cow's milk to the extent of approximately 0.1 per cent., roughly three times as much as in human milk.

Studies of the rate of growth of rats have demonstrated that there are in milk certain materials which belong to the group of accessory substances or vitamines. Milk contains fat-soluble A and water-soluble B and the anti-scorbutic vitamine. It apparently contains a smaller proportion of the last two vitamines than is found in some vegetables and fruits.

The constituents of the milk of any species are qualitatively the same. Slight quantitative differences exist due to individuality, the course of lactation, the change of seasons, and the time of milking, night or morning, the first milk drawn, or the last, etc. Variations in the diet have little effect upon the composition of milk. However, the composition of milk fat may be affected by feeding foreign fat; the fat tends to acquire the characteristics of the ingested fat. Milk of different species differs chiefly in amount rather than in kind of the constituents present.

The composite milk of a herd of cows, or from a city dairy is quite uniform in composition, although showing slight seasonal variations. Protein and fat are higher in the autumn and winter than in the spring and summer. Lactose remains fairly constant throughout the year. Generally the predominating breed of cow influences the percentage of fat. Individual variations within a given herd, however, have been shown to be as great as the variations between breeds of cows. The following table gives the composition of cow's milk.[1]

COMPOSITION OF MILK.

	Water = 87.1			
		Fat = 3.9	Nitrogen compounds = 3.2	Casein = 2.5
	Solids = 12.9			Albumin = 0.7
Milk = 100	100.0			3.2
		Solids not fat = 9.0		
		12.9	Milk-sugar = 5.1	
			Ash (salts) = 0.7	
	Gases { Carbon dioxide Nitrogen Oxygen		9.0	

Substances foreign to milk appear in it when fed to a lactating animal. Thus strong flavors occur in milk as the result of certain diets; the peculiar taste of milk when the cows begin to graze in the spring is due to certain foreign constituents derived from the green food which have been transferred to the milk. Drugs and narcotics have been shown to appear in milk following their ingestion.

Variations in Composition.—Milk of different kinds of animals shows very striking variations in the proportions of

[1] United States Public Health and Marine Hospital Service, 1900, Bull. 56.

their constituents. The accompanying table shows the composition of human and cow's milk.

	Water.	Protein. Caseinogen.	Albumin.	Fat.	Lactose.	Salts.
Human milk .	88.5	1.2	0.5	3.3	6.0	0.2
Cow's milk .	87.1	3.0	0.53	3.7	4.8	0.7

A consideration of this table, with its many differences and the favorable growth of all young, emphasizes the fact that there is an elaboration of milk best adapted to the young of the particular species. Milk of one species when fed to the young of another may, as we know is the case in infant feeding with cow's milk, prove deficient in one constituent and excessive in another and thus be entirely unsatisfactory.

The adaptation of milk to the young of a species has been shown to be pertinent in the case of the inorganic constituents as well as in the organic constituents. The similarity of the composition of the ash of the young and the ash of the milk has been shown by Bunge and others. The following table gives the ash constituents of the young and milk of the rabbit, dog, and man, and the milk of the cow.

COMPARISON OF THE COMPOSITION OF THE ASH OF MILK WITH THAT OF THE NEWBORN YOUNG FOR WHICH IT IS INTENDED.

	Human milk.	Infant.	Cow's milk.	Rabbit's milk.	Rabbit 14 days old.	Bitch's milk.	Puppy few hrs. old.
Potassium (K_2O) .	35.2	6.2	22.1	10.1	10.8	15.0	11.1
Sodium (Na_2O) .	10.4	8.1	13.9	7.9	6.0	8.8	10.6
Calcium (CaO) .	14.8	40.5	20.0	35.7	35.0	27.2	29.5
Magnesium (MgO) .	2.9	1.5	2.6	2.2	2.2	1.5	1.8
Iron (Fe_2O_3) .	0.18	0.39	0.04	0.08	0.23	0.12	0.72
Phosphorus (P_2O_5) .	21.3	35.3	24.8	39.9	41.9	34.2	39.4
Chlorine (Cl) . .	10.8	4.3	21.3	5.4	4.9	16.9	8.4

It will be seen that the species which rapidly increases in weight, a milk is secreted with ash constituents that are quite similar to those of the young, while for the more slowly growing organisms, as man, there is a discrepancy between the two.

Condensed Milks.[1]—Milk is condensed (*a*) thorough evaporation in a vacuum, condensed (sweetened) milk and evaporated milk and (*b*) by drying. The products of the first class retain a considerable quantity of their moisture and depend upon canning and sterilization for their preservation while the milks of the second class are sufficiently dry to keep for long periods of time without further sterilization. A

[1] For a discussion of condensed milk and its relation to infant feeding see bulletin on "Milk," by Mendenhall, U. S. Dept. Labor, Children's Bureau.

further advantage of the dried milks is that when the container is once opened it is not imperative to make immediate use of the product to prevent spoilage. The relative value of any of the condensed milk products depends upon the manner in which the original milk is handled, and this is particularly so of the dried milks.

Evaporated (unsweetened condensed milk) milk has had from one half to three fifths of its water removed by evaporation. It must contain 25.5 per cent solids and 7.8 per cent fat. This milk is put up in cans and sterilized. The degree of sterilization varies; it appears that very few evaporated milks are actually sterile. Most brands of this class of milk will keep for long periods particularly if kept in a cool place.[1] Condensed (sweetened) milk depends upon the addition of approximately 40 per cent of cane sugar to assist in its preservation. The high sugar content is objectionable for many purposes. Condensed milk must contain 28 per cent. of total milk solids and 8 per cent. of fat.

Dried milks have been prepared on an extensive scale for only a comparatively short time. They may now be had in the form of skimmed milk, half-skimmed milk and whole milk. These milks particularly skimmed milk have been used extensively in the manufacture of candy, milk chocolate and bakery products. The value of milk powders varies considerably according to the method of manufacture The best powders are made from fresh milk and are subjected to the influence of heat for a very short time. Such milks when mixed with water "dissolve" readily and are hard to tell from fresh milk. Skimmed milk powder mixed with butter in a special machine was found to be very satisfactory in the hospitals in the army where fresh milk could not be obtained. The following table gives the composition of condensed milks.

COMPOSITION OF CONDENSED MILKS—IN PER CENT.

		Condensed (sweetened).	Evaporated.	Dried whole	Skimmed milk.
Milk solids	fat	9.0	8.3	28.5	1.0
	protein	8.5	7.5	24.3	33.9
	lactose	13.3	9.7	36.8	55.0
	ash	1.8	1.5	5.6	....
Cane Sugar		40.9	....	....	....
Water		26.5	73.0	4.8	....

In condensing milk most of the biological properties are retained. The value of the protein remains practically

[1] Evidence of spoilage is easily detected through the swelling of the can. Occasionally spoilage occurs without swelling due to the growth of an organism without the production of gas; this is called "flat sour."

unchanged. Fat-soluble A and water-soluble B **are only** partially destroyed. What the effect of storage **may be is** not known. The anti-scorbutic vitamine is app**arently** destroyed. There is a possibility that dried fresh **raw milk** may retain a part at least, of its anti-scorbutic pro**perties**. If any of these products are to be used for infant **feeding it** is well to supplement it with fruit or vegetable juice to **supply** the anti-scorbutic vitamine. For infant feeding, milk **powder** has been found very satisfactory and likewise evap**orated** milk. The condensed milk contains too much cane-**sugar** for infant feeding.

Influence of Temperature — Bacteria.—Milk when **drawn** from the mammary gland contains, in addition to the **food**-stuffs, organisms and substances, such as leukocytes, **bac**-teria, and enzymes. If raw milk be permitted to stand **at** ordinary temperatures, particularly when exposed to **the** air, physical and chemical transformations take place. These are chiefly bacterial; changes caused by leukocytes and the enzymes secreted with the milk are of little practical importance.

The bactericidal properties of milk prevent the initial rapid growth of bacteria. Raw milk exhibits, at room temperature, an apparent inhibition of bacterial growth; in some cases a destruction of bacteria has been demonstrated. The restraining action of raw milk extends over a period of from twelve to twenty-four hours; after this time a rapid multiplication of bacteria takes place. This increase is retarded at low temperatures, 15° C. and below. When heated to 80° C. or above milk loses its power to restrain bacterial growth. There is a more profound change in the latter case, for such milk permits a rapid growth of the bacterial organisms. Heated milk may therefore become more dangerous than unheated milk unless care is taken to prevent reinoculation of the heated product, otherwise a greater number, and perhaps more virulent types, of bacteria may develop than would have developed in unsterilized milk.

The presence of pathogenic organisms in a heterogeneous milk supply, however, demands some means of killing them or restraining their growth, such as sterilization or pasteurization. In pasteurization milk is heated to 60° to 70° C. (140° to 160° F.) for from ten to twenty minutes. As the result of this treatment practically all of the bacteria are destroyed. Such a temperature does not affect the spores, hence milk must be cooled and kept at a temperature which will inhibit or restrain their development. Heating to a temperature of 60° C. for twenty minutes has been shown to have little effect upon the germicidal power of milk or upon the enzymes present in it. Sterilization is the process of destroying *all* of the organisms present, both bacteria and their spores. Complete sterilization can only be accomplished by long-continued boiling or intermittent heating below the boiling point. Such a procedure also destroys the enzymes and the germicidal property of milk. In both pasteurization and sterilization the water-soluble accessory substance is destroyed.

Action of Bacteria.—Bacteria, which produce unusual and abnormal products, find their way into milk as the result of carelessness in handling. They cause alterations in the color, odor, and taste of milk. The formation of blue milk, or red milk, of slimy or ropy milk, and the development of a bitter taste are the result of bacterial action. Certain yeasts cause alcoholic fermentation.

Lactic acid is the most important of non-pathogenic bacterial action in milk; it is the predominating substance formed in the souring of milk. With the accumulation of the lactic and other acids the reaction of milk changes from approximately neutral to distinctly acid. Caseinogen is insoluble in this medium as shown by its precipitation, ordinarily called curdling. The precipitated caseinogen settles to the bottom of the liquid, leaving the "whey." Whey contains all of the constituents of milk except the caseinogen and a portion of the fat with the addition of lactic acid, the loss of some lactose, and the transformation of a portion of the protein into its cleavage products. The physical evidence of souring is often the secondary result of bacterial action rather than the direct consequence.

Action of Heat.—The first evidence of the effect of heat upon milk is the formation of a pellicle or skin upon its surface. If this skin is removed another immediately takes its place. An examination of this film shows it to consist chiefly of protein and fat. The evidence favors the view that the pellicle consists of protein (caseinogen) which has entangled the fat, for solutions of caseinogen when heated give the same kind of film. Surface evaporation and fat facilitate the formation of the skin but are not essential. If the milk be slightly acid, such as following bacterial action, heat does not produce a film but coagulation occurs. It is the presence of a small quantity of acid which causes the coagulation of apparently fresh milk in the process of pasteurization.

When milk is heated to between 60° and 70° C. most of the bacteria present in it are destroyed. Such heating has little effect upon the other constituents of milk. If the temperature be raised above 70° C., however, the composition, color, odor and taste are affected according to the extent of heating. The accessory substances or vitamines are at least in part, if not entirely, destroyed by heating.[1] The caseinogen is apparently affected by boiling when judged from its retarded coagulation with rennin. Pure solutions of caseinogen are not affected by heating, hence the retardation of coagulation may be due in part to the altered state of a portion of the calcium salts which have probably been precipitated as tricalcium phosphate. Experimental evidence indicates that there is no change in the digestibility of caseinogen as the result of heating, and it may even be an advantage for the curd of heated milk tends to be more flocculent than that of raw milk. The biological properties of milk—enzymes, etc.—are destroyed by heating.

The albumins are coagulated in the process of heating. Studies on the change in the viscosity of milk when heated have shown that permanent coagulation takes place at 70° C. The liberation of ammonia and of volatile sulphide, probably hydrogen sulphide, are indications of changes in the proteins. These last factors are probably partially concerned in the taste and odor of heated milk. If the boiling be sufficiently long continued, milk acquires a brownish color from the modification of the milk-sugar, lactose. This change is similar to the browning of sugar or caramelization. The influence of heat upon the digestibility of milk will be considered later.

Refrigeration of milk retards the growth of bacteria and the action of enzymes but these processes are not entirely inhibited. The changes in the composition of refrigerated milk are due principally to bacterial action. They consist in a gradual proteolysis or digestion of the casein, the fermentation of lactose, and the hydrolysis of fat. Proteolytic changes in the albumin are due to enzyme action; such changes are negligible in the ordinary period during which milk is kept.

Digestion of Milk.—The coagulation of the milk protein, caseinogen, through the action of rennin, is the distinctive difference between the digestion of milk and that of other substances. Practically all other proteins are ingested in a solid state. Milk when swallowed passes into the stomach which contains the acid gastric juice. Under such conditions we might expect the caseinogen to be precipitated. This is not the case, however, for it has been shown that

---

[1] The addition of orange or potato juice will tend to prevent the development of scurvy when pasteurized milk is used by infants.

milk is coagulated, clotted by the rennin, before acid precipitation takes place. The cause of this is to be found in the nature of milk, in its ability to absorb a considerable amount of acid without changing its reaction appreciably, and in the fact that the gastric juice is not secreted fast enough to furnish sufficient acid to precipitate the caseinogen before the rennin has transformed it into casein.

The reason for the coagulation of milk before digestion is not clear. Milk can be digested completely in a test-tube without the formation of the insoluble casein. It may be that if the caseinogen were not coagulated, the milk would pass on into the intestine more rapidly than that organ could take care of it and digestive disturbances would result. Coagulated caseinogen must pass through the usual stages of gastric digestion; the intestinal juice continues and completes its digestion.

The coagulation of milk apparently concerns but two of its constituents, the caseinogen and the calcium salts. According to the views of Hammarsten, caseinogen is hydrolyzed through the action of rennin into two constituents, soluble casein and a peptone-like substance called whey protein. Soluble casein unites with calcium ions (soluble calcium salts), forming the insoluble calcium compound usually called casein, or calcium caseinate. More recent work has failed to discover the formation of this peptone-like substance in the process of hydrolysis by rennin. The present conception of the changes in the hydrolysis is the splitting of the caseinogen into two equal molecules of casein, which, being insoluble in the presence of soluble calcium salts precipitate out of solution, forming the clot. In the absence of soluble calcium salts hydrolysis occurs, but the formation of the insoluble clot does not take place until they are added. There is a tendency to ascribe to pepsin the changes we have assigned to rennin, *i. e.*, to assume that rennin and pepsin are identical and the hydrolysis just described is the first step in the gastric digestion of caseinogen.

The physical nature of the clot is influenced by the conditions under which it is produced. In the test-tube cow's milk gives a firm, tough, clot which finally contracts, squeezing out the whey. If the milk be agitated slightly, a fine flocculent precipitate is formed. This is probably the type of clot which is produced in the stomach rather than the tough clot usually described. The presence of fat influences the nature of the coagulum. Fat becomes entangled in the precipitated casein, causing it to form rather dense masses which show a tendency to coalesce; a distinction from the flocculent, finely divided coagulum obtained with skimmed milk. This fact is of importance in the feeding of infants, and will be discussed later. Boiled milk is held to give a more flocculent clot than unboiled milk.

Various methods are employed, particularly in the feeding of infants, to ensure a light flocculent clot and to increase its digestibility, such as the addition of barley water, dilution with water or lime water, the addition of citrates, or heating. The addition of cream and coagulation before eating (butter milk) also ensures a finer curd, but these methods are restricted to adults.

The intestine completes the digestion of milk. Here the proteoses, caseoses, are reduced to simpler complexes by the trypsin of the pancreatic juice and the erepsin of the intestinal juice. Erepsin has the ability of converting caseinogen into amino-acids, although it is unable to act on most other natural proteins. This is probably an important factor in digestion by infants who, it is affirmed, receive a part of the ingested milk from the stomach without its first having been acted upon by the gastric juice. Lactose and the fats are first acted upon extensively in the intestines,

CHAPTER VIII

PROTEIN FOODS

THE protein requirement of the human body is supplied from both the animal and the vegetable kingdoms. A closer analysis of the facts shows the latter to be the ultimate source of protein; for, at least so far as our present knowledge extends, only the plant is able to synthetize this essential food-stuff from inorganic matter. With one or two exceptions, however, we find that protein predominates in animal foods and that the latter are the chief source of this food-stuff in the human diet.

In our previous discussion we considered the need for protein, the general products of its digestion, the forms in which its decomposition products are excreted, and the quantity of protein necessary for the functioning of the body. These considerations have been confined so far as possible, to protein in general. The consideration of the differences among proteins has been postponed until a discussion of the various kinds of protein food could be concluded.

The various proteins in one organism differ from those in another. The proteins in the individual organisms are also of different kinds. Even proteins of the same kind from various sources are different in composition. These differences are exhibited in the physical properties as well as in the chemical composition. The processes of metabolism are concerned with the utilization of these varied proteins for the maintenance of the supply of the various body proteins.

A determination of the elements present in proteins shows them to consist of carbon, hydrogen, oxygen, nitrogen, and sulphur. These elements are combined to form amino-acids, the structural units of the protein. Phosphorus is also present in some proteins, while others contain traces of certain of the metallic elements, such as iron, copper, iodine, manganese, and zinc. A protein is, then, a combination of amino-acids as such, or in combination with certain non-protein substances, such as carbohydrates, lipins (fatty acids) purine bases, phosphoric acid, etc. In digestion the protein molecule is split by hydrolytic cleavage into simpler complexes—proteoses and peptones; these in turn give rise to less complex compounds, peptides, and finally amino-acids. It is through studies of the products of these hydrolytic cleavages that we have gained our knowledge of the constitution of protein.

Consideration of the kinds and quantities of amino-acids present in proteins of various kinds and from different sources is not only instructive but necessary, for recent invesgations have indicated the importance of relative quantities of amino-acids in the diet.

The table on page 165 gives the proportions of the different amino-acids obtained from certain proteins. It is important to remember that every protein food is composed of a number of proteins and that the mass of total food at any meal is seldom deficient in any particular amino-acid.

The protein content of food is usually estimated from the amount of nitrogen in it by multiplying this value by 6.25. This calculation is based on the fact that the average nitrogen content of protein is approximately 16 per cent. This procedure is not entirely correct, for in different kinds of protein variations from 15 to 18 per cent. of nitrogen have been observed. Vegetable proteins are particularly high in nitrogen. The average for wheat protein is 17.55 per cent., which would give a factor of 5.7 instead of 6.25.

Another error in the use of the value 6.25 is due to the fact that not all nitrogen in a food is present as protein; a certain proportion is present as extractive nitrogen. Calculations of the protein content of foods based upon determinations of protein itself as compared with the calculated values for protein (N x 6.25) show that on the latter basis the flesh of different animals contains various amounts of protein, whereas actually they differ but little in their percentage protein content.

Species.	Protein. (N. x 6.25).	Determined by Janney.[1]
Chicken	19.3	16.6
Fish (halibut)	18.6	16.5
Ox	21.6	16.6
Rabbit	20.8	16.3
Cat	21.1	17.8
Dog	20.2	17.4
Man	19.7	16.4

The body proteins differ from one another and from the food proteins. Some proteins are entirely lacking in certain amino-acids. In our discussion of the protein requirement (p. 76) we saw that the effect of the absence of particular

[1] Janney: Jour. Biol. Chem., 1916, xxv, 85.

	Salmine (protamine).	Globin of hemoglobin, horse (histone).	Egg.	Horse serum.	Lactalbumin.	Legumelin (pea).	Leucosin (wheat).	Horse serum.	Fibrin.	Edestin.	Legumin (pea).	Wheat.	Maize.	Wheat.	Maize Zein.	Caseinogen (milk).	Vitellin (egg).	Colein.	Keratin, sheep horn.	Chicken.	Fish (halibut).	Scallops.	Ox.
			Albumins.					**Globulins.**				**Glutens.**		**Gliadins.**		**Phospho-protein.**				**Flesh or muscle.**			
Glycine			0	0	0	0.5	0.9	3.5	3.0	3.8	0.4	0.4	0.3	0.0	0.0	0	0	16.5	0.5	0.7	0.0	0.0	2.1
Alanine		4.2	8.4	2.7	2.5	0.9	4.5	2.3	3.6	3.6	2.1	0.3		2.0	9.8	1.5	0.8	0.8	1.6	2.3	0.8		2.7
Valine	4.3				0.9	0.7	0.2	+	1.0	+				3.4	1.9	7.2	1.9		4.5				0.8
Leucine		29.0	15.2	20.0	19.4	9.5	11.3	18.7	15.0	20.9	8.0	4.1	6.2	6.6	19.6	9.4	9.9	2.1	15.3	11.3	10.4	8.8	11.7
Phenyl alanine		4.2	5.2	3.1	4.8	4.8	3.6	3.8	2.5	2.1	3.8	1.0	1.8	2.4	3.6	3.2	2.6	0.4	1.9	3.6	3.1	4.9	3.2
Tyrosine		1.8	1.0	2.1	0.9	1.6	3.3	2.5	3.5	0.8	1.6	1.9	3.8	1.2	3.6	4.5	8.4		3.6	2.3	2.4	2.0	2.3
Serine	7.8	0.6		0.6					0.8	1.7	0.5			0.2	1.0	0.5		0.4	1.1				
Cystine			0.4	2.5										0.5					7.5				
Proline	11.0	2.8	1.1	1.0	4.0	4.0	3.3	0.9	1.2	2.0	3.2	4.0	5.0	13.2	9.0	6.7	4.2	7.7	3.7	4.3	3.2	2.3	5.8
Oxyproline																		3.0					
Aspartic acid		4.4	1.7	3.1	1.0	4.1	3.4	2.3	3.6	4.5	5.3	0.7	0.7	0.6	1.7	1.2	2.2	0.6	2.5	3.2	2.8	3.5	4.5
Glutamic acid		1.7	8.5	7.7	10.1	13.0	6.7	8.5		1.8	17.0	24.0	12.7	43.7	26.2	11.4	16.5	0.9	17.2	16.5	10.1	14.9	15.5
Arginine	87.4	5.4	2.1		3.2	5.5	5.9	8.5	2.0	11.7	11.7	4.4	7.1	3.2	1.6	15.8	7.5	7.6	2.7	6.5	6.4	7.4	7.5
Tryptophane			+	+		+	+	+	10.4	+	+	+	+	1.0	0.0	1.5	+		0.2	+	+	+	+
Lysine	0	4.2	2.3		9.2	3.0	2.8			1.0	5.0	2.2	2.0	0.6	0.0	5.8	4.8	2.8		7.3	7.6	5.8	7.6
Histidine	0	11.0	0		2.1	2.3	2.3		1.3	1.1	2.4	1.2	2.0	5.2	0.8	2.5	1.9	0.4		2.5	2.6	2.0	1.8
Ammonia					1.3	1.3	1.4				2.1	2.5	2.1		3.6	1.6	1.3	0.4		1.7	1.4	1.1	1.1

amino-acids from the protein molecule, when used as the sole source of protein, was a failure to grow. In a previous chapter the inability of the body to synthetize protein and certain amino-acids was discussed (p. 76). The necessity for a liberal supply of the different amino-acids in the form of a varied selection of proteins, and for a kind of digestion that converts these structural elements in protein into readily available substances either as the amino-acids or simple complexes of these is therefore evident. Such a variety is obtained in the ordinary mixed diet; in special diets it is a factor to be considered. The influence of the ingestion of proteins homologous to those present in the body upon the minimum protein requirement has been discussed (p. 78).

Proteins are not ordinarily distinguished by their amino-acid content, however, but chiefly by their physical properties. Differences in chemical composition are, however, the basis of distinction between the members of one group—the conjugated proteins.[1]

The following outline of the kinds of proteins and their characteristics, the classification adopted by the American Physiological Society and the American Society of Biological Chemists, will be adhered to in our discussion. This classification differs from that of the English societies in a few instances; in most matters they are essentially identical.

1. Simple Proteins.—Protein substances which yield only α-amino-acids or their derivatives on hydrolysis:

(a) *Albumins.*[2]—Soluble in pure water and coagulable by heat. Albumins are present in all cells and in the important fluids of the body. Ovalbumin is the predominating protein of egg white. Other important albumins are serum-albumin present in blood plasma, lymph and other body fluids; lact-albumin of milk; the vegetables albumins, leucosin of wheat, and legumelin of the pea.

[1] The terms *protein* and *proteid* are often used together. The present-day German writers use the word protein to designate simple albuminous substances, and proteid for combinations with other complexes. The simple proteins and the conjugated proteins of the American classification are proteins and proteids respectively in the German classification. A distinction is sometimes made between protein and proteid among English-speaking writers. Proteid designates definite chemical compounds, or isolated albuminous substances (our proteins), while protein is used to denote the mixture of proteids in a food, the measure of which is the quantity of nitrogen which the food yields upon analysis times 6.25, the average percentage of nitrogen in pure proteid. Protein has been adopted by English-speaking scientists as the generic term for the class of substances which we are discussing—and we will use this term in that sense.

[2] A distinction is sometimes made between the pure individual substances albumin and a mixture of proteins occurring naturally together, or albumen, as the white of egg. The term albumen is used very little and is now practically restricted to the expression "egg albumen."

(*b*) *Globulins.*—Globulins are insoluble in pure water but soluble in neutral solutions of salts of strong bases with strong acids. Globulins are present in blood, serum globulin; egg, ovoglobulin; milk, lactglobulin; seeds, edestin (hemp seed); legumin (pea).

(*c*) *Glutelins.*—Glutelins are simple proteins insoluble in all neutral solvents but readily soluble in very dilute acids and alkalies, *e. g.*, the vegetable protein, glutenin, from wheat.

(*d*) *Alcohol Soluble Proteins (Prolamines).*—Simple proteins soluble in 70 to 80 per cent. alcohol, insoluble in water, absolute alcohol, and other neutral solvents, *e. g.*, zein, corn; gliadin, wheat; hordein, barley.

Gluten, readily obtained from wheat flour by washing away the starch, albumin, etc., is a mixture of members of the last two classes of proteins, glutenin and gliadin.

(*e*) *Albuminoids.*—Simple proteins possessing a similar structure to those already mentioned, but characterized by a pronounced insolubility in all neutral solvents. The proteins concerned in the framework of the body are the most important members of this group, *e. g.*, elastin and collagen; connective tissue; keratin—hair, nails and horn; and fibroin from silk. Acids or prolonged boiling with water convert collagen into gelatin. Gelatin is not, however, classed as an albuminoid. The English nomenclature aptly designates the albuminoids as scleroproteins.

(*f*) *Histones.*—Soluble in water and insoluble in very dilute ammonia and, in the absence of ammonium salts, insoluble even in excess of ammonia; yield precipitates with solutions of other proteins and a coagulum on heating which is easily soluble in very dilute acids. On hydrolysis they yield a large number of amino-acids among which the basic ones predominate. In short, histones are basic proteins which stand between protamines and true proteins, *e. g.*, globin, one of the constituents of hemoglobin; thymus histone and scrombrone from sperm.

(*g*) *Protamines.*—Simpler polypeptides than the proteins included in the preceding groups. They are soluble in water, uncoagulable by heat, have the property of precipitating aqueous solutions of other proteins, possess strong basic properties and form stable salts with strong mineral acids. They yield comparatively few amino-acids, among which the basic amino-acids predominate. These proteins are obtained from spermatozoa in which they occur in combination with nucleic acid. The various members of this class are designated according to the animal from which they are obtained, as salmin from the salmon sperm; sturin from mackerel sperm, etc.

II. Conjugated Proteins.—Substances which contain the protein molecule united to some other molecule or molecules otherwise than as a salt.

(*a*) *Nucleoproteins.*—Compounds of one or more protein molecules with nucleic acid. This type of protein is the principal constituent of cell nuclei and is found in practically all protein-rich foods. Milk and the white of egg are important exceptions. Nucleoprotein is a very complex substance yielding upon hydrolysis first protein and nuclein. Nuclein then disintegrates into a second protein, usually basic, as histone or protamine, and nucleic acid. Nucleic acid may consist of one or more combinations of phosphoric acid, carbohydrate, and one of the purine or pyrimidine bases called nucleotids. Upon hydrolysis of a combination of nucleotids, the various nucleotids result. The phosphoric acid is next split off from the nucleotids leaving the purine- or pyrimidine-carbohydrate complex, nucleosid, which finally yields carbohydrate and the base. The following scheme shows the disintegration of nucleoprotein:

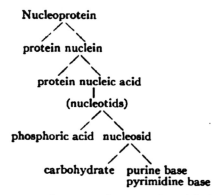

The purine bases from nucleoprotein are the chief source of the uric acid which appears in the urine of mammals.

(*b*) *Glycoproteins.*—Compounds of the protein molecule with a substance or substances containing a carbohydrate group other than a nucleic acid, *e. g.*, mucins and mucoids (osseomucoid from bone, tendomucoid from tendon, ichthulin from carp eggs, helicoprotein from snail).

(*c*) *Phosphoproteins.*—Compounds of the protein molecule with some, as yet undefined, phosphorus-containing substances other than a nucleic acid or lecithin, *e. g.*, casein from milk, ovovitellin from egg yolk.

(*d*) *Hemoglobins.*—Compounds of the protein molecule with hematin, or some similar substance, *e. g.*, hemoglobin from red blood cells, hemocyanin from blood of invertebrates.

(*e*) *Lecithoproteins.*—Compounds of the protein molecule with lecithin.

III. Derived Proteins.—A. Primary Proteins Derivatives.— Derivatives of the protein molecule apparently formed through hydrolytic changes which involve only slight alteration of the protein molecule.

(*a*) *Proteins.*—Insoluble products which apparently result from the incipient action of water, very dilute acids or enzymes, *e. g.*, myosan from myosin, edestan from edestin.

(*b*) *Metaproteins.*—Products of the further action of acids and alkalies whereby the molecule is so far altered as to form products soluble in very weak acids and alkalies but insoluble in neutral fluids, *e. g.*, acid metaprotein (acid albuminate), alkali metaprotein (alkali albuminate).

(*c*) *Coagulated Proteins.*—Insoluble products which result from (1) the action of heat on their solutions, or (2) the action of alcohol on the protein.

B. Secondary Protein Derivatives.—Products of the further hydrolytic cleavage of the protein molecule.

(*a*) *Proteoses.*—Soluble in water, non-coagulable by heat, and precipitated by saturating their solutions with ammonium—or zinc sulphate, *e. g.*, protoproteose, deuteroproteose.

(*b*) *Peptones.*—Soluble in water, non-coagulable by heat, but not precipitated by saturating their solutions with ammonium sulphate, *e. g.*, antipeptone, amphopeptone.

(*c*) *Peptides.*—Definitely characterized combinations of two or more amino-acids, the carboxyl group of one being united with the amino group of the other with the elimination of a molecule of water, *e. g.*, dipeptides, tripeptides, tetrapeptides, pentapeptides.

Influence of Heat.—The effect of heat upon simple proteins is to cause them to coagulate. Such changes are continually occurring in the preparation of food for the table. The boiling of an egg, or the roasting of meat is accompanied by the coagulation of the protein, and it is to a large extent the coagulation of the protein among expanded gas bubbles which keeps bread and cake "light." Two changes take place in the coagulation of protein: there is first a reaction between the hot water and the protein as the result of which the protein loses certain of its characteristic properties, such as solubility, *i. e.*, the protein is denatured. Secondly, the altered particles of protein agglutinate into visible masses or coagula which separate from the solution. When the protein is held in the meshes of connective tissue, etc., the denatured protein shrinks or contracts so that water and dissolved salts are squeezed out. This phenomenon is called syneresis. The accumulation of beef juice around a roast when cut on the platter is the result of syneresis. The presence of acid and small quantities of salt facilitates the coagulation of protein. An excess of acid or alkali results in a solution of the protein and prevents coagulation.

Certain proteins of the albuminoid class, such as collagen, are readily hydrolyzed (rendered soluble) particularly so in the presence of small quantities of acid. The long-continued cooking (usually just below the boiling point) of tough cuts of meat accomplishes the hydrolysis of the connective tissue (rich in collagen) which tends to free the muscle fibers and permit their ready separation, *i. e.*, makes the meat tender. The use of veal for soup stock and the ease with which the fibers of fish are separated is due to the large proportion of easily hydrolyzed connective tissue which they contain. Acid facilitates hydrolysis; it also tends to cause protein material to swell. The value of acid in cooking fish and tough meat is, then, self-evident.

Protein combines with both acid radicles and basic radicles to form protein salts; the insoluble curd formed in the coagulation of milk occurs because the calcium salt of casein is insoluble in water; the sodium or potassium salts are soluble, and it is in this form that certain soluble casein preparations are placed on the market. Certain proteins of the legumes form insoluble calcium and magnesium salts, which is the reason for the objection to the use of hard water in preparing legumes for the table. The use of egg white, etc., as an antidote for poisons is due to the insoluble salts which are formed by the protein with the heavy metals.

Effect of Low Temperatures.—Low temperatures have no direct effect upon protein. Its properties may be altered, however, as the result of changes produced in the medium in which it is suspended. The crystallization of the intracellular water results in a concentration of the salts. This causes the precipitation of some proteins and the solution of others. Upon the return to the normal temperature the original state is restored. Long-continued low temperatures produce a change in the precipitated proteins so that they will not redissolve. The change just noted has been shown to occur in plants.

During refrigeration protein food-stuffs undergo considerable modification as the result of predominant enzyme action, autolysis, rather than of bacterial action which shares in the transformation at room and body temperatures. Low temperatures inhibit both bacterial and enzyme action, the former more than the latter, however. The changes which occur at low temperatures are analogous to those which take place in aseptic or sterile tissues, either in the body or out of it. The "ripening" of flesh is due to these autolytic changes brought about by the intracellular enzymes. The action of the intracellular proteases is quite similar to that of the digestive enzymes, particularly trypsin. Protein passes gradually through the various stages of proteolytic digestion, finally yielding amino-acids. Examination of refrigerated meat, for instance, shows an increase in the quantity of water-soluble proteins, indicating a partial digestion. Other enzymes produce changes in the fats and carbohydrate. The changes which result in foods preserved with certain chemical substances, without the use of heat, are the result of autolysis.

Bacterial growth is not entirely checked at comparatively low temperatures and changes undoubtedly occur as the result of their action. At higher temperatures, room temperatures and above, the activities of bacteria increase. The products of their action on proteins are in part similar to those produced in enzymatic digestion. The harmful effects of bacteria from a dietary point of view are not in the bacteria themselves so much as in the products (ptomaines) produced in the food, protein, during their growth. These substances are produced by non-pathogenic as well as by pathogenic organisms. The ptomaines are soluble basic substances closely related to the amino-acids; not all are toxic.

The changes which proteins undergo in the course of digestion and absorption have already been discussed (p. 38). The rate with which they are made available for absorption depends upon their physical properties, whether they are in solution or solid, dense or finely divided, will imbibe water easily or with difficulty; and upon their chemical properties, such as acidic or basic, complex or simple. Preparation of food for use is often accompanied by change in the digestibility as well as in the availability of the foodstuffs. This is particularly true with regard to protein. The total available quantity of the protein is often increased in the course of preparation. The effect of grinding vegetable food-stuffs very fine is to increase their total digestibility. The influence of heat upon the connective tissue of animal food-stuff is to cause a partial conversion of collagen into glatin; hence the ease of digestion is increased. In vegetable food-stuffs the indigestible cellulose structure is ruptured through the combined action of heat and water, thus promoting the action of the digestive enzymes upon the contained protein and carbohydrates.

CHAPTER IX

MEAT OR FLESH FOOD

THE dietary value of meat is due chiefly to its protein content. It contains in addition a varying quantity of lipin or fat, a small amount of carbohydrate, salts, and certain nitrogenous derivatives related to the proteins called extractives. The palatability, variety, ease with which the flavor may be modified, facility of preparation, concentration of protein, and digestibility are factors which have made meat the most important protein of the adult human dietary. With regard to its biological value meat contains adequate protein and the water-soluble and anti-scorbutic vitamines. It is relatively poor in the fat-soluble vitamine, calcium, sodium and chlorine. The use of meat in the diet, therefore, requires the correction of these deficiencies through the use of vegetables, particularly the leafy vegetables. Cereals, grains and seeds will not serve to correct the deficiencies of meat.

The dietary and economic advantages and disadvantages of animal and vegetable protein have been discussed (p. 144).

Meat is derived almost entirely from the skeletal or striated muscles. Such muscles are composed of fibrils enclosed in sheaths known as sarcolemma (fibers) and bound together in the form of bundles by connective tissue. The fibers terminate in bundles of white fibrous connective tissue, the tendons, by means of which they are attached to the bones. Embedded in the connective tissue of the muscle bundles are cells more or less rich in fat, while between the various muscles comparatively large masses of fatty tissues are found. Living muscle is practically neutral in reaction, but after death lactic acid is formed and the reaction rapidly changes to acid. An alkaline reaction in meat is an indication of putrefaction.

The important proteins of muscle plasma are myogen (a globulin) which predominates, and myosin. After death these proteins become coagulated to form the muscle clot;[1] this is the form in which the greater portion of the protein of meat exists. Immediately after death autolytic changes commence with the formation of lactic acid and protein di-

[1] Myosin is the name given to muscle clot by some investigators.

gestion products and are attended by an increase in the quantity of soluble proteins. These are the processes concerned in "ripening."

The connective tissue contains a large percentage of the albuminoid collagen, which is a source of gelatin—the base of the jelly of cooked meat. The flesh of young animals, *e. g.*, veal and lamb, is particularly rich in connective tissue and their bones in collagen. The readiness with which meat from such animals yields gelatin makes it valuable as the basis of soup. Fish are also rich in gelatin-yielding tissues. Blood remaining in the capillaries and bloodvessels and in the blood plasma surrounding the cells, contains serum albumin, globulin, fibrin, etc.

The hemoglobin in muscle and the residual blood give meat its red color. The identity of the coloring substance in blood and in muscle is not generally admitted, although the close relation is acknowledged. The quantity of hemoglobin varies; it is greatest in muscles concerned in long-continued and powerful contractions and least in the more passive muscles. The dark and light meat of the birds show this relation. Certain species, *e. g.*, the rabbit, are poor in hemoglobin. The muscle of the young of most species is low in hemoglobin, hence their light color. The decided red color of meat preserved with nitrates appears to be due to the presence of nitrous oxide hemoglobin.

The small amount of glycogen normally present in muscle is almost entirely changed to glucose after death. The comparatively large quantity of glycogen in fresh horse meat is one of its distinguishing characteristics. Fat varies in quantity kind, and color with the condition of the animal, the food ingested, and the cut (portion of the carcass).

Flavor in meat is due to the presence of the extractives—substances soluble in water, alcohol, or ether. In addition to the carbohydrates and fat just mentioned these include certain non-protein nitrogenous constituents, such as creatin, xanthin, hypoxanthin, inosin, etc.; the latter are the chief source of the exogenous uric acid. It is the latter extractives which the gouty patient should avoid and to which vegetarians and certain food cults object, holding them to be waste products and a burden to the excretory system.

The presence of purine compounds in the diet under certain pathological conditions, such as gout, is objectionable. It is important to know, therefore, the relative quantity of these substances in various foods. A table giving the purine contents of various kinds of flesh and of certain other foods will be found in a subsequent discussion of diet in disease.

Meat often contains certain substances characteristic of the food ingested which give to it the flavor so prized by epicures: these are particularly evident in game.

Flesh or meat is ordinarily composed of about three-fourths water, but there is less water in fat than in lean meat and likewise in old than in young animals. In the ash of muscle the salts of potassium and phosphoric acid predominate. Traces of sodium, calcium, magnesium, iron, sulphur, and chlorine are also found. The following table gives the approximate proportions in which the inorganic constituents occur in meat.

COMPOSITION OF THE ASH OF TYPICAL FLESH FOODS.

	$CaO.$	$MgO.$	$K_2O.$	$Na_2O.$	$P_2O_4.$	$Cl.$	$S.$	$Fe.$
Beef, lean .	0.011	0.04	0.42	0.09	0.50	0.05	0.20	0.0038
Veal, lean .	0.16	0.045	0.46	0.12	0.50	0.07	0.23	
Lamb, me-ium fat .	0.0039	0.04	0.29	.0.093	0.42	0.12	0.23	
Pork, lean .	0.012	0.046	0.34	0.13	0.45	0.05	0.20	
Poultry .	0.015	0.06	0.56	0.13	0.58	0.06	0.216	
Fish . .	0.03	0.04	0.40	1.30	0.40	2.40	0.22	0.0003

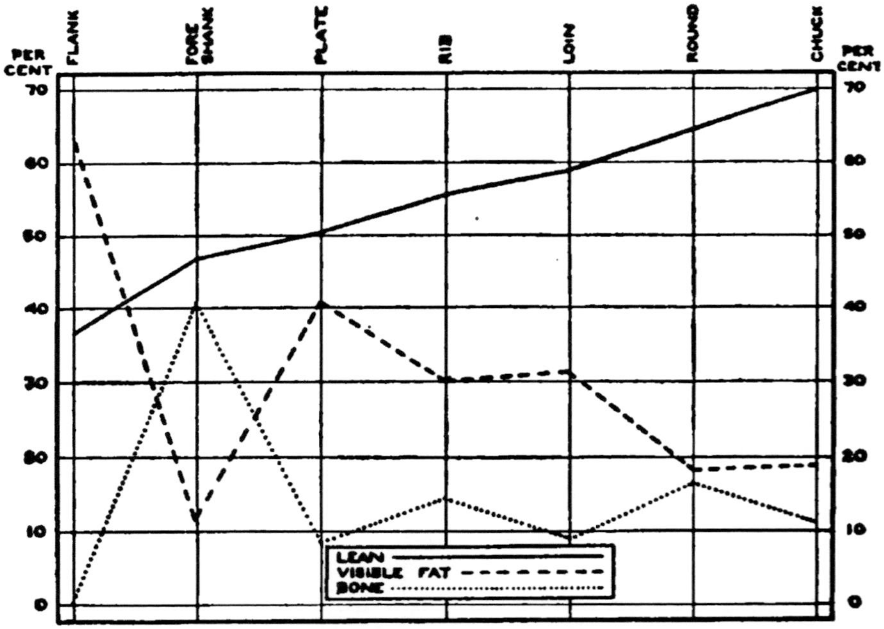

FIG. 3.—Percentages of lean, visible fat and bone in the straight wholesale cuts.[1] (Courtesy of the Illinois Agricultural Experiment Station.)

Some meats when purchased contain inedible parts, such as bone, the exterior portions of the carcass, large blood-vessels, connective tissue, gristle and tendon. In consider-

[1] Hall and Emmett: Univ. Ill. Agr. Exp. Sta., Bull. 158, 1912.

ing a particular piece of meat from a purely dietary point of view allowance should be made in the calculation for the waste which these portions represent. From an economic standpoint it is essential to know the quantity of edible material likely to be derived from a given piece of meat. Fig. 3 gives the percentages of lean, visible fat, and bone in the straight wholesale cuts of beef.

An inspection of this chart reveals in general an inverse relation between the percentage of lean meat and that of visible fat; the relative weight of bone is more variable.

The proportions of the various food-stuffs in meat varies according to the kind of animal and the portion of the anatomy from which it is obtained. The same "cut" of meat from different animals varies according to its age and nutritive condition. The relative differences in the protein content of the various cuts of beef is shown in the following chart (Fig. 4) prepared by Hall and Emmett, which gives the percentage of the total protein in the boneless meat of wholesale cuts.

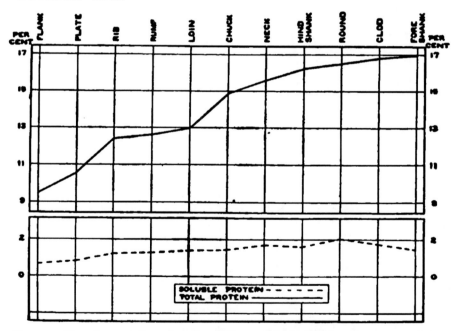

FIG. 4.—Percentages of total and soluble protein in the boneless meat of the wholesale cuts.[1] (Courtesy of the Illinois Agricultural Experiment Station.)

The curves show a relative increase in the quantity of protein as we consider the cuts from the left to right. Calculated on the basis of the dry, moisture-free, substance an

[1]Hall and Emmett: Univ. Ill. Agr. Exp. Sta., Bull. 158, 1912.

even greater increase is found, because the cuts on the right contain more lean and less fat and also because the lean meat has a greater water content. When the fat is excluded from consideration, the protein content of the various cuts is quite similar. In other words, the difference in the various cuts of beef is due to the varying quantities of fat and water.

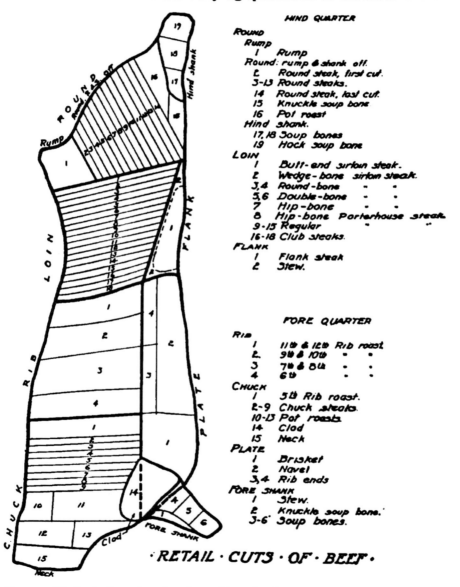

FIG. 5.—Method of cutting the three sides, showing retail cuts. (Courtesy of the Illinois Agricultural Experiment Station.)

COMPOSITION OF TYPICAL FLESH FOODS.[1]

	Water, per cent.	Protein N x 6.25, per cent.	Fat, per cent.	Ash, per cent.	Fuel value per pound.
Beef	70.0	21.3	7.9	1.1	709
Veal	70.3	21.2	8.0	1.0	711
Lamb	63.9	19.2	16.5	1.1	1022
Pork	60.0	25.0	14.4	1.3	1042
Poultry	63.7	19.3	16.3	1.0	1016
Fish	81.7	17.2	0.3	1.2	324

The differences among the percentages of the food-stuffs in the various kinds of meat are likewise due to similar variations; this is shown in the accompanying table taken from a compilation of analyses by Atwater and Bryant.

PERCENTAGES OF WATER-SOLUBLE, INSOLUBLE, AND TOTAL PROTEIN IN THE BONELESS MEAT OF THE WHOLESALE CUTS.[1]

Wholesale cuts.	Soluble.	Insoluble.	Total.
Fore shank	1.42	15.56	16.98
Clod	1.81	14.88	16.69
Round	2.08	14.42	16.50
Hind shank	1.59	14.67	16.26
Neck	1.65	13.94	15.59
Chuck	1.47	13.40	14.87
Loin	1.37	11.59	12.96
Rump	1.26	11.30	12.56
Rib	1.20	11.12	12.32
Plate	0.83	9.76	10.59
Flank	0.66	8.78	9.44

Fig. 5 p. 176 enables one to locate the portion of the animal under consideration.

Effect of Heat on Meat.—*Cooking.*—The objects to be accomplished by cooking meat are the improvement of its flavor and appearance; the modification of its texture, and the destruction of parasites and bacteria. Digestibility of protein is not increased by cooking; it is diminished in many cases. Such changes as the hydrolysis of connective tissue and comminution increase the ease of digestion.

The flavor acquired by meat through cooking is due to changes, probably oxidative, in the soluble, extractive, portions of the flesh and in the fats.[2] A study of the development of flavor in which the juices were separated from the insoluble portions (fiber) of beef showed the flavors to develop in the juice more than in the residue, and in the extract not coagulable by heat more than in the coagulable portion. A study of the effect of various temperatures showed the flavor to develop most at temperatures above 100° C.; below this the taste is more or less insipid. The pronounced flavors developed by dry heat are thought to be due to the

[1] Hall and Emmett: Univ. Ill. Agr. Exp. Sta., Bull. 158, 1912.
[2] Grindley and Emmett: U. S. Dept. Agr., Office Exp. Sta., Bull. 162.

12

higher temperatures attained.   The fat of meat when heated sufficiently high also gives rise to characteristic flavors.

The appearance of meat is improved by cooking as the result of the coagulation of the proteins and the transformations in the hemoglobin whereby the more or less objectionable reddish-purple color of uncooked, raw meat is changed to the light red or brown color of cooked meat.   These changes in appearance are most evident in roast beef and are enhanced by the crisp outer layer of fat.

Three methods are employed to make a piece of meat tender: (1) Cooking for a long time at low temperature; simmering at approximately 80° C. (this is sometimes incorrectly designated boiling) whereby the insoluble collagen of the connective tissue is changed to gelatin, thus loosening the fibers.   (2) The mechanical separation of the fiber from the connective tissue by scraping, a tedious process practised in the preparation of a readily digestible protein food for the sick.   (3) Grinding, mincing, or pounding by which means the connective tissue is mechanically severed.

In the cooking of meat two general methods are employed which differ in the mode of application of the heat: (a) The direct application of radiant heat, as in roasting and broiling and (b) the application of heat through the medium of a liquid, as boiling in water and frying in deep fat.

Roasting and baking are used synonymously by the average cook.   A distinction should be made, however, between so-called roasting or baking and true roasting.[1]   *True roasting* is cooking by radiated heat from glowing coals, but one side of the food being exposed to the heat at a time.   *Broiling* is essentially the same in principle as true roasting, but the food is brought into direct contact with radiant heat.   The length of time of the two processes differs for a thinner cut of meat is used for broiling.   *Baking* is cooking in a ventilated oven.   Although frying in deep fat belongs properly, as indicated, to the indirect method of cooking, the results obtained are more like those obtained with the direct application of dry heat.

The changes produced in meat by cooking, aside from slight differences in flavor, are of two kinds, those characteristic of roasting and of boiling.   Combinations of these, as in pot roasting, so admirably adapted to the preparation of tough cheap cuts, yield some of the advantages of each method. In this case the tenderness of boiled meat is combined with the flavor of roasted meat.   Grindley and Emmett have

[1] Bevier and Sprague: Univ. Ill. Agr. Exp. Sta., Circular 71, 1903.

shown the effect of roasting (baking) to be similar to that produced in broiling, parboiling, sauteing, and frying.

Roasting is practised principally for the development of flavor and appearance. The application of a high heat sears the surface of meat and immediately coagulates the proteins, the hemoglobin being changed from bluish red to brown. Such treatment also causes changes in the surface fat, thus developing an additional flavor. The preliminary searing, usually conducted at a higher temperature than the subsequent cooking, serves to retain the water and the extractives. The subsequent changes which occur within the roast are gradual for muscle fibers are very poor conductors of heat, and the internal temperatures never reach those of the air surrounding the meat.

Precise Method of Roasting Beef.—As the heat gradually penetrates inward the proteins are coagulated at a low heat, and the hemoglobin is changed in color, assuming first the pink color characteristic of rare meat, and finally becomes brownish gray—"well done." This last color is common to all meats heated to a temperature above 70° to 75° C. and is due to the complete coagulation of the hemoglobin. At these higher temperatures the coagulated protein, and consequently the piece of meat shrinks. Careful studies of the physical changes occurring during roasting have emphasized these points and established the conditions necessary to obtain the desired kind of roast—rare, medium, or "well done" (Sprague and Grindley). The inner temperature of the meat determines the degree of the roast regardless of the external temperature. When a thermometer placed in the middle of a roast registers a temperature of approximately 43°C., 55° C., or 70° C., if the roast be removed from the oven, the final temperature will be approximately 55° C., 65° C., or 70° C., and the meat will be respectively rare, medium, or well done. These temperatures hold with the external temperature of the average roasting oven (175° to 195° C.). At lower oven temperatures the temperature at which the meat is removed will more nearly approximate the final one desired.

The most desirable conditions for successful "boiling" of meat are long continued heating at a temperature below the boiling-point, 80° to 85° C. Under such circumstances the connective tissue is softened and the protein coagulated without becoming hardened (toughened) characterized by the shrinking of the meat. Long experience in cooking has demonstrated the advisability of searing the outside of the meat or plunging it into boiling water and keeping it at this temperature for a few minutes before beginning the cooking at the lower temperature. Such a practise is held to assist in the formation of a more or less impervious layer by the coagulation of the surface proteins which retains the extractives and soluble proteins, and thereby improves the nutritive value and flavor. If a rich broth is desired the opposite method is used, beginning with cold water which is gradually heated. The work of Grindley and his associates, studies on the losses in cooking meat (see below for further discussion), has shown, however, that when meat is cooked at 80° to 85° C. there is practically no difference in the quantity of nutrients (protein, extractives, and ash) which pass into the broth when the cooking is begun in hot or cold water. The length of time and the fat content have a much greater effect upon the losses than the method of cooking.

Chemical Changes in Meat as the Result of Cooking.—The chemical changes which occur in meat during cooking, whether by roasting or boiling, consist in an increase of insoluble (coagulated) protein and in the removal of water and extractives (nitrogenous, non-nitrogenous, fat and ash). Boiling causes a removal of a greater proportion of these substances than does roasting. Fat meats lose less water, protein, and mineral matter, but more fat, than do the lean cuts. Prolonged cooking at higher temperatures is accompanied by greater losses than at lower temperatures. Under like conditions the larger the piece of meat the smaller are the relative losses. As already mentioned, when "boiling" at 80° to 85° C., the effect of such preliminary treatment, as placing in cold or hot water has little effect upon the quantity of material found in the broth. It is interesting to note that the beef used in the preparation of beef tea or broth loses little of its nutritive value, although it loses much of its flavoring material. The work of Grindley and his associates has been verified and extended by that of other investigators, particularly with regard to the changes in the protein and extractives under various conditions. The table on page 181 taken from their results shows the influence of cooking upon the composition of meat.

Digestibility of Meat.—Many conflicting statements are made with regard to the digestibility of meats of various kinds and as prepared by the various methods of cooking. The observations upon which the conclusions regarding the digestibility of meat are commonly based are of two general types (1) the time the food remains in the stomach and (2) the degree of digestion, *i. e.*, the amount absorbed, measured by the quantity of nitrogenous substances excreted in the feces.

Changes in Composition of Meat during Cooking.

	Water	Protein			Extractives			Fat	Ash	Protein	Nitrogen. Non-protein	Total
		Insoluble.	Soluble.	Total.	Nitrogen-ous.	Non-nitro-genous.	Total.					
Beef:												
Fresh	69.13	15.52	2.29	17.81	1.08	1.62	2.70	10.95	1.03	2.85	0.35	3.20
Boiled	57.50	31.57	0.38	31.95	0.60	0.75	1.35	9.34	0.66	5.12	0.19	5.31
Roasted	66.14	22.54	0.82	23.36	1.35	1.65	3.00	6.96	1.24	3.74	0.43	4.17

LOSSES OR GAINS IN COOKING EXPRESSED IN TERMS (PERCENTAGE) OF TOTAL WEIGHT OF UNCOOKED MEAT.

	Water	Insoluble.	Soluble.	Total.	Nitrogen-ous.	Non-nitro-genous.	Total.	Fat.	Ash.
Boiling	-39.09	...	...	-0.63	-0.83	-1.07	...	1.24	0.61
Roasting	-35.31	...	...	+3.87	-9.02	-16.64	...	6.87	11.68

COMPOSITION OF EXTRACTS AND BROTHS.

	Water	Insoluble.	Soluble.	Total.	Nitrogen-ous.	Non-nitro-genous.	Total.	Fat.	Ash.	Protein.	Nitrogen. Non-protein	Total.
Cold-water extract:												
Fresh meat	...		...	2.29	1.08	1.62	2.70	...	0.83	0.37	0.35	0.71
Broth:												
Complete maximum	97.8		...	1.56	1.06	1.36	2.42	6.48	0.77	0.34	0.57	0.25
Complete minimum	91.1		...	0.19	0.56	0.73	1.30	0.06	0.44	0.18	0.25	0.03
Average	95.62		...	0.58	0.83	1.07	1.90	1.26	0.61	0.27	0.36	0.09
Broth, clear (filtered):												
Maximum	98.0		...	0.96	1.07	1.37	2.44	...	0.79			
Minimum	96.6		...	0.15	0.60	0.74	1.39	...	0.46			
Average	97.1		...	0.33	0.85	1.09	1.94	...	0.62			

The first method is open to the objection that it measures the activity of the stomach and tells nothing of the processes which go on in the intestines. Stomachic processes involve chiefly the swelling of the protein under the influence of the hydrochloric acid and a partial hydrolysis by the pepsin, resulting in the reduction of the food to a semifluid mass, but there is little absorption through the gastric mucosa. Moreover, so many variables must be taken into consideration accurately to measure the time required for food to leave the stomach that the results obtained by such experiments must, unless they are very striking, be considered as merely suggestive. For example, the ease of swelling and the degree of peptic activity are modified by the mode of preparation. Fat particularly tends to retard gastric digestion; there is no lipolytic activity of importance in the stomach. The composition of the flesh likewise affects gastric digestion, very fat meats being less digestible than lean meats. The presence of large quantities of connective tissue, particularly in partially cooked food, serves to hinder peptonization. Finely divided meat is more easily attacked by the gastric juice than large masses. Foods which are acid remain a shorter time in the stomach than do alkaline foods. The quantity, strength, and acidity of the gastric juice have a very pronounced effect upon the rate of ejection from the stomach.

The second method of measuring digestibility—the completeness of absorption of the ingested food—indicates only the extent of absorption and does not enable us to judge of the length of time required for its digestion. Food which is completely absorbed leaves little residue and is likely to lead to constipation, while that which is poorly absorbed may (a) be subject to extensive bacterial action in the large intestine, (b) increase the rate of peristalsis, or (c) lead to the accumulation of large masses of food residues in the intestines. In a well-selected diet, foods which are completely digested are accompanied by some of those which are difficult of digestion, particularly foods low in protein and rich in cellulose, such as vegetables and fruits. In the treatment of pathological cases it is particularly necessary to take into consideration the degree of digestibility of the foods prescribed. The extent to which a food is absorbed depends quite as much upon the nature of food as does the ease of digestion. Foods that contain material in quantity which is not acted upon by the digestive enzymes are not only poorly absorbed but retard the digestion and absorption of other foods which are ordinarily completely digested and absorbed. The mode of preparation also influences the extent of absorption, for by its proper preparation connective tissue and cellulose structures are partially or completely hydrolyzed or disintegrated and thus become more readily and completely digested.

Conventional consideration of the relative digestibilities of various kinds of meat is based, then, upon data which are not entirely satisfactory. Clinical observation is an aid in determining the digestibility of food in its most general sense, but here there may be influences of personal idiosyncrasies as the result of pathological conditions in the patient under observation, and this is particularly true of protein foods. Some individuals show distinct reactions to certain foods. Many cases are known, however, in which the inability to eat eggs, fish or milk is a psychical factor and that the ingestion of such foods is not attended by metabolic disturbances.

In feeding persons whose condition necessitates prompt emptying of the stomach, food must be selected which will pass out readily, just as in certain intestinal diseases food must be taken in such a form that complete absorption occurs without extensive intestinal digestion or in which little residue results. These factors are discussed on p. 52. It seems to us that the method of the preparation and the consistency of the food are more important factors in the treatment of nutritional diseases in which a specific food substance is not involved, such as a specific idiosyncrasy or disease, than the selection of a few from among a number of foods compatible with the patient.

MEAT PREPARATIONS

Certain products prepared from meat, particularly from beef flesh, such as digested beef, beef juice, beef broth, beef extracts, and gelatin, contain less insoluble material than meat itself and are therefore held to be desirable not only for general use but for use in the sick-room and for convalescents. Such products are either readily soluble in water or yield fine aqueous suspensions. It is the possibility of furnishing protein or its digestion products in a fluid or soluble form which makes these preparations attractive for the special diets of therapeutics.

The nutritive value of meat preparations as compared with meat depends upon the mode of preparation. They are prepared from lean meat through the action of digestive enzymes, with the aid of heat, or by simple water extraction. Beef extract and some beef broths contain only small pro-

COMPOSITION OF TYPICAL MEAT PREPARATIONS (EXTRACTS, POWDERS, BROTHS).

| | Water. | Forms of nitrogen. | | | | | | | | | | Ash. | | |
| | | Total nitrogen. | Protein (coagulable nitrogen). | Ammonia nitrogen. | "Proteose² peptone." | Meat bases difference. | Meat bases. | | | | | Chlorine. | Phosphoric acid. | Potash. |
							Creatinine.	Creatine.	Purine.	Undetermined.	Total.			
Paste . . .	20.5	9.41	....	0.37	4.51	4.44	0.86	1.30	0.76	1.50	17.60	1.90	5.00	7.60
Extracts (fluid) .	42.0	4.01	0.10	0.42	1.50	1.99	0.43	0.48	0.35	0.72	21.60	6.80	2.70	5.50
Meat juice . .	55.7	3.13	....	0.26	0.90	1.92	0.22	0.13	0.37	1.20	11.60	0.90	2.70	5.20
Fluid proprietary preparations .	74.3¹	0.50	....	....	0.31	0.19	0.02	0.02	0.03	0.12	0.38	0.30	0.02	0.10
Beef powder .	11.2	12.64	0.05	0.14	12.20	0.26	0.00	Trace	0.04	0.23	6.10	0.02	1.47	0.13
Fresh beef . .	69.1	3.20	2.85	....	....		0.346	....	....	....	1.08			
Beef broth:														
Complete .	96.8	0.58	0.58	....	....	0.83		....	....	....	0.61			
Filtered . .	97.1	0.33	0.33	....	....	0.35		....	....	....	0.62			

¹ Contains alcohol, 12.52 per cent. by weight.
² Products non-coagulable and precipitated by tannin-salt, chiefly proteose, peptone and gelatin.
Compiled from Conn. Agr. Exp. Sta., Food Products Report, 1908, and Emmett and Gindley, loc. cit. Values of protein related substances are expressed in terms of nitrogen. Coagulable protein and the proteose-peptone can be expressed in their approximate protein equivalent by multiplying by 6.25. (See p. 164.)

portions of nutritive protein material, whereas cold pressed beef juice, gelatin, and broths prepared with gelatin-yielding meats and flesh in which the proteins have been partially digested are highly nutritious. The table on page 184 gives the comparative composition of such products.

Meat Extracts.—Beef extract, the most common meat extract, contains the water-soluble, non-coagulable substances in meat in a concentrated form. These consist essentially of non-protein, nitrogenous extractives such as creatine, purine bases, etc.; non-coagulable products of protein hydrolysis, amino-acids, proteoses, peptones, and gelatin, and the salts of muscle, a large proportion of which are salts of potassium and phosphoric acid; sodium chloride is sometimes added in the preparation of the extract. Extracts prepared from meat containing considerable quantities of connective tissue are more likely to contain greater quantities of gelatin. Gelatin, digested meat, and yeast extract are sometimes used as adulterants of meat extracts. Yeast extract is being used not only as an adulterant but also as a substitute for meat extract.

Meat extracts are particularly valuable as stimulants, for their salt content, and as flavoring materials for otherwise unpalatable dishes. The extractives of meat have been shown to stimulate the flow of the gastric juice: in this way they tend to increase the digestibility of foods. Extracts to which have been added gelatin or finely divided protein— made more or less soluble by digestion or solution in acid— increase the food value of such preparations. The use of beef juice is, from a nutritive point of view, to be preferred to such preparations.

Meat Juice.—Meat juice, particularly beef juice, is often prepared and used in the diet of the sick-room and for feeding infants. Such extracts are prepared by pressing out the water and soluble proteins from raw or half-broiled lean meat, preferably from finely divided meat. Preparations of this kind contain a certain proportion of the water soluble, coagulable proteins in addition to the ordinary extractives obtained by a method which involves heating to a temperature above the coagulation temperature of protein. They have, therefore, considerable nutritive value and may be used for the administration of protein in a liquid form.

Commercial preparations of meat juice can be obtained but they are never as satisfactory as the freshly prepared juice and broths.

Meat Broths.—Meat broths are of two kinds: (*a*) those that have been prepared by boiling beef, mutton, veal, chicken, etc., with water and straining off the protein material; (*b*) those prepared by extracting the juice from finely hashed meat with a small quantity of cold water, and expressing the water retained by the meat. The latter process removes a greater proportion of the soluble protein constituents of the meat and is therefore more economical. The product is, of course, more dilute than in the case of meat juice, above, but the greater proportion of protein it contains makes the two products comparable. The composition of the water extract varies of course with the quantity of water used. Such products contain from 2 to 5 per cent. of protein and a fraction of 1 per cent. of fat. (See table, p. 181.) Meat broths, method (*a*), are similar to meat extracts except that they have not been concentrated.

Beef tea is essentially beef broth which has been prepared according to the second method and carried to the boiling point to bring about the flocculent coagulation of the dissolved protein. This procedure is sometimes modified by slowly coagulating the proteins, extracted with cold water, with the finely divided meat after which the resultant liquid, including the flocculent coagulum and small particles of meat, is poured from the more solid residual meat. Beef tea contains approximately the same constituents as beef juice except that the soluble proteins are coagulated and a flavor has been developed by cooking. The finely divided coagulum is readily digestible.

Broths are often prepared by the slow cooking of meat containing considerable connective tissue and the liquid poured off without straining. Such preparations are intermediate between the ordinary broths and teas; they contain considerable gelatin.

Gelatin.—Gelatin is prepared from collagen-containing material, such as connective tissue, tendons, bones, etc., by hydrolysis with water (steam). A slight chemical change probably takes place in the formation of gelatin. The purified product is used for food, while impure gelatin is the basis of glue.

When gelatin is treated with water it swells. In hot water it forms a colloidal solution which sets as a jelly upon cooling. To such jelly-like masses fruits, fruit juices, etc., are added in the preparation of desserts. When heated with acid-containing substances gelatin is gradually hydrolyzed into non-gelatinizing material; this accounts for its failure to "jell" at times. Gelatin is also used in the manufacture of ice cream because of the smoothness it imparts to the finished product.

Gelatin differs chemically but little from the protein from which it is derived. The amino-acids, tryptophan and tyrosine, are not present, or at least they are present in very minute quantities; consequently gelatin cannot be used exclusively as the protein part of the diet. It has been shown, however, to be capable of replacing other protein to the extent of approximately 60 per cent. When taken with proteins rich in tryptophan or tyrosine it might replace an even greater proportion of other proteins.

CHAPTER X

FISH AND SHELL FISH—POULTRY AND GAME.

FISH AND SHELL FISH

FISH are an important and an economic source of protein. When properly prepared they are fully as palatable as meat and in many ways more delicate in texture. The short muscle fibers of fish, surrounded as they are by connective tissue which is readily hydrolyzed under the ordinary conditions of cooking, are easily broken apart, and this fact, together with their generally low fat content, has placed fish among the flesh foods which are easily digested. With the increasing facilities for cold storage and the realization that when properly stored fish show little change in their composition or in their palatability, they should become more widely used throughout the year than they now are.

A large number of fish are used for food; a choice between them is, largely, a matter of taste and economy. When consideration must be given to their digestibility, the fat content becomes the controlling factor, although such fish as cod and carp are held to be "coarser" than others. Variety in fish is not limited to those freshly caught, for processes of preservation have been so developed that fish may be had in many forms: those in which they approximate fresh fish in every way such as the cold storage and canned fish, or those that have been modified in texture or flavor, by drying, salting (dried or moist), smoking or preserving in oil.

Shell fish are another source of protein. They are not, however, as important economically as fish. The more important kinds of shell fish are (a) mollusks—oysters, clams, mussels, and scallops; (b) crustaceans—lobsters, crabs, shrimps, and crawfish. Shell fish are used more extensively as a delicacy than as a primary source of protein. Oysters, however, are often used as a means of modifying the diet of invalids, for they are held to be easily digested.

Fish differs from meat in its chemical composition particularly in the relative proportions of fat and water. The fattest of the fresh fish commonly used for food contain roughly the same proportion of fat as the lean cuts of meat (10 to 12 per cent. fat),[1] while the lean types of fish contain but a

---

[1] Certain cuts of meat, particularly the cheaper ones, are very low in fat, 1 or 2 per cent.

fraction of 1 per cent. of fat. Associated with this lower fat content of fish we find a higher percentage of water than in meat. Fish have in general, therefore, weight for weight, a lower caloric value than meat. The percentage of protein is approximately the same in both meat and fish, but it tends to be slightly higher in fish. When the extractives are omitted from our calculation the nitrogen value of fish and meat protein is essentially the same.

Our knowledge of the qualitative composition, particularly of the amino-acid content, of fresh fish is very limited. In general it appears to be quite similar to that of other kinds of flesh (see table, p. 165). Fish contain a relatively greater proportion of gelatin-yielding tissue, collagen, and a smaller proportion of extractives than do meats.

The fat of fish is relatively richer in the low melting-point fats; it has more of the properties of oils than of "fat" as we ordinarily think of fat.

Carbohydrate is present as glycogen in considerable amounts in certain of the fish foods—oysters, clams, scallops. It is the glycogen which is in part responsible for the opalescence of the liquor which surrounds oysters.

The following table contains the composition of certain of the more common varieties of fish arranged according to their fat content.

COMPOSITION OF TYPICAL FISH (EDIBLE PORTION).

LOW IN FAT.

Kind.	Water, per cent.	Protein N x 6.25, per cent.	Fat, per cent.	Ash, per cent.	Fuel value per pound, Calories.
Bass	76.7	20.6	1.7	1.2	455
Blue fish	78.5	19.4	1.2	1.3	410
Cod	82.6	16.5	0.4	1.2	325
Flounder	84.2	14.2	0.6	1.3	290
Trout (brook)	77.8	19.2	2.1	1.2	445
Weakfish	79.0	17.8	2.4	1.2	430

HIGH IN FAT.

Kind.	Water, per cent.	Protein N x 6.25, per cent.	Fat, per cent.	Ash, per cent.	Fuel value per pound, Calories.
Butter fish	70.0	18.0	11.0	1.2	800
Halibut	75.4	18.6	5.2	1.0	565
Herring	72.5	19.5	7.1	1.5	660
Mackerel	73.4	18.7	7.1	1.2	645
Salmon	64.6	22.0	12.8	1.4	950
Shad	70.6	18.8	9.5	1.3	750
White fish	69.8	22.9	6.5	1.6	700

This classification is based, in some cases, upon the analysis of but one or two fish, and it must be remembered that the fat content of fish varies at the time of spawning, different seasons of the year, and with changes in feeding conditions. Fish are found to have deposited the maximum amount of fat just before the spawning season and to have a minimum fat content a few weeks afterward. Analyses of shad,[1] a comparatively fat fish, illustrate this point.

	Fat wet basis, per cent.
Shad, roe not very ripe, April 2	14.43
Shad, roe ripe, April 13	13.93
Shad, roe ready to spawn, May 22	5.87
Shad, after spawning, June 19	2.95

The same variations have been found to hold for salmon. The spawning season for shad is early in April and that for king salmon about August and September. The food supply also affects the composition of fish; when forced away from their accustomed feeding grounds by storms or natural enemies, they often arrive on our shores in a very lean condition.

The following table indicates the time of year in which fish are in season.

FISH AND SEA FOODS IN SEASON.

Variety.	Season.
Black bass.	All year.
Blue fish.	April to December.
Blue points (shell oysters).	September to May.
Buffalo.	All year (except in time of low water).
Butter fish.	March to December.
Cod.	All year.
Cape Cod (large shell oysters).	September to May.
Crappie.	All year.
Cat, channel.	All year.
Cat, bull head.	All year.
Cat, slicing (spoonbills).	All year.
Ciscoes (white).	March to November.
Carp.	All year (except in time of low water).
Crab meat.	All year.
Crab flakes.	All year.
Crabs, hard shell.	All year (best season April to October).
Crabs, soft shell.	March to October.
Clams, bulk.	All year.
Clams, shell and soft.	All year.
Crawfish.	April to November.
Eels.	All year (scarce during winter).
Frogs.	February to October.
Flounders.	All year.
Grass pike.	All year.
Halibut.	All year (more plentiful in summer).
Haddock.	All year.
Jack salmon.	February to November.
Lobsters.	All year.
Mackerel, Spanish.	May, June, October, November, December.
Oysters.	September to May.
Pompano.	May, June, October, November, December.
Perch, yellow.	All year.
Perch, white.	All year.

[1] Clark and Almy: U. S. Dept. Agr., 1917.

FISH AND SEA FOODS IN SEASON—(Continued).

Variety.	Season.
Roe, shad.	January to September.
Red snapper.	All year (except in stormy weather).
Salmon, California.	March to December.
Salmon, silver.	March to December.
Smelts.	November to June.
Sun fish.	All year.
Shrimp, fresh.	September to December; March to July.
Shad.	January to September.
Scallops.	October to May.
Turtle, soft shell.	All year.
Trout.	April to February.
White fish.	April to December.

The restriction of the fishing industry to certain seasons of the year and the difficulties of shipping have resulted in the extensive preservation of fish.

Cold Storage Fish.—Fish are frozen and placed in cold storage in this condition (dry packed) or coated with ice. It has been found that fish placed in cold storage soon after they were caught and analyzed later, shortly after removal from the refrigerating plant, showed practically no change which could be detected chemically. Results of investigations of refrigeration in general indicate, however, that food kept in cold storage undergoes a slight modification which is not of a harmful nature. Studies of the palatability of cold storage fish as compared with fresh fish have showtn tha where the subjects were entirely unbiased, cold storage and fresh fish were practically indistinguishable. We may conclude, therefore, that cold storage fish which have not been kept in the market for more than a day or two are fully as palatable as fresh fish.

Preserved Fish.—Canned fish are subjected to the usual process of cooking in the can and sterilizing. With the care observed at present in canning fish this form of preservation is most satisfactory. The flesh retains most of the characteristics of cold, cooked, fresh fish. Some fish, particularly sardines, are preserved in oil or mustard sauce. In this method of canning, the fish are pickled in brine to toughen them and to add flavor, cooked with steam, dried, and finally packed. In the preparation of dried fish the drying is accomplished by the use of salt, by pressure, or by simply drying in the sun or artificially. Dried cod fish are used to a considerable extent and are often sold in a shredded form. Preserved fish are held to be less readily digested than fresh fish.

Cooking of Fish.—Fish flesh is rich in connective tissue. The process of cooking hydrolyzes this with the result that the short muscle bundles and fibers are easily separated.

Fish is often boiled in water acidulated with vinegar or lemon juice, which tends to toughen the fibers and to coagulate the protein on the outside portions and thus keep the fish intact. Other processes are employed to the same end, such as slow, quiet boiling and wrapping in cloth.

Digestibility of Fish.—Fish are as thoroughly digested as other types of flesh food and meats. Estimations of its digestibility show that the protein is absorbed to the extent of approximately 96 per cent. and fats 97 per cent. There is practically no carbohydrate. Considered from the point of view of the ease of digestibility, fish, particularly the lean fish, are held to be more readily digested than the lean meats, while the fat fish are of the same digestibility as fat meats. Cooked fish is more easily masticated and consequently more rapidly digested than meat. Oysters are fully as digestible as lean fish.

Comparative studies of the digestibility of certain types of fish in which the rate of nitrogen excretion and retention of nitrogen are taken as indices of digestibility showed that absorption appeared to be most rapid in the following order: Boiled meats—fresh cod, beef, tantog, eel, weak fish, mussel, salt cod, periwinkle. When the quantity of nitrogen retained was considered, the order was reversed. Comparison of freshly boiled or fried cod and salt cod showed in general that while the fish prepared by the former method of preparation was absorbed more rapidly it was not retained as well as the latter. Such data indicate that foods which are absorbed at a slower rate furnish the body with protein over a longer period of time, the excess at any moment is not so great and consequently the body retains a greater proportion for its use. From these facts it would appear that fish is fully as digestible as meat, and, when we consider that it is poorer in fat than meat and that the fat of fish has a lower melting-point than that of meat, it would seem that fish should be, perhaps, more readily digested than most meats.

POULTRY AND GAME

Poultry differs but little in its composition from other types of meat. It has in many cases a more delicate flavor and the fibers of the flesh are, to a certain extent, more tender. Its place in the diet is in the nature of a delicacy rather than as a staple form of food.

The greater ease of digestibility attributed to poultry is to be ascribed to tradition more than to fact. Young poultry is comparatively low in fat and for that reason undoubtedly passes more rapidly from the stomach than foods containing a greater proportion of fat. Poultry rich in fat, as the goose or duck, are, in this respect, much less digestible than chicken or turkey. The tenderness of the cooked flesh and the ease with which it is masticated, because of the short fibers, also contribute toward ease of digestion. Studies of the utilization of poultry show, however, that it is not any more completely absorbed in the course of normal digestion than other kinds of flesh, nor does it pass more readily from the stomach than lean meats.

The low purine content attributed to the flesh of poultry as compared with other meats has been shown to be erroneous, for beef and mutton contain very little more purine than chicken. The extractive nitrogen in the white muscle has been shown to be higher than that of red muscle. Tables showing the composition of poultry are to be found on page 177.

13

CHAPTER XI.

EGGS AND CHEESE.

EGGS

THE egg occupies as does milk, an important place in the human dietary. It belongs primarily with protein foods—although by simple mechanical separation it may be divided into a portion containing protein, egg white, and into a portion rich in lipins, or fat, egg yolk. The protein of egg is of good quality. The yolk is particularly rich in fat-soluble A and water-soluble B but deficient in the anti-scorbutic vitamine.

The egg is prepared for the development of the fertilized embryo up to the time that a fully formed chick is capable of breaking the shell and continuing its growth with food obtained by its own effort. The nutritive material for this restricted growth, which includes the formation of the skeletal, muscular, and organic systems as well as the maintenance of the growing tissues, is contained in the yolk, white, and shell. Its constituents are therefore both highly nutritious and concentrated; its dietary usefulness is self-evident.

Eggs are important not only as a simple food, but also as an essential constituent of certain prepared foods—cakes, custards, and confectionery.

Since eggs[1] contain quantities of iron and calcium and are also easily digested, they are a desirable supplementary food for young children, and an acceptable food for convalescents and invalids.

The egg consists grossly of three parts—shell, white and yolk. The relative proportion of these in the egg varies somewhat with different breeds of hens; in general they are shell, 11 per cent.; yolk, 32 per cent.; and white, 57 per cent. of the total weight of the egg. These parts may be mechanically separated with relative ease. Only the white and yolk are used for food. The average weight of the edible portion of an egg is 50 grams.

The following table gives the composition of the various parts of the hen's egg.

---

[1] In this discussion we restrict our remarks to the egg of the hen, unless otherwise stated. The egg of the duck, goose, turkey, guinea fowl, many wild fowl, and certain amphibians, as turtle and alligator, are used for food, but seldom to the extent to which the hen's egg is utilized. Their properties are very similar.

COMPARATIVE COMPOSITION OF THE EDIBLE PORTIONS OF THE EGG.[1]

Constituents.	Edible portion (whole egg), per cent.	White, per cent.	Yolk, per cent.
Water	73.7	86.2	49.5
Protein	13.4	12.3	15.7
Fat	10.5	0.2	33.3
Ash	1.0	0.6	1.1
Potassium, K_2O	0.165	0.19	0.13
Sodium, Na_2O	0.2	0.21	0.1
Calcium, CaO	0.093	0.015	0.2
Magnesium, MgO	0.015	0.015	0.02
Phosphorus, P_2O_5	0.37	0.03	1.0
Chlorine, Cl	0.10	0.15	0.1
Sulphur, S	0.19	0.20	0.16
Iron, Fe	0.003	0.0001	0.0085
Weight of average egg, grams	50.0	33.0	17.0
Weight of average egg, ounces	1.8	1.2	0.6
Fuel value, average egg, calories	74.0	17.0	60.0
Weight, 100-Calorie portion, grams	68.0	194.0	28.0

Egg White.—Egg white, when raw, is a viscous, semiliquid mass having a slightly greenish tinge and practically no flavor; the reaction of the egg, when fresh, is very slightly alkaline. It consists almost entirely of protein, water and salts; though a small amount of carbohydrate is present. Water predominates, as it does in all animal tissue or products. There are several proteins in egg "albumen," ovalbumin, conalbumin, ovoglobulin, ovomucin, and ovomucoid. The albumins which predominate and comprise approximately 90 per cent. of the total protein are similar in composition. They differ in their ability to crystallize from a solution of ammonium sulphate. Ovoglobulin exists to the extent of about 6.5 per cent. of the total protein; it is probably not an individual protein but a compound. The glycoproteins, mucin and ovomucoid, are present in small amounts. Egg white is practically free from fat. The inorganic constituents of the egg white are chiefly phosphorus and calcium. The sulphur in albumen is the source of the hydrogen sulphide in the spoiled egg.

Egg Yolk.—Egg yolk is particularly rich in lipins (fats and lipoids). The relatively high caloric value of egg yolk, approximately seven times that of egg white, is to be ascribed to its lipin content. The lipin constitutes approximately 20 per cent. of the solid constituents of the yolk. The glycerides of palmitic acid, 38 per cent.; stearic acid, 15 per cent.; and oleic acid, 40 per cent., are the principal fats present. Of the lipoids, lecithin is present to the extent of

[1] Compiled from Sherman: Food Products, 1914.

approximately 11 per cent. and cholesterol 1.5 per cent. The composition of egg fat varies with the diet of the hen; certain characteristics of ingested food are often transferred to the egg and modify the color, odor, or taste. The color of eggs particularly varies with the nature of the ingested food; green vegetables, etc., tend to produce a darker colored yolk than do other foods. The feeding of fish affects the taste of eggs and it has been shown that benzoic acid when fed to hens appears in the egg. The lipins exist in egg yolk as a fine emulsion. The low melting-point of egg fat and the fact that the fat is highly emulsified make the yolk easy to digest and therefore valuable as a food for the sick.

Of the proteins in egg yolk, the phosphoprotein, vitellin, is the most important. It has been shown that vitellin exists in the yolk as a lecithin-nucleovitellin compound or mixture containing from 15 to 30 per cent. of lecthin combined with a lecthin-free substance which has been designated nucleovitellin. Purine bases are practically absent from the egg; they are contained only in the nucleus of the yolk.

Eggs and particularly egg yolk are a good source of phosphorus, iron, and calcium. The phosphorus occurs almost entirely as organic phosphorus—lecithin and vitellin; certain other phosphorus-containing lipoids are also present. Iron is in organic combination. It exists in a complex molecule which contains in addition to carbon, hydrogen, oxygen, and nitrogen: iron, 0.455 per cent.; calcium, 0.352 per cent.; and magnesium, 0.126 per cent. This compound has been called hematogen because it is supposed to be the precursor of hemoglobin. The composition of the compound has not been found to be the same under different methods of preparation; it may be a mixture of substances. The ash of egg is predominantly acidic.

The table on page 195 shows the quantity of the more important mineral constituents of egg in the percentage of the total ash.

Cooking of Eggs.—Eggs are prepared for the table by boiling in the shell, dropping into hot water (poaching), or frying over a hot plate. The degree of coagulation of both white and yolk in boiled eggs is a matter of great personal taste and habit. There are three average degrees of hardness to which an egg may be boiled—*soft-cooked*, in which the white resembles a soft, thick curd and the yolk is fluid; *medium-cooked*, in which the white is firmer though still soft and tender, and the yolk is thickened, and *hard-cooked*, in which both the white and yolk are completely coagulated and quite firm. A certain flavor is developed upon cooking which is best in the medium-cooked egg. Of the three methods of boiling eggs: cooking in continuously boiling water for a certain length of time; or placing in cold water and bringing it to a boil; or placing in boiling water which is no longer heated, the last, which involves cooking below the boiling point, is the best, both for the consistency of the white and yolk and, as we shall see, for its digestibility. With this procedure the texture of the egg can be readily controlled. It has been found that an egg taken from the ice-chest, when placed in one pint of water, in a quart stew pan, which has been brought to a boil over a gas flame and allowed to remain six minutes was soft-cooked; the temperature of the water dropped from (212° F.) the temperature of boiling water to 185° F. upon the addition of the egg, and then steadily to 170°F. If the egg remained in the water eight minutes it was medium-cooked and the temperature of the water had fallen to 162° to 164° F. These data relate to one egg. For a greater number of eggs the amount of water must be increased proportionately or the time lengthened. A little experience will fix the time required for conditions which differ from those outlined above.

Poached eggs are similar in consistency to boiled eggs. In this case the yolk and white are coagulated in the water instead of in the shell and there is undoubtedly a slight but negligible loss of mineral matter.

Fried eggs are cooked at a relatively high temperature with the use of fat of some kind, factors which increase the flavor of the eggs but which tend to decrease the ease with which they are digested.

The function of the egg in cakes, in addition to its fuel value, is to ensure lightness. Egg protein plays the most important role in the process. As the result of whipping or beating fine bubbles of air are incorporated into the viscous egg. When this beaten mass is mixed with the other ingredients and cooked, the expansion of these air bubbles and other gas bubbles formed by the leavening agents and the coagulation of the surrounding protein produce the comb-like structure indicative of "lightness" in such foods.

Digestibility of Eggs.—From a quantitative point of view egg protein is as digestible as meat or milk protein; the protein and fat of eggs show a high degree of absorbability. Egg white, raw or soft-boiled when fed alone tends to leave the stomach more rapidly than other protein material. Raw egg white has been observed to begin to pass from the stomach, without becoming acidified, almost immediately after ingestion. Later the remaining food becomes acid and passes out more slowly. It is interesting in this connection to know that raw egg white does not excite the flow of the gastric juice any more than water does.

Cooked egg white passes from the stomach at a rate which appears to depend more upon its consistency than on the extent to which it is cooked. Particles of "hard-boiled" eggs leave at a slower rate than soft-boiled eggs, although thorough mastication tends to increase the rate of evacuation.

In a comparative study of the digestibility of eggs cooked in various ways it was found that eggs when eaten raw, or after being soft or hard-boiled had completely left the stomach at the end of periods as follows:

Raw	1 hour, 10 minutes
Soft-boiled	1½ hours
Hard-boiled	2½ hours

The amount of gastric juice poured out in each case was:

Raw	399 c.c.
Soft-boiled	372 c.c.
Hard-boiled	481 c.c.

While raw egg leaves the stomach much more rapidly than soft-boiled egg it has been repeatedly shown that it is not so rapidly or completely digested in a given time in the stomach or upper part of the small intestine as soft-boiled eggs. Large quantities of raw egg white may cause diarrhea. The indigestibility of raw egg white is related to its chemical constitution, or perhaps to the presence of antitrypsin, than to its physical texture. When considered on the basis of the rate of elimination of nitrogen, raw and hard-boiled eggs are not as rapidly absorbed as other protein substances, e. g., meat, gelatin, or casein. This has been ascribed for raw egg to the short time which it stays in the stomach and to the possibility that its digestion is difficult in the intestine. In the case of coagulated egg white the slowness of absorption has been ascribed to the compactness and impermeable character of the particles.

Preserved Eggs.—The fact that a greater number of eggs are produced at certain seasons of the year than at others has led to the practise of storing them in the refrigerator and otherwise preserving them in salt, water-glass, etc., and by desiccation and freezing. Eggs kept in cold storage change slightly, as do all cold storage products according to the length of time they are kept there. They gradually develop a taste and odor different from that of a fresh egg. Water passes from the white to the yolk with a resultant increase in the size of the yolk and, if the increase be sufficiently great, the yolk membrane is weakened or ruptured. Moisture is lost through evaporation. There is an alteration in the properties of the white, upon which its value for cooking depends, perhaps as the result of autolysis. These changes do not develop sufficiently in a period of a month or six weeks to alter the characteristics of the egg from those of a moderately fresh egg. Eggs kept for a greater time show proportionately greater change.

One of the most important objections to cold-storage eggs is that they are usually sold for fresh eggs. Good cold-storage eggs are very useful in cooking and are often nearly as palatable as fresh eggs. When eggs are sold as "cold-storage" eggs they are an important economic factor in the diet. Present methods of rapid drying yield dried-egg preparations which are satisfactory for cooking and general use where the intrinsic character of fresh eggs is not an essential consideration. The objection to dried eggs has been that they are sometimes prepared from decayed eggs. When it is known that they are properly prepared from fresh eggs they are satisfactory for use as indicated above.

Egg Substitutes.—Preparations which consist of some form of protein and a small amount of coloring matter are placed on the market as substitutes for eggs. Custard powders are offered which are essentially starch and seldom contain egg and often no protein.

CHEESE.

Cheese is a preparation made from milk or cream by coagulating the caseinogen with rennin. The casein thus formed is subjected to the action of bacteria, moulds or enzymes which "ripen" the cheese, producing changes in the flavor, consistency, and composition of the product. Cheese, without any designation to indicate a modification, contains approximately one-third each of water, protein, and fat; that is, roughly, 50 per cent. of the solid matter is butter fat. The designations, "cream," "full cream," "whole milk," and "milk," although used more or less interchangeably in this country, indicate that the cheese is made from whole milk or sometimes from milk and cream. Some cheeses are made from skimmed milk "filled" with fat other than butter fat, as lard, cotton-seed oil, etc. Goat's milk is sometimes used in preparing cheese, The greater proportion of American cheeses are, however, made from cow's milk. Cheese, from the mode of preparation, is then a combination of the greater portion of the protein, caesinogen and the fat of milk. It contains a large proportion of calcium and phosphorus combined with the casein and a smaller proportion of the other salts and lactose present in milk; salt (sodium chloride) is added in the process of manufacture of cheese.

There are two types of cheese: the hard cheeses of the Cheddar, "American cheese," type (Cheddar, Edam, Emmental (Swiss), Parmesan, and Roquefort) and the soft cheeses (brie, camembert, gorganzola, Limberg, Neufchatel, and Stilton). These cheeses vary in their consistency and flavor according to the manner of preparation. Cottage cheese is a term applied to "unripened" casein and is usually prepared at home from sour milk, although it can be obtained from dairies in many cases.

In the process of ripening there is an increase in the soluble protein (proteose, peptone and amino-acids), indicating a partial digestion of the protein; while the fat is not so completely emulsified as in milk, it does not appear to undergo any extensive modification.

The composition of cheeses of various fat content in comparison with other milk products is given on page 152.

Digestibility of Cheese.—Cheese is as completely utilized as other protein foods. Its digestibility has been shown to be approximately equal to that of meat, eggs, etc. The general opinion that cheese is indigestible is due to the fact that the casein of cheese is associated roughly with an equal quantity of fat which tends to prolong its stay in the stomach and that the volatile fatty acids and certain of the protein cleavage products formed during the ripening process may be irritating to the stomach. Careful chewing of cheese when eaten alone should increase the "ease" of digestibility, for the finely divided particles will tend to leave the stomach more rapidly than the larger pieces of cheese.

Cheese should be served with starchy foods and vegetables, for it is rich in protein and fat and very poor in carbohydrate. When so served it is a most desirable article of diet. Since cheese is comparatively cheap it may be used to advantage in the variation of the protein part of the diet in place of meat and fish.

Casein Preparations.—A number of specially prepared foods can be obtained whose base is chiefly casein. These may be the dried calcium caseinate obtained from milk with additional food-stuffs, or the water soluble salt, or salts of the stronger alkalies, sodium or potassium; glycerophosphates are sometimes added. The nutritive value of these preparations is approximately that of casein. The therapeutic value which is claimed for many of them is probably overestimated for the same quantity of casein taken as milk or freshly coagulated skimmed milk or even as soft cheese (cottage cheese) undoubtedly possess all the advantages of these preparations and in addition the constituents of milk, fat, salts, lactose, and accessory substances, which have been shown to be in many ways desirable. The prepared products are desirable in diets which are too low in fat and sugar, or where the protein content is to be increased without an increase in bulk. For further discussion, see section on Clinical Dietetics.

CHAPTER XII.
PROTEIN–RICH VEGETABLE FOODS.

LEGUMES

CERTAIN vegetable foods, particularly the legumes, are rich in protein, and are at the same time comparatively poor in carbohydrate; others, such as nuts, contain considerable quantities of fat. It is desirable to classify these foods as protein-rich foods. The grains, wheat, barley, oats, corn, etc., are likewise comparatively rich in protein (10 to 12 per cent.). Carbohydrate predominates, however, and this fact together with the place of these foods in the average diet, serves to differentiate them into the class of carbohydrate foods. The legumes and nuts are preserved in a semidried state in which they may be kept almost indefinitely. Their low water content and comparatively high protein content make them a valuable source of protein when transportation is a problem, as in hunting and campaigning in war. These foods are relatively cheap and are therefore a valuable source of protein in diets of low cost.

The legumes are of lower biological value when used as the chief constituent of the diet; their proteins are of lower value than those of milk; they are relatively poor in fat-soluble A and the anti-scorbutic vitamine, and they are poor in calcium, sodium and chlorine. When corrected for these deficiencies by the inclusion of the proper foods the legumes are a valuable and economical constituent of the diet.

The vegetable and animal proteins are in many ways similar in both their physical and chemical properties. In general, vegetable proteins yield more glutamic acid and in some cases proline, arginine and ammonia than do the animal proteins. Many of them are deficient in one or more essential amino-acids but they do not differ in this respect from certain animal proteins (gelatin). In seeds, the form of vegetable protein food with which we are particularly concerned, most of the protein is found in the endosperm, as reserve protein surrounding the embryo. Proteins of the globulin, glutelin and prolamine type predominate in the endosperm. Legumes are particularly rich in globulins, the legumins. These proteins form salts with calcium which are insoluble in water. It is the formation of these com-

202

pounds which accounts for the difficulty encountered in cooking peas and beans in hard water—the failure to soften. The use of water poor in calcium, as distilled water, or water softened with sodium carbonate, overcomes the difficulty. In addition to these proteins the embryo contains others which are more varied in character and apparently similar to the physiologically active animal proteins, as albumin, nucleoprotein. The following proteins have been found by Osborne to be present in wheat:

	Spring wheat, per cent.	Winter wheat, per cent.
Glutenin	4.68	4.17
Gliadin	3.96	3.90
Globulin	0.62	0.63
Albumin	0.39	0.36
Proteose	0.21	0.43

It is from the nucleoprotein in the embryo that the greater proportion of the small amount of purine bases contained in the legumes and nuts is obtained. The following table gives the quantity of purine bases in certain of these foods.

PURINE BASES IN VEGETABLE FOODS.

Practically absent.	Present percentage of purine base nitrogen.	
White bread	Oatmeal	0.021
Rice	Pea meal	0.016
Tapioca	Beans	0.025
Cabbage	Lentils	0.025
Lettuce	Potatoes	0.0008
Cauliflower	Onions	0.0031
	Asparagus (cooked)	0.0086

The difference in composition between fresh and dried legumes is to be ascribed to variations in the water content. Fresh shelled beans and peas contain a large proportion of water. The removal of water in drying is accompanied by a relative increase in the nutritive constituents. The table on page 240 gives the composition of typical fresh and dried legumes rich in protein.

In the preparation of the dry legumes for consumption a considerable amount of the water lost in drying is restored, thus yielding a food of considerable bulk in proportion to its protein content. This comparatively large bulk of legumes which must be ingested to furnish the requisite amount of protein constitutes one of the chief objections to a vegetarian diet.

The fat content of legumes is low. There are, however, one or two exceptions; soy beans and peanuts are comparatively rich in fat. Accompanying the high fat content of these legumes we note a smaller proportion of carbohydrate.

The legumes have a relatively high ash content.   Potassium, phosphate, and iron are abundant: the proportions of these and of other ash constituents will be found below.

COMPARATIVE COMPOSITION OF PROTEIN-RICH VEGETABLE FOOD WITH OTHER FOODS (EDIBLE PORTION).

	Water, per cent.	Protein (N x 6.25), per cent.	Fat, per cent.	Carbo-hydrate, per cent.	Calories per pound.	100-Calorie portion, gm.
Legumes, dried .	12.6	22.5	1.8	59.6	1567	29
Legumes, fresh .	68.5	7.1	0.7	22.0	557	82
Nuts . . .	2.4	18.4	64.4	13.0	3182	14
Cereals . . .	12.0	11.4	1.0	75.1	1610	28
Lean meat . .	70.0	21.3	7.9	. .	652	64
Dried beef . .	54.3	30.0	6.5	0.4	840	56
Fish, lean . .	75.4	18.6	5.2	. .	550	83
Milk . . .	87.1	3.3	4.0	5.0	314	145
Cheese . . .	35.0	27.7	36.8	4.1	2080	22
Eggs . . .	73.7	13.4	10.5	. .	672	68

Soy Bean.—The soy bean is particularly rich in protein, contains a high percentage of fat, and is poor in carbohydrate. The sugar content is relatively high.   In China and Japan the soy bean is prepared in various ways in the form of cheeses and sauces in which the beans are cooked, mixed with various grains and subjected to the action of bacteria—shoyu, natto, miso—or precipitated and, after removing most of the water, pressed into cakes or tablets (tofu).   Because of its low starch and high fat and protein content the soy bean has assumed an important place in the diet of the diabetic.   The carbohydrate is chiefly in the form of sucrose, hemicellulose, and cellulose.   The following data give the result of the analysis of a soy bean:

SOY BEAN (HOLLYBROOK).[1]

	Per cent.
Water	12.67
Ash	4.64
Protein (N x 6.25)	36.69
Ether extract	14.92
Nitrogen-free extract	31.08

CONSTITUENTS IN NITROGEN-FREE EXTRACT.

Galactan	4.86
Pentosan	4.94
Raffinose	1.13
Starch	0.50
Cellulose	3.29
Undetermined hemicelluloses	0.04
Dextrin	3.14
Sucrose	3.31
Invert sugar	0.07
Organic acids (as citric)	1.44
Waxes, color principles, tannins, etc. (by difference) . . .	8.60

[1] Street and Bailey: Jour. Ind. and Eng. Chem., 1915, vii, 853.

The quantity of sucrose and starch present in the soy bean varies chiefly with the manner in which the bean is allowed to ripen or the time at which it is gathered. Those which are not permitted to ripen thoroughly or which are allowed to ripen after the vine is cut are more likely to contain starch than others. Beans which are permitted to become thoroughly ripe are practically free from starch.

Peanut.—The peanut, like the soy bean, is rich in protein and fat and poor in carbohydrate, and is therefore a most satisfactory diabetic food. Peanut butter, prepared from peanuts by grinding, is even richer in protein and fat than the untreated peanut itself.

Preparation of Legumes.—Legumes are prepared for the table by boiling in water, baking, or roasting. Partially broken or ground into flour the legumes are used in soups: split-pea soup, for example, is a most palatable and nutritious dish. The effect of cooking legumes is to soften the cellulose structures, hydrate the starch, coagulate the protein and develop flavor. Fresh peas and beans are cooked without other preparation than the removal of their pods. Since the cellulose is still soft, the time required for cooking is comparatively short. Dried legumes, however, must be soaked in water, swollen, before they are cooked, and, because of the hardened condition of the cellulose must be heated for a long time to ensure the complete softening of the cellulose and the rupture of the starch granules. Soaking of dried legumes in some cases permits the removal of the indigestible skin surrounding the bean or pea. Certain bitter constituents are also removed in the soaking process. To prevent the formation of insoluble calcium-protein compounds, which occurs when hard water is used, legumes should be soaked and cooked in soft or distilled water.

The digestibility of dried legumes, even after cooking, is slightly lower than that of the flesh foods. Digestion experiments show that while the carbohydrate and fat—usually added to them in preparation—are readily digested and absorbed, the protein is not completely digested; the degree of digestion is estimated at approximately 80 per cent. for legumes, as compared with 95 per cent. for meat. That the low digestibility of legumes is due largely to the cellulose structures which prevent digestion and absorption is shown by the greater digestibility of the cooked food and the fact that the protein of finely ground legumes is practically as well absorbed as meat protein.

The general contention that legumes are indigestible has been ascribed to the consciousness of the digestive processes experienced following the ingestion of these foods. Such indications are heightened in some people by the flatulence which often occurs during digestion. The economic importance and food value of legumes have been discussed on page 145.

Nuts.—Nuts are seldom used as a staple article of diet. They might well be so used, for they are particularly rich in both protein and fat. Studies of the digestibility of nuts are few. It has been shown that in a fruit-and-nut diet the food constituents are practically as digestible as those of a mixed diet.

DIGESTIBILITY OF FRUITS AND NUTS.

	Fruits and nuts.	Mixed diet.
Protein	90	94
Fat	85	92
Starch and sugar	96	96
Crude fiber	54	49
Ash	68	
Energy	86	88

The protein is, however, slightly less digestible. Nuts are generally held to be, physically, indigestible because they often produce a feeling of discomfort upon ingestion. This is no doubt largely due to excessive ingestion and poor mastication. The high fat content of nuts will tend to retard the passage of food from the stomach and this delay may also be a contributing factor to the conception of indigestibility. When eaten properly, nuts are a digestible and valuable food. A diet of nuts and cereals and vegetables has recently been shown to be a satisfactory diet for the production of milk by women. The accompanying table gives the composition of the more important nuts.

COMPOSITION OF TYPICAL FRUITS AND NUTS (EDIBLE PORTION).

	Water, per cent.	Protein (N x 6.25), per cent.	Fat, per cent.	Carbohydrate, per cent.	Calories per pound.	100-Calorie portion, gm.
Almonds	4.8	21.0	54.9	17.3	2940	15
Brazil nuts	5.3	17.0	66.8	7.0	3162	15
Chestnuts, fresh	45.0	6.2	5.4	42.1	1097	43
Chestnuts, dried	5.9	10.7	7.0	74.2	1828	25
Cocoanut	14.1	5.7	50.6	27.9	2675	17
Hickory nuts	3.7	15.4	67.4	11.4	3238	14
Peanuts[1]	9.2	25.8	38.6	24.4	2490	18
Pecans	2.7	9.6	70.5	15.3	3330	14
Walnuts, California	2.5	18.4	64.4	13.0	3200	14

[1] Legume

CHAPTER XIII.

CARBOHYDRATE–RICH FOODS.

CARBOHYDRATES are one of the two important classes of energy-yielding food-stuffs. Studies of the respiratory quotient of men have demonstrated repeatedly that when the body has a choice between fat and carbohydrate to be used in the production of energy or work, particularly when there is a sudden call upon the body resources, carbohydrate (glucose) is the first to be utilized and, when this is gone, the fats. When carbohydrates are entirely lacking in the diet, or have been withdrawn from the body, marked disturbances in metabolism occur, particularly in fat metabolism. The chief disturbance is evidenced by an incomplete oxidation of the fats, resulting in a condition known as acidosis. The evidence is, for man at least, that carbohydrate is essential to the normal continuance of body functions, and that when this is not supplied in the food, it must be formed from protein.

In considering carbohydrate foods we will include those foods in which carbohydrates predominate. Such a classification includes some foods, such as cereals, which are comparatively rich in protein; their chief place in the diet is, however, as a source of carbohydrate. This classification also excludes the legumes which contain a rather large proportion of carbohydrate, but their place in the diet justifies their classification with the protein-rich foods. The potato and banana will also be considered here, for even though they might be classed with the succulent vegetables and fruits, they serve as valuable sources of carbohydrate.

For dietetic purposes, carbohydrates are quite often classified as sugars, starches, and cellulose. Such a division is sufficient for most practical purposes; it does not, however, serve for differentiation on the basis of their chemical composition. The following classification is based upon the relative complexity of the carbohydrate molecule:

I. Monosaccharides.
1. Pentoses, $C_5H_{10}O_5$: (a) Arabinose; (b) xylose (c) rhamnose (methyl-pentose), $C_6H_{12}O_5$.
2. Hexoses, $C_6H_{12}O_6$: (a) Glucose; (b) frutose; (c) galactose.

II. Disaccharides, $C_{11}H_{22}O_{11}$: (1) Maltose; (2) lactose; (3) isomaltose; (4) sucrose.

III. Trisaccharides, $C_{11}H_{1}O_{16}$: (1) Raffinose.

IV. Polysaccharides $(C_6H_{10}O_5)_x$: (1) Gum and vegetable mucilage group: (a) Dextrin; (b) vegetable gums. (2) Starch group: (a) Starch; (b) inulin; (c) glycogen; (d) lichnin. (3) Hemicellulose group: (a) Cellulose; (b) hemicellulose. (1) Pentosans, gum arabic; (2) Hexosans, galactans, agar agar.

The carbohydrates of particular dietetic importance are the monosaccharides, having six carbon atoms, the hexoses, or compounds whose molecules are multiples of these, such as the starches.

SUGARS.

The term sugar is, by convention applied to the disaccharide sucrose obtained chiefly from the juice of the sugar-cane, sugar-beet, and maple tree. Other simple mono- and disaccharides, such as glucose (dextrose or grape-sugar), fructose (levulose or fruit-sugar), lactose (milk-sugar), maltose (barley or malt-sugar) are also classed among the sugars. The sweetness of various fruits and vegetables is due either to sugar, its products of hydrolysis or a combination of these. Unless it is specifically defined or inferred, the term sugar applies, in the following discussion, only to sucrose.

Sucrose.—Sugar (cane-sugar, beet-sugar, sucrose) is widely distributed in the vegetable kingdom. Upon digestion or hydrolysis it yields one molecule each of fructose and glucose. The combined effect of these two sugars upon polarized light is to rotate it in the opposite direction from that produced by the solution of sucrose from which it was obtained. For this reason the hydrolyzed mixture is called invert sugar.

The sugar of commerce is obtained almost exclusively from the sugar-cane and the sugar-beet. There is often a discrimination between the two. Cane-sugar is supposed to be purer and more satisfactory for certain culinary processes, such as canning and jelly making. As far as the sucrose is concerned there is no difference, and between the highest commercial grade of each there is no distinction. The cheaper grades of beet-sugar may have a bitter taste or an odor suggestive of glue.

In the manufacture of sugar the juice is expressed (cane-sugar) or extracted (beet-sugar), treated with lime to clarify it, filtered, and evaporated *in vacuo*. Upon standing the first crop of crystals separate from the concentrated liquid.

The mother liquid or first molasses is removed by draining or by centrifugal force. This liquid is then diluted and a second lot of sugar and molasses obtained. This process is often carried out for a third time. The yellowish or brown sugar obtained by crystallization from the molasses is usually refined by redissolving, clarifying, decolorizing, and finally recrystallizing. Crude cane-sugar is often sold as brown sugar. Crude beet-sugar, however, has a rather unpleasant flavor, and is not usable.

In addition to the final product, sugar, the molasses or mother liquid remaining after the *first* crystallization from the juice of the sugar-cane and the mother liquor from the crystallization of the refined sugar are used as food. The latter is often mixed with glucose, or corn syrup, and sold as "corn syrup with cane flavor."

Glucose.—Glucose (dextrose or grape-sugar) is found most widely distributed in the plant and animal kingdom. It occurs in the free state and in combination with other sugars. It is the end-product of the digestion of starch, glycogen and maltose, and one of the products of the hydrolysis of sucrose and lactose. In the body it is the form of carbohydrate present in the blood. Glucose is assuming an important place in the manufacture of syrups and confections and is often used by manufacturers in place of cane-sugar. It is prepared from starch by the action of acids which hydrolyze it, yielding a product known as "commercial glucose," or "corn syrup," a viscid liquid mixture of glucose, maltose, and dextrin. The complete hydrolysis of starch yields practically pure glucose which upon recrystallization, is sold as starch-sugar or grape-sugar.

Glucose is often used in the preparation of preserved fruit products and as such it is considered an adulteration. Many artificial jams or fruit butters are prepared from apple pulp which, when flavored and colored, are sold as jams of different kinds. The present pure food laws require such preparations to be labelled as artificial. As far as their food value is concerned they are as satisfactory as the true products.

Lactose.—Lactose, the sugar in milk, yields galactose and glucose upon hydrolysis. It is not as sweet as cane-sugar and is therefore often a valuable food in cases where it is desired to raise the caloric value of the diet. It is a concentrated form of carbohydrate, and is readily absorbed. Further, it has been shown that fermentation in the stomach does not take place as readily with lactose as with sugar. Coleman has used lactose successfully to increase the caloric value of the diet of typhoid fever patients.

14

Maltose.—Maltose, one of the digestive products of starch, is composed of two molecules of glucose. It occurs in the diet usually as the result of special preparation, as in the preparation of malt or the preliminary digestion of food.

Maple-sugar.—Maple-sugar is obtained from the sap of the sugar-maple. The sap is evaporated in open kettles and the sugar allowed to crystallize into a solid mass. Maple-sugar is seldom refined; it contains in addition to the sugar certain ethereal substances and organic acids which give to it the characteristic flavor. When the concentrating process is not carried far enough for the sugar to crystallize, maple syrup is obtained; the greater part of the sugar from the maple tree is sold in this form.

Invert Sugar.—Invert sugar, a mixture of equal parts of glucose and fructose, is seldom sold as such. It is found in ripe fruits and vegetables, molasses from cane-sugar, and often in jellies and confections as the result of hydrolysis.

Fructose.—Fructose (levulose or fruit-sugar) is found in fruit associated with glucose, as invert sugar (see above). Inulin, the starch-like substance in the roots of the dandelion, chicory and the tubers, and of artichokes yields fructose upon hydrolysis.

Candy, Jams and Jellies.—The sugars are important constituents of confectionery, preserves and jams. Candy is essentially cane-sugar or glucose to which certain flavoring and coloring substances and sometimes a filling material has been added. In the commercial preparation of many candies sugar is partially hydrolyzed to invert sugar, which gives them a greater smoothness.

Preserves, jams, and jellies are essentially fruit pulp or juice to which sugar has been added and the whole boiled to the proper consistency. Their food value is largely due to the sugar. The gelatinizing constituent of jellies is the pectin of the fruit. When pectin is deficient it is often obtained from other fruits, giving the mixed jellies. Acid is also necessary in the preparation of jellies, for it aids in the gelatinization of pectin and in the inversion of the sugar. In the latter process a large proportion of the added cane-sugar is "inverted" into non-crystallizing invert sugar. This is an important consideration in preparing such products for otherwise the cane-sugar would crystallize and the jelly or jam would be physically unpalatable. The table on page 211 gives the comparative composition of the expressed juice and pulp and of the jelly and jams prepared from them.

Digestion and Utilization of Sugar.—We will confine our discussion to the utilization of sucrose and its products of hydrolysis, for the quantities of the other sugars ingested are comparatively small. The only important exception is the lactose in milk, the source of carbohydrate in the diet of infants. The digestion of sugars takes place wholly in the intestines. They are there transformed, in the processes of digestion, into monosaccharides and in that form are completely absorbed.

COMPOSITION OF JAMS AND JELLIES AND THE JUICES FROM WHICH THEY WERE PREPARED.

	Water, per cent.	Ash, per cent.	Acid calc. as H_2SO_4, per cent.	Protein (N x 6.25), per cent.	Reducing, per cent.	Sugars. Cane-sugar added, per cent.	Cane-sugar found, per cent.	Added cane-sugar, inverted, per cent.
Grape:								
Juice	91.2	0.57	0.902	0.237	5.10	...	0.89	
Jelly	36.3	0.45	0.524	0.175	32.29	60.29	30.52	49.33
Pulp	87.5	0.75	...	...	6.11	...	0.29	
Jam	43.4	0.48	0.744	0.525	33.44	42.45	11.33	73.38
Orange:								
Juice	93.9	0.36	0.297	0.581	1.52	...	2.29	
Jelly	31.4	0.30	0.171	0.418	3.95	65.59	62.62	4.91
Pulp	86.9	0.61	0.686	0.985	4.13	...	3.33	
Jam	19.5	0.44	0.433	0.944	13.61	69.13	54.23	21.55

Under certain conditions, however, sucrose may be absorbed into the system without being first inverted. When excessive quantities of a sugar are ingested, absorption takes place more rapidly than digestion, *i. e.*, the *assimilation limit* is exceeded. Sucrose which gains access to the blood stream in this way is not utilized, however, for it immediately appears in the urine. This fact has also been proved by the injection of sucrose into the blood when it is excreted almost quantitatively. The appearance of sugar in the urine under such conditions is termed "glycosuria." An alimentary glycosuria may occur upon the excessive ingestion of any of the readily absorbable sugars. The quantity which may be ingested at one time without causing glycosuria is a rather definite quantity for each individual. The following are average figures:

	Grams.
Lactose	120
Cane-sugar	150–200
Levulose	200
Glucose	200–250

When the ingestion of a sugar is distributed over long periods of time and particularly when it is taken with other food, greater quantities than these can be given without causing glycosuria. Taylor has suggested that the assimilation limit of glucose is not as definite a quantity as formerly supposed but that it depends upon the capacity of the individual to retain it without regurgitation.

Cane-sugar, when taken in concentrated solution, has a disturbing effect upon the digestive processes. These disturbances are likely to arise from the ingestion of candies or sweet syrups except when accompanied by food or sufficient water. The effect has been shown to be a direct irritation of the gastric mucosa due to the rapid withdrawal of water, causing inflammation and excessive secretion of mucus and a highly acid gastric juice. The repeated irritation of the stomach may lead to serious gastric disturbances. Investigations have shown that with too large an ingestion of sugar (120 grams) the emptying of the stomach is delayed. Invert sugar does not have as pronounced an effect upon the digestive processes as sucrose.

Since sugars are not absorbed in the stomach, when their passage is delayed fermentation often takes place. The products of such fermentation vary—there may be lactic, butyric, or alcoholic "fermentation" according to the conditions which exist. Lactose has been shown to be less likely to give rise to fermentation.

Sugar is the most concentrated form of carbohydrate food, for, in the form in which it is usually ingested it contains very little water. For this reason and because they are easily digestible and assimilable sugars are valuable when it is desired to supply food for the performance of work involving a sudden outburst of effort; they become available to the tissues in a comparatively short time. Experiments with soldiers have shown that they are able to perform a greater amount of work without fatigue after the ingestion of sugar than without it. Since continued effort is accompanied by a depletion of the carbohydrate stores, it is necessary, when sugar is being taken for an increase of efficiency, to ingest it at intervals during the whole period. The fact that sugars are completely absorbed is of importance in the construction of a diet in which it is desired to supply the energy requirements without producing a large fecal mass.

Valuable as sugar is in certain cases, from a dietetic standpoint there is a certain danger in its use. Von Bunge has pointed out that the excessive use of sugar in the diet is likely to lead to a decrease in the ingestion of vegetable foods and to a consequent failure to obtain the inorganic elements, such as iron, calcium, phosphorus, etc., which are necessary for continued good health. The average diet has been shown to be comparatively low in these food constituents and any tendency to lower the quantity taken is to be guarded against.

STARCH

Starch is the principal form of carbohydrate in the food of man. It is the form in which the plant stores the soluble carbohydrate formed in the processes of photosynthesis against the future demands of the embryo or plant itself. It is a member of the group of carbohydrates designated as polysaccharides. A starch molecule is composed of a number of molecules of glucose which have been united into a complex structure in which one molecule of water has been removed in the union of two molecules of glucose.

Upon digestion (hydrolysis) starch is broken down into simple compounds—soluble starch, dextrin, maltose, glucose—according to the nature and intensity of the digestive process. The final product, glucose, is absorbed and used in the body or synthetized into a compound, glycogen, which is similar in structure and serves as a reserve carbohydrate to the same end in the animal economy that starch does in the plant. In the plant, starch is stored in the form of fine grains or granules. These consist of alternate layers of particles of starch and of cellulose, a more dense and complex compound similar to starch, arranged in concentric rings. The shape of the granule and arrangement of the rings is characteristic of the plants in which they are formed. The microscopic appearance of the starch granule thus becomes a valuable means of determining its origin and of detecting the adulteration of foods.

Raw starch is insoluble in cold water. Under the influence of heat (or acids) it takes up water, becomes hydrated, swells, and becomes semitransparent, forming an opaque solution. This is not a true solution but one in which the starch particles are suspended in water—a colloidal solution. Careful treatment of starch with acids gives a partially hydrated product known as *soluble starch*, the dried form of which is soluble—a colloidal solution—in cold water. The hydration of starch under the influence of heat and in the presence of water causes the starch grains to swell and rupture the surrounding cellulose layers. This is the object sought in the cooking of vegetables.

Dextrin is one of the first products of hydrolysis of starch, formed by the action of enzymes (digestion), of acids, or of heat. Although it still retains the complex structure of starch, it is more soluble in water. The carbohydrate of the crust of a loaf of bread is composed largely of soluble starch and dextrin formed during the baking process.

The readily soluble and diffusible products of the hydrolysis of starch, maltose and glucose, have already been considered in our discussion of sugars.

Starch itself is readily digested and absorbed. Glucose is the end-product of its digestion—the form of carbohydrate present in the blood stream. The digestion and absorption of starch extends over a considerable length of time being delayed by the associated indigestible cellulose. The result is that starchy foods yield glucose to the body over a much longer period of time than those containing soluble carbohydrates, sugars. This is in most cases an advantage, particularly where severe muscular work is to be performed. The gradual absorption of the carbohydrate keeps the body continually supplied with the most efficient food for the performance of work yet without depleting the store of glycogen before the next meal.

The digestibility of the various prepared foods, particularly bread and potatoes, will be discussed later (pp. 223 and 226).

GRAINS AND THEIR PRODUCTS.

This group of foods includes the seeds of various plants such as barley, buckwheat, corn or maize, oats, rice, rye, and wheat, and the products manufactured from them. Grains are harvested in the partially dried state and contain, therefore, a lower percentage of water (10 to 12 per cent.) and a higher percentage of carbohydrate, protein and fat than the fresh grain. Starch is the predominating food-stuff (65 to 75 per cent. of the dried grain). Small quantities of sugar and cellulose are present. The protein content is rather high (10 to 12 per cent.) and a number of different kinds are present. The predominating proteins, such as the alcohol-soluble protein, gliadin, and the glutelin, glutenin of wheat, are of a different type from those found in flesh foods. The nutritive value of vegetable proteins has been discussed (p. 144). The fat content of grains may be rather high, oats and corn contain as much as 8 per cent.; the values average between 0.5 and 8 per cent., according to the kind of grain. The fat of the grains has a low melting-point and exists as an oil. Approximately 2 per cent of ash is present in grain. This is distributed chiefly in the outer layers of the kernel and the germ. The tables on page 215 give the composition of the various whole grains and of the flours prepared from them.

COMPOSITION OF VARIOUS WHOLE GRAINS AS MARKETED BY THE FARMER.

	Water, per cent.	Protein (N x 6.25), per cent.	Fat, per cent.	Carbohydrate, per cent.	Fiber, per cent.	Ash, per cent.
Barley .	10.85	11.00	2.25	69.55	3.85	2.50
Corn . .	10.75	10.00	4.25	71.75	1.75	1.50
Oats . .	10.06	12.15	4.33	57.93	12.07	3.45
Rye . .	10.50	12.25	1.50	71.75	2.10	1.90
Wheat .	10.60	12.25	1.75	71.25	2.40	1.75

COMPOSITION OF PREPARED CEREALS.

	Water, per cent.	Protein (Nx6.25), per cent.	Fat, per cent.	Carbohydrate, per cent.	Fiber, per cent.	Ash, per cent.	Fuel value per pound, Calories.	Grams for 100 Calories.
Barley, pearled .	11.9	10.5	2.2	72.8	6.5	2.6	1603	28
Buckwheat flour .	13.6	6.4	1.2	77.9	0.4	0.9	1577	29
Cornmeal, granular .	12.5	9.2	1.9	75.4	1.0	1.0	1620	28
Oatmeal	7.3	16.1	7.2	67.5	0.9	1.9	1811	25
Rice	12.3	8.0	0.3	79.0	0.2	0.4	1591	29
Rye flour	11.4	13.6	2.0	71.5	1.8	1.5	1626	28
Wheat flour . . .	12.0	11.4	1.0	75.1	0.3	0.5	1610	28

With few exceptions the grains are rolled or milled before they are used in the preparation of food. In the various processes certain portions of the grain are removed, particularly the outer layers of the kernel and the germ. The accompanying data related to the polishing of rice gives the important changes in chemical composition during milling.

CHEMICAL COMPOSITION OF THE HONDURAS TYPE OF RICE AFTER VARIOUS MILLING PROCESSES OF MODERN RICE MILLS.[1]

Constituents (per cent.).

	Moisture.	Ash.	Ether extract.	Crude fiber.	Protein.	Pentosans.	Protein.[2]	Pentosans.[2]
Rough rice	11.27	5.40	1.58	8.67	7.48	5.90	8.43	6.65
After removal of hulls .	12.32	1.18	1.79	0.99	8.57	2.42	9.78	2.75
After removal of bran and most of the germ . .	12.56	0.53	0.40	0.39	7.79	1.90	8.91	2.17
After further removal of bran (pearling) . .	12.50	0.47	0.28	0.30	7.88	1.53	9.00	1.75
After polishing . . .	11.89	0.36	0.25	0.30	8.06	1.80	9.15	2.04
Coating	12.02	0.40	0.21	0.26	7.75	1.66	8.81	1.88
Total loss[2] . . .	. . .	66.00	85.00	73.00	10.00	32.00	10.00	32.00

[1]Bulletin 330, U. S. Dept. Agr., 1916.   [2]On a moisture-free basis.

Barley.—Barley is not used extensively for human food in this country. As "pearled barley," prepared by removing the germ and the greater portion of the bran, it is used in soups. Barley water, prepared from "patent" barley flour, is used in infant feeding and in the diet of the sick room. "Patent" barley flour is finely ground pearl barley or barley which has been more thoroughly polished than pearl barley.

Buckwheat.—Buckwheat, although ordinarily classed with the cereals, does not belong with them according to its botanical classification. Its use is confined chiefly to the preparation of pancakes, a hot breakfast cake. In the preparation of buckwheat flour the outer covering is removed and the remaining portion rolled and bolted as in the preparation of wheat flour. A rather coarse bolting cloth is used which permits a certain amount of the middlings (see *flour*) to pass through. A white grade of flour, bolted over a finer cloth, is poorer in protein and fat. Buckwheat is rich in "gluten" the water-insoluble, elastic protein mixture which is the basis of a batter capable of considerable expansion; thus giving a light cake when baked.

Corn.—Indian corn or maize differs in composition from the other grains with the exception of the oat, in that it has a high percentage of oil. Corn products are not readily leavened because of their low gluten content; wheat flour is often added to rectify this defect. Corn and corn products show the same digestibility as other grains. There are a number of varieties of corn. From a dietetic stand-point distinctions are made among them chiefly on the basis of their use for food: the variety used for cornmeal flour or hominy is field corn; for "popping," popcorn; for use in the green state, green or sweet corn. Field corn is harvested in the semidry state; it is marketed for human food as cornmeal, corn flour, hominy, and corn starch.

Cornmeal or corn flour is prepared from the whole grain. "Old process" cornmeal is made by grinding the entire kernel and then separating the larger particles of bran with a sieve; this method gives a flour containing the germ and a certain amount of bran in addition to the starchy portion of the kernel. This product is rich in oil and protein. It is difficult to keep such meal, for the oil tends to become rancid. By more careful milling and bolting both the germ and bran are removed, yielding a product which is low in protein, ash, and particularly oil. This flour may be kept for a longer time than the "old process" cornmeal without becoming rancid. But the advantage is gained at the expense of nutritive value and accessory substances.

Yellow and white cornmeal are prepared from yellow and white varieties of corn respectively. Any preference shown for one or the other of these meals is a matter of taste, for there is essentially no difference between them.

Corn starch is also prepared from maize. In its prepaiation the corn is steeped in warm water; the swollen grain is passed through coarse mills to disintegrate the kernel without breaking the germ; the germ is removed by a process of differential sedimentation in which the oily germ floats off at the top while the starch granules and other particles settle to the bottom of the separator; the sedimented starch granules and associated hulls are reground and passed over a fine sieve to remove the hulls, and the starch finally purified by fractional sedimentation. Purified starch is sold as such or after being hydrolyzed with acids and steam under pressure, as glucose (p. 209).

Green or sweet corn is characterized by its high sugar content. It is eaten in the green state, hence its place in the diet is with succulent vegetables. Large quantities of sweet corn are canned, thus making it available throughout the year.

Oats.—Oats, like corn, have a high fat content. The products prepared from oats usually contain the whole kernel and are therefore highly nutritious. The use of oatmeal by the Scotch has won for it a reputation as a stimulating and muscle-building food which is perhaps overestimated in comparison with other grain products of a similar character. Oat preparations do not leaven readily, since little gluten is present. Oatmeal is used largely in the preparation of porridges and to a smaller extent in bread and cakes. Because of the presence of the germ in oat products the percentage of purine bases is higher than in products prepared from the other cereals in which the germ is removed; for this reason they are excluded from a purine-free diet. Studies of the digestibility and availability of oats show them to be fully as well utilized as bread.

Rice.—Rice is particularly rich in carbohydrate. It is used among certain people as the principal constituent of the diet, which is therefore deficient in protein and fat. The lack of protein accompanying a rice diet has been assigned by certain investigators as the cause of the inferior physical and mental development of these races.

Rice is supplied in three forms: unhulled; "cured," free from the husk but still retaining the bran; and polished. The polished rice is sometimes coated with talc, paraffin or glucose to improve its appearance. In the processes of pol ishing the outer layers of bran are removed and in so doing a large portion of the mineral matter, particularly phosphorus, is lost. In polishing rice some important dietary constituents (accessory substances) are also removed. People who use polished rice as the major constituent of the diet tend to develop beriberi, a disease which affects then ervous system. The ingestion of unpolished rice or the addition of foods containing the accessory food substances will cure beriberi.

Rice is as readily and thoroughly digested as other grains. The small amount of cellulose it contains makes it a desirable food when the fecal residue is to be kept as low as possible. This applies particularly to polished rice. Because of the low protein and fat content it is advisable to eat protein-rich foods, such as eggs, cheese, and milk, with it. Vegetables should be used with rice, particularly with polished rice, because of its low content of ash and accessory food substances.

Rye.—Rye is used extensively in the preparation of bread. In composition it closely approaches wheat. Its proteins are in slightly different proportions; it has considerable protein corresponding to the gliadin of wheat, but the other constituent of gluten, glutenin, is lacking. Bread made from rye flour is darker, the texture is more dense, and it contains rather more nourishment than wheat bread. The digestibility of rye bread is approximately equal to that of white bread. Bread made from flour from which the bran is not removed is not as thoroughly digested as the bolted flour.

Wheat.—Wheat is used more extensively in the human dietary than any other grain. Chemical analysis does not indicate any particular superiority of wheat over other grains, nor is it found to be more digestible. It is the appearance of the prepared product and the ease with which it may be leavened that makes wheat prized above the other grains. The fact that wheat flour is comparatively rich in the water-insoluble proteins present in the gluten, the alcohol-soluble gliadin and the alkali-soluble glutenin, makes it the preëminent bread-making grain. For the elastic adherent mixture, gluten, stretches and holds the expanding bubbles of gas produced by the leavening agents. It is the coagulation around these bubbles which gives to bread the porous structure in the baked product. With wheat or its products as the basis, the addition of various substances enables the housewife to prepare an endless variety of dishes, and thus use this valuable food without creating a distaste for it because of the monotony of the diet.

In spite of its general adaptability to variety in preparation wheat is consumed largely in one form, bread. Rye is the only other grain which approaches wheat in its bread-making properties. Rye bread is, however, a less attractive product for it is darker and slightly more sticky than wheat bread.

Wheat is seldom eaten without a certain amount of mechanical preparation and modification. The majority of the wheat is consumed in the form of products made from flour. The crushed or whole kernel is often used as a breakfast food after it has been swollen and the starch partially cooked by boiling. A recent preparation has been put on the market in which the whole wheat kernel is subjected to pressure, heated, then allowed suddenly to expand, producing a change in the structure similar to that obtained in popped popcorn.

Flour is prepared by a process of grinding and sieving by which the kernel is pulverized and the outer coverings or bran and the germ are separated from the inner portion, which is rich in starch and gluten. ·Formerly the wheat was ground in one process and the resulting products sifted and graded according to their fineness of division. This gave three general grades: white flour (finest), middlings (which contain some fine particles of the coarse outer material) and bran. Middlings obtained from the roller process differ from the above in that they contain very little bran. The present method is to crush the grain between a series of rollers which reduce the size of the particles gradually until the desired texture is obtained. Between the different sets of rollers are sieves to separate the finely divided flour from the coarser bran and germ. Early in the rolling process a white flour poor in gluten, called "break" flour is separated; as the grinding becomes finer more and more of the gluten-rich flour with a yellowish color, or the middlings is obtained. A mixture of these two general classes of flour, "breaks" and middlings give a flour containing the proper amount of gluten for bread-making. The highest grades of flour are known as "patent," "standard patent flour," "straight grade flour," "first clear." The lower grades of flour are designated "second clear," "baker's flour" and the lowest grade is called "red dog." The highest grades of flour are light in color and contain more gluten and show a better granulation than the lower grades. In the latter, the protein content is higher, but the gluten is less elastic and not as satisfactory for bread-making purposes. The .best test of a good flour is its baking properties.

ANALYSIS OF WHEAT AND THE PRODUCTS OF ROLLER MILLING (UNITED STATES DEPARTMENT OF AGRICULTURE).

Milling products.	Water, per cent.	Protein (N x 5.7). per cent.	Fat, per cent.	Carbohydrate, per cent.	Ash, per cent.
First patent flour . . .	10.55	11.08	1.15	76.85	0.37
Second patent flour . .	10.49	11.14	1.20	76.75	0.42
First clear grade flour . .	10.13	13.74	2.20	73.13	0.80
Straight or standard patent flour	10.54	11.99	1.61	75.36	0.50
Second clear grade flour .	10.08	15.03	3.77	69.37	1.75
"Red dog" flour . . .	9.17	18.98	7.00	61.37	3.48
Shorts	8.73	14.87	6.37	65.47	4.56
Bran	9.99	14.02	4.39	65.54	6.06
Entire wheat flour . . .	10.81	12.26	2.24	73.67	1.02
Graham flour	8.61	12.65	2.44	74.58	1.72
Wheat ground in laboratory	8.50	12.65	2.36	74.69	1.80
Germ	8.73	27.24	11.23	48.09	4.71

There are a number of varieties of wheat: spring, winter, soft, and hard. By the use of these and by different methods of manipulation a number of grades of flour is produced which vary chiefly in their gluten content. In baking these differences assume more or less importance. From a nutritive point of view, however, it is the relative proportion of the inner portion of the kernel, bran, the outer covering, and the germ which is of importance.

Certain grades of flour have distinctive names under which they are sold in commerce. Graham flour is composed of the carefully ground, unbolted entire wheat kernel. As such it contains all the constituents of the wheat, the bran, the germ, and contents of the endosperm (starch and gluten). This flour derives its name from Sylvester Graham who advocated the ingestion of the whole wheat for both economical and dietetic reasons. The greater cellulose content of the bran renders bread from such flour less digestible. The added intestinal irritation, the bulk derived from the particles of indigestible bran, and certain substances present in the bran and germ have mild laxative properties.

Entire wheat flour is made of wheat from which the greater part of the outer covering, or bran, has been removed. It contains the germ with its added fat and protein content in addition to the usual constituents of flour. The increased nutritive value protein—fat and ash—of the flour is of economic importance.

Gluten flours are prepared by removing the greater part of the starch from ordinary flour and are supplied in various grades, according to the quantity of gluten present. They are of particular value as food for diabetics. Gluten flours are discussed further in connection with diabetes.

Bread.—The term bread is usually applied to the baked, leavened preparation of wheat flour. It may, however, include similar preparations of all forms of finely divided grains, such as rye bread or corn bread. When the added ingredients used with flour assume importance with regard to flavor and texture, the mixture is no longer distinguished as bread. Thus sugar, butter, eggs, milk, spices, are used with flour in the preparation of cakes, puddings, and pastries.

Bread in the sense ordinarily used is a combination of white flour, water, salt, and yeast which have been leavened as the result of the growth of the yeast. In this process carbon dioxide is formed and the mixture "rises," assuming a spongelike structure. This "sponge" is kneaded with the addition of flour, divided into appropriate masses, permitted to rise again and, at the proper time, baked. In the process of baking heat causes a further expansion of the carbon dioxide and air and by coagulating the proteins retains the sponge-like structure. Various changes take place in the chemical composition of the flour during the leavening process. A certain amount of sugar is converted into carbon dioxide and alcohol; during baking there is a loss of water and fat, the protein is coagulated, the starch grains are broken, and at the outer surface particularly starch is converted by dry heat into soluble starch and dextrin. The partial caramelization of the starch and dextrin produces the delicate brown color of a well-baked loaf.

Leavening may be accomplished in a number of ways—with yeast (enzymatic) which is supplied in both moist (compressed yeast) and dried condition; by mechanical incorporation of air; or by the evolution of gas as the result of chemical action (baking powder). When yeast is used the carbon dioxide is produced at the expense of the constituents of the flour, the starch is partially converted into simpler products in addition to alcohol, and certain amounts of organic acids, such as lactic or acetic, which in quantity are said to injure the flavor of bread.

The simplest form of aëration with mechanical incorporation of gas is that produced by "beating up" a mixture of flour and water. The entrapped bubbles of air swell and produce, when baked, porous though rather dense biscuit or bread. Unleavened bread is used in certain religious festivals. In the commercial preparation of bread, water saturated, under pressure, with gas is sometimes mixed with flour. When the pressure is released the dough swells; it is then baked. This is called aërated bread.

Baking Powders.—Baking powders will leaven dough more quickly than will yeast, in a few minutes, instead of in six to ten hours. All baking powders depend in principle upon the interaction between a carbonate and an acid. Sodium bicarbonate (saleratus or baking soda) is the most common source of carbon dioxide. The old method of making certain breads with sour milk and soda often resulted in a semifailure because of the varying degrees of acidity of the milk. The baking powders now supplied have the acid and alkali so balanced that there is complete neutralization. Preparations vary chiefly in the nature of the acid constituent or its equivalent; thus we have the "tartrate" (tartar), acid potassium tartrate or tartaric acid powders; the phosphate (calcium acid phosphate) powders, and the alum powders (a sulphate of aluminum). These salts when mixed with bicarbonate are relatively inert in the dry state but in the presence of water react readily to yield carbon dioxide.

There are certain objections to the use of baking powders in that the salts resulting from their reactions may be deleterious to the health through their action on the system in general or to their laxative effect. While it is certain that excessive doses of these salts are harmful it is difficult to determine whether or not small amounts, such as are ingested in breads, are detrimental.

Rolls, Biscuits, Muffins, etc.—Rolls are similar to bread except that they usually contain more added fat in the form of lard or butter and sometimes more sugar. They differ little in composition from bread. In baking they are ordinarily made into small loaves or "rolls" and have more crust in proportion to their size than bread. Such breads are often used while hot or warm.

The ordinary baking powder biscuit differs from the roll in that it is leavened with baking powder and contains more shortening, as lard or butter. The effect of the shortening is to render the gluten less tenacious. Biscuits are, therefore, readily broken into pieces when hot.

Muffins are similar to biscuits; they usually contain egg in addition to other ingredients.

Rolls, biscuits and muffins are often referred to as indigestible. This indigestibility is ascribed in part to the added fat and in part to the fact that since they are served hot, they are eaten rapidly and without sufficient mastication, thus yielding a sodden mass which does not pass readily from the stomach. Experiments have shown the relative availability of the protein, fat, and carbohydrate of these foods to be fully as complete as those of bread.

Biscuits, Crackers.—The term biscuit is used commonly to designate the hard, dry breads baked in thin layers and prepared with the addition of little or no baking powder. These are sold in various forms depending upon the ingredients used in their manufacture. They are held to be very digestible, no doubt because of their dryness and to the complete salivation and mastication necessary in eating them.

Cakes.—Cakes are sweetened breads in which eggs, milk, flavoring and spices and considerable shortening, such as butter and lard, are used. They are very "rich" foods in that they contain more fat and protein than the breads.

Breakfast Foods.—Certain specially prepared grains are sold as breakfast foods. These are usually patented preparations. Among them will be found representatives of all the more important grains. The changes produced are chiefly of a mechanical nature associated with a certain amount of chemical change resembling the natural processes of digestion. The changes are in general of a fermentative nature, such as those produced by the action of malt or yeast and the action of heat upon either the moist or dry grain. Condiments, such as sugar and salts, are sometimes added. Those foods which are cooked are sold for direct consumption; the others must be subjected to prolonged cooking before they are ready for the table.

Macaroni.—Macaroni is a preparation of a highly glutenous wheat flour and water. It is molded into various forms and sold under different trade names, as spaghetti, macaroni, and noodles. A special type of wheat, durum wheat, is used. The relative composition of macaroni will be found in the accompanying table.

The composition of some wheat preparations is given in the following table:

COMPOSITION OF TYPICAL WHEAT PRODUCTS.

	Water, per cent.	Protein (Nx6.25), per cent.	Fat, per cent.	Carbohydrate, per cent.	Fiber, per cent.	Ash, per cent.	Fuel value per pound.	Grams per 100 Calories.
Breakfast food:								
Cracked Wheat .	10.1	11.1	1.7	75.5	1.7	1.6	1635	28
Shredded Wheat .	8.1	10.5	1.4	77.9	1.7	2.1	1660	27
Macaroni . . .	10.3	13.4	0.9	74.1	..	1.3	1625	28
Rolls, Vienna . .	37.1	8.5	2.2	56.5	0.4	1.1	1270	36
Bread:								
White	35.3	9.2	1.3	53.1	0.5	1.1	1182	38
Whole wheat .	38.4	9.7	0.9	49.7	1.2	1.3	1113	41
Crackers, soda . .	5.9	9.8	9.1	73.1	0.3	2.1	1875	24
Cake, cup . . .	15.6	5.9	9.0	68.5	0.3	1.0	1716	26

The digestibility and nutritive value of bread, particularly the comparative digestibility of white bread and the whole wheat or Graham bread assumes considerable economic importance with regard to the diet of the poor and there has been a great deal of controversy over the question. Comparative studies of the two forms of bread have demonstrated a lower digestibility of the protein and carbohydrates of entire wheat and Graham flours.

Celluloses.—Celluloses form a large portion of the cell wall of plants. They are polysaccharids having a more complex structure than the starches. Celluloses differ according to whether they are composed of glucose or some other sugar, as pentose or galactose. These carbohydrates are very insoluble in water and more difficult to hydrolyze than starch, and are practically indigestible for man. It is the indigestibility of the celluloses which makes vegetable and fruits a valuable means of adding bulk to the intestinal mass with the resultant stimulation of peristalsis. Cellulose is also largely responsible for the low utilization of vegetable foods.

Hemicelluloses differ from true celluloses in that they are hydrolyzed by dilute acids. Of this class the sea-weed, agar agar and Iceland moss are of dietetic and therapeutic importance. Because of their comparative indigestibility and their ability to absorb and hold water they yield a soft fecal mass which may be easily evacuated.

Potatoes.—The true, "Irish," potato, as well as the sweet potato, is used to a large extent as one of the important sources of carbohydrate. We will therefore discuss these foods here, although they possess properties which might place them with the succulent vegetables, more valuable for their salts and water. Bananas are, from a nutritive point of view, comparable with potatoes; they are, however, ordinarily classed with fruits.

COMPOSITION.

	Water, per cent.	Protein (N x 6.25), per cent.	Fat, per cent.	Carbohydrate, per cent.	Fiber, per cent.	Ash, per cent.	Fuel value per pound, Calories.	Grams per 100 Calories.
Potatoes:								
Irish . . .	78.3	2.2	0.1	18.4	0.4	1.0	378	120
Sweet . . .	69.0	1.8	0.7	27.4	1.3	1.1	558	81
Bananas . . .	75.3	1.3	0.6	22.0	1.0	0.8	447	101

The chemical composition of potatoes varies somewhat according to the different varieties, and to the portion of the country in which they are grown. The average potato contains 18 to 20 per cent. carbohydrate (largely starch); 2 to 2.5 per cent. protein; practically no fat—0.1 per cent.; and 75 to 80 per cent. water. The greater proportion of the carbohydrate present in potatoes is starch; but there is also a small proportion—0.3 to 0.2 per cent. of sugars and glucose. The sugar content of young or early and old, sprouted potatoes is greater than that of the mature potato. The tuber receives carbohydrate as glucose and converts it to starch; later as the potato sprouts the starch is reconverted into glucose for the use of the growing shoots. The protein of potatoes is usually expressed as the nitrogen value times 6.25. We know that in the case of the potato this does not entirely represent protein, for there is a considerable quantity of non-protein, nitrogenous-containing material, particularly asparagin. The ash of potato contains considerable quantities of calcium, phosphorus and iron. The total ash is predominantly basic.

Potatoes are rich in the water-soluble accessory substances (vitamines). The use of potato water as an anti-scorbutic has been suggested for infants in place of the more expensive orange juice.

The sweet-potato plant does not belong to the same botanical family as the Irish potato. This tuber resembles the latter, however, in its general chemical composition and is usually associated with it dietetically. The sweet potato is roughly similar in composition to the Irish or white potato; it contains a little less water—averaging 70 per cent.—and a slightly higher percentage of starch, sugar and protein, averaging 24 per cent., 5 to 8 per cent., and 1 per cent., respectively. The effect of the storage of sweet potatoes is to increase the sugar content. The material designated as "sugars" is chiefly sucrose with a small amount of invert sugar (glucose and fructose).

Because potatoes are an important source of mineral matter it is essential to conserve this as much as possible. In the process of paring as much as 20 per cent. of the potato is lost; furthermore, a large proportion of the protein and mineral matter is in the layers beneath the skin. The skin tends to prevent the loss of protein and salts. Peeled potatoes when soaked in water and then boiled in water lose a considerable proportion of their salt content, approximately ten times as much as when they are cooked without removing the skins. When they are baked or steamed the loss is

15

comparatively small. If the cooking is begun in hot water the loss of material is less than when the cooking is commenced in cold water.

Potatoes when properly cooked are quite digestible; approximately 92 per cent. of the carbohydrate and 70 per cent. of the protein is absorbed. They have been found to leave the stomach quite rapidly—more so than bread. The ease with which potatoes are digested varies with the mode of preparation. Boiled or baked mealy potatoes pass more readily from the stomach than waxy potatoes or potatoes which have been fried or prepared with fatty substances as in salads. Finely divided pieces of potatoes pass out of the stomach more readily than larger pieces. The low fat content of potatoes indicates the addition of fatty substances after they are cooked when they are used as the principal source of food.

Because of the low cost of potatoes they have been advocated as the chief article of diet in some countries. There is a certain amount of objection to this because of the quantity which must be eaten to supply the necessary energy and protein—approximately 6.5 pounds or 3 kilos. Such quantities would contain a smaller proportion of protein than is deemed necessary by some. The energy value is, moreover, roughly a third that of white bread. Hindhede, of Sweden, who has advocated the adoption of a potato diet, has shown that the body may be maintained in perfect health over long periods of time on a diet of potatoes, milk, oleomargarine, green vegetables, and fruit, provided the total diet has an energy value in proportion to 3000 Calories for a man of 70 kilos (164 pounds).

CHAPTER XIV.

FAT-RICH FOODS.

FATS are important in the diet in that they supply energy in a concentrated form and certain of them carry the fat-soluble vitamine. In general, organ fat as distinct from body fat is rich in fat-soluble A; thus butter fat, kidney fat and cod liver oil are valuable sources of this food factor. Beef fat is relatively poor in fat-soluble A, while in lard, and the vegetable fats it is practically absent. Considerations of the relative value of butter, and the hydrogenated vegetable fats, and the margarines must take these facts into consideration.

Animal or plant fat is a mixture of true fats and lipins. The true fats are glycerol esters of fatty acids; they are named according to the acid from which they are derived by substituting "in" for "ic" of the name given the fatty acid, thus: Butyrin, olein, stearin, or tributyrin, triolein, tristearin for fats formed from butyric, oleic and stearic acids. Fats are widely distributed in the plant and animal kingdom and are one of the most valuable sources of energy to the body. Associated with fat are the lipins, or fat-like substances related by composition and solubility. In their chemical constitution lipins may differ entirely from fats as cholesterol, or may be compounds of fat with other radicles as in the case of lecithin. The lipins are constituents of all cells and particularly of the highly organized nervous tissue. Our knowledge of their occurrence and functions is, however, very limited.

The fats most commonly found in food are those derived from the saturated fatty acids, butyric acid, caproic acid, caprylic acid, capric acid, lauric acid, myristic acid, palmitic acid and stearic acid, and from the unsaturated fatty acids, oleic, linoleic, and linolenic acids. Of the saturated fatty acids, the first members, butyric and caprylic acids, are liquid at ordinary temperatures, while the others are solid: the melting-point increases with the complexity of the molecule. The unsaturated fatty acids and the glycerol esters, fats, are liquid at ordinary temperatures.

Food fats are mixtures of these individual fats. Those of animal origin are composed largely of olein, palmitin, and stearin. The fluidity or solidity of any particular fat depends upon the relative proportion of these. The more solid fats contain a greater amount of palmitin and stearin, while the softer fats contain more olein.

The fat of various animals is more or less characteristic for each species. Warm-blooded animals have harder fat than cold-blooded animals, such as fishes; and of the land animals herbivora have, as a rule, harder fats than carnivora. The composition of subcutaneous fat appears to be determined in part by the external temperature of the air surrounding the body. The facial fat of individuals exposed to the weather is richer in olein and has a lower melting-point than of those less exposed. The fat of those portions of animals which have a poor blood supply, such as the back, is richer in olein and has a lower melting-point than fat in other parts thoroughly warmed by the blood. The fat of beef animals has been found to become richer in olein with age, fatness, and nearness to the surface of the body.

Butter contains a variety of fatty acids—all of those mentioned above in the saturated fatty acid series and oleic and butyric acids. The latter acid, while not the *most* important from a quantitative point of view, is most characteristic. The vegetable oils contain more of the unsaturated fat compounds than animal fats.

Certain fats—milk fat and the fat of egg yolk in particular—occur in a finely divided state or emulsion. Such fats are readily digestible because of the size of the fat particles and great surface exposed to the action of the digestive enzymes. Emulsification may be produced artifically by thorough agitation of fat with water or by the addition of protein material, certain carbohydrates, gum tragacanth, or of soaps. Alkalis when added to fats form soaps which in turn aid in emulsification. Mayonnaise dressing, in which comparatively large quantities of oil are changed from the liquid state to a semi-solid form, is a case of emulsification in the presence of protein material.

Fats are as easily digested and absorbed as proteins and carbohydrates. In the process of digestion and absorption they are emulsified and broken down into fatty acids and glycerol, absorbed into the intestinal wall and in part at least resynthetized into fat. The presence of fat tends to delay the passage of food from the stomach. The "indigestibility" of fatty foods in the sense of the "ease" of digestion is to be ascribed in part to this fact. The presence of fats in food, particularly of those having high melting-points which are not liquefied in the stomach at body temperature, tends to retard peptic and salivary digestion. Fats form a protective coating over the particles of protein and starch and prevent their partial digestion, thus increasing the extent of digestion necessary in the intestine. The effect of cooking foods in fat is to form a similar layer of fat over the surface of the food particles. This applies particularly to the ordinary process of frying, in which heavy fats are often used; cooking in deep fat results in the formation of an impervious layer on the outside of the food which prevents the further entrance of fat. The partial oxidation of fats which takes place in cooking, particularly in frying, leads to the formation of substances which may be irritating to the alimentary tract.

The retarding action which fats exert upon the passage of food from the stomach has been found to be beneficial in the case of the relatively indigestible vegetables, for by subjecting them to a more prolonged contact with the digestive juices their digestion is more complete. Vegetables to which a soft fat, such as butter, has been added, *after* cooking, have been found to be more thoroughly digested than those cooked *in* fat. Studies of the utilization of fat have shown that ordinary fats are readily absorbed, approximately 97 per cent. of the ingested fat.

Feces obtained from a fat-poor diet may contain more fat than is found in the food ingested. On a milk diet under normal conditions the fecal fat melts at 50° to 51° C., while the fatty acids of butter melt at 43° C.; in diarrhea the fecal fat has the same melting-point as milk fat. These facts indicate that considerable fat is excreted or secreted into the intestines from the body in the process of digestion.

The melting-point of fat affects its digestibility. Those fats whose melting-points are close to the temperature of the body are liquefied in the alimentary canal, readily emulsified and digested in the intestines, and show practically complete absorption. The more solid fats, are, on the other hand, emulsified with greater difficulty and their digestion is less complete. Certain fat-like substances, such as paraffin oil and lanolin, are not absorbed at all; it is for this reason that paraffin oils are used to relieve constipation. These facts have been brought out in the following table (Munk and Arnshink):

Fat	Melting-point, °C.	Percentage loss in feces.
Stearin	60	91–86
Stearin and almond oil	55	10.6
Spermaceti	53	31.0
Mutton fat	50–51	9.2
Mutton, fatty acids	56	13–20
Lard	43	2.6
Pork fat	34	2.8
Goose fat	25	2.5
Olive oil	fluid	2.3

Langeworthy and Holmes[1] compared the relative digestibility of butter, lard, beef and mutton fat when fed with a uniform mixed diet of blanc mange, wheat biscuit, fruit and sugar. In general the digestibility decreased with an increase in the melting-point of the fat. The following table contains data demonstrating this:

COMPARISON OF DIGESTIBILITY AND MELTING-POINT.

Fat studied	Coefficient of digestibility, per cent.	Melting-point. °C.
Butter fat	97	32
Lard	97	35
Beef fat	93	45
Mutton fat	88	50

In the processes of metabolism both fat and carbohydrate are used chiefly in the production of energy. Their role in the structure of the body, while little understood, is highly important; this is particularly true of the lipins, lecithin and cholesterol, which are constituents of the outer surface of all cells. As a source of energy fats and carbohydrates may, in general, be used interchangeably. It seems necessary, however, that a certain amount of carbohydrate be present in the food for the normal continuance of the metabolic processes. The entire absence of carbohydrate tends to produce certain disturbances, among which acidosis is the most prominent indication. The minimum quantity of carbohydrate needed is not known; that it may be comparatively low is illustrated in the case of the Eskimo whose diet is essentially fat and protein and in which practically the only source of carbohydrate is the glycogen contained in meat.

Although carbohydrate appears to be indispensable in the diet, the presence of fat (lipins) is also essential. Studies of growing animals have shown that certain animal fats, e. g., kidney fat, egg yolk fat, butter fat, are more satisfactory than others or than plant fats for the continuance of growth. The advantage apparently does not reside in the purified fat itself, such as tristearin, or triolein for these are without effect. It is known that there are substances associated with fat which are important for growth and that the absence of these from the diet result in pathological conditions. Such substances as the accessory food substances, "fat-soluble A" of McCullum, which the body apparently cannot synthetize and must therefore obtain them from the food are present and necessary. It is the absence of these substances which in part explains the failure of some fats to promote growth. The necessary amount of natural fat required per day is not known—the minimum has been estimated at from 25 to 50 grams of fat per day.

[1] U. S. Dept. Agr., 1915, Bull. No. 310.

Fat is a much more concentrated food than carbohydrate or protein in the sense that it yields, because of its lower state of oxidation, a greater amount of energy for a given weight:

	Calories per gram.	Calories per pound.
Fat	9.0	4082
Carbohydrate	4.0	1814

It is therefore the most economical means available to the body for storing energy against future need. But not all the fat of the body comes from fat; it may be formed from carbohydrate (glucose). Protein yields complexes which may be built up into fat.

Fat is present in the human diet in two forms: (*a*) that associated with the food as it occurs naturally and (*b*) that which has been extracted from the medium in which it was deposited—flesh, milk, fruits—and which is ingested as such or added to food in the process of preparation. Prepared fats are similar to the unextracted fats, for the processes of manufacture are essentially physical ones: the fatty substance is separated from its surrounding medium by means of pressing, churning, or heat or a combination of these; very little chemical change takes place except perhaps in some forms of rendering or heating in which there is a partial hydrolysis and slight oxidation of the original fats. We shall therefore confine our discussion largely to the manufactured fats and oils, indicating occasionally the relative fat content of certain particularly fatty natural foods when discussing the particular prepared fat which it would yield.

Two types of fat-rich foods are obtained from milk: cream, in which the finely emulsified fat is concentrated by gravity or centrifugal force and which contains a small proportion of all the constituents of milk, and butter, in which the fat droplets are made to coalesce. Butter contains very little of the milk constituents other than the fat.

CREAM

Cream is obtained from milk in two ways, both depending upon the difference in specific gravity between the fat and the other constituents. Formerly milk was placed in a cool place for six or eight hours and the fat or cream permitted to rise to the top; it was then removed or "skimmed off." The separation of the cream from the milk is hastened by the use of a centrifuge or separator which throws the heavier portions of the milk, water, protein, insoluble salts and cells to the periphery from which it is removed while the lighter

fat is drawn off from the center. With the separator varying concentrations of butter fat can be obtained in the
cream.

BUTTER

Butter is obtained from cream by the process of churning,
i. e., by mechanical agitation the natural emulsion of milk
is destroyed and the fat droplets made to coalesce. This process is facilitated by the slight changes produced in the cream
as the result of fermentation or souring. The crude butter
collected in the process of churning is separated from the
rest of the cream—the butter milk—washed and worked into
the final product which we know as butter. The process
of working removes most of the particles of curd remaining
and the soluble constituents of milk. This gives pure, uncolored sweet butter. Salt is usually added to sweet butter
to give it a flavor; it also acts as a preservative. The
amount added varies according to the market for which it
is intended—from 0 to 4 per cent. In salting a very good
grade of sodium chloride is used. Salted butter is then
worked to distribute the salt, to remove the excess of water,
to press the particles of fat together into a compact mass,
and to give it the texture characteristic of the butter of commerce.

The color of butter will vary according to the nature of the
diet of the cow, for the coloring matter of the body fat and
milk has been shown to be derived from the coloring matter
of plants. Butter made from the milk of cows receiving certain green foods is particularly rich in the yellow color commonly associated with butter; thus butter made in the spring
usually has a deeper yellow color than that made in the winter. To ensure a butter of uniform color throughout the
year dairymen resort to the use of coloring matter.

The presence of bacteria in butter is a matter of fully as
great importance as their presence in milk. The processes of
butter-making tend to increase the number of bacteria:
centrifulgalization so generally employed for the separation
of cream from milk tends to leave the bacteria in the cream
and the conglomeration of the particles of fat in the process
of churning results in a concentration of bacteria in the butter. The result is that butter often contains many more
bacteria than the cream from which it is prepared. The
souring of cream before its use in butter-making results in an
accumulation of lactic-acid-producing bacteria with an accompanying decrease in the rate of growth of certain other
types. The Bacillus tuberculosis has been found in butter

prepared from milk containing this organism; cold storage does not result in the death of the bacillus.

The following table gives the composition of American creamery butter:

	Per cent.
Fat	82.41
Water	13.90
Lard	2.51
Curd	1.18

Vaıiation from these figures will occur, depending upon the process of manufacture. Dividing the samples of butter into classes according to the fat content, the following general variations were observed in the case of the data given above: butter fat 5.0 per cent., water 2.9 per cent., salt 1.74 per cent., and curd 0.39 per cent.

Butter fat is a mixture of the glycerides of various fatty acids with small amounts of lipoids—lecithin and cholesterol—and coloring matter. The relative proportions of these individual fats, or as they are usually expressed in analysis, "fatty acids," varies with the food, particularly with the fat content of the food, the individuality of the cow and stage of lactation. The taste and odor of butter is influenced by the food given the cow; garlic, for instance, gives to milk and butter a decided odor characteristic of the plant.

The following table gives the distribution of the more important fatty acids found in a particular sample of butter:[1]

Acid.	Percentage of triglycerides.
Dioxystearic	1.04
Oleic	33.94
Stearic	1.91
Palmitic	40.51
Myristic	10.44
Lauric	2.73
Capric	0.34
Caprylic	0.53
Caproic	2.32
Butyric	6.23

Butter fat is practically completely absorbed. The average caloric value of butter, based upon an 85 per cent. fat content, is approximately 3500 Calories per pound or 7.7 Calories per gram.

Renovated Butter and Butter Substitutes.—When butter which has become rancid is treated to restore its sweetness the product is designated as "processed or renovated" butter. The rancid butter is melted, the curd and brine drawn off,

[1] Browne: Jour. Amer. Chem. Soc., 1899, xxi, 807.

the fat separated and aërated and then rechurned with milk or cream to restore the texture and flavor. Such butter is in many respects as satisfactory as the average grade of butter; it is not equal in quality to the better grades of butter.

Oleomargarine.—A fat product prepared from various animal and vegetable fats and oils which resemble butter in its consistency is sold under various names, of which oleomargarine or margarine are the most common. Its manufacture is restricted by the government; a tax is levied against it, a fourth cent per pound for the uncolored product and ten cents per pound for oleomargarine artifically colored to resemble butter. Yet oleomargarine is a satisfactory substitue for butter; it is often more desirable than some good grades of butter. One objection to oleomargarine is that it is many times sold as butter with the intent to deceive. Containing as it does a higher percentage of stearin, we might expect to find oleomargarine less readily absorbed than butter; experience has shown, however, that the losses in digestion are nearly the same for the two products. But-ter is, however, in many ways a finer product and more palatable. It is much richer in the accessory substances or vitamines than oleomargarine and is from this point of view a much more desirable food.

The materials used in the manufacture of oleomargarine are chiefly neutral lard, "oleo oil," and cotton seed oil. Neutral lard is prepared from the fresh "leaf lard" of the hog. This is ground up, worked with water, and rendered at a temperature of 40° to 50°.C. Only a portion of the lard is removed from the fat. The product obtained is almost neutral in reaction and practically free from taste or odor. Oleo oil is prepared by a somewhat similar process. Fat from the abdominal cavity of beef or caul fat is thoroughly worked in water, chilled, the hardened fat ground up and finally rendered at a low temperature. The liquid fat ob-tained by this process is permitted to cool, when stearin and palmitin partially crystallize out. The fluid portion is pressed out of the semisolid mass, run into cold water and allowed to solidify. This product is designated as "oleo" or "oleo oil." The cotton seed oil used is especially prepared for the purpose. Cocoanut fat and peanut oil are also used. The nut margarines do not have the same biological value as butter or the oleomargarines, since they lack the fat-soluble vitamines. In the final stage of preparation the fats and oils are mixed in the desired proportion; the quantities of the various constituents used depends upon the market for which the oleomargarine is intended. For warm climates more of the oleo oil and lard are used than for cold climates. The properly mixed fats are then churned with milk or cream, or with an emulsion of milk and butter to give the flavor of butter to the product. This yields a coarse emulsion which, upon cooling, is washed, salted, and worked into the final product. The following is the composition of oleomargarine, given by Koenig, in per cent.: Water, 9.07; fat, 87.59; nitrogenous extractives and lactose, 0.99; ash, 2.35; sodium chloride, 2.15.

Lard.—Lard is the rendered fat of the hog. The fat is extracted by means of heat which liquefies it and gradually frees it from the connective tissues. Lards are designated according to the portion of the animal from which they are prepared and the mode of rendering. "Neutral" and "leaf" lard are obtained from the fat surrounding the kidneys. The preparation of the former has already been indicated (p. 234). "Leaf lard" is obtained by heating the leaf fat or the residue from neutral lard to a higher temperature with steam. Kettle-rendered lard is made from leaf and back fat by heating in open jacketed kettles. Steam lard is made from the remaining portions of the hog not used for direct consumption by the direct application of steam.

Various substitues for lard are prepared and sold under trade names. They are ordinarily mixtures of cotton seed oil and beef fat or specially treated cotton seed oil.

VEGETABLE OILS

Cotton Seed Oil.—Cotton seed oil is used extensively as a substitute for olive oil or in the preparation of substitutes for animal fats. In the preparation of cotton seed oil the cotton seeds are cleaned and ground, the meal heated under pressure to 210° to 215° F. and the oil expressed with hydraulic presses while still warm and the crude oil refined. The best grades of cotton seed oil are practically free from any characteristic flavor and are suitable substitutes for olive oil. As with the butter substitute, oleomargarine, the real objection to its use is the economic one, that it is often sold as olive oil. However, it lacks the characteristic natural flavor of olive oil.

By a process of chilling and pressing the higher melting-point fats of cotton seed oil are partially separated from the more liquid ones. The former are used as substitutes for lard while the latter becomes a satisfactory oil for cold climates.

Cotton seed oil is used extensively in the preparation of lard substitutes in which the fatty acids of the liquid unsaturated fats are transformed, reduced, into their corresponding saturated compounds which are solid at the ordinary temperatures. These transformations are brought about by heating with hydrogen in the presence of finely divided nickel. The nickel is added as a catalyst to hasten the reaction between hydrogen and the fatty acid. Small quantities of nickel remain in the final product and there is a possibility that they may be detrimental to health. This point has not as yet been determined. Such prepared products are as well utilized as lard and other fats and might well be substituted for them when cheaper were it not for the nickel present.

Olive Oil.—Olive oil is prepared by pressing the flesh of the ripe olive. The selection of the olive and the mode of preparation determine in general the grade of oil. The highest grade of oil, virgin oil, is from selected hand-picked olives. The product is obtained by slight pressure of cold olives. Subsequent pressure of the mass, first cold and then later heated with water, gives the various more or less inferior grades of oil. In some processes the olives are macerated and crushed before being subjected to pressure. The various oils obtained are subjected to a refining process in which foreign particles are removed by filtration and by gravity in settling tanks. Of the fatty acids present in fats of olive oil palmitic and oleic are the most important: there is little, if any, stearic acid. Other fatty acids are present but only in small quantities. Practically all of these fatty acids occur as neutral fat or glycerides; the small percentage which exists as free fatty acids varies with the ripeness of the fruit and the mode of preparation; most of the high grades of oil contain less than 3 per cent. Olive oil is eaten principally in salads; it is used to some extent in cooking. Other vegetable oils are used for food, such as peanut oil, sesame oil, cocoanut oil, etc. Vegetable oils have been found to be fully as digestible as animal fats.

Corn Oil.—Corn oil is a by-product of the starch and glucose industry. It is obtained from the germ of the corn seed. The oil is golden yellow in color and has a pleasant taste and odor. It is satisfactory as a salad oil.

COD-LIVER OIL

Cod-liver oil is prepared by means of pressure from the raw fresh livers of codfish. It has been used extensively because it is apparently assimilated under conditions in which other fat foods are not effective. It contains a number of low melting-point saturated fats in addition to olein, which is present to the extent of approximately 70 per cent., cholesterol, a small amount of iodine, and a number of basic substances are also present. The presence in cod-liver oil of specific substances necessary for growth and maintenance, such as are found in butter and egg yolk, may be one of the reasons for its successful use in therapeutics. Cod-liver oil is sometimes adulterated by the admixture of other fish oils which results in an inferior product. Preparations are also sold which purport to have all of the therapeutic properties of cod-liver oil without the peculiar oily taste which is repugnant to some persons. Those preparations from which the fat has been entirely or largely removed are practically useless as substitutes for cod-liver oil since the therapeutic value rests as much in the readily assimilable oils as in any other factor.

CHAPTER XV.

FOODS VALUABLE FOR THEIR SALTS, VITA-MINES, WATER, AND BULK.

In addition to those foods which furnish primarily protein, carbohydrate, or fat is a group of foods which, while supplying these food-stuffs to a certain extent, are not sufficiently rich in them to be valuable sources of such material. They form, however, an important part of the diet because they are valuable sources of inorganic salts (particularly the salts of organic acids), of water, and of certain accessory food-stuffs essential for a satisfactory diet. They are comparatively indigestible. It is the indigestible residue which serves to give bulk to the intestinal contents and thus promotes peristalsis. Some of these foods contain a certain amount of soluble material which in itself stimulates peristalsis—laxatives. These water-rich, indigestible foods are then a means of adding salts, accessory substances and bulk to the diet without markedly increasing the energy or protein portion of the regimen. In addition to these purely material advantages they are in most cases appetizing and are in this way valuable as aids to digestion. To this class of foods belong the succulent plant foods—the vegetables and fruits. A clear-cut classification is difficult in a few cases. To classify dried legumes as protein foods, and fresh and canned varieties of the same food as valuable chiefly for their salts and their value as appetizers may appear illogical. A consideration of their usual place in the diet, however, makes this the most desirable classification. Our discussion will confine itself, therefore, unless otherwise stated, to the succulent fruits and vegetables.

Fruits and vegetables are composed largely of water; cellulose, the chief structural material; starches; sugars; organic acids; gums; mineral matter; protein, and a small amount of fat. So far as nutritive value is concerned, the quantities of the food-stuffs present are so small as to be practically negligible. The small amount of protein is poorly absorbed; carbohydrate, exclusive of cellulose, and fat are almost completely digested, but the small quantity ingested is very seldom of practical importance. This is particularly true of the fat.

The indigestibility of fruits and vegetables as a whole is due to the cellulose content. Cooking will increase the digestibility of this carbohydrate to a certain extent, particularly in the case of raw fruit and the starchy vegetables for it softens the cellulose structures and ruptures the starch grains. The accompanying table gives the composition of some of the more important fruits and vegetables.

CHEMICAL COMPOSITION OF TYPICAL FRUITS (PER CENT.).

FRESH.

Fruits.	Water, per cent.	Protein (N x 6.25), per cent.	Fat, per cent.	Carbohydrate, per cent.	Crude fiber (cellulose), per cent.	Ash, per cent.	Fuel value, Calories per pound.	Grams yielding 100 Calories.
Apples	84.6	0.4	0.5	14.2	1.2	0.3	285	159
Bananas . . .	75.3	1.3	0.6	22.0	1.0	0.8	447	101
Blackberries . .	86.3	1.3	1.0	10.9	2.5	0.5	262	173
Cherries . . .	80.9	1.0	0.8	16.7	0.2	0.6	354	128
Grapes . . .	77.4	1.3	1.6	19.2	4.3	0.5	437	104
Huckleberries . .	81.9	0.6	0.6	16.6	..	0.3	336	
Lemons . . .	89.3	1.0	0.7	8.5	1.1	0.5	201	226
Muskmelons . .	89.5	0.6	..	9.3	2.1	0.6	180	252
Oranges . . .	86.9	0.8	0.2	11.6	..	0.5	233	195
Peaches . . .	89.4	0.7	0.1	9.4	3.6	0.4	188	242
Strawberries . .	90.4	1.0	0.6	7.4	1.4	0.6	177	256

DRIED.

	Water, per cent.	Protein (N x 6.25), per cent.	Fat, per cent.	Carbohydrate, per cent.	Crude fiber (cellulose), per cent.	Ash, per cent.	Fuel value, Calories per pound.	Grams yielding 100 Calories.
Apples	28.1	1.6	2.2	66.1	..	2.0	1318	34
Dates	15.4	2.1	2.8	78.4	..	1.3	1575	29
Figs	18.8	4.3	0.3	74.2	..	2.4	1437	
Prunes	22.3	2.1	..	73.3	..	2.3	1368	33
Raisins	14.6	2.6	3.3	76.1	..	3.4	1562	29

CHEMICAL COMPOSITION OF TYPICAL VEGETABLES (PER CENT.).

Vegetables.	Water, per cent.	Protein (N x 6.25), per cent.	Fat, per cent.	Carbohydrate, per cent.	Crude fiber (cellulose), per cent.	Ash, per cent.	Fuel value, Calories per pound.	Grams yielding 100 Calories.
Asparagus . . .	94.0	1.8	0.2	3.3	0.8	0.7	101	450
Beans, fresh:								
Lima . .	68.5	7.1	0.7	22.0	1.7	1.7	557	82
String . .	89.2	2.3	0.3	7.4	..	0.8	189	241
Cabbage . . .	91.5	1.6	0.3	5.6	1.1	1.0	143	317
Carrots . . .	88.2	1.1	0.4	9.3	1.1	1.0	205	221
Celery . . .	94.5	1.1	0.1	3.3	..	1.0	84	540
Lettuce . . .	94.7	1.2	0.3	2.9	0.7	0.9	87	524
Potatoes:								
White . .	78.3	2.2	0.1	18.4	0.4	1.0	378	120
Sweet . .	69.0	1.8	0.7	27.4	1.3	1.1	558	81
Pumpkins . . .	93.1	1.0	0.1	5.2	1.2	0.6	117	389
Spinach . . .	92.3	2.1	0.3	3.2	0.9	2.1	109	418
Tomatoes . . .	94.3	0.9	0.4	3.9	0.6	0.5	104	439

Fresh vegetables and fruits have long been known for their anti-scorbutic properties. These have been ascribed to the predominance of the basic elements in the ash. While this may be a factor, recent work has shown the presence of the accessory food-stuffs, vitamines, which may be of much more importance.

The constituents of vegetables and fruits which make them so desirable as foods are the salts and in fruits, the acids or acid salts, soluble sugars, and the essential oils, esters and ethers which give the pleasant taste. Cellulose is important for its laxative effect. The pleasing appearance of fresh and cooked vegetables and fruits has some esthetic value. Most fruits and many vegetables are palatable even in the raw state, in which form it is the crispness of the pulp or leaf which is particularly attractive. The delicate coloring matter which these foods contain is not only attractive to the eye but serves to stimulate the appetite. When cooked with sugar, as preserves or jellies, these coloring matters and flavors are the means of increasing the appetite not only for the conserve itself but for insipid foods, chiefly carbohydrates, to which they are added. In this way they are valuable in the diet of the sick room.

Vegetable foods are comparatively tasteless. To make them palatable it is necessary to add fats, usually in the form of oil or butter, and condiments, particularly acids, *e. g.*, vinegar. The addition of salt to vegetables is also necessary.

The importance of vegetables and fruits as sources of salts is indicated by the following table which gives the percentage of individual ash constituents of typical vegetables and fruits:

COMPOSITION OF THE ASH OF TYPICAL FRUITS (PER CENT.).[1]

FRESH.

Fruits.	CaO.	MgO.	K_2O.	Na_2O.	P_2O_5.	Cl.	S.	Fe.
Apples . . .	.014	.014	.15	.02	.03	.004	.005	.0003
Bananas . .	.01	.04	.50	.02	.055	.20	.013	.0006
Blackberries .	.08	.035	.20	..	.08	..	.01	
Cherries . .	.03	.027	.26	.03	.07	.01	.01	.0005
Grapes . . .	.024	.014	.25	.03	.12	.01	.024	.0013
Huckleberries .	.035	.025	..	..	.07	.02	.013	.0011
Lemons . .	.05	.01	.21	.01	.02	.01	.012	.0006
Muskmelons .	.024	.02	.283	.082	.035	.041	.014	.0003
Oranges . .	.06	.02	.22	.01	.05	.01	.013	.0003
Peaches . .	.01	.02	.25	.02	.047	.01	.01	.0003
Strawberries .	.05	.03	.18	.07	.064	.01	..	.0009

DRIED.

	CaO.	MgO.	K_2O.	Na_2O.	P_2O_5.	Cl.	S.	Fe.
Dates . . .	.10	.13	..	..	.12	.32	.066	.003
Figs . . .	.299	.145	1.48	.064	.332	.056	.056	.0032
Prunes . . .	.06	.08	1.2	.1	.25	.01	.03	.0029
Raisins . .	.08	.15	1.0	.19	.29	.07	.06	.005

[1] Sherman: Food Products, 1914, p. 347.

COMPOSITION OF THE ASH OF TYPICAL VEGETABLES (PER CENT.).

Vegetables.	CaO.	MgO.	K_2O.	Na_2O.	P_2O_4.	Cl.	S.	Fe.
Asparagus . .	.04	.02	.20	.01	.09	.04	.04	.001
Beans:								
Lima . .	.04	.11	.7	.12	.27	.009	.06	.0025
String . .	.075	.043	.28	.03	.12	.018	.04	.0016
Cabbage . .	.068	.026	.45	.05	.09	.03	.07	.0011
Carrots . .	.077	.034	.35	.13	.10	.036	.022	.0008
Celery . . .	.10	.04	.37	.11	.10	.17	.025	.0005
Lettuce . .	.05	.01	.42	.04	.09	.06	.014	.001
Potatoes:								
White . .	.016	.036	.53	.025	.14	.03	.03	.0013
Sweet . .	.025	.02	.47	.06	.09	.12	.02	.0005
Pumpkins . .	.03	.015	.08	.08	.11	.01	.02	
Spinach . .	.09	.08	.94	.20	.13	.02	.041	.0032
Tomatoes . .	.02	.017	.35	.01	.059	.03	.02	.0004

Green vegetables and fruits are an important source of iron. Investigations have shown that combined iron, such as occurs in nature is in a readily assimilable form, probably in the most desirable state. The iron of meat is chiefly in the form of hemoglobin, which is comparatively indigestible. The iron compounds of vegetables and fruits are, however, quite readily digested and absorbed. It is the availability of the iron which makes plant foods desirable in the diet for the iron they contain.

The tables indicate only the relative amounts of the various elements, or their oxides, present in fruits and vegetables. If we consider them with regard to the form in which these elements exist we find the basic elements combined with both inorganic and organic radicles. The organic acids exist in many cases as the acid salts, chiefly the acid potassium salts. As the organic acids occur in the fruit or vegetable they exhibit in some cases a considerable degree of acidity, as is the case of lemons or apples. After absorption in the body the organic acid is oxidized and the base, associated with the acid, combines with carbonic acid to form the carbonate which functions as a potential base. An examination of the ash of fruits and vegetables shows it to contain an excess of base over the acid-forming elements. In our discussion of inorganic salts it was noted that animal food is, with the exception of milk, potentially acid-yielding. Vegetables are then important in the dietary, for their ability to neutralize the acids produced in metabolism. In the case of fruits and vegetables it is the small amount of nutritive material associated with the salts which makes it possible to balance the diet with regard to its acid and alkaliforming properties, so as to aid in the maintenance of the neutrality of the blood. For the same reason, vegetables are important when it is desired to reduce the potential

16

acidity of the blood and urine. An excess of base-forming elements is not as objectionable as an excess of acid-forming elements because of the ever-present excess of carbon dioxide to form bicarbonate with the base. The natural tendency to ingest plant food with meat in a mixed diet has had, therefore, a scientific foundation. The greater solubility of uric acid in an alkaline urine, resulting from the ingestion of an excess of basic material, than in a neutral or acid urine is also an advantage.

The sugars of fruits and vegetables are chiefly sucrose (cane-sugar), dextrose, and levulose. Some fruits, such as the grape, often contain a high proportion of sugar.

The more important plant acids are citric (lemon), malic (apple), tartaric (grape), and in some oxalic acid. The acids occur in varying proportions in the different fruits and vegetables. The fruits designated in parentheses above are representative of the class of fruit in which the particular acid predominates; other acids are also present. The relative proportion of starch, sugar and acid in fruits varies during the process of ripening. The following table gives the variation in the composition of an apple at various stages of its growth.

COMPOSITION OF BALDWIN APPLE AT DIFFERENT PERIODS IN ITS GROWTH,[1]
PER CENT.

Condition.	Water.	Solids.	Invert sugar.	Sucose.	Total sugar.	Starch.	Free malic acid.	Ash.
Very green	81.5	18.5	6.4	1.6	8.0	4.1	1.2	0.27
Green . .	79.8	20.2	6.5	4.1	10.5	3.7		
Ripe . . .	80.4	19.6	7.7	6.8	14.5	0.17	0.65	0.27
Overripe .	80.3	19.7	8.8	5.3	14.1	..	0.48	0.28

Green fruit, in general, contains considerable starch. As the fruit ripens there is a gradual reduction in the quantities of the starch and acids and an increase of sugar. Pectin, the carbohydrate which forms the basis of jellies, gradually decreases as the fruit ripens.

Cooking of Vegetables and Fruits.—Vegetables and fruits are cooked to soften the cellulose structure, rupture the starch grains, improve the texture and flavor, and thereby increase digestibility and palatability. Many fruits and vegetables which are also eaten in the raw form are cooked to add variety to the diet and for purposes of preservation. Heat converts the water in the cells into steam, the expansion of which ruptures the cells, freeing the enclosed starch; an exaggerated example of the expansive action of steam is seen in the popping of corn, in which expansion takes place

[1] Browne: Penn. Dept. Agr., Bull. 58.

suddenly throughout the whole mass of starch cells when internal pressure is sufficient to rupture the tough outer layer of the kernel. During the process of cooking hydrolytic changes occur: the starch and cellulose are partially hydrated, take up water, and are transformed into simpler products—glucose and sugars; protein is coagulated; the mineral salts are only slightly affected.

Since inorganic salts are, from a dietetic point of view, one of the important food factors in fruit and vegetables, it is desirable then, to conserve them as much as possible. In boiling, the method usually employed for cooking vegetables, a large proportion of the salts and also protein may be lost; by direct removal before cooking, as in peeling; by extraction in the water used in washing and soaking, or discarded with the water poured off at the end of the cooking process. Methods which will avoid these losses should be used. Baking or steaming, with the least removal of outer coverings, is the most desirable. Some vegetables, such as spinach and chard, which are cooked by steaming in the water contained in them, are found to lose a large proportion of their salts when the liquor is poured off before they are served.

LOSSES IN COOKING VEGETABLES (PERCENTAGE OF FRESH EDIBLE PORTION).[1]

Kind of vegetable.	Solids.	Ash.	P_2O_5.	CaO.	MgO.
Spinach:					
Boiled	31.59	51.65	52.33	6.89?	60.38
Steamed	0.18	9.34	5.23	8.69	7.85
Cabbage:					
Boiled	32.86	42.62	33.93	27.66	26.71
Steamed	2.54	11.47	1.79	9.31	4.23
Carrots:					
Cut up and boiled . .	10.05	11.48	22.88	10.88	19.19
Boiled whole	6.28	7.38	17.97	8.77	19.19

Fruits and vegetables may be kept at ordinary temperatures for a considerable length of time before they begin to decay, wilt, or dry up. With proper refrigeration many of them can be kept for a comparatively long time. Such a method of preservation is becoming more prevalent, and some vegetables and fruits may be had throughout the year. Apples in particular are commonly preserved in cold storage.

The process of canning fruit and vegetables has long been used by the housewife to preserve them for use when out of season. Canned foods can now be purchased in the stores in great variety, tomatoes, corn, and peas being supplied in the greatest quantity. Since canned fruits and vegetables

[1] Berry: Jour. Home Economics, 1912, iv.

retain most of the properties of the freshly cooked food they are excellent sources of this type of food in the winter when green vegetables are generally "out of season." In canning vegetables and, to a certain extent fruit, are heated only enough to sterilize them. This is done after the can is sealed. Sugar is often added to fruit to aid in their preservation and increase the flavor. The juice of fruits is also sterilized and kept for use as beverages or mixed with sugar and made into jellies. It is the pectin of fruit which gelatinizes and forms the basis of jellies.

FOOD ADJUNCTS.

Food which is entirely satisfactory, in its quantitative composition, with regard to proteins, fat, carbohydrate, salts, and even the accessory substances or vitamines, may be in such a form that it is not relished; we have no desire to eat it. This distaste may be due to the appearance or taste of the particular food, or to a lack of interest in food in general. Such conditions are not confined to man alone. These factors do not affect the ultimate absorption of food so much as is sometimes thought, for food-stuffs which are ingested with much effort have been found to be just as thoroughly digested as those which are appetizing. The extent of variation in the diet is a matter largely of personal taste. Some people relish the same diet day after day, while others require frequent changes. Animals fed artificial diets of similar composition from day to day often refuse to eat. If to the same diet small amounts of flavoring substances, having no nutritive value, be added and the flavor changed from time to time, it will be eaten readily during long periods of time. There are also experiments on the flow of gastric juice which show that when there is desire for food, the mere sight of food results in a flow of highly acid and strongly active gastric juice which starts the process of gastric digestion, the products of which are capable of causing a continued secretion. Certain food constituents, such as the extractives of meat and some condiments, are capable of stimulating such a flow of gastric juice, and this in turn affects the secretion of the other digestive juices. The garnishing of food when served likewise has through the increased attractiveness of the dish a beneficial effect upon the digestion of food. There is a fundamental reason, therefore, for the use of condiments and for different methods of preparing food.

Spices.—Spices are used almost exclusively for their flavor. Such spices as allspice, cloves, cinnamon, ginger, caraway, etc., are used chiefly in cooking. The peppers (black and white), paprika, mustard, and horse-radish are often added to food after it has been prepared.

Flavoring Extracts.—Many alcoholic extracts of various plants of which vanilla, lemon, orange, peppermint, spearmint, and wintergreen are the most common, are used to add an agreeable flavor or taste to foods.

Meat Extracts.—Meat extracts are to be classed with the food adjuncts (see p. 183).

Vinegar.—Vinegar is the product of the alcoholic and acetic acid fermentation of fruit juices; its distinguishing constituent is acetic acid. It may also be prepared from the products of alcoholic fermentation of grain or is compounded from acetic acid and substances to give a flavor and color which will simulate the natural vinegars. Vinegar is used with more or less insipid foods to intensify the flavor, and to soften food somewhat; for colloidal material tends to swell in acid solutions.

Sugar and Salt (Sodium Chloride).—Sugar and salt may both be classified differently but may, for convenience, be included here as condiments, for they are used to add flavor and stimulate the appetite.

Sugar Substitutes.—Saccharine, dulcin, granatose and saxin, benzene derivatives, are sometimes used in place of sugar to sweeten food. These products are used particularly to sweeten the food of diabetics and of the obese to increase its palatability without increasing the carbohydrate content. When taken in sufficient quantity these substitutes for sugar are harmful. It is the contention of manufacturers that small quantities are not deleterious to the health. While this may be true during short periods of time, it is doubtful whether their continued ingestion may not cause serious disturbances in the body. Their use in diabetes is defensible on the basis that the harmful effects are overweighed by the possibility of reducing the carbohydrate content of the food.

BEVERAGES.

Many foods are ingested in a liquid or semiliquid form. There are, however, liquids which possessing a certain amount of food value, are taken for their stimulating effects upon the nervous and digestive systems. The pleasurable conditions under which they are ordinarily ingested should not be neglected in considering the effect of these beverages.

Those beverages most commonly taken with food and most properly considered a part of the diet are tea, coffee, cocoa, chocolate, and the malted and spirituous (and carbonated) liquors.

Tea.—Tea is prepared from the leaves and leaf buds of various varieties of hardy shrubs, *Thea*. Two general types of tea are used, green and black. This classification refers particularly to the general method of preparation. Green tea is prepared by steaming the withered leaves and then drying them in the sun or artificially, thus retaining the green color. Black tea has undergone a fermentation (or oxidation) process which darkens the color of the leaves and reduces the quantity of tannin. Numerous varieties of both kinds of tea may result from the selection of leaves from different parts of the shrub or twig or from the country or locality from which they are obtained.

The active constituent of tea is theine or caffein, but certain volatile oils and tannin contribute to the aroma and taste of the prepared beverage. In the preparation of the beverage it is the relative proportion of these three constituents to which most attention is given. The end commonly believed to be desirable is the extraction of the maximum amount of caffein and volatile oils, with the minimum quantity of tannin.

From a study of the nature of the products extracted from tea leaves the *Lancet* has come to the conclusion that it is the relative proportions of caffein and tannin extracted which determine the quality of tea. They show that when caffein and tannin are present in the proportion of one part of caffein to three parts of tannin they may be precipitated completely by acidification in the form of caffein tannate. Caffein tannate has neither the astringent taste of tannin nor the bitter taste of caffein, and it is precipitated by acids. It has been suggested that the caffein of tea, unlike the caffein complex of coffee, is precipitated in the stomach and is not absorbed until it reaches the alkaline intestine. A comparison of the valuation of tea by tea-tasters and the proportion of caffein to tannin in the tea shows that the infusion of those teas classed as "good" contain these two substances in the proportion in which they exist in caffein tannate, and that inferior teas yield an excess either of caffein or of tannin in the infusion, usually the former.

The following table shows the extractives from teas of three different types and the relative proportion of caffein and tannin contained. It will be seen that the high-priced teas contain a greater proportion of tannin and caffein (caffein tannate).

TEA INFUSIONS (5 GRAMS OF TEA TO 400 C.C. BOILING WATER).

Tea.	Caffein tannate. Determined.	Tannin combined with caffein.	Caffein combined with tannin.	Total tannin.	Total caffein.	Caffein not combined.	Tannin not combined.	Price. cents.
India	8.54	6.41	2.13	6.80	2.56	0.43	0.39	15
	13.36	10.02	3.34	10.92	4.32	0.98	0.90	46
Ceylon	8.88	6.66	2.22	6.30	2.80	0.58	..	17
	• 12.00	· 9.00	3.00	8.40	3.60	0.60	..	33
China	5.36	4.02	1.34	3.02	1.92	0.58	..	13
	6.48	4.86	1.62	4.60	2.80	1.18	..	35

The chemical composition of the water used in making tea may affect the composition of the infusion, for, should the water be rich in calcium, the calcium will tend to precipitate the tannin and leave an excess of caffein. The period of extraction affects the composition of the infusion; continued extraction of good tea results for a time in a proportionate increase in both caffein and tannin so that the balance is but little disturbed; inferior teas, on the other hand, yield an excess of either caffein or tannin. Prolonged boiling of tea tends to extract a greater proportion of tannin. The *Lancet* believes that caffein and not tannin is the injurious constituent of tea, for tannin is rarely in excess of the ratio in which it exists in caffein tannate. Studies of the quantity of caffein and tannin present in tea steeped for varying lengths of time have shown that practically all of the caffein is extracted in the first three to five minutes. A longer period of extraction results in an increased proportion of tannic acid in the infusion. For those, then, who desire to obtain the maximum aroma and exhilarating effect of the caffein without the bitter, stringent tannin, tea should be extracted for a short period.

The total quantity of caffein and tannin present in the average cup of tea after an infusion of five minutes varies with the kind of tea—it has been found to be roughly 1 grain (0.07 gram) of caffein and three or four times as much tannin. The effects of tea are discussed with those of coffee on p. 250.

Coffee.—The beverage coffee is prepared from the roasted bean, of the *Caffea arabacia*. The coffee berry contains a bean composed of two elongate, hemispherical halves enclosed in a thin membranous sheath, which is surrounded by an outer layer of pulp. The berries are separated and roasted to preserve them, to render them brittle and readily ground, and to develop certain flavors and aroma. In the roasting process a large proportion of the sugar is caramelized and there are losses of water and to a certain extent of caffein. Caffeol is the name given to a mixture of substances present in the roasted product which gives to coffee its characteristic flavor and aroma. The alkaloid of coffee is, as in tea, largely caffein.

The caffein of coffee is combined in a different manner from that of tea; it is almost entirely extracted by cold water while that of tea is not. It appears to be combined with an acid designated as caffetannic acid related to tannin but exhibiting properties different from those of the tannic acid of tea. The caffein of coffee is soluble in both an acid and an alkaline medium, while that of tea is precipitated by acids. This fact may account for the greater stimulatory effect of coffee than of tea, for the caffein being in solution may be absorbed by the stomach, while that of tea must pass to the intestines for solution and absorption.

The several kinds of coffee vary chiefly according to the country from which they are obtained. As with tea the advantage of the different kinds is to a considerable extent a matter of taste.

The coffee bean contains roughly one-third the quantity of caffein present in dry tea. The greater quantity of coffee used gives approximately the same quantity of caffein in both prepared beverages. Coffee contains a greater amount of total extracted material.

In the process of preparing coffee for its most pleasurable effects the caffein and the aroma are the two constituents which it is desirable to extract. It has been found that when 2 ounces (60 grams) of coffee are used, a teacupful of coffee will contain approximately 1.7 grains (0.1 gram) of caffein, a value which is slightly higher than that of tea; the smaller quantity of infusion taken when cream or milk is used will make this value slightly lower. The quantity of caffein and caffetannic acid extracted in the preparation of coffee varies considerably with the mode of preparation. Cold water extracts approximately the same weight of material from coffee as does hot water, but hot water extracts oils which improve the odor and taste of the beverage.

Four general methods of preparing the beverage coffee are used: boiling, steeping, percolation, and filtration.

Boiled coffee is prepared by heating medium-ground coffee placed in cold water to the boiling-point and maintaining it at that temperature for five minutes. This method gives the greatest proportion of extract, and one which is rich in caffein and caffetannic acid.

Steeped coffee is similar to boiled coffee except that the infusion is poured off soon after the boiling-point is reached. This method yields the lowest caffein content.

Percolation consists in passing warm water through finely **ground** coffee in a specially constructed coffee pot. The **temperature** of the water which is forced over the coffee **seldom** reaches the boiling-point. A low total extract high **in caffe**tannic acid and caffein is obtained.

Filtered coffee is made from finely pulverized coffee which **has been** placed in a muslin bag and over which vigorously **boiling** water is poured. The product is lower in total ex-**tractives** and contains less caffetannic acid than boiled coffee. **If the** water be poured through more than once a darker **liquid** is obtained which has a less agreeable flavor because **of the** additional tannin and other objectionable substances. **This** method of preparing coffee is in many ways the most **satisfactory.**[1] The cloth used should not be allowed to dry **but** should be kept in clear cold water.

A comparison of the relative quantities of caffein and tan-nin extracted by the various methods is given below.

TANNIN AND CAFFEIN EXTRACTED BY VARIOUS METHODS OF PREPARATION (7 TABLESPOONFULS (80 GRAMS) COFFEE TO 6 CUPS (750 C.C.) WATER).

Method of preparation.	Tannin, grains.	Caffein, grains.
Boiled	2.44	2.5
Steeped	2.40	{ 0.5 medium ground { 1.75 finely ground
Percolated	2.21–2.90	2.75
Filtered	0.2 –0.25	2.50

Specially prepared coffees are sold for the use of those who cannot take coffee because of its caffein content, usually with the implied statement that some or most of the harm-ful ingredients of coffee have been removed. After a com-parison of some of these with three types of pure coffee the following statement has been made:[2]

"'Kaffee Hag' is almost caffein-free but contains the normal amount of caffetannic acid. 'George Washington Coffee' (a soluble concentrated coffee) contains about four times as much caffein and caffetannic acid as normal coffee. 'Cafe des Invalides' contains about 80 per cent. as much caffein as ordinary coffee, the decrease being due to its dilu-tion with other vegetable substances; its caffetannic acid is somewhat higher than in normal coffee. 'Richelieu Vacuum Coffee' contains practically the same amount of caffein and caffetannic acid as ordinary coffee."

Certain coffee substitutes prepared from roasted grains are sold for the use of those who desire a beverage simulating coffee but who do not wish to ingest the alkaloid caffein.

[1] Aborn: Tea and Coffee Trade Jour., 1913, xxv, 568.
[2] Food Products and Drugs, Report of Conn. Agr. Exp. Sta., 1911, Pt. 5.

These products accomplish this end more or less satisfactorily although their action is chiefly that of a warm beverage.

The general effect of tea or coffee is to produce wakefulness and relief from fatigue, increased strength and rapidity of the heart beat and increased blood-pressure. In some people drowsiness rather than wakefulness is induced by coffee: this is usually followed by a period of wakefulness. These effects are to be ascribed chiefly to the caffein contained in them; caffein also has a diuretic effect. The feeling of well-being which accompanies the ingestion of coffee after a meal has been ascribed to the local action of the contained oils.

The effect of coffee upon digestion is to increase the period of gastric digestion without affecting it quantitatively. Since the direct effect of water when taken with food is to delay evacuation of the stomach, the best results are obtained when water and other liquids are taken after food rather than when mixed with it. On the other hand, the ingestion of bread or cake with coffee is desirable, for it prolongs the feeling of satiety and delays diuresis. Coffee infusion has been found to tend to inhibit the coagulation of milk and to inhibit peptic activity outside the body while tea has a less retarding action on coagulation and appears to promote peptic activity.

The harmful effects of tea and coffee are sometimes referred to the tannin content because tannic acid precipitates protein, simple protein cleavage products, and digestive enzymes. The work performed for the *Lancet* tends to show for tea, at least, that in good teas the tannin is so combined with caffein that it will be precipitated out by the gastric juice and only become absorbable in the intestine in which the alkaline tannate would not have the precipitating power of tannic acid. They are therefore inclined to ascribe the harmful effect of tea to caffein.

The slight laxative effect of hot drinks is probably to be ascribed chiefly to the hot water.

Cocoa and Chocolate.—Cocoa and chocolate are prepared from the seed or bean of the tree *Theobroma cacao*. The beans are removed from the pod, fermented in boxes or in holes in the ground, and then dried in the sun until they assume the characteristic brown color of the beans shipped to the market. In the preparation of the products cocoa and chocolate the dried beans are cleaned, roasted, crushed, and finally ground, after which the ground mass is molded or specially treated according to the nature of the final product—chocolate or a special variety of chocolate such as milk chocolate or cocoa. It is during the fermentation processes just after picking and the subsequent roasting processes that care must be taken if the product is to develop the most desirable flavor.

Ground cocoa nibs, obtained by crushing the roasted beans, constitute the ordinary chocolate of commerce. Sugar, dried milk, flavoring extract (particularly vanilla), etc., are added to the ground mass in the preparation of sweet chocolate, milk chocolate, etc.

In preparing cocoa a portion of the oil or fat is removed from the ground seeds. This fat is removed by pressure—usually when warmed slightly; the residue is the finely pulverized cocoa of commerce. The expressed fatty material is cocoa butter, a semisolid fat used in the manufacture of chocolate and particularly in pharmaceutical preparations. Alkaline salts, sodium, potassium or ammonium carbonate, are often added to the ground cocoa ostensibly to increase the solubility of the product; such products are sometimes designated as "Dutch process" cocoa. The addition of alkali neutralizes any fatty acid present. Tests of these preparations in comparison with untreated preparations have failed to show any marked increase in solubility; such treatment would tend, however, to aid in the emulsification of the cocoa fat and thus produce an apparent increase in solubility.

Specially prepared cocoas are sold which have been treated with alkali as indicated above or with the addition of sugar, starch, etc.

COMPARATIVE COMPOSITION OF PRODUCTS OF THE COCOA BEAN.[1]

	Cocoa nibs.		Chocolate.		Cocoa.	
	Original material.	Fat-free.	Original material.	Fat-free.	Original material.	Fat-free.
Ash . . .	3.32	6.66	3.15	6.59	5.49	7.49
Soluble ash	1.16	2.33	1.41	2.95	2.82	3.85
Sand . .	0.02	0.04	0.06	0.13	0.24	0.32
Nitrogen .	2.38	4.77	2.26	4.73	3.33	4.54
Fat . . .	50.12	..	52.19	..	26.69	
Fiber . .	2.64	5.29	2.86	5.98	4.48	6.11
Starch . .	8.07	16.18	8.11	16.75	11.14	5.20

Cocoa and chocolate differ, as indicated above, particularly in the quantity of fat present. Cocoa contains roughly one-half as much fat as chocolate. The fat is largely a mixture of the glycerol esters of palmitic, stearic, lauric and arachidic acids, melting-point 38° to 33° C.

The active principle of cocoa and chocolate is theobromine, or trimethylxanthin, and is closely related chemically

[1] Winton: Conn. Agr. Exp. Sta. Report, 1902, p. 282.

to the caffein of tea and coffee. There is roughly about as much theobromine in cocoa as there is caffein in tea or coffee, between 1 and 2 per cent., less in the specially prepared products because of the dilution with other substances; a small amount of caffein is present. Tannin is also present; the reddish color of the finished product has been held to be an oxidation product of the tannin present in the raw bean.

Cocoa and chocolate contain theobromine which does not have the stimulating power of caffein, and these drinks are therefore less objectionable from that point of view. Because of the high fat content they tend to retard the passage of food from the stomach. While these beverages are prepared from substances with a high food value the prepared liquid is comparatively low in such value because of the relatively small quantity of material used; the added milk is often of more importance.

Mineral Waters.—Water may be roughly divided for convenience into three classes: hard, soft and "mineral" water. The presence of considerable quantities of the salts of the alkaline earth metals, particularly calcium and magnesium, is the chief characteristic of a hard water. Water analysts recognize two degrees of hardness: temporary and permanent. The quantity of calcium and magnesium present in water as the bicarbonate which may be precipitated through the removal of carbon dioxide by boiling or by the addition of lime is an index of the temporary hardness of water. When combined with the chloride or sulphate radicle calcium and magnesium are not precipitated readily by heating and the water is said to be permanently hard.[1]

Soft waters are comparatively free from dissolved inorganic matter. Distilled water is an artifically prepared soft water and is free from inorganic salts; it may contain a certain amount of ammonia. Rain water, when properly collected is virtually free from inorganic salts. It often contains a certain amount of organic material, particularly when collected from the roof.

The term "mineral water" is applied to those naturally occurring (and also artificially prepared) waters rich in particular salts or gases as distinguished from the usual table water poor in such constituents and having no specific effect.

[1] The temporary hardness of water may be removed by adding to it a saturated solution of calcium hydroxide,"lime water." In the presence of calcium hydroxide the calcium bicarbonate is changed into normal calcium carbonate which precipitates, and in this way both the calcium of the water and the calcium of the added lime water are removed. The quantity of lime water to be added to any water must be determined by experiment or it may be approximated from published analyses of the water under consideration.

The name has developed particularly in conjunction with the therapeutic use of such water. The classification of mineral waters has not been standardized. Since they are ordinarily used for their medicinal effect it is perhaps best to classify them according to the nature of the substance contained, as lithium water (lithia); sulphurous water; sulphate water (aperient); iron water (chalybeate); radio-active water. To these should be added the alkaline waters, a type which may include one or more of the types of water just named. Many waters are rich in sodium chloride and are sometimes designated as saline waters. Some waters are naturally charged with carbon dioxide while others are sold artificially charged. The classification indicated above recognizes only the most characteristic constituent of mineral water; it may contain one or all of the other constituents.

Lithium waters, or lithia waters, are waters which have been advocated because of the supposed solvent effect of lithium upon uric acid in the body. Consideration of the ionic equilibrium in the body makes it appear very improbable that the ingested lithium salts could dissolve uric acid to any considerable extent. Since most lithia waters are comparatively poor in lithium, large amounts of water would need to be taken to produce even a slight effect.

Sulphurous water contains hydrogen sulphide gas as the most characteristic constituent. The gas is liberated readily unless properly bottled; to obtain hydrogen sulphide, therefore, the water should be taken at the spring. The curative power of such waters is probably due to other constituents than the gas itself. It may be in the sulphur, sometimes "used as a blood purifier." Sulphurous waters are found at the Anderson Sulphur Springs in California, French Lick Springs, Richfield Springs, and Cold Sulphur Springs.

Sulphate waters are rich in alkali and alkali earth sulphates, such as sodium sulphate (Glauber's salt) and magnesium sulphate (Epsom salt); these two salts usually occur together. Such waters are laxative and purgative, the efficiency varies with the amount of magnesium and sodium present. Many of these waters are concentrated by evaporation and are to be diluted or dissolved before using. Salts (sulphates) are sometimes added to the natural water to increase its concentration. Some American waters rich in sulphates are found at the Mendenhall Springs, Isham and Nuvida Springs in California; the Warm Springs, Hot Springs and Healing Springs in Virginia. Foreign waters such as Hunyadi Janos, Kissengen, Seidlitz and Friedrichs-hall are of this type.

Iron waters usually contain other mineral constituents which may have as great an effect as the iron itself, such as carbonates, sulphates, lithium, and arsenic. Many waters used as table waters are rich in iron. The presence of the associated salts must be considered in prescribing iron waters; a water containing bicarbonates is preferable as a tonic. The Berkely Springs, West Virginia, and the Round Spring at the Aurora Springs, Missouri, are examples of American iron-containing bicarbonate springs. Similar foreign waters are to be found at Spa, Belgium; St. Moritz, Switzerland; Schwalbach, Germany; Trubridge Wells and Flitwick Well, England.

Radio-active Water.—The presence of traces of radium in certain waters has led to their use in therapeutics. It has been found that such waters lose their radio-activity with time. Springs which have been advocated for their healing properties because of the presence of various salts have been found to be, in addition, radio-active. Many waters, such as those at Hot Springs, Arkansas, the mineral springs of Yellowstone Park in America, and the foreign waters at Carlsbad, Gastein, Wiesbaden, Kissengen and Bath have been found to be radio-active. Radio-active water is artificially prepared and sold or may be prepared with suitable apparatus.

Alkaline waters include particularly those of the lithium, sulphate and iron types. They are valuable as a means of administering alkaline salts. The alkalinity of these waters is due to the presence of bicarbonates, primarily of sodium, potassium, or lithium and secondarily of magnesium and calcium. Many alkaline waters are effervescent. Vichy water is perhaps the most generally used alkaline water. Some American alkaline waters are: White Rock and Clysmic (Wakeshau, Wisconsin); Vichy (Saratoga Springs, New York); Londonderry Spring (New Hampshire); Hot Springs (Arizona). Vichy (France), Carlsbad (Austria), and Fachingen (Germany) are alkaline European waters.

An analysis of the various medical data with regard to the use of mineral water has brought out the following facts.[1] (*a*) many patients are improved in health under mineral water treatment; (*b*) waters of widely different composition have been recommended for the same disease; (*c*) curative properties are ascribed to many waters whose mineral content is the same as, or lower than, the city supplies used

[1] R. B. Dole: The Production of Mineral Waters in 1911, U. S. Geol. Survey, advance chapters for Mineral Resources of United States, 1912. This discussion of water is taken in part from this paper.

daily by many people without peculiar physiological effects; (*d*) treatment at resorts is often recommended for those afflicted with chronic organic diseases, many of which are obscure in nature or are caused by failure of nutrition. Such facts lead to the conclusion that the beneficial effects are to be ascribed more to the free use of water itself, augmented by dietetic treatment, exercise, and other hygienic restrictions and possibly change of climate and freedom from business and household cares than to the contained mineral constituents.

The demonstration of the value of various waters will depend upon the concentration of the dissolved constituents. The determination of the effects of a particular water is difficult to accomplish because of the difficulty in controlling the physiological factors associated with its ingestion. The specific action of salts may occur in three ways: as stimulants to (*a*) increase or (*b*) depress the activities of an organ or function or (*c*) as irritants which cause a change in form, growth, and nutrition, rather than of activity. The action of mineral waters is due to the contained ions rather than to the undissociated salt. The effect of any particular ion will depend upon its associated acidic or basic radicle and the presence of other ions in solution. When two ions occur together one ion may neutralize the effect of the other. Such an effect is apparently specific and not necessarily in the ratio of the combining power of the ions; thus, roughly, one part of calcium chloride will neutralize or antagonize the effect of one hundred parts of sodium chloride in its effect upon the permeability of membranes. This antagonistic action of ions may be the explanation of the tolerance of comparatively large quantities of some mineral waters. We know that a tolerance for water is acquired; the development of diarrhea in some persons upon moving from one locality to another may be looked upon as of this nature.[1]

The fact that an individual dose of a salt is not harmful does not mean that its continued ingestion may not be injurious, for small repeated doses of a salt will in some cases induce symptoms which are more marked than from a single dose, such as in lead poisoning, or an abnormal tolerance may be acquired as in the case of arsenic.

Analyses of water do not tell the manner in which the various ions are combined but only their proportionate distribution. From such analytical data we say by inference that the ions exist in certain combinations. These combinations are hypothetical, for the complex combinations of

[1] Diarrhea may be due to infection from a water new to the individual.

various salts and the effect of loss of dissolved gases, particularly carbon dioxide, alter the molecular and possibly ionic complexes actually present in the original water analyzed.

The results of water analyses are usually expressed in parts per million.

The following equivalents of certain methods of expressing analytical results will aid in understanding the significance of this expression.

	Equivalent in parts per million.
1 part in 100	1 part in 10,000
1 part in 1000	1 part in 1,000
1 gram in a liter	1 part in 1,000
1 milligram in a liter	1 part
Grains per imperial gallon ÷ 0.07 gives parts per million.	
Grains per U. S. gallon ÷ 0.058 gives parts per million.	

Dole has suggested the use of the quantity of a specific salt in four kilograms of water (the water intake for a day) as the basis of differeniation between medicinal and common water with reference to the minimum dose of the individual constituent in the absence of other ions which have a pharmacological effect, ignoring as difficult of demonstration the effect of associated ions.

The following table of the minimum dose of constituents common to mineral waters has been prepared by Dole:

Radicle.	Average minimum dose, grams.	Equivalent concentration, mg. per kg.
Arsenite (AsO_3) ⎰ Arsenate (AsO_4) ⎱	0.0002[1]	⎰0.2 ⎱0.3
Fluoride (F)	0.002	0.5
Barium (Ba)	0.003	0.7
Hydroxide (OH)	0.013	3.0
Aluminum (Al)	0.011	3.0[2]
Iron (Fe)	0.024	6.0
Lithium (Li)	0.075	15.0
Ammonium (NH_4)	0.078	20.0
Manganese (Mn)	0.12	30.0
Metaborate (BO_2) ⎰ Pyroborate (B_4O_7) ⎱ ([3])	0.035	⎰30.0 ⎱30.0
Iodide (I)	0.12	30.0
Calcium (Ca)	0.2	50.0
Magnesium (Mg)	0.2	50.0
Orthophosphate (PO_4)	0.23	50.0
Carborate (CO_3)	0.281	70.0
Sulphite (SO_3)	0.315	70.0
Thiosulphate (S_2O_3)	0.300	70.0
Nitrate (NO_3)	0.5	100.0
Bromide (Br)	0.53	100.0
Sulphate (SO_4)	0.60	150.0

In preparing the table care was taken that the concentration expressed should represent a minimum below which

[1]Equivalent as arsenic (As); [2]in acid solution; [3]equivalent as boron (B).

therapeutic activity could not logically be attributed to the radicle in question.

The significance of the last column may be illustrated as follows: If the average quantity 0.53 gram of bromine were in four kilograms of water the concentration of the radicle would be 132 milligrams per kilogram (reduced to 100 in the table), that is, a person who drank 4 kilograms of water containing 132 milligrams per million by weight of bromide might exhibit symptoms produced by bromides, if the water did not contain some other radicle which was antagonistic. 530 kilograms, roughly quarts, of bromide water containing one part per million of bromine would have to be ingested to obtain a similar effect.

Alcoholic Beverages.—Beverages containing alcohol are used chiefly for their psychological effects. They have, as a rule, a pleasant taste, often a fragrant odor, and are usually cooled, factors which make their consumption a pleasure. In sufficient quantities their use is accompanied by pleasurable after-effects, a sense of exhiliration, relief from fatigue, and warmth, followed, however, in many cases by depression. The effect of moderate quantities, 30 to 40 c. c., of alcohol, is to quicken the heart beat without materially raising the blood-pressure; larger quantities produce a fall in blood-pressure except in certain abnormal conditions of the circulatory system, a result which is due to a depressant action on the nervous centers and in part to a weakened heart. The general effect is that of a narcotic rather than of a stimulant. There is an increased rate of respiration, disturbed heat regulation, and secretion of saliva and gastric juice. While alcohol produces, for the time being, a feeling of well-being, and ability to work, these are more or less subjective effects. The true result appears to be a lowered capacity for work, particularly work requiring thought, and lessened endurance.

A thorough and far-reaching study of the effect of alcohol upon the body processes is being undertaken by Benedict in the nutrition laboratory of the Carnegie Institution of Washington. This series of investigations has only been started. The results of a psychological study indicate that the period of response in the simple reflex arcs in the lumbar cord, the patellar reflex, and the protective-lid reflex and to more complex cortical arcs, certain eye reactions to peripheral stimuli, speech reactions to visual word stimuli, and free associations were increased following the ingestion of doses of alcohol containing 30 c.c. and 45 c.c. of absolute alcohol; memory and free association were only slightly affected.

17

As a food, alcohol is of the type of the energy-yielding food-stuffs, fats and carbohydrates. It can be substituted for them at least to a limited extent and is capable of exerting a similar sparing effect upon protein. Its use must, however, be considered in connection with the fact that alcohol has also a toxic effect foreign to fat and carbohydrate. It is not converted into sugar by the diabetic and may then become a source of energy. It is not, however, an antiketogenic substance. The use of alcoholic beverages as food is of only secondary importance. Alcohol or even beverages fortified with sugar, such as some wines, are not economical sources of energy and there is no proof that alcohol itself is more efficient than carbohydrate in the body economy. The trend of the evidence is rather against such a possibility. Discussion of the use of alcohol as food has therefore little practical dietetic value; the food or fuel value of alcohol is a bone of contention between those advocating its use in general and their opponents.

Studies of the food value of alcohol have shown that from 90 to 98 per cent. of alcohol ingested in small quantities is oxidized; that the effect of the addition of the equivalent of 500 calories in the form of alcohol, 72 grams, to a standard diet was practically identical with the addition of an equivalent amount of sugar, and that alcohol is not as efficient in sparing protein as carbohydrate or fat. Certain investigations have demonstrated in short experiments that for small amounts of alcohol there is an increased protein metabolism. Experiments of longer duration have shown that there is an initial rise in the nitrogen excretion (loss of protein) but that in the course of a few days the metabolism returns to the normal, or there may be a retention of nitrogen. The utilization of foods is unaffected by the ingestion of *small* amounts of alcohol. These observations, which apply only to small quantities of alcohol, have demonstrated quite clearly that it may serve as a food. Large doses of alcohol exert a toxic effect, increase protein metabolism, and also the respiratory exchange; as the result of the restlessness of partially intoxicated persons. With complete intoxication the energy exchange is decreased.

The desirability of using alcohol as a food under all circimstances is doubtful; the associated danger of excessive consumption should certainly bar it as a constituent of the diet. While it can replace in part fats and carbohydrates it does not serve as a reserve food in the sense that these foods do, for it is oxidized immediately.

The therapeutic use of alcoholic beverages in medicine, such as in the treatment of fevers on the basis that it is a readily assimilable and oxidizable type of food in a condition in which food is more or less contraindicated, loses its importance somewhat in the light of our present knowledge of the effect of food in such cases. With regard to the combined stimulating and food value of such beverages and their effect upon the appetite, little of a definite nature can be said.

Alcoholic beverages are products obtained as the result of the alcoholic fermentation of sugar or prepared from fermented products. They are of two types, fermented and distilled. Fermented liquors are the result of naturally occurring fermentations. Of these there are (a) the products of direct spontaneous fermentation of saccharine fruit juice such as wine and cider, and (b) beverages produced from starch-bearing grains in which alcoholic fermentation takes place after the conversion of starch into sugar, such as the malted and brewed liquors, beer, ale, etc.

Distilled liquors, sometimes designated as "spirits," such as whiskey, brandy and rum, etc., are obtained by the distillation of naturally fermented products.

COMPOSITION OF ALCOHOLIC LIQUORS.

| | Carbon dioxide. | Alcohol | | Extract. | Nitrogenous material. | Sugars. | Gums and dextrin. | Acidity | | | Ash. | P_2O_5. |
		By weight.	By volume.					Fixed.	Volatile.	Total.		
Beer, lager	0.4	4.3	5.6	4.2	0 5	1.10	1.6		....	0 06	0 20	0.06
Porter	0.4	6 1	7 7	5.9	0 8	0.57	2.8	....	....	0 15	0.37	0.05
Ale	0.5	5.7	7.1	4.4	0.5	0.49	2.2	....	....	0 12	0.31	0.07
Malt extract.[1]												
U. S. P.	....	....	....	76.6	3.1	65.40	6.9	....	0 02	0 26	1.20	0.56
Claret	....	9.7	....	....	....	0.24	...	0.89	0.17	0.60	0.21	
Sherry	....	17 8	....	....	....	3.00	...	0 29	0.16	0.49	0.50	
Port	....	18.1	....	....	....	2.54	...	0 81	0.09	0.43	0.23	
Champagne	....	....	18.7	8.67	....	1.92	...	....	....	0.40		
Whiskey	....	43.6	51 2	0.11	...	....	...	....	....	3.36		
Brandy	....	41.1	48.5	0.67	...	....	...	....	....	3.75		
Gin	....	40.2	47.5	0.05	...	....	...	....	....	1.92		
Liqueur	....	38.5	52.0	36.00	....	32.60	...	....	....	....	0.41	
Cider:												
Hard	trace	5.2	6.5	....	....	0.04	...	....	....	0 40[2]	0.38	
Sweet	...	1.4	1.7	....	0.06	....	..	....	....	0.21	0.32	

Fermented liquors, cider and wines, are beverages in which the alcohol is formed as the result of direct fermentation of fruit juices. Cider is the fermented juice of the apple. It contains from 3 to 8 per cent. of alcohol. Sweet cider is the freshly expressed juice and contains only small amounts of alcohol. Perry, or pear cider, is made from the pear.

[1] Diastatic action complete in ten minutes.　　　[2] As malic acid.

Wines.—The term wine is customarily used to designate the fermented juice of the grape. A number of wines are to be had which differ particularly in their method of preparation and to a certain extent according to the country or locality in which they are prepared.

Classification of Wines.—A number of terms are used to express the type or quality of wines.[1] With regard to the method of preparation we have: *Natural wines*, wines which are prepared from the juice of the grape as expressed and to which no sugar or alcohol has been added, *e. g.*, hock and claret; and *fortified wines*, to which alcohol has been added, usually before the natural fermentation is completed, *e. g.*, Madeira, sherry, port. According to the intrinsic properties of wines we have the *non-effervescing* or *still wines* which contain little dissolved carbon dioxide; *effervescing* or *sparkling wines*, more or less heavily charged with carbon dioxide (*a*) from natural fermentation of added sugar in the corked bottles—champagne; or (*b*) artifically charged with carbon dioxide; *red wines*, Burgundy and Bordeaux wines or claret; *white wines*, *e. g.*, Rhenish and Moselle wine and sauternes; *dry wines*, in which the sugar has been exhausted by fermentation; and *sweet wines*, which possess a considerable amount of unfermented sugar and to which sugar is often added.

Of the different varieties of wines champagne is an effervescing selected, sweet, white wine fortified with sugar mixed with brandy. It contains 8 to 10 per cent. of alcohol; claret is a light red wine somewhat acid and astringent, contains very little sugar, is high in volatile ethers, alcohol 8 to 13 per cent.; Madeira is a strong white wine generally fortified with alcohol and possesses a rich, nutty, aromatic flavor, alcohol 17 to 20 per cent.; sherry, a Spanish wine, is a sweet wine sometimes fortified with alcohol, deep amber colored, slightly acid and possesses much fragrance, alcohol 8 to 20 per cent.; hock, German wines, are white wines mildly acid, alcohol 9 to 12 per cent.; port, an astringent wine, always fortified with alcohol, dark purple in color, alcohol 15 to 18 per cent.

Malt Liquors (Beer, Ale, Porter, Stout).—Malt liquors are made by the alcoholic fermentation of malt with hops; other grains are sometimes added. To obtain the sugar from which the alcohol is to be formed, grain is malted; that is, it is permitted to sprout. In the process of sprouting,

[1] The particular mode of preparation and more specific details of their composition may be found by consulting such books as, Leach: Food Inspection and Analysis, New York, 1913.

starch is transformed in part into soluble sugars, particularly maltose; the quantity of the enzyme, diastase, formed is often sufficient to change the starch of added grains, rice, corn, etc., to a considerable extent. The sprouting process is stopped at the proper point and the germinating mass is dried. The temperature at which the malt is dried determines to a large extent the depth of color of the final product; higher temperatures give the darker beers. In some cases caramelization of the starch is permitted as in stout. To complete the conversion of the starch the dried malt and admixed grain, if there be any, are crushed and mixed with water to permit the diastase to continue its action. The saccharine liquor or wort is concentrated, mixed with hops and a selected yeast and permitted to ferment. The nature of the yeast added for the alcoholic fermentation is a matter of great importance in the production of good malted liquors. After fermentation has proceeded to the proper stage the beer is drawn off from the greater portion of the yeast and stored in casks or vats for an after-fermentation. When this process is completed the liquor is clarified and stored in casks or bottles.

Of the different varieties of malt liquor we have beer, prepared as above without special modification; ale, essentially a light colored beer which usually contains more hops than beer; porter, a dark ale, and stout. The latter are prepared from roasted, partially caramelized malt. Such liquors are dark colored, usually heavy, and contain considerable quantities of dextrin and starch.

Malt liquors contain in addition to water, alcohol, and sugar, a variety of substances formed in the processes of malting and fermentation. Of these the carbon dioxide, which produces the effervescence, the volatile oils and the bitter principles which contribute to the taste are the most important; certain nitrogenous substances, chiefly peptone and amino-acids are also present.

Malt Extracts.—True malt extracts are free from alcohol and contain the soluble principles of malt. Such extracts have a high percentage of sugar, maltose, 48 to 70 per cent., a certain proportion of dextrin, 2 to 16 per cent., and a high diastatic activity. Many of the malt extracts sold have been found to have the general characteristics of beer. Some have been analyzed which contained approximately from 2 to 9 per cent. of alcohol. Such extracts have no diastatic activity and their nutritive value depends essentially upon the sugar content, which is in many cases low. These extracts should not be compared with the U. S. P. malt extract described above.   The following table gives the composition of commercial malt extracts in comparison with the U. S. P. extract.

Analyses of twenty-one samples of commercial preparations sold as malt extract gave the following maximum and minimum values:[1]

COMMERCIAL PREPARATIONS.

	Maximum.	Minimum.	U. S. P. (for comparison).
Alcohol	9.11	2.52	
Extract	15.32	5.39	76.6
Ash	0.37	0.14	1.2
Nitrogenous constituents, protein	1.09	0.34	3.1
Sugar solids	14.04	4.84	
Maltose	11.17	1.41	65.4
Dextrin	5.80	2.03	6.9

Distilled Liquors.—Distilled liquors, as the name implies, are the product of the distillation of fermented liquors.   By this process a liquor is obtained which is high in alcohol and contains in addition certain of the higher boiling-point alcohols, their esters, and acids which pass over with the alcohol. The distillation process is usually repeated and the intermediate portions taken for the best liquors, while the first and last distillates yield inferior products.   The liquor obtained is harsh to the taste and must be stored for a time in casks and aged, to soften and refine the flavor.

Whiskey is the product of the distillation of fermented grains, usually mixtures of corn, wheat, and rye, which has been stored in casks for at least four years, alcohol content approximately 30 to 50 per cent.   Brandy is the aged product of the distillation of fermented grape juice or wine.   The term is sometimes applied to the distillation of the fermented juice of other fruits, alcohol 20 to 50 per cent.   Cognac is a brandy distilled in certain parts of France.   Rum is the distillation from fermented molasses or cane juice, usually distilled twice and stored for a long time.   Gin is an alcoholic liquor flavored with the volatile oil of the juniper berry; other aromatic substances are sometimes used, such as coriander, anise, cardamom, orange-peel, fennel.   Gin is water-clear and is kept in glass and not wood as are the other distilled liquors, alcohol 27.5 to 42.5 per cent.

Liqueurs and cordials are manufactured beverages containing a large proportion of alcohol, sugar, and essential oils.   They are often highly colored.

[1] Conn. Agr. Exp. Sta. Report, 1914, p. 254.

PART III.

FEEDING IN INFANCY AND CHILDHOOD.

CHAPTER XVI.

BREAST FEEDING—FEEDING NORMAL AND ABNORMAL CHILDREN

WOMAN'S MILK.

MILK is a secretion of the mammary glands, but a few of its normal constituents are the result of transudation from the mother's blood. The composition of human milk is qualitatively similar to cow's milk, but quantitatively quite different. Furthermore, women's milk varies in amount and composition at different times, depending upon the length of time which has elapsed since the labor, upon the health of the mother, and upon whether or not the breasts are completely emptied at each nursing.

Colostrum.—Colostrum is the term applied to the milk secreted during the first few days (1 to 12) postpartum, before lactation is well established. Czerny and Keller include under this term all milk that shows evidence of absorption. Colostrum is deep yellow in color, has an average specific gravity of about 1.040, a strongly alkaline reaction, and is coagulated by heat. Its composition varies considerably. The following table gives the average composition of five early colostrums compiled by Holt, Courtney and Fales:[1]

AVERAGE COMPOSITION OF FIVE COLOSTRUMS (1 TO 12 DAYS).

Fat	2.83
Lactose	7.59
Protein	2.25
Ash	0.3077
Total solids	13.42

The fat droplets of colostrum are more unequal in size than those of milk. Colostrum contains, besides the usual constituents of milk, many large nucleated granular bodies, called "colostrum corpuscles," which are about five times as large as ordinary leukocytes, contain many small fat drop-

[1] Amer. Jour. Dis. Child, 1915, x, 229.

lets and have ameboid motion. They are present in large numbers for the first few days, rapidly disappear after lactation is well established, but reappear when lactation is interrupted. Czerny considers them leukocytes that appear when the breasts are not sufficiently emptied of milk and help in the absorption of fat.

General Characteristics of Woman's Milk.—Woman's milk is bluish-white in color, odorless and sweet to taste. Microscopically it shows many fine fat droplets which are smaller than most of the fat droplets in cow's milk. It contains a few epithelial cells and leukocytes. The number of the latter is greatly increased when there is any inflammation of the breast. Its average specific gravity is 1.031, but it may vary between 1.026 and 1.036.

Woman's milk is neutral or slightly alkaline in reaction; and is amphoteric. The latter condition is due to the presence of both mono- and diphosphates, the former being acid and the latter alkaline in reaction.

The casein of woman's milk does not coagulate in such large clots as the casein of cow's milk. On the addition of acetic acid a fine flocculent precipitate is formed. Rennin alone does not coagulate it.

Quantity.—The quantity of milk secreted increases rapidly for the first six to eight weeks, after this more slowly. To a certain extent the quantity is governed by the demands of the infant. A large vigorous infant will obtain more milk than a smaller, less vigorous infant. Furthermore, a wet-nurse will secrete more milk while nursing two or three infants than while nursing only one.

The following table gives the average daily amount of milk drawn by an infant (from Czerny and Keller):[1]

Age in weeks.	Average weight of breast-fed infants according to Camerer.		The calculated day's amount of milk.		Age in weeks.	Average weight of breast-fed infants according to Camerer.		The calculated day's amount of milk.	
	gm.	lb. and oz.	gm.	oz.		gm.	lb. and oz.	gm.	oz.
1	3410	7 2	291	9.7	14	5745	11 15	870	29.0
2	3550	7 6	549	18 3	15	5950	12 6	878	29.3
3	3690	7 11	590	19.7	16	6150	12 13	893	29.8
4	3980	8 5	652	21.7	17	6350	13 4	902	30.1
5	4115	8 9	687	22.9	18	6405	13 5	911	30.4
6	4260	8 14	736	24.5	19	6570	13 11	928	30.9
7	4495	9 6	785	26.2	20	6740	14 1	947	31.6
8	4685	9 12	804	26.8	21	6885	14 5	956	31.7
9	4915	10 4	815	27.2	22	7000	14 9	958	31.9
10	5055	10 9	800	26.7	23	7150	14 14	970	32.3
11	5285	11 ..	808	26.9	24	7285	15 3	980	32.7
12	5455	11 6	828	27.6	25	7405	15 7	990	33.0
13	5615	11 11	852	28.4	26	7500	15 10	1000	33.3

[1] Des Kindes Ernährung, Ernährungsstörungen und Ernährungstherapie. Leipzig und Wien, x. 353.

Composition.—Woman's milk varies widely in its composition. Its principal ingredients are the same as those in cow's milk: namely, fat, lactose, protein, salts and water. The average composition is as follows:

AVERAGE COMPOSITION OF WOMAN'S MILK.

Fat .	3.50
Lactose	7.00
Protein	1.50
Salts	0.21
Water	87.29

Holt, Courtney and Fales[1] divide lactation into four periods: the colostrum period (1 to 12 days), the transition period (12 to 30 days), the mature period (1 to 9 months), and the late period (10 to 20 months), and give the following figures as averages for these periods:

PERCENTAGE COMPOSITION OF WOMAN'S MILK.

Period.	No. of analyses.	Fat.	Sugar.	Protein.	Casein.	Albumin.	Ash.	Total solids.
Colostrum, 1–12 days	5	2.83	7.59	2.25	..	..	0.3077	13.42
Transition, 12–30 days	6	4.37	7.74	1.56	..	..	0.2407	13.39
Mature, 1–9 mos.	17	3.26	7.50	1.15	0.43	0.72	0.2062	12.16
Late, 10–20 mos.	10	3.16	7.47	1.07	0.32	0.75	0.1978	12.18

The sugar content remains practically constant throughout the entire period of lactation. Protein and ash are highest in the colostrum period and fall quite rapidly to the mature period, after which they vary little. The fat content is lowest in the colostrum period, rises rapidly in the transition period, and then falls in the mature period. These analyses of Holt, Courtney and Fales are particularly important, because many of their specimens were entire twenty-four-hour amounts.

Fat.—The fat in human milk is held in permanent emulsion. The average percentage of fat is 3.5 or 4 per cent., but it may vary from 0.75 to 10 per cent. As a rule the amount of fat in the milk increases from the beginning to the end of each nursing.

Volatile fatty acids form 2.5 per cent. of the total fat of woman's milk and 27 per cent. of the total fat of cow's milk. Oleic acid forms about 50 per cent. of the non-volatile fatty acids, the remainder being composed of myristic, palmitic and stearic acids.

Lactose.—The percentage of lactose in woman's milk is more constant than that of the other constituents, being about 7 per cent. which is nearly twice that of cow's milk. It is in solution.

[1] Loc. cit., 239

Protein.—The proteins of woman's milk comprise casein, which is insoluble in water, and lactalbumin and globulin, which are soluble in water. Besides these there are some nitrogenous substances which do not give the protein reactions. A large part of the latter is supposed to be urea. There is considerable difference of opinion as to the proportions of these substances. According to Talbot the probable division of the total nitrogen is as follows: "Casein 41 per cent., lactalbumin and globulin 44 to 39 per cent., residual nitrogen 15 to 20 per cent." Thus the lactalbumin and globulin form a much larger part of the total protein in woman's milk than they do in cow's milk.

Salts.—The average ash content of woman's milk is less than a third that of cow's milk, being only 0.21 per cent. The following table gives the average salt content of 100 c.c. of woman's milk according to Holt, Courtney and Fales:[1]

AVERAGES FOR THE DIFFERENT PERIODS.

	No. of analyses.	Total ash.	CaO.	MgO.	P_2O_4.	Na_2O.	K_2O.	Cl.
Colostrum, 1–12 days	5	.3077	.0446	.0101	.0410	.0453	.0938	.0568
Transition, 12–30 days	6	.2407	.0409	.0057	.0404	.0255	.0709	.0580
Early mature, 1–4 months	9	.2056	.0486	.0082	.0342	.0154	.0539	.0351
Middle mature, 4–9 months	8	.2069	.0458	.0074	.0345	.0132	.0609	.0358
Late milk, 10–20 months	10	.1978	.0390	.0070	.0304	.0195	.0575	.0442

The average percentage composition of the ash by the same investigation is as follows:

AVERAGE PERCENTAGE COMPOSITION OF ASH FOR THE DIFFERENT PERIODS.

	CaO.	MgO.	P_2O_4.	Na_2O.	K_2O.	Cl.
Colostrum	14.2	3.5	12.5	13.7	28.1	20.6
Transition	17.0	2.4	16.9	10.9	30.8	22.9
Mature	23.3	3.7	16.6	7.2	28.3	16.5
Late	19.8	3.6	15.5	10.1	18.8	22.3

Iron.—The iron content of woman's milk is about three times that of cow's milk. This makes the iron intake of an infant fed on diluted cow's milk much lower than that of a breast-fed infant.

Phosphorus.—Woman's milk contains much less phosphorus than cow's milk. About three-fourths of the phosphorus of woman's milk is in organic combination, as against one-fourth of that of cow's milk.

Salts of Woman's and Cow's Milk.—The total ash content of cow's milk is about three and one-half times that of woman's milk. The proportion of the different salts is quite

[1] Am. Jour. Dis. Child., 1915, x. 243, 245.

similar, the chief differences being in the larger amount of iron and the smaller amount of phosphorus in woman's milk. Holt, Courtney and Fales[1] give the average composition as follows:

COMPARISON OF THE PERCENTAGE COMPOSITION OF THE ASH OF WOMAN'S AND COW'S MILK.

	CaO.	MgO.	P_2O_5.	Na_2O.	K_2O.	Cl.
Mature woman's milk	23.3	3.7	16.6	7.2	28.3	16.5
Cow's milk	23.5	2.8	26.5	7.2	24.9	13.6

Bacteria.—A few bacteria, usually staphylococci, are found in the milk of healthy women. Typhoid bacilli have been demonstrated in the milk of a woman ill with typhoid fever. Syphilis can probably be transmitted by the milk even when the breasts are apparently normal. Pathogenic bacteria may be present in the milk when the mother is suffering from a local infection of the breast or a general sepsis.

Drugs.—Some drugs are excreted in woman's milk. They are alcohol, bromides, iodides, salicylates, mercury, calomel, antipyrin, arsenic, urotropin, the saline cathartics and salvarsan. Probably morphine and atrophine also are excreted in woman's milk. Most of these are found in very minute amounts.

Nervous Impressions.—Any severe, acute or prolonged nervous strain may so alter the mother's milk as to seriously upset the infant. For this reason it is important that a nursing mother should lead a quiet life and avoid all nervous strain and excitement. Women that are prone to nervous disturbances, as hysteria, are seldom able to nurse their infants successfully.

Menstruation.—Menstruation does not, as a rule, seriously affect the milk supply. Not infrequently the infant is uncomfortable and has undigested stools at the onset. Only rarely is the disturbance more serious and prolonged.

Pregnancy.—If a nursing mother becomes pregnant her milk rapidly deteriorates both in quantity and quality. Weaning is imperative.

Transmission of Immunity.—A mother, who is immune to one or more of the infectious diseases, usually transmits a varying degree of immunity to her offspring. Some of the immune bodies enter the fetus by way of the placenta but the work of Famulener[2] would seem to show that a greater number pass from the mother to the infant in the colostrum which is secreted in the first few days. He, as well as others, demonstrated immune bodies in the colostrum of immune

[1] Am. Jour. Dis. Child., 1915, x. 246.
[2] Studies from Research Lab. Dept. Health of New York City, 1911, vi, 199.

mothers. Furthermore the concentration of immune bodies in the colostrum was greater than in the mother's blood serum at the same time. Milk of a later period contained a much smaller number of immune bodies. After taking the colostrum of such mothers for several days, the concentration of immune bodies in the blood serum of the young animals was greatly increased. There seems to be no reasonable doubt but that new born infants can absorb such immune bodies from the digestive tract. Immune bodies with homologous proteins, such as are present in milk of the same species, are more readily absorbed than those associated with heterologous proteins as in milk of other species. These facts would emphasize the importance of young infants nursing at least for a few days.

Diet.—Within narrow limits the amount and composition of the milk may be altered by changes in the diet. The best results are obtained when the mother has been underfed, and the milk is abundant but poor in quality, especially in fat. Increasing the diet generally, but especially the fat and carbohydrate, will usually increase the fat content of the milk. When the fat is too high, reducing the fat and carbohydrate in the diet and increasing the mother's exercise will usually reduce the fat. Low protein can be overcome by increasing the diet when the mother has been underfed, but is rarely influenced when the mother is already receiving a plentiful diet. Reducing the diet and increasing the exercise will sometimes reduce a too high protein. The percentage of lactose in woman's milk is more constant than that of either the fat or the protein and is little influenced by diet. An increase in the fluid intake will often increase the quantity of milk.

BREAST FEEDING.

The simplest and best way to feed an infant is to nurse it. No artificial food has been evolved which gives nearly as uniformly good results. Therefore every mother that can do so should nurse her infant. The great value of breast feeding as compared with artificial feeding is proved by the much higher mortality rate among artificially fed infants. Another factor of importance is the greater frequency of rickets among the artificially fed. With premature infants, full-term infants that are feeble and under-developed, and the occasional infant that is unable to digest cow's milk, breast milk is essential. Among the poor there is very little opposition to breast feeding, unless the mother is the wage-earner and has to be away from home during the day, and even these mothers usually nurse their infants night and morning. Among the well-to-do the mothers are less frequently able to nurse their infants and they find the frequent nursings and especially the restrictions which nursing places upon their time very irksome.

Contra-indications for Breast Feeding.—The most frequent contra-indication is insufficient milk, but every effort should be made to increase the amount of milk before resorting to artificial feeding.

Another important contra-indication is serious illness of the mother, as tuberculosis, typhoid fever, puerperal fever and mastitis. When a nursing mother develops an infectious disease of short duration, as tonsillitis, she may stop nursing during the febrile stage and resume it later. The breasts should be emptied two or three times a day by massage and the breast pump. Many women resume nursing in this way after intervals of as long as two weeks.

Frequently an infant is taken from the breast of a healthy mother and given a cow's milk mixture because he does not thrive or has indigestion. If the amount and quality of the mother's milk is insufficient and cannot be improved by diet and regulation of her mode of living, there is nothing else to do. When, however, the supply of milk is ample and the quality good, every effort should be made to adapt it to the infant before beginning artificial feeding, and in only rare instances is this impossible.

Occasionally a nursing mother will become pregnant. When this occurs her milk deteriorates rapidly in amount and quality. At first the infant stops gaining, later he loses weight. Artificial feeding should be begun at once.

Intervals of Nursing.—Formerly an infant was nursed whenever he cried and appeared hungry, and this is today the usual procedure among the ignorant. Many such infants thrive and gain steadily, but they are usually irritable and frequently upset the entire household. Habits are soon formed by infants, and regularity is an important one. Six to eight hours after birth the infant is allowed to nurse for five minutes. After this the nursings are repeated every six hours for the first two days. When the breasts begin to secrete milk, which usually occurs on the third or fourth day, the intervals are shortened to three hours, with one nursing omitted at night. At the same time the length of time that the infant is allowed to nurse is increased to ten or fifteen minutes.

From this time to the third month the infant should nurse at 6, 9, 12, 3, 6, 9, and once during the night, usually about

2 A. M. Always after the fourth month and occasionally earlier the night feeding may be stopped. It is well to stop this feeding as soon as possible, as the long undisturbed sleep is good for both the mother and infant. After the fifth month the intervals may be lengthened to four hours and the number of nursings reduced to five. The hours will now be 6, 10, 2, 6, 10. During the day the time of feeding should be strictly adhered to. At night, however, the time may be varied considerably to suit the convenience of the mother. For example, occasionally an infant will wake at 5 A. M. He may be fed then instead of at 6 A. M., but he should not receive his second bottle before the regular time, that is at 9 or 10 A. M., depending on whether he is on a three or four hour schedule. The time for giving the evening bottle may vary between 9 and 12 P. M. When the night feeding is dropped, it shortens the interval between the last evening feeding and the first morning feeding if the evening feeding is given at 11 P. M., instead of 9 or 10 P. M. The infant is, therefore, more apt to sleep until the usual time for the morning feeding.

These intervals are somewhat longer than those frequently recommended for the first few months. Feeble and premature infants frequently do better when nursed every two or two and one-half hours. Normal infants, however, gain just as rapidly on three-hour intervals, which have the advantages of allowing the stomach to empty more completely between nursings, giving the mother more freedom and lessening the likelihood of cracked nipples. Even four-hour intervals from the beginning are recommended by some physicians.

Length of Each Nursing.—After lactation is well established, most infants will nurse fifteen to twenty minutes each time for the first few weeks. Later they will frequently be satisfied in ten minutes. An infant should never be allowed to nurse a few minutes, play a few minutes and then nurse again. They should be taught from the beginning to nurse steadily, with an occasional rest, until they are through. An infant should never be allowed to sleep in the same bed with his mother, as this encourages him to nurse frequently during the night. An infant should seldom be allowed to nurse more than twenty minutes. If he is not satisfied by this time, he is either taking too much or the supply of milk is scanty. Weighing him before and after nursing will settle this point.

Mother's Diet and Exercise.—A nursing mother should take a plentiful diet of easily digested food, with some extra fluid, as milk, egg and milk, cocoa or gruel in the middle of the morning and afternoon and before going to bed at night. If preferred the extra milk may be taken after each meal. Besides this she should drink a plentiful supply of water. She should avoid all articles of diet that are highly spiced, very rich or difficult of digestion, such as peppers, pickles, relishes, vinegar, rich puddings and sauces, lobster, crabs, Welsh rarebit, and excessive amounts of coffee, tea and alcohol. Most nursing mothers can take moderate amounts of raw or cooked fruits and vegetables. Occasionally, however, even moderate amounts of fruit, especially the more acid ones such as grapefruit or green vegetables, particularly tomatoes and onions, will cause colic and indigestion in the infant. When this happens the particular fruit or vegetable causing the trouble should be omitted from the diet. If it is impossible to determine which fruit or vegetable is causing the trouble, it is well to omit all fruit and green vegetables until the infant is normal again. Then they may be resumed one at a time, the infant being watched for any return of the symptoms. In this way the cause of the disturbance can usually be identified and so eliminated.

A nursing mother should be relieved, as far as possible, of all strenuous work and exercise. Moderate exercise, on the other hand, is essential for her health and counteracts the tendency to too rich milk. Walking in the open air is one of the best forms of exercise.

More essential even than exercise is sufficient rest. She should have at least one long period of sleep during the night, and at least two hours of sleep during the day. The longer intervals between nursings and the early stopping of the night feeding all help toward this end.

It is possible to influence the quantity and composition of the mother's milk to a considerable extent by altering her diet and mode of living.

If the quantity is too small the mother's diet should be increased, especially the amount of milk, eggs, and meat. Also her water intake should be increased. Her exercise should be limited and sufficient rest assured. Frequently relieving her of the physical and mental strain of caring for the infant helps a great deal. If she is anemic, run down or unable to take sufficient food because of lack of appetite, appropriate medication is indicated.

If the milk is too rich, which usually means a high fat and protein content, lessening the mother's diet (especially meat, eggs and milk), increasing the amount of water which she takes, and increasing her exercise will usually reduce the fat content of the milk. At the same time the infant may be given one-half ounce of sterile water before each breast feeding and the length of the nursing reduced or the interval between nursings increased.

When the milk is poor in quality, that is, has a low fat content, the procedure is the same as when it is insufficient, except that it is more important to increase the solids in the mother's diet than the fluids.

It is easier to correct an abundant supply of overrich milk than an insufficient supply of milk which is poor in quality.

Vomiting.—Most infants, whether breast or bottle fed, will occasionally regurgitate small amounts, from a few drops to a teaspoonful or two. This is to be expected and need cause no alarm. When, however, a breast-fed infant vomits large amounts after a good many feedings, something is wrong either with the milk or the method of handling the infant. The possibility of pyloric stenosis must always be kept in mind. Not infrequently it is due to the infant's efforts to rid himself of air swallowed during the nursing. This is apt to happen when the infant is placed in his bed immediately after nursing. C. H. Smith[1] has demonstrated that under these circumstances the gas is water-locked in the stomach, and an endeavor to belch it on the part of the infant is sure to cause some vomiting. If the infant is held erect for a minute or two after nursing he will belch the gas without losing any milk.

Too much milk or too high fat will cause vomiting. The amount can be determined by weighing before and after nursing. If the infant is taking too much, the length of the nursing should be shortened. If analysis of the breast milk shows a too high fat content the mother's diet should be cut down slightly, especially the solid food, and her water intake and exercise increased. Also the infant may be given one-half ounce of sterile water before each nursing.

Gas and Colic.—Both gas and colic occur much less often when an infant is breast fed than when he is artificially fed. The usual cause of gas has been explained in the previous section on vomiting. Occasionally certain articles in the mother's diet will cause colic in the infant. The most frequent are the raw acid fruits and green vegetables. The method of handling this situation has been explained in the section on the mother's diet.

Normal Stool.—A normal breast fed infant usually has from one to four stools a day. The stools are soft, almost never formed, and yellow in color. They are not uniform

[1] Am. Jour. Dis. Child, 1915, ix, 261.

in consistency, like the stool of an artificially fed infant, but contain a varying number of small, soft masses, each about a millimeter in diameter, which are light in color. Their reaction is slightly acid. Not infrequently an infant, that is gaining regularly and is comfortable, will have decidedly abnormal stools. This in itself is not an indication for stopping nursing.

Abnormal Stools.—Constipation is unusual in the breast-fed infant unless the milk is insufficient either in quality or quantity.

Loose, too frequent stools, often containing considerable mucus accompanied by colic may occur when the mother is menstruating, after an indiscretion in diet on the mother's part, when the mother is suffering from an acute infection, or when the milk is not adapted to the particular infant. All but the last condition are transient and easily righted. If the milk is at fault the first thing to do is to determine the quantity taken by the infant and the composition of the milk. The quantity taken can be determined by weighing the infant before and after nursing. If the quantity is too great the length of each nursing should be shortened.

If the composition of the milk is wrong an endeavor should be made to correct the fault by changing the mother's diet and routine as is explained in the section on the mother's diet. This is at times impossible, especially when the milk is both scanty and poor in quality. Unless some improvement is made within two weeks it is rarely wise to persist any longer.

MIXED FEEDING.

When a woman has an insufficient supply of milk for her infant, supplementary feedings of cow's milk may be used. This is mixed feeding, and it is indicated whenever the breast milk is of good quality but insufficient in amount to properly nourish the infant. One of two procedures may be employed, either small bottle feedings may be given after each breast feeding, or bottle feedings may be substituted for some of the breast feedings. If the former method is followed the infant is given only one breast at a nursing. The amount of breast milk obtained is calculated by weighing the infant before and after nursing. Then a sufficient bottle feeding is given to make up the proper amount. As a rule it is not necessary to weigh the infant before and after nursing for more than a few days. If the second method is chosen, one, two or three of the breast feedings are omitted and a full bottle feeding given at these times. At the breast feedings

18

it is best to give the infant both breasts each time, **as other-**wise the long intervals between nursings tend to **diminish** the amount of milk secreted. It is rarely possible **to keep** up the supply of milk if the infant nurses less **than four** times in each twenty-four hours. There is a distinc**t advan-**tage in always giving one bottle feeding a day to all **breast-**fed infants after the third month. By so doing they **become** accustomed to taking the bottle and their digestion **becomes** adapted to cow's milk. Furthermore it allows the **mother** one long interval during the day in which she may **rest or** be out of doors. If at any time it becomes necess**ary to** wean the infant suddenly it can be accomplished with **much** less likelihood of disturbance.

In beginning mixed feeding a relatively low formula **should** be used at first. A three-months-old infant should **begin** with about a 6 in 20 and a six-months-old infant with **an 8** in 20 mixture. The full amount for the infant's age may **be** given from the beginning. The strength of the formula **may** be increased quite rapidly, about an ounce of milk being **added** every three days, provided there are no evidences of **indi-**gestion, until the strength of the formula is proper for **the** infant's age.

The advantages of mixed feeding over artificial feeding **are** that it gives the infant a considerable amount of breast **milk,** that it allows the infant to become accustomed to cow's milk gradually, and that it simplifies weaning.

WEANING

Few women can nurse their infants to advantage after the eighth or ninth month, and many have to give supplementary feedings long before this. Where it is possible to obtain good cow's milk it is a distinct advantage to give the infant one bottle feeding a day after the third or fourth month. This accustoms the infant to the bottle and greatly lessens the difficulty of weaning if the latter, becomes necessary at any time. Infants that have never had a bottle feeding until they are six months of age or older will frequently refuse it absolutely as long as they are given the breast at all and sometimes for several days, even after the breast feedings have been entirely stopped. During this time they lose weight rapidly and not infrequently develop considerable fever. Little is gained by forcing them to take the bottle under these circumstances. The best method is to offer the bottle at the regular intervals and take it away if refused. They always give in finally. No serious results follow this method. A three-months infant, on the other hand, soon becomes accustomed to taking one feeding from the bottle.

The indications for early weaning are insufficient milk, severe illness of the mother, and pregnancy. When possible it is better to wean gradually. If the infant has been taking one bottle a day another of the same strength is added and after a few days another until all of the breast feedings have been stopped. The rapidity with which this is done will depend upon the cause of the weaning and the amount of milk which the mother has. If the infant is already taking a bottle feeding, the other feedings should be of the same strength. If the infant has never taken any cow's milk the first formula should be considerably weaker than a normal artificially fed infant of the same age would be taking. After the first few days the strength of the formula should be gradually increased until the food is sufficient for the infant. When it is necessary to stop all breast feedings at once it is more important to begin with a relatively weaker formula than when the bottle feedings can be gradually substituted.

When the mother is able to nurse the full eight or nine months the process is much simpler. The various foods other than milk are added to the diet in the same order and amounts as with the artificially fed infant, except that it is not necessary to make these additions quite as early. When cereal is begun, a small amount of cow's milk (1 or 2 ounces) diluted with an equal volume of boiled water is given with the cereal. As the cereal is increased the strength and amount of milk is increased. Then one feeding of diluted milk is substituted for a breast feeding. If the mother is well and strong and has an abundant supply of milk she may be allowed to nurse to the twelth or thirteenth month. When this is possible it may not be necessary to use bottles at all, the infant being weaned directly to the cup. In no normal case should bottles be continued after the eighteenth month.

CHAPTER XVII.

ARTIFICIAL FEEDING

FOOD REQUIREMENTS OF THE ARTIFICIALLY FED INFANT.

Energy.—Repeated efforts have been made to formulate some law or laws by which the caloric requirements of a given infant could be calculated. The first work was based entirely upon the body weight. It was soon found that the caloric requirement per pound was considerably larger for thin infants than for well-nourished infants. Then it was suggested that the surface area, and not the body weight, was the governing factor. As it is obviously impossible actually to measure the surface area of all infants, different investigators have worked out formulæ by which the surface area of infants can be calculated. The results obtained by this method are more uniform than those obtained where the weight alone is considered, but the calculations are too complicated to be of practical use in every-day practice. Recently it has been suggested that the caloric requirement of an infant varies directly with the mass of active protoplasmic tissue in the body. This would explain why a thin infant requires more calories than a fat infant of the same weight. Unfortunately we have no means of calculating the mass of active protoplasmic tissue in any living infant.

Muscular exertion has a marked influence upon the requirements of the infant. Hard crying may increase the energy output by 100 per cent. Thus a very active infant always requires more energy than a quiet passive infant.

For practical use the body weight must be the guide at present. The usually accepted requirement is 100 calories per kilo or 45 calories per pound of body weight for each twenty-four hours from the end of the second week to the ninth month. At the same time we must remember that a very thin infant will frequently require considerably more than 100 calories per kilo, while a very fat infant may gain and do well on considerably less. During the first two weeks the caloric requirement is considerably less than 45 calories per pound, averaging only about 30 calories. After the eight month the requirement falls to about 40 calories per pound.

Protein.—Protein is required by the infant to replace that lost in tissue waste and for the formation of new tissue in growth. This double demand makes the protein requirement of a growing infant relatively greater than that of an adult. Furthermore, as the most rapid growth takes place during the early months, the protein requirement is greatest during these months. Morse and Talbot[1] say, "The average protein need of infants is at least 1.5 gram per kilogram, or 0.7 gram per pound of body weight." In order to obtain this amount an infant must take nearly an ounce of cow's milk per pound of body weight. The generally accepted rule of one and a half ounces of cow's milk per pound of body weight furnishes considerably more than this amount.

Almost all cow's milk mixtures contain more protein than woman's milk. This is especially true of whole-milk mixtures. The low fat content of the latter makes it necessary either to use a very high sugar content or to raise the protein considerably above the theoretical requirement in order to furnish the necessary calories. Thus the whole milk mixtures which are commonly used, contain about 1¾ ounces of milk per pound of body weight.

Animal protein is more easily digested and more completely absorbed than vegetable protein. The protein of milk is most readily digested by infants, that of woman's milk more easily than that of cow's milk.

Formerly most of the digestive disturbances of infants were attributed to the protein, but of late the tendency has been to minimize the importance of protein as a cause of indigestion. Some justification for the larger amounts of protein frequently fed in cow's milk mixtures is found in the smaller amounts of some essential amino-acids in the protein of cow's milk.

Fat.—As fat furnishes approximately twice as many calories per gram as carbohydrate or protein, it is a very important element in the food, and small variations in the fat content of the food have a marked influence upon its energy value. In health from 90 to 98 per cent. of the fat in the food is absorbed. In digestive disturbances, especially those conditions which are associated with diarrhea, a much smaller portion of the fat ingested is absorbed. Holt, Courtney and Fales,[2] found that from 90.3 to 99.2 per cent. of the fat intake was absorbed in healthy breast-fed infants, and an average of 91.3 per cent. by healthy infants fed on modified cow's milk. In normal infants they found the

[1] Diseases of Nutrition and Infant Feeding, 1915, p. 201.
[2] Am. Jour. Dis. Child., 1919, xvii, 241, 423.

average fat per cent. of the dried stool to be 34 per cent. whether the infant was taking woman's or cow's milk. The fat in the stools of breast-fed infants was divided as follows: soap fat 43.1 per cent., free fatty acids, 36.7 per cent., neutral fat 20.2 per cent.   In the stools of healthy infants fed on modified cow's milk the fat was divided as follows: soap fat 60.5 per cent., neutral fat 12.1 per cent.   In both groups of infants suffering from diarrheal conditions the fat retention fell markedly.   At the same time the percentage of soap fat in the stools fell and the percentage of free fatty acids and neutral fat rose.

There is considerable difference of opinion as to the amount of fat which a normal infant's food should contain.   Many physicians use top milk mixtures and thus keep the fat content of the food about twice that of the protein.   Others use whole-milk mixtures which make the fat content of the food only slightly greater than the protein.   Both methods have their advantages and disadvantages.   An infant fed on the higher fat mixtures will gain more rapidly and be satisfied with smaller amounts of food, especially during the early months, than one fed on whole-milk mixtures.   Furthermore, the higher fat content permits the use of smaller amounts of sugar, which is necessary in feeding infants with an intolerance for sugar.   The disadvantage is that infants fed on high fat mixtures are more apt to have digestive disturbances.   For this reason whole-milk mixtures with their lower fat contents are safer in the hands of those with comparatively little experience.

Carbohydrate.—Sugar.—All milk contains lactose or milk-sugar.   The sugar content of woman's milk is about 7.5 per cent., which is nearly twice that of cow's milk.   When cow's milk is diluted its sugar content is still further reduced so that a considerable amount of sugar has to be added to cow's milk mixtures in order to bring their sugar content up to the required amount.   As a rule sufficient sugar is added to make the sugar content of the mixture about 6 per cent., never more than 7 per cent.   An infant fed on woman's milk receives slightly more calories in fat than in sugar, while an artifically fed infant taking cow's milk mixtures receives a rather large part of his calories in the form of sugar.

Three sugars are used in infant feeding, lactose (milk sugar), saccharose (cane-sugar), and maltose.   All of these sugars are disaccharides and in the process of digestion they are broken down into monosaccharides.   The rapidity with which they are absorbed differs and hence their effect upon intestinal fermentation and peristalsis.

Lactose is more slowly absorbed than either maltose or saccharose. Its longer stay in the intestinal canal is supposed to favor the normal fermentation processes and thus to hold in check excessive putrefaction. Furthermore, it is slightly laxative. For these reasons it is the sugar of choice for feeding normal infants. Pure maltose is never used in feeding because of its cost. The maltose used is always a mixture of maltose with dextrin, the maltose forming about 50 per cent. of most of the preparations. The dextrin content is more variable. The following table taken from Morse and Talbot[1] gives the percentage of maltose and dextrin in the more common preparations used:

Food.	Maltose, per cent.	Dextrin, per cent.
Löflund's nährmaltose	40.00	60.00
Mead's dextrimaltose	51.00	47.00
Neutral maltose (Maltzyme Co.)	63.00–66.00	8.00–9.00
Löflund's malt soup extract	58.91	15.42
Maltose (Walker-Gordon laboratory)	57.10	30.90
Mellin's food	58.88	20.69
Malted milk	49.15	18.80

In digestion one molecule of maltose is split into two molecules of dextrose. For this reason it is more rapidly absorbed than either lactose or saccharose. This rapidity of absorption and the fact that some infants that have developed a fermentative diarrhea while taking lactose will digest maltose easier than lactose are the chief reasons for its use.

Saccharose (cane-sugar) is split into dextrose and levulose in the process of digestion. As the levulose has to be changed into dextrose before being absorbed, cane-sugar is more slowly absorbed than maltose. Cane-sugar is somewhat less laxative than lactose. Furthermore it is much cheaper than either of the other sugars. Many normal infants will thrive as well on cane-sugar as on lactose or maltose. Its cheapness is its chief recommendation.

Starch.—Starch is used for two purposes in infant feeding, first to prevent the formation of large casein curds in the stomach, and second, to increase the strength of the food. For the first purpose only a small amount of starch is necessary, 0.75 per cent. of starch in the food being as effective as larger amounts. This amount of starch may be added to the food of very young infants.

After the second month some form of starch is usually added to most artificial mixtures. At first a cereal water, made by boiling one level tablespoonful of either oat or bar-

---

[1] Diseases of Nutrition and Infant_Feeding, 1915, 194.

ley flour and a pinch of salt in a pint of water for three-fourths of an hour, is used. After the fifth month two level table-spoonfuls of flour may be used. Barley water is generally believed to be slightly more constipating than oat water.

Inorganic Salts.—The salt content of cow's milk is about three and one-half times that of woman's milk. The result is that the ordinary infant fed on diluted cow's milk receives a considerably greater amount of salts than a breast-fed infant. Furthermore, the relative proportions of the various salts differ somewhat in the two feedings, the chief difference being in the phosphoric acid. These differences are believed to have a considerable influence upon the growing infant, especially in disturbances of digestion.

The following table from Holt[1] gives the relative percentage of the different salts in both cow's and woman's milk.

	Cow's.	Woman's.
CaO	22.8	23.3
MgO	2.8	3.7
P_2O_5	27.4	16.6
K_2O	24.7	28.3
Na_2O	10.9	7.2
Cl	15.5	16.5

Water.—The amount of fluid required by an infant in-creases rapidly during the first three months and more slowly after that. A normal infant usually requires about 12 ounces at the end of the first week, 24 ounces at the end of the first month, 30 ounces by the end of the third month, 36 ounces by the fifth month, and 40 ounces by the eighth month. As a rule the fluid intake is about one-seventh of the body weight. As long as all the food is fluid, little addi-tional water need be given, but as soon as part of the food is solid additional water must be given.

PROPRIETARY FOODS.

There are many so-called "infant foods" on the market. While these differ greatly in composition they all have cer-tain common characteristics. Almost all contain large amounts of carbohydrate and small amounts of fat and pro-tein. It is well to remember that similar mixtures can be produced with the usual ingredients of infant's food without using these proprietary preparations.

They may be divided into four classes: first, those con-taining cow's milk; second, those containing considerable amounts of maltose and dextrins; third, farinaceous foods; and fourth, miscellaneous preparations.

[1] Diseases of Infancy and Childhood, 7th ed., 1916, 150.

Preparations Containing Cow's Milk.—This group includes the malted milks, Allenbury's milk food No 1. and No. 2, and Nestlé's food. The basis of all these is milk that has been evaporated to dryness. All have considerable quantities of carbohydrate added. Their fat content is considerably higher than that of any of the other classes.

Preparations Containing Large Amounts of Maltose.— Mellin's food which contains about 60 per cent. of maltose, is the best example of this group. Mead's dextrimaltose No. 1 contains about 53 per cent. of maltose. The malted milks are usually included in this group but their fat content is a great deal higher, due to the milk used in their manufacture. These foods may be used when maltose is indicated but should never be used without milk.

Farinaceous Foods.—This group includes imperial granum, Ridge's food, Robinson's barley and oat flour, Brook's barley flour, and the Cereo Company's flours. The group differs from the first in that they contain almost no fat, and from the second in that they all contain considerable amounts of unchanged starch. They may be used when it is desirable to add some carbohydrate partly in the form of starch to the food. The Cereo Company also furnish an enzyme preparation called cereo. By its use from 70 to 98 per cent. of the starch is converted into soluble carbohydrates.

Miscellaneous Foods.—Eskay's albumenized food is made from egg albumen and cereals. Peptogenic milk powder is largely milk-sugar.

The following table[1] gives the composition of most of the foods mentioned:

Name.	Fat, per cent.	Sugar, per cent.		Protein, per cent.	Starch, per cent.	Ash, p. c.
Horlick's malted milk	8.10	67.95	milk, malt 49.15 dextrin 18.80	15.00	.....	4.00
Allenbury's food No. 1	13.80	66.55	milk 42.00 malt 14.00 dextrin 10.00	9.88	.....	3.98
Allenbury's food No. 2	14.20	70.90	milk 36.00 malt 20.00 dextrin 13.00	9.75	.....	3.70
Nestlé's food	5.70	58.93	milk 6.57 cane 25.0 malt, dextrin 27.36	11.94	20.25	1.45

[1]The figures for fat, protein, starch and ash in the above table are taken from the Report of the Connecticut Agricultural Experiment Station, 1916, 328. Those for sugar are for the most part from Morse and Talbot: Diseases of Nutrition and Infant Feeding, 1915, 230.

Name	Fat, per cent.	Sugar, per cent.			Protein, per cent.	Starch, per cent.	Ash, p. c.
Mellin's food . . .	1.80	79.57	malt	58.88	11.31	.....	4.45
Mead's dextrimaltose No. 1	.....	93.00	dextrin	20.69	.....	.....	2.00
			malt	52.00			
			dextrin	41.00			
Imperial granum . .	0.50	1.80	dex-trose	0.42	13.88	72.79	0.50
			dextrin	1.38			
Ridge's food . . .	0.33	2.96			10.31	70.93	0.75
Robinson's barley .	1.40	2.92			6.75	70.20	0.85
Brook's barley .	1.03	3.48			8.69	68.51	0.88
Cereo barley . . .	2.03	5.20			14.88	58.39	1.48
Cereo oat	6.40	2.36			16.44	56.31	2.53
Eskay's food . . .	1.28	55.82	milk	54.12	7.75	31.95	1.58
			dextrin	1.70			

ARTIFICIAL FEEDING.

None of the rules for the artificial feeding of infants so far advanced apply to the newborn, because these infants are unable to digest cow's milk in sufficient strength or amount to satisfy completely their theoretical requirements. Hence we are forced to begin with such dilutions and amounts as experience has taught us are safe, and increase them as rapidly as the infant's digestion will allow, until a sufficient amount of food is taken. After that the food may be calculated with reference to the caloric requirement.

For the first twenty-four to forty-eight hours many infants vomit repeatedly, especially when given any fluid. During this time it is best to give boiled water or a 5 per cent. solution of lactose in boiled water. One or two ounces should be given every three hours. After thirty-six hours, provided the vomiting has ceased, a weak solution of milk may be given. Although many still use top-milk mixtures, it is safer to use whole-milk dilutions with a small amount of lactose added. Infants fed on whole-milk mixtures do not gain as rapidly at first as those fed on top-milk mixtures. On the other hand, they are much less likely to become upset.

The intervals between feedings should now be three hours, with one feeding omitted at night. The first formula[1] should be

Milk	2 ounces
Milk-sugar	2 level tablespoonfuls
Boiled water	18 ounces

[1] All formulæ in this section are made up to 20 ounces. This method has been adopted because it is simpler and more widely understood than the other methods. As soon as the total twenty-four-hour amount exceeds 20 ounces, one and a half times or double the formula is made up, depending upon the total amount of food required.

Method of Preparing Formula.—To make up a formula of whole milk the following articles are needed:

Bottles—As many as there are feedings in twenty-four hours. They should be graduated in ounces.

Measure—The best is an enamelware vessel marked on the inside in ounces and large enough to hold the entire twenty-four-hour amount. A glass graduate may be used but they break easily, especially if they are boiled.

A small enamelware funnel. A tablespoon. Non-absorbent cotton. Milk. Lactose (milk sugar). Boiled water.

The bottles, measure, spoon and funnel should have been washed and boiled.

The bottle of milk is well mixed so that the cream is evenly distributed and the desired amount of milk poured into the graduate. The desired amount of sugar is measured (three level tablespoonfuls equal one ounce), dissolved in part of the boiled water and added to the milk. Then boiled water is added to the mixture to make up the desired amount. It is now mixed and poured into the bottles, the proper amount for one feeding into each bottle. Finally the bottles are stoppered with cotton and placed in the ice-box.

Increasing Formula.—The amount of milk and sugar in the formula can usually be increased every second or third day until the infant is taking 7 ounces of milk in each 20 ounces of food with two and one-half level tablespoonfuls of lactose added. After this the increase has to be slower. By the time the infant is two and a half months old he will usually be taking equal parts of milk and diluent with two and one-half tablespoonfuls of lactose added to each 20 ounces of food. While this increase in strength is taking place the amount is also gradually increased. It is best to begin by offering the infant 1 or 2 ounces at each feeding. Thus after the second day he will receive seven feedings of 2 ounces each, making 14 ounces in each twenty-four hours. As soon as he is not satisfied with 2 ounces he may have more. The best method is to increase each feeding ½ ounce at a time. Such increases can usually be made about every five days until the infant is receiving 4 ounces at each feeding, making 28 ounces in each twenty-four hours. Most infants will reach this point about the fifth or sixth week. After this the amount may be slowly increased, reaching 5 ounces about the end of the third month, when the night feeding is usually dropped. At this time the infant will be receiving six feedings of 5 ounces each, making 30 ounces in each twenty-four hours.

The strength and amount of the food is still gradually increased so that by the fifth or sixth month the infant is taking 36 ounces of a mixture containing two-thirds milk and one-third diluent with 1 ounce of sugar added to the twenty-four-hour amount. It is well at this time to increase the intervals between feedings, so that the total twenty-four-hour amount is not lessened. Thus an infant who has been receiving six feedings of 6 ounces each, 1 every three hours, will receive five feedings of 7 ounces each, one every four hours.

From the sixth to the twelfth month the strength and amount of the food are increased very slowly. Most infants are taking whole milk undiluted and with no additions when they are ten to twelve months old. Delicate infants and those who have had digestive upsets frequently cannot digest whole milk until they are fifteen months old. The amount of each feeding is increased about an ounce each month until the infant is taking 40 to 45 ounces of food in each twenty-four hours. Usually this point is reached at eight or nine months. After this the increase is in the form of other food, the total amount of formula given being gradually reduced as the proportion of milk is increased.

Cereal.—Frequently some cereal, usually barley water, is added to the food from the start. It is best to omit the cereal for the first two or three months in most cases, as its addition complicates the formula and adds one more factor which has to be considered when the food disagrees. After the third month it should be added, as it seldom disagrees by this time and, furthermore, it increases the carbohydrate content of the food slightly. The cereal most frequenty used is barley, either as a flour or pearl barley. The desired amount of barley flour and a pinch of salt are brought to a boil in an amount of water slightly less than that used in the formula, and then simmered for three-quarters of an hour. It is then strained, partly cooled and added to the milk. After the fifth month a stronger cereal mixture is used. If pearl barley is used it has to be cooked much longer. In other respects its preparation is similar.

If the infant is inclined to be constipated, oat water is preferable. There are several oat flours on the market. They are prepared exactly like barley flour. If oatmeal is used it should be cooked at least four hours.

Some infants do better with imperial granum water prepared in the same way. It may be tried when barley and oatmeal cause colic or indigestion. A considerable portion of its carbohydrate content is in the form of dextrins. Many infants like its taste better than that of either oat or barley water.

The table on page 286 gives the composition of a series of formulæ such as have been described with the approximate age at which they should be used. While this table will serve as a guide it cannot be followed absolutely, as some infants will take more food or stronger food at the respective ages than that given in the table, and others will not be able to keep up to the schedule. Each infant has to be fed according to his individual needs and any schedule can serve as an approximate guide only.

Dr. F. H. Bartlett has devised a ready method of compounding a formula for older infants. The caloric requirement of the infant is calculated by multiplying 45 (the required calories per pound) by the weight of the infant in pounds. From this he subtracts 120 (the calories furnished by 1 ounce of sugar). The remainder he divides by 20 (the calories furnished by 1 ounce of whole milk). This gives the number of ounces of whole milk which the formula must contain. The only remaining factors to be decided are the amount of food for each twenty-four hours, and the number and amount of the feedings.

Suppose the formula required is for a healthy infant weighing 16 pounds. The calculation is as follows:

$$16 \times 45 = 720. \quad 720 - 120 = 600. \quad 600 \div 20 = 30.$$

Such an infant would take 40 ounces in twenty-four hours, divided into five feedings of 8 ounces each. So our formula would be

Whole milk	30 ounces
Milk-sugar	1 ounce
Barley water	10 ounces
	40 ounces

five feedings of 8 ounces each, one feeding every four hours.

This method is easy to remember and is very satisfactory for infants after the third month. In the early months it allows more milk than most infants can take.

Higher Fat Mixtures.—A good many healthy infants are able to take mixtures which contain more fat than the formulæ given in the table on page 286. There are certain advantages in using such mixtures in some cases. They furnish the necessary number of calories with less milk than the whole milk formulæ. Infants taking more fat are more easily satisfied and usually gain more rapidly. Furthermore, the tendency to constipation is less marked with infants taking more fat. The chief disadvantage is that they

WHOLE-MILK FORMULÆ FOR FIRST YEAR.

Age.	3rd day.	5th day.	7th day.	9th day.	12th day.	15th day.	25th day.	40th day.	70th day.	3 mos.	3½ mos.	4 mos.	5 mos.	6 mos.	7 mos.	8 mos.	9 mos.
Milk (ounces)	2	3	4	5	6	7	8	9	10	11	12	13	14	15	16	17	18
Lactose (level tablespoonfuls)	2	2	2½	2½	2½	2½	2½	2½	2½	2½	2½	2	2	2	1½	1	½
Boiled water (ounces)	18	17	16	15	14	13	12	11	10	9	8	7	6	5	4	3	2
Starch (level tablespoonfuls)	..	..	..	..	..	..	..	..	..	½	½	1	1	1	1	1	1
Number of feedings	7	7	7	7	7	7	7	7	7	7	7	6	6	6	5	5	5
Amount of each feeding (ounces)	2	2	2	2½	2½	3	3½	4	4	4½	4½	5	5½	6	7	8	9
Total 24-hour amount (ounces)	14	14	14	17½	17½	21	24½	28	28	31½	31½	30	35	36	35	40	45
Fat, per cent.	0.40	0.60	0.80	1.00	1.20	1.40	1.60	1.80	2.00	2.20	2.40	2.60	2.80	3.00	3.20	3.40	3.60
Sugar, per cent.	3.80	4.00	5.10	5.35	5.60	5.82	6.07	6.30	6.55	6.80	7.05	6.45	6.70	6.90	6.35	5.75	5.15
Protein, per cent.	0.35	0.52	0.70	0.87	1.05	1.22	1.40	1.57	1.75	1.92	2.10	2.27	2.45	2.62	2.80	2.97	3.15
Starch, per cent.	..	..	..	..	..	..	..	..	..	0.80	0.80	1.60	1.60	1.60	1.60	1.60	1.60
Calories in 20 ounces	..	140	180	200	220	240	260	280	300	335	370	375	395	415	415	415	415

are much more apt to upset the infant's digestion and to lead to a fat intolerance. Such an intolerance when once established may persist for a long time, necessitating the use of little fat over this period.

By using the upper half of the milk in a quart bottle milk containing 7 per cent. of fat may be obtained. Before removing the top milk the milk should stand in the bottle at least four hours. Then the top milk should be removed with a small dipper. It should not be poured off. After being removed it is mixed and the desired amount used to make up the formula just as with whole milk.

It is seldom wise to use these top milk mixtures for very young infants, but after the third month a vigorous infant will usually thrive on them. A formula containing slightly less milk than the appropriate whole milk formula should be used. Each ounce of 7 per cent. milk in the formula furnishes 0.35 per cent. of fat, while each ounce of 4 per cent. milk furnishes only 0.2 per cent. of fat. By using these higher fat mixtures the sugar content of the food can be reduced without lessening the caloric value of the food. This is desirable when feeding an infant with sugar intolerance.

Food Other than Milk.—Orange Juice.—Artificially fed infants do better if given food other than milk earlier than breast-fed infants. This is especially true of those who are fed on pasteurized or sterilized milk. By the fifth month some fruit juice should be added to the diet. Orange juice is most frequently used. At first one teaspoonful of the juice diluted with an equal quantity of water is given one hour before one of the bottle feedings; usually the second feeding in the morning. The amount is gradually increased so that four to six weeks later the infant is taking 1½ to 2 ounces of orange juice each day. It does not have to be diluted after the first few days. Many infants do not like orange juice at first, but they soon take it readily. Its laxative qualities must be borne in mind and the number and character of the stools considered before increasing the amount. Often slight constipation can be controlled in this way.

Beef Juice and Broth.—At seven months beef juice and broth are given, usually just before the noon bottle. At first one teaspoonful of beef juice diluted with an equal amount of warm boiled water and salted to taste is used. The amount may be gradually increased so that by the end of six weeks the infant is taking 1 or 1½ ounces of beef juice every other day. Broth, either lamb or chicken, can be given on the alternate days. At first only ½ or 1 ounce at a time, but later as much as 4 or 5 ounces, should be given.

Beef Juice.—Beef juice is made by searing a piece of lean beef, usually what is called "top round," and then squeezing out the juice in a small meat press. The fat will rise to the surface and may be skimmed off after it has stood a few minutes. A little salt is added and frequently an equal volume of warm boiled water. Boiling or the addition of too hot water coagulates the soluble proteins and therefore should be avoided. It should be freshly prepared.

Cereals.—At eight months some cereal, besides that in the formula, should be added to the diet. Oatmeal is the one of choice in most cases, especially when the infant is constipated. It should be cooked in water at least four hours and then strained. Cream of wheat or farina may be used when there is a tendency to loose stools. They are prepared like oatmeal except that they do not need to be cooked more than two hours. At first a teaspoonful with a little of the formula poured over it is given at the time of the second bottle. The balance of the bottle is given immediately afterward. A few days later the same amount may be given with the 6 P. M. feeding. The amounts are gradually increased so that by the ninth month the infant is taking ½ or 1 ounce of cereal (1 or 2 tablespoonfuls) twice a day.

Egg.—At nine or ten months egg is given. The egg should be soft-boiled (two minutes) or coddled. At first only a little (1 teaspoonful) of the white should be given. The amount is gradually increased and after a few days part of the yolk as well as the white is given. Some infants that cannot take soft-boiled or coddled eggs will take very finely grated hard-boiled eggs. The latter should be boiled thirty minutes. A few infants cannot take eggs in any form. Soon after ingestion they vomit and frequently they develop an erythematous or urticarial eruption and fever. All egg should be withheld from these infants, until they are older when they may be immunized to egg as Schloss has suggested.

Vegetables.—Vegetables may be given after the ninth month. The best vegetables to begin feeding are spinach, summer squash, asparagus, or celery. Later string beans, carrots and lettuce may be added. All should be thoroughly cooked and then strained through a fine wire sieve. The resulting vegetable will resemble apple sauce in consistency. Of this one teaspoonful is given with the broth and egg at noon. The amount of the bottle feeding at this time should be gradually lessened as the other food is increased. The amount of vegetable may be gradually increased, so that the infant will be taking about a tablespoonful by the eleventh month.

Rice and Potato.—By the tenth month rice or baked potato may be added to the noon feeding. The rice should be boiled at least four hours. The potato should be dry and mealy, never soggy. At first only a teaspoonful is given but this may be increased to one and one-half tablespoonfuls by the eleventh month. If the rice is given on the same day with the broth, it may be added to the latter and on the alternate days the beef juice may be mixed with the potato.

Bread.—Bread or hard crackers, such as the Huntley and Palmer breakfast biscuits, may be given by the ninth or tenth month. The bread should be at least a day old, cut into thin slices and then dried on top of the stove until it is crisp and brittle. At first a small piece may be given with the 2 P. M. feeding, and later with the 10 A. M. and 6 P. M. feedings also.

In the above schedules solid food has been added earlier than has been customary. The tendency of late, however, has been to feed solid food much earlier than formerly and certainly the results seem to warrant the change. While many of the infants do not gain as rapidly as when they are fed larger amounts of milk, especially when top-milk mixtures are used, they develop earlier and their bones and muscles are better formed and stronger. Furthermore, the tendency to rickets is much less marked in such children.

The daily diet at twelve months of an infant fed in this way would be as follows.

6 A. M. 8 ounces of milk.

9 A. M. 1 or 2 ounces of orange juice.

10 A. M. Cereal, 1 ounce (2 tablespoonfuls); 8 ounces of milk (part on cereal and balance in bottle); dry bread, 1 small piece.

2 P. M. Beef juice, 1 or 2 ounces, or broth, 4 or 5 ounces, or egg; boiled rice or baked potato, 1 ounce (2 level tablespoonfuls); green vegetable, ½ ounce (1 level tablespoonful).

6 P. M. Cereal, 1 ounce (2 tablespoonfuls); dry bread, 1 small piece; 8 ounces of milk.

10 P. M. 8 ounces of milk.

ABNORMAL SYMPTOMS.

While the great majority of breast-fed infants go through the first year without any nutritional disturbance many artificially fed infants have more or less trouble. In some cases the difficulty is easily rectified, in others it is more severe and

19

may lead rapidly to death, or as more frequently happens, to a long chronic illness. These differences are those of degree rather than of kind, as they all depend upon the inability of the infant to digest one or more of the several ingredients of the food in the strength or amount furnished. Formerly the protein of cow's milk, especially the casein, was considered the most frequent cause of these disturbances of digestion, but recent evidence places the responsibility more frequently upon either the fat or the sugar. The condition is complicated by the fact that an infant who develops an intolerance for fat is likely soon to develop an intolerance for sugar, and vice versa, unless the first difficulty is promptly corrected. In many cases a carefully taken history will reveal the error which is at the bottom of the trouble. If this is corrected at the beginning an immediate cure may be effected. Where the history reveals no such error and after the disturbance has persisted for some time the best method is to reduce markedly the strength of those ingredients that appear to be at fault. While the logical way to classify these cases is according to the particular food-stuff which causes the disturbance, the difficulties of following this scheme are so great that it has seemed wiser to discuss different symptoms and their treatment.

Vomiting.—The occasional regurgitation of small amounts, one or two teaspoonfuls, is of little importance. Holding the infant erect for a few minutes after he has finished taking his bottle enables him to belch what air he has swallowed with the feeding, and so eliminates the usual cause of regurgitation.

Large amounts are vomited when the feedings are too large or the intervals between feedings too short. A normal infant should seldom be fed more frequently than every three hours and even longer intervals are more successful with infants that are inclined to vomit.

Too high a content of fat in the food is a frequent cause of vomiting. In these cases it is necessary to reduce the fat content of the food considerably below that proper for an infant of corresponding age and development. This is accomplished by using partly or wholly skimmed milk in making up the food. After the vomiting has ceased the amount of fat in the food is gradually increased, but it is usually necessary to keep the fat slightly lower than normal for several weeks.

Maltose preparations are more apt to aggravate vomiting than either lactose or cane-sugar. As a rule lactose is the best sugar.

When the vomiting consists of large curds the addition to the formula of some alkali as sodium citrate (one grain for each ounce of milk is usually sufficient), or the use of a cereal water as diluent instead of plain boiled water will help to prevent the formation of large curds and lessen the vomiting.

Gas.—All infants swallow more or less air while taking their feedings. In order that the infant may get rid of this it is well to hold him erect for a few minutes after the feeding is finished.

Gas in the intestine is either air that has been passed on from the stomach or the result of fermentation. The first is prevented by the precedure mentioned above. The second is controlled by reducing the amounts of sugar and starch in the food or by changing to another kind of sugar.

Colic.—Colic is a symptom of indigestion. Not infrequently even a slight increase in the strength of the food will cause colic. In mild cases dropping back to the previous formula will stop the colic. When the strength of the food is next increased a smaller addition should be made. In more severe cases the food should be diluted with an equal part of water, or even more, until the symptoms subside, and then gradually increased. Constipation is a frequent cause of colic. Its treatment is considered in a later section.

Loose Stools.—Loose stools are the result of the infant's inability to digest one or more of the ingredients of the food. The sugar is the most frequent cause. From the previous history and an inspection of the stools a conclusion as to which is at fault can frequently be arrived at. The formula should be made up without sugar, except what is in the milk, for a few days. As soon as the consistency of the stools has improved a small amount of sugar may be added to the food and gradually increased. If lactose has been used previously it is well to substitute cane-sugar or one of the dry preparations of maltose.

At times the fat is the cause of the diarrhea. In these cases it should be reduced temporarily and gradually increased as the condition improves but the amount of fat in the food should be kept below the previous point for some time.

Diarrhea.—All recent cases should have all food withheld for twelve to twenty-four hours. During this time boiled water or a thin cereal water should be given. The water may have a very little tea added and be sweetened with saccharine if the infant takes it better this way. At least as much fluid as the infant usually takes should be given each twenty-four hours. If the infant will not take sufficient fluid, enteroclysis or hypodermoclysis may be used. For the latter an o.8 per cent. salt solution is used; 150 to 200 c.c. may be given two or three times in each twenty-four hours.

After twelve to twenty-four hours food should be given. In the less severe acute cases a formula made up of boiled skimmed milk without any additional sugar is frequently successful. The strength of the formula will depend on the age and condition of the infant. At first the amount of skimmed milk in the formula should not be more than one-third that of the milk in the previous formula. In the more severe cases better results are usually obtained by using buttermilk or protein milk. The buttermilk is diluted with water or cereal water and later may have fat and sugar added to it. It should not be boiled.

Protein Milk.—Protein milk (Eiwess-Milch) is prepared as follows: One quart of whole milk is heated to 98° F. Two rennet tablets are dissolved in an ounce of cold water and mixed with the milk. The milk is now allowed to stand at room temperature until it has coagulated, which takes about twenty minutes. It is cut and allowed to drain through two thicknesses of gauze until the curd is very dry. The curd is then washed twice with cold boiled water. The dry curd is mashed in a mortar and then forced through a very fine wire sieve. This may have to be repeated several times. One pint of buttermilk is then gradually added to the curd. Finally sufficient boiled water is added to make one quart. The composition of protein milk made in this way is about as follows: fat, 3.25 per cent.; sugar, 1.8 per cent.; proteins, 3.75 per cent.; salts, 0.65 per cent. Each ounce furnishes about 15 calories. Protein milk may be made from 2 per cent. milk when it will contain about 1.5 per cent. fat. For very young infants it may be diluted. That with the lower fat content is preferable for young infants. The advantages of protein milk are its low sugar content (1.8 per cent.) and its high protein content (3.5 per cent.). For this reason it cannot be used for long periods without the addition of some sugar. The best sugar to give in this condition is maltose. It should be begun as soon as the stools are semisolid, at first only one teaspoonful in each twenty-four hours' food. Another teaspoonful may be added every second or third day.

It is seldom wise to keep these infants on protein milk for long periods. In changing them back to milk mixtures it is safer to begin with a formula containing less fat than the protein milk. Even then considerable difficulty is frequently experienced. Some of these infants will take unsweetened condensed milk better than ordinary milk. The unsweetened condensed milk is about two and one-fifth times as strong as ordinary milk and has to be diluted accordingly. Sugar has to be added to it as to ordinary milk.

Constipation.—Constipation may be due to a too high fat content of the food, in which case the stools are large, dry and crumbly. Reducing the fat and increasing the carbohydrate, especially the starch content of the food, rectifies the condition. On the other hand, a food which contains too little fat will cause constipation. In this case the stools are not so large and more normal in consistency. If the infant is strong and healthy a moderate increase in the fat will frequently relieve the condition.

One or two ounces of orange juice daily will help. Lime water should be omitted from the food and milk of magnesia used if an alkali is necessary. Furthermore, lactose and maltose are more laxative than cane-sugar and oat flour is more laxative than barley flour.

CHAPTER XVIII.

FEEDING OF THE PREMATURE INFANT. FEEDING AFTER THE FIRST YEAR. FEEDING DURING ACUTE ILLNESS AND IN NUTRITIONAL DISTURBANCES

FEEDING OF THE PREMATURE INFANT.

FOR the first twenty-four to thirty-six hours a premature infant should receive only small amounts of a 3 per cent. solution of lactose at regular intervals. One or two drams (teaspoonfuls) is given every hour to a three-pound infant, and a slightly larger or smaller amount to a larger or smaller infant. As these infants are at first unable to suck they have to be fed with a medicine dropper or with a Breck feeder. The latter is a glass tube with a perforated nipple on one end and an unperforated nipple on the other end. The tube is filled with food, the perforated nipple held in the infant's mouth and the other nipple gently squeezed. This method is useful for the larger, better developed infants, but is of no use for the very small infants. The latter have to be fed by gavage, and great care must be used in feeding them, as they are apt to regurgitate and aspirate part of the food, especially when it is given too rapidly or in too large quantities.

The best food for a premature infant is diluted breast milk. As the mother's milk secretion is usually insufficient for the first two or three weeks the milk must be obtained from another woman. It is not essential that her infant should be of the same age. At the same time everything possible should be done to stimulate the mother's milk secretion. Her breasts may be massaged and pumped at regular intervals. A better method is to have the mother nurse a vigorous infant.

Breast milk diluted with an equal amount of a 4 per cent. lactose solution is given after twenty-four to thirty-six hours. For very small infants the breast milk should be diluted with two parts of lactose solution. At first only two drams are given every hour. The amount is gradually increased to a half-ounce every hour, then an ounce every one and a half or two hours. At the same time the strength of the food is gradually increased. By the end of the second or third week the infant will be fed every two hours—12 times in each twenty-four hours, the total amount of food for twenty-four hours being about 12 ounces. By this time the breast milk should be little, if any, diluted.

As soon as the infant is able to suck, it should be given the breast for a few minutes, but if insufficient food is obtained from the breast the necessary amount should be given afterward. When the infant obtains sufficient from the breast the other feedings may be stopped.

When it is impossible to obtain woman's milk, cow's milk mixtures must be used. At first 1 ounce of milk and 19 ounces of a 4 per cent. lactose solution may be given. For very small infants the milk had best be partly skimmed at first. The amounts and intervals are the same as when breast milk is used, but the strength of the food has to be increased much more slowly.

In feeding a premature infant it is important to remember that the food requirement is probably considerably less than that of a normal infant.

FEEDING DURING THE SECOND YEAR.

From the eleventh to the fifteenth month the schedule remains practically the same except that the 10 P. M. bottle can be stopped during the thirteenth or fourteenth month. It is often difficult to do this suddenly, but if water is gradually substituted for milk the change is scarcely noticed. A good method is to pour off 1 ounce of the milk and add 1 ounce of water, the next night pour off 2 ounces of milk and add 2 ounces of water. After eight or nine days the entire feeding will consist of water. The amount of water may now be gradually reduced.

At fifteen months the 6 A..M. bottle may be stopped and the breakfast given at 7:30 A. M., a small milk feeding being given just before the nap about 10:30 A. M. The orange juice may be given on waking or with the breakfast. At the same time the amounts of the different articles are slightly increased, and a greater variety of vegetables allowed. The daily schedule will now be as follows:

6.30 A. M. Orange juice, 2 ounces (may be given with 7.30 A. M. feeding).

7.30 A. M. Cereal, 1 or 1½ ounces (2 or 3 tablespoonfuls); dry bread, 1 small slice; milk, 8 or 9 ounces.

10.30 A. M. Milk, 7 or 8 ounces.

2.00 P. M. Beef juice, 2 ounces, or broth, 5 ounces; egg; boiled rice or baked potato, ½ ounce (1 tablespoonful); green vegetables, ½ ounce (1 tablespoonful); stewed fruit (prune pulp or apple sauce) ½ or 1 ounce (1 or 2 tablespoonfuls); no milk.

6.00 P. M. Cereal, 1 or 1½ ounces (2 or 3 tablespoonfuls); dry bread, 1 small slice; milk, 8 or 9 ounces.

About the fifteenth or sixteenth month all bottle feedings can usually be stopped, all fluid being given from a cup. The 6 A. M. bottle is stopped when the schedule is changed. A little later the breakfast bottle can be stopped, then the supper bottle and finally the 10.30 A. M. bottle. It is easier to stop them one at a time, rather than all at the same time. The 10.30 A. M. milk feeding can be stopped at about the sixteenth or seventeenth month. Many women, who are busy, find it a great convenience to continue one or two bottles during the second year. As a rule the infants do better if all bottles are stopped by the eighteenth month.

Meat is begun about the fifteenth month. At first only a half-teaspoonful with the 2 P. M. feeding. The amount is gradually increased so that by the eighteenth month about one-half ounce (1 tablespoonful) is being taken. It is well to alternate meat and egg at first, meat and broth being given every second day, and egg and beef juice on the alternate days. Later the egg may be given with breakfast and meat given every day at 2 P. M.

As the amount of solid food is increased during the second year, the quantity of milk is gradually reduced. Infants fed in this way rarely take much over 20 ounces of milk a day after the eighteenth month. This is important, as they will sometimes refuse to take sufficient solid food as long as they are given large amounts of milk. This is especially true when the milk is given in a bottle.

FEEDING AFTER THE SECOND YEAR.

By the end of the second year, a normal child should be taking only three meals a day, with at times a cup of milk in the middle of the forenoon, before the nap. Between meals only water should be given, but this may be given freely especially in hot weather. It may be cool but it should not be iced. About 20 ounces of milk should be taken each day equally divided between breakfast and supper. Up to the fourth or fifth year it should be warmed, but after that it may be given at room temperature. Dinner at 1.30 P. M. is the main meal and consists of 5 or 6 ounces of soup (broth or purée), or 2 or 3 ounces of beef juice, meat (lamb chop, steak, chicken, roast beef or lamb), potato (baked or mashed), or boiled rice, some green vegetable (asparagus tips, stewed celery, spinach, string beans, carrots, summer squash, or fresh peas), and some dessert—either cooked fruit (apple sauce, baked apple, stewed prunes, peaches or plums), or rice pudding, junket, custard, apple pudding, tapioca pudding or occasionally vanilla ice-cream, and one or two slices of bread and butter. No milk but only water should be given at dinner. Breakfast and supper are simple meals. Breakfast consists of some cooked cereal (oatmeal, Pettijohn, cream of wheat or farina), a soft egg (soft-boiled, poached or scrambled), bread and butter and 8 to 10 ounces of milk. If desirable some cooked fruit may be given at breakfast. Supper consists of cereal, bread or toast and butter, and 8 to 10 ounces of milk.

The daily schedule would be about as follows:

7.30 to 8.00 A. M. Breakfast:
>Cooked fruit (1 or 2 tablespoonfuls), if desired; cereal (3 or 4 tablespoonfuls); soft egg; bread or toast and butter; milk, 8 to 10 ounces.

1.00 P. M. Dinner:
>Soup, 6 ounces, or beef juice, 2 or 3 ounces; meat (1 or 2 tablespoonfuls); baked potato or boiled rice, 2 or 3 tablespoonfuls; green vegetable, 2 or 3 tablespoonfuls; dessert or cooked fruit, 2 tablespoonfuls; water.

5.30 P. M. Supper:
>Cereal, 3 tablespoonfuls; bread or toast and butter; milk, 8 to 10 ounces; occasionally a soft-boiled egg or cooked fruit.

FEEDING DURING ACUTE INFECTIONS.

In feeding infants and young children during acute infectious diseases the important facts to be borne in mind are: first the great need of water, second the impairment of digestion, and third the fact that fats are not digested as readily as carbohydrates and proteins.

Infants.—The total amount of fluid ingested should be kept up to the amount usually taken. More may be allowed if desired. It should be given in small amounts at frequent intervals between feedings. The food should be weaker than during health. For short illnesses which last only a few days, simple dilutions of the previous food is usually sufficient.   At first the previous formula may be diluted one-half with boiled water or some cereal water.   As the infant's condition improves the strength of the food may be gradually increased, but the full strength should not be reached until the temperature has been normal for two or three days. If the illness is of long duration the formula may be made up with partly skimmed milk and two-thirds or even all of the usual amount of sugar.   In this way the fat may be reduced as much as desired while the protein and carbohydrate content of the food is only slightly reduced.

Regular intervals of feeding are just as important with ill infants as with well infants. They should seldom be fed oftener than every three hours.   Water, however, may be given freely between the feedings.

Gavage.—Infants that are extremely prostrated, delirious or comatose frequently will not take sufficient food.   If the condition persists more than a few hours forcible feeding becomes necessary.   Such infants may be fed by gavage.

Children Over One Year.—Regular intervals of feedings are just as important as with infants.   During the febrile stage they should be fed every three hours during the day and if ill for any length of time once during the night, making five or six feedings in each twenty-four hours.   Water should be given freely between the feedings.   It is important to keep the total twenty-four-hour amount of fluid well up to the usual intake or even above the same.   A child of two years should take at least 30 ounces, and one of four or five years 40 ounces in each twenty-four hours.   If plain boiled water is not well taken, an alkaline water, as Vichy or Seltzer, may be given.   During the febrile stage the diet may include broth, thin gruel, milk (diluted with water, Vichy or lime water), and albumen water (which may be flavored with orange juice).   The gruels and milk furnish the most nourishment.   Later cereals and dried bread may be added, then soft-boiled eggs and potato, and finally vegetables and stewed fruits.

Gavage.—Delirious and comatose children may have to be fed by gavage.   This can be done almost as easily as with infants by wrapping the child in a sheet.   The food given may be predigested if advisable.   Gavages should not be repeated oftener than four times in each twenty-four hours.

Long Illness.—In illness associated with prolonged fever as tuberculosis the same general rules for diet apply as with adult patients.

PYLORIC STENOSIS.

In mild cases of pyloric stenosis dietetic treatment may be tried for a short time. If, however, some improvement is not quickly shown the case should be treated surgically. The best food according to Holt[1] is breast milk with a low fat content. If necessary the breast milk may be skimmed. If breast milk cannot be obtained a low skimmed-milk formula should be tried. As the condition improves the amount of skimmed milk in the formula may be gradually increased until the formula is sufficiently strong for the infant's age except that the fat content is low. Then the fat may be slowly increased, but it should be kept lower than normal for several weeks or months. As a rule these infants do best on long intervals between feedings, usually four hours. The amount of each feeding should be small, at first not more than two ounces. Later it may be gradually increased to the proper amount for the infant's age. Small amounts of water should be given between the feedings. Holt says that occasionally a case does better on small amounts at frequent intervals, as one-half ounce every hour. This is especially true when breast milk is used.

Morgan[2] has given the best detailed statement of the postoperative treatment of these cases. His work is based on 50 cases treated at the Babies' Hospital where the present routine is as follows.

"The patient is given, an hour after operation, provided the recovery from the anesthetic has been complete, 16 c.c. of water, and an hour later 12 c.c. of breast milk mixed with 4 c.c. of water. It may be necessary at first to use a medicine dropper for the administration. The breast milk is repeated every three hours, eight feedings a day, and is alternated with water. Both are gradually increased so that twenty-four hours after operation 16 to 24 c.c. of undiluted breast milk is being given every three hours and a similar amount of water between feedings. At the end of forty-eight hours the child is usually taking 20 to 30 c.c., at the end of seventy-two hours 30 to 45 c.c. at a feeding. The administration of water by mouth during the first three or four days is of the greatest importance. The time required to increase the milk to meet the caloric requirements of the child has been on an average of five days; in small babies three days may be sufficient, and in the well nourished as much as eight to ten days."

[1] Jour. Am. Med. Assn., 1914, lxii, 2014.
[2] Am. Jour. Dis. of Child., 1916, xi, 245.

Morgan emphasizes the importance of breast milk for these cases, at least for the first ten to twelve days after the operation. If the mother has been nursing the infant before the operation every effort should be made to keep up her supply of milk. The best method is to have her nurse a strong, healthy infant until her own infant is able to nurse again. If this is impossible her breasts should be massaged and emptied by means of a breast pump several times each day. Downes[1] says that the infant may be given the breast forty-eight hours after operation. Morgan advises a longer delay of not more than seven days. If the mother is unable to nurse her infant a wet-nurse should be obtained when this is possible. When this cannot be done modified cow's milk may be gradually substituted for the breast milk, beginning on the twelfth day. At first the formula should be considerably weaker than that proper for the infant's age.

CYCLIC VOMITING.

The cause of periodic vomiting is probably some error in metabolism, but until the cause has been determined, the diet cannot be so regulated as to exclude it. The one factor common to all cases is a well-marked acetonuria. In some cases the acetonuria appears very early, if not before the actual vomiting, in others the acetonuria does not appear until later, when it may well be the result of starvation.

The dietetic treatment can best be considered under two headings: first that during an attack, and second, that during an interval. During an attack no food should be given by mouth. Water should be given freely either by mouth, by rectum or by hypodermoclysis. Small amounts may be tried by mouth, but if this aggravates the vomiting, as it usually does, it shculd be stopped. The best way is to give colon irrigations of one or two quarts of water every six to eight hours. The water should run in slowly, great care being taken not to overdistend the colon. A good method is to use an inlet and an outlet tube, the outlet tube being slightly larger and introduced two or three inches higher than the inlet. The amount of water retained can be calculated by measuring the amount allowed to flow in and the amount returning. At least 30 ounces should be retained in twenty-four hours. If insufficient water is retained from the irrigations, hypodermoclyses should be given. In mild attacks normal saline may be used, but in severe attacks the use of

[1] Jour. Am. Med. Assn., 1914, lxii, 2019.

a 2 or 3 per cent. solution of sodium bicarbonate helps to counteract the acidosis. As the sterilization of solutions of sodium bicarbonate changes the latter into sodium carbonate, which is very irritating, it is necessary to change the carbonate back to the bicarbonate before using the solution. This is best accomplished, according to Howland and Marriot, by passing a current of carbon dioxide under aseptic precautions through the cold sterilized solution, to which a few drops of a phenolphthalein solution have been added, until all the pink color disappears.

Alkali should be given in all cases, best as sodium bicarbonate. It may be added to the water ingested, to the irrigations, or to the hypodermoclysis fluid. The endeavor should be to keep the urine alkaline.

In protracted cases rectal feeding may be advisable. Four to 6 ounces of peptonized skimmed milk with 2 or 3 drams of sugar (dextrose) may be given every eight hours.

When the vomiting has ceased for twelve hours, water may be given by mouth, at first in small amounts, ½ ounce every hour. If this is retained, a thin cereal gruel may be tried, beginning with a teaspoonful every half-hour and gradually increasing the amount. The kind of gruel used may be varied: arrowroot, cream of wheat and farina are all good. Later thick cereal and either Huntley and Palmer breakfast biscuits or dried bread may be added. Then broth, white of egg, fat free milk, strained vegetables and scraped meat. All fat should be withheld for some time.

Between attacks the plan which has proved most successful in our hands has been to withhold all fats for long periods. The child is allowed the usual diet for his age, except that the milk is fat-free and no butter, olive oil or meat fat is allowed.

Occasionally these patients show sensitization to some foreign protein. Such proteins should be excluded from their diet, or an effort made to immunize the patient by feeding him gradually increasing amounts of the offending protein, according to the method devised by Schloss.[1]

Sufficient alkali, usually in the form of sodium bicarbonate, should be given to keep the urine barely alkaline.

After several months have elapsed without an attack, small amounts of fat may be added to the diet, but such additions should be considered experimental and should be stopped at the first evidence of a return of the trouble.

[1] Am. Jour. Dis. of Child., 1912, iii, 341.

FEEDING IN NUTRITIONAL DISTURBANCES.

Rickets.—Rickets is an extremely common disease, regarding the cause of which very little is known. The one known fact common to all cases of rickets is a very low calcium content of the body, but why this occurs is not known. The amount of calcium in the food appears to be of little importance, as all the ordinary cow's milk mixtures contain an abundance of calcium, much more than breast milk.

Breast-fed infants develop rickets under two conditions: first, when they are kept on the breast exclusively much longer than usual; second, among the very poor, especially the Italians and negroes in the large cities of America. Much has been written about the poor surroundings of such infants, especially the lack of sunlight and fresh air. Of possibly greater importance would seem to be the diet of the mothers, who eat very little fresh meat, milk, green vegetables and fresh fruit. Is it not possible that such a restricted diet deprives the mother's milk of something necessary to the infant for his proper growth?

Artificially fed infants are particularly apt to develop rickets when fed on the various proprietary foods, especially those that are made up without milk. A prolonged digestive disturbance in the first few months often precedes rickets in an infant that otherwise may be doing very well when the rickets develop. Finally many artificially fed infants develop rickets, usually of a mild type, in spite of having had proper cow's milk mixtures and without having experienced any digestive disturbance.

These facts would suggest that even good cow's milk mixtures are frequently insufficient in some particular. Furthermore cases of rickets are self-limiting, and begin to recover about the time they receive a liberal mixed diet. Funk's suggestion that rickets is the result of a lack of certain accessory factors or vitamines in the diet, would seem to offer a possible explanation, but it needs more proof than has been brought forward. At least it gives us a rational theory on which to base our treatment, and fortunately this coincides with the results of the best empiricism.

The best prevention of rickets is breast feeding, but the mother's health should be watched and she should receive a liberal mixed diet, containing a fair amount of fresh meat, eggs, milk, green vegetables and fruit. When rickets develops very early good breast milk will probably do more to check its progress than any artificial feeding.

With artificially fed infants all proprietary foods, especially those that are to be used without milk, should be avoided. Raw cow's milk mixtures, when it is possible to obtain a safe raw milk, are the best substitutes for human milk. Condensed milk should be avoided. When the milk supply is questionable it may be pasteurized, but it should not be boiled. If the infant's digestion is deranged he may be unable to take raw or pasteurized milk at first but he should be changed to them as soon as possible.

Fortunately rickets rarely appears before the sixth month, and by that time the infant can be fed fruit juice and beef juice and a little later, egg, potato and green vegetables. All these articles should be begun in small quantities and gradually increased as is explained in the section on feeding (p. 287), but they may be begun considerably earlier in a case of rickets than with a normal infant.

PART IV.

FEEDING IN DISEASE.

INTRODUCTION.

THE intelligent use of foods in disease should become more and more a matter of interest, not only to the specialist but to the practioner as well, and the time is far past when the conscientious physician can afford to turn over the diet regulation to the nurse, prompted by the patient's appetite or lack of it. As time has gone on we have come to recognize the importance of an adequate diet for the sick and the dangers which unnecessarily accrue to the patient from an insufficient supply of proper nourishment. With the tables of food values so generally at hand, the correct proportion of food elements, as well as the total food value necessary in a given case, may at least aproximately be easily calculated. When the illness is slight or of short duration it is of course not so essential to go into minute details, but at least a general supervision should be kept of what the patient takes, even if a good deal of latitude is allowed in the choice ot particular foods and drink.

A sick person is proverbially difficult to please and when it comes to a matter of providing suitable food in a form that will appeal to such a patient, the difficulties are often nearly insuperable. Some simple rules might well be formulated to express the requirements of food and feeding in sickness.

1. Food should all be as daintily prepared and served as possible, as much of the pleasure in food, as well as its proper digestion, lies in its manner of presentation to the patient.

2. Food should be hot or cold as the patient prefers, iced, if necessary, but almost never served lukewarm.

3. The seasoning of food should be carefully done, using preferably only the simplest condiments in minimal amounts, salt, pepper, celery salt.

4. It should be served at regular intervals as nearly as possible.

5. Only the easily digestible parts of foods should be presented to a patient, as tender meats, young vegetables, etc. Avoidance of all well-known indigestible foods.

6. All food should be thoroughly chewed and insalivated.

7. The teeth and mouth should be kept in the best possible condition by tooth brush, mouth washes and cleaning of the tongue.

8. Unless there is some special contra-indication, as in peptic ulcer, water should be regularly and freely given to the patient and a pitcher of water kept by the bedside for them to help themselves from when they are able to do so.

9. A feeding cup or feeding spoon should be used in giving food to patients flat in bed, or if too ill to use the cup, fluids may be sucked through a glass tube.

10. The physician, giving due regard to the patient's preferances and appetite whenever possible, should be absolutely definite in his direction, preferably writing down intervals for feeding, definite quantities at each feeding, the foods to be used and whether they are to be given hot or cold. When the illness is apt to be prolonged and the patient's appetite no guide, feedings on a definite nitrogen and caloric basis should be prescribed in order to conserve the patient's strength and weight as much as possible.

11. The services of a good nurse who is personally agreeable to the patient must be insisted upon, whenever the illness is prolonged and finances permit. Such a nurse will be tactful in the care of the sick-room and feeding utensils.

In any discussion of foods for sick people cognizance must be taken not only of the individual kinds of foods, but also that of their general type and preparation. Thus for example we might well divide foods for patients into—

1. A normal general diet, meaning the diet usual for normal people and applicable to patients who are more or less confined by incapacities other than illness, *e. g.*, a broken leg, etc.

2. Soft diet, meaning a diet which is either put through a colander or capable of having this done, excluding vegetables and fruits.

3. Fluid diet, meaning a diet confined to liquid foods of various sorts.

4. Milk diet, either as whole milk, buttermilk, skimmed milk, modified milk, malted milk, cream and milk mixtures alone or with alkaline additions.

5. Convalescent diet which usually refers to a diet rich in easily assimilable proteins of delicate texture, made especially nourishing and appetizing by various food accessories, jellies, condiments, etc.

6. Diets to meet special mechanical or chemical body needs. Of these one may designate—

    A. Diets which have in view the power to neutralize excessive gastric acidity, as in peptic ulcer, by offering a large amount of non-stimulating albumin, which readily combines with the gastric juice, *e. g.*, lactalbumin and egg albumin.

B. Diets particularly rich in basic salts useful in conditions where the hydrogen ion concentration of the blood is increased, as in chronic nephritis, cyclic vomiting, and the later stages of diabetes mellitus. These are the so-called alkaline diets useful in any condition characterized by an acidosis.

C. Diets especially poor in salts, *e. g.*, sodium chloride and calcium. The former being of use in almost any type of edema, especially that due to salt water retention in nephritis. The latter of doubtful value in chronic arthritic conditions or for experimental purposes where a low calcium diet is needed.

D. Diets especially rich in certain other salts, *e. g.*, iron in anemic conditions, calcium in tuberculosis, (although it is doubtful if any excess of calcium in the diet is retained).

E. Diets, poor in purine bases of use in gout and chronic nephritis and possibly in cancer.

F. Diets low in protein, useful in chronic nephritis where we wish to spare the renal tissues as much work as possible. Also in certain types of intestinal disease accompanied by putrefaction.

G. Diets high in protein, useful in convalesence and in fevers to a limited extent, also in all conditions accompanied by a rapid destruction of body protein, *e. g.*, cancer, pernicious anemia, hyperthyroidism (non-stimulating proteins only).

H. Diets rich in carbohydrates, for fattening purposes and in intestinal putrefaction.

I. Diets poor in carbohydrates where they are badly metabolized, *e. g.*, diabetes mellitus and obesity.

J. Diets rich in fats for fattening purposes and where a prolonged muscular effort is needed. Also in constipation.

K. Diets poor in fats in obesity, in acidosis in any of its manifestations.

It can be seen from the foregoing incomplete classification of diets in general that a good deal can be done on a definite scientific basis to select a diet suitable for many different conditions of varied body chemistry, either in normal or diseased persons.

CHAPTER IX.

DISEASES OF THE CIRCULATORY ORGANS.

DIET in relation to diseases of the heart and bloodvessels is many-sided in that it must of necessity vary according to the particular condition under consideration, thus, for example, in acute infections affecting the heart, the diet should be in accordance with the principles of diet in fever or acute infections. In myocarditis, coronary sclerosis or decompensation of the heart from any cause, diet may be of extreme importance by virtue of its possible adverse mechanical effects, giving rise to dangerous or even fatal symptoms by pressure on the heart from the bulk of the food or from fermentation of the wrong kind of food or undue distention from gastric atony. In arteriosclerosis food may act as a cause, in that overeating has a distinct etiological relation to this disease and by the increase in blood-pressure caused by certain foods and drink, either from quantity or quality, a cerebral hemorrhage may be precipitated. These specific effects must be noted in addition to the usual nutritive role of foods.

FUNCTIONAL CARDIAC DISTURBANCES.

Functional cardiac disturbances are frequently purely matters of dietary regulation. Here the disturbance takes the form of either a tachycardia or an arrhythmia, and analysis of the diet may show the patient to be an excessive tea or coffee user or else to have a marked idiosyncrasy for these drinks. Gastro-intestinal disturbances are frequently at fault, usually accompanied by fermentation or confined gas, giving rise to a cardiac reflex through the vagus, producing extra systoles.

Sutherland[1] puts it well when he says "more patients come to a doctor complaining of heart trouble when the digestion is at fault, than do those whose hearts are actually diseased."

DIET IN ORGANIC CARDIAC DISEASE.

Organic cardiac lesions may be acute or chronic, compensated or decompensated to varying degrees, and require special dietary consideration based upon these facts.

[1] System of Diet and Dietetics.

308

In the acute infections (endocardial or pericardial) the requirements are much alike, and one tries to furnish the needed food requirements in such form that they will be easily assimilated and promote excretion. Milk mixtures modified in various strengths, as often given in typhoid fever, are useful and fulfill the essential necessities, or a soft diet restricted as to amount.

In compensated chronic valvular or myocardial disease, individuals need food in the same proportion and amounts as do normal persons, provided they are in other respects normal. It is often a fact, however, that these people have other concomitant conditions which must be taken into account such as chronic renal disease, with or without hypertension, obesity, arteriosclerosis, etc., any one of which complications must be the determining factor in prescribing a diet. In such cases the food must be ordered in obedience to the limitations set to the diet for these conditions. Overfeeding any case of chronic cardiac disease would be manifestly a mistake, as the resulting increase in body weight might completely change compensation to decompensation. On the other hand, these cases must be fully nourished in order to obtain the best mechanical result from a diseased organ and special attention given to preventing indigestion.

Cardiac Decompensation.—In conditions of decompensation whether due to valvular lesion or myocarditis, diet is of great importance as already pointed out, and many systems of diet have been arranged for such cases. In the uncomplicated cases of mild or only very moderately severe decompensation, much the same rules hold true as for the compensated hearts, stress being laid on the fact that *indigestion in all its forms must be prevented*, as an acute attack of indigestion may change the prognosis from a favorable one to a prompt exitus, particularly in large, full-blooded individuals. The moderate restriction of fluids to prevent overfilling of the vascular system must also be kept in mind, particularly at meals only small amounts of fluid should be allowed. When marked decompensation supervenes we are at once in the presence of complications. All the internal organs are congested functionate at a disadvantage and often imperfectly; there is usually more or less subcutaneous edema and often collections of fluid in one or other of the body cavities; hence the indication is imperative that we should do nothing to further handicap the patient. It is for this state of things that most of the so-called dietary cures for cardiac diseases have been devised, and among these there are some worthy of more detailed discussion.

The Karell Cure.—The Karell Cure[1] is perhaps the oldest of these, although as originally published by Karell it is rather indefinite as to details. The idea of this diet and its many modifications is the same, namely, to furnish only a fraction of the daily food requirements by giving small quantities of milk for a time, then gradually increasing by adding other articles of food, keeping the total fluid intake down to 800 c.c. (27 oz.).

For the first five to seven days: 8, 12 A. M.; 4, 8 P. M.; milk 200 c.c. (7 oz.). No other fluids.

Eighth Day: Milk as above.
    10 A. M. 1 soft-boiled egg.
    6 P. M. 2 pieces of dry toast.
Ninth Day: Milk as above.
    10 A. M. 1 soft-boiled egg and 2 pieces of dry toast.
    6 P. M. 1 egg and 2 pieces of dry toast.
Tenth Day: Milk as above.
    12 Noon. Chopped meat, rice boiled in milk, vegetables.
    6 P. M. 1 soft-boiled egg.
Eleventh and Twelfth Days: Same as tenth day.

No salt is used throughout the diet. Salt-free toast and butter used. A small amount of cracked ice is allowed with the diet. All meats can often be advantageously omitted.

He explains the good effect of the Karell cure on the following grounds:

1. The limitation of fluids.
2. The low salt content of the diet.
3. The elimination of toxins.
4. Antitoxic effect (against uremia).
5. Mechanical (no distention).

N. B. Potter tried the effect of the Karell cure diet modified in various ways, keeping the total quantity at about 800 c. c. (27 oz.) for the twenty-four hours, and found that the results were almost, if not quite, as good as the original Karell diet, with the added advantage that it is less monotonous.

Potter's Modifications of the Karell Diet.[2]

		Calories.	Protein.	Fat.	Carbohydrates
1. Skimmed milk	800 c.c.	303.0	27.2	2.4	41.8
2. Whole milk	800 c.c.	570.7	26.4	32.0	40.0
3. Whole milk	700 c.c.				
30% cream	100 c.c.	806.9	25.6	58.0	39.5
4. No. 2 + Lactose	oz. j (30 gm.)	685.4	26.4	32.0	68.0

[1] Karell Diet, modified as used at New York Hospital.
[2] Potter, New York Med. Jour., 1916, ciii, 450; Arch. Gen. de méd., 1866, ii, 513.

					Calories.	Protein.	Fat.	Carbohydates.
5.	No. 2 + Lactose	oz. iij (90 gm.)			915.0	26.4	32.0	124.0
6.	No. 2 + Oatmeal	oz. j	(cooked)		588.7	27.1	32.1	43.3
7.	No. 2 + "	oz. iij			624.9	28.7	32.4	49.9
8.	No. 3 + Lactose	oz. j			921.7	25.6	58.0	67.5
9.	No. 3 + Oatmeal	oz. j			825.0	26.4	58.1	42.8
10.	No. 8 + "	oz. j			939.8	26.4	58.1	70.8
11.	No. 3 + "	oz. iij			1205.6	28.0	58.4	133.4
	Lactose	oz. iij						

While on this diet the patients often lose their edema and compensation is restored, but the great disadvantage is, of course, that so little of real food value is given that the patients are insufficiently nourished and a considerable loss of body protein results—a thing in itself often disastrous when the patient is already undernourished. Its usefulness cannot be denied in certain cases, particularly of the sthenic type, but it must be used with caution, never forgetting that we are at the same time starving the patient and probably at longest it should only be used for a few days. There are various forms of restricted fluid intake, particularly as urged by Oertel and again by von Noorden, the former instituting practically a thirst cure and the latter recommending "thirst days" comparable to the "green days" in his diabetic dietary regimen.

Strauss[1] recommends a moderate amount of protein, 72.8 gm., and warns against the extreme reduction as seen in the Karell diet, except for a very short time. He also restricts, but only moderately, the fluid intake and advises against Kraus's routine of reducing the daily amount to 1500 c.c., then 1000 c.c. and later 800 c.c., which amounts to a thirst cure. These restrictions are all more advantageous when the decompensation is accompanied by high arterial tension,—obesity or both. Many cases of decompensation when accompanied by general anasarca do well on one of the salt-poor diets as recommended in renal edema, great good often resulting from the limitation of the sodium chloride intake (see Salt-poor Diets) unless the decompensation is extreme and the general internal congestion excessive. This is often more generally and successfully used than the Karell diet, as the patients do not lose strength and muscle substance while on it. As one would naturally infer, its greatest usefulness is seen when there are renal complications.

Carter[2] published the results of Gaulston's sugar treatment for decompensation and a year later Dingle[3] also reported a case. Both were cases of marked and progressive

[1] Veröffent. d. balneol. Gesellsch. in Berlin, 1912, xxxiii, 2, 27-37.
[2] Brit. Med. Journal, 1911, No. 1401.   [3] Ibid, 1912, i, 66.

decompensation in which all the usual forms of diet and drugs had been tried without result. In each the success was marked and under similiar conditions is certainly worth consideration. Carter recommends that the cane-sugar be given as follows: First week, 2 ounces daily. Second week, 3 ounces daily. Third and fourth weeks, 4 ounces, then gradually reduce to 3, 2 and 1 ounce. His diet is as follows:

> *Breakfast:* Coffee, ham, tongue, boiled egg, two pieces thin toast. No fat of any kind.
>
> *Luncheon;* One piece dry toast, spring cabbage(?), broccoli or asparagus with boiled fish, boiled meat or boiled chicken (no fat or sauces). Rice boiled in a little milk or water, sugar being taken on the rice. No fruits or acid taken. A tumbler of hot water to be taken one hour before luncheon and dinner and nothing to drink at either meal.
>
> *Afternoon Tea:* Two pieces of dry bread with sugar on it and a little sugar in a cup of tea.
>
> *Dinner:* Much the same as luncheon, only a flaked cereal instead of rice on which to take the sugar. No fats, fruits or sauces.

Physiologically this method of increasing the efficiency of the cardiac muscle seems reasonable, as the heart obtains[1] at least one-third of its energy from carbohydrates. It is, however, difficult to produce any hyperglycemia by means of the oral exhibition of sugar, so Büdingen[2] has tried rectal and intravenous injections of an isotonic (5.4 per cent.) solution of glucose, with surprisingly good results in some instances. It is at least a method that deserves further trial, although hypodermic use of the glucose solution would seem a much simpler method to employ.

Mackenzie insists that the food for cardiac cases shall be appetizing, nutritious, of small bulk, easily digested and thoroughly masticated, and it might be added that in all cases, particularly in decompensation, the evening meal should be especially light.

Fatty Heart.—Fatty heart is usually a part of a general adiposis, the heart being surrounded by an overcoat of fat with strands of fat even dipping in between the muscle bands. This gives a heart which has to work at a mechanical disadvantage, often with the resulting symptoms of decompensation, *e. g.,* dyspnea on exertion, edema and palpitation.

In the dietary treatment of this, the first object to be sought is a general reduction in body fat, which is best ac-

[1] Jour. Am. Med. Assn., 1914, p. 1895.
[2] Deutsch. Arch. f. klin. Med., 1914, cxiv, 534.

complished by one of the reduction cures. In these cases the *Karell diet* is especially useful and gives great satisfaction. Other methods are in accordance with the diets as suggested for reduction.

Combined with any dietary routine there must go hand in hand a definite plan for the strengthening of the heart muscle by physical exercises, passive and active, for without this the reduction diets will leave the patient thinner, but with an entirely inefficient heart muscle, so that the second state is as bad as the first. For this purpose a sojourn at Nauheim is of great benefit if one can go abroad, or in this country much the same result can be obtained at home by artificial Nauheim baths and resistance exercises if given under expert direction. This regimen may be obtained at many of the American bathing resorts, among which may be mentioned Watkins Glen, The Chamberlain, Old Point Comfort, White Sulphur Springs, Battle Creek, etc.

In many cases merely the resistance exercises strengthen the heart muscle satisfactorily and at the same time add to the general muscular improvement.

Diet in Adolescent Heart and Cardiac Myasthenia following Infectious Disease.—This condition is seen not infrequently in young people who grow rapidly in a very short time, there being a disporportion between the circulatory organs and the more rapidly developing bones and muscles. The result is a heart which is not well up to the ordinary strain of daily life or slight increase in activities.

A condition of real disease does not exist, but an asthenia affecting the heart, accompanied by palpitation, breathlessness after exertion, or a feeling of weakness and lassitude. The dietary regulations designed to overcome this state are merely such as would meet the conditions of malnutrition following a prolonged disease, which has left the entire organism myasthenic, and include the giving of foods that are primarily nourishing, with the exclusion of all fancy dishes, salads and unnutritious foods. The food should be simply prepared, giving three meals a day with a small extra feeding between meals and at bedtime, if the appetite allows. Milk, cream and butter are valuable and a fair increase in protein should be insisted upon. With a regulation of the diet should be combined good hygiene and light exercise gradually increasing always keeping below the patient's capacity. The use of the Nauheim resistance exercises does much to strengthen these hearts.

Senile Heart.—The senile heart has received considerable attention at the hands of various authors, notably Balfour, who goes so far as to prescribe an absolute diet. It would seem, however, that the rules laid down for cardiac conditions in general would apply equally well to the senile heart, remembering that elderly people require actually less food than younger individuals, as their metabolism goes on at a so much lower rate. The necessity of a light evening meal should also be emphasized.

DIET IN DISEASES OF THE BLOODVESSELS.

Arteriosclerosis.—When we come to consider the question of diet in arteriosclerosis we find almost everybody has something to say, most of it based on individual clinical evidence (?) and much on speculation. As a matter of fact little is known of the specific action of food-stuffs on the various organs and whether this or that article of food causes or favors arteriosclerosis must yet be worked out experimentally in the biochemical laboratories.

There seems, however, very direct evidence that persistent overeating in general is responsible for many cases and as we know experimentally that artificially raising the blood-pressure apparently causes arteriosclerosis (adrenalin injections in rabbits), all foods which raise pressure presumably favor its production. Longcope[1] showed that in animals after having been sensitized by previous injection, repeated inoculations of protein produced in the organs changes analogous to those seen in general fibrosis, whether of vessels, heart, liver, kidney, etc. Broughton[2] also showed by experiments that repeated anaphylactic shocks caused lesions of a degenerative type in the smaller arteries most marked in the liver (100 per cent.; kidneys (66 per cent.); heart (66 per cent.); spleen (100 per cent.) This fact may have great bearing on the production of arterial changes. Clinically Bishop[3] arrived at much the same conclusion. considering arteriosclerosis, chronic nephritis, cardiosclerosis, etc., to be caused by the pathological reaction between the animal cell and some particular protein ingested or derived from bacterial growth, to which the organism had been sensitized, analogous to anaphylaxis. To combat this he recommends a diet in which all animal protein but one is excluded; cheese is the one usually given first, then later adding other proteins one by one to see if any one causes symptoms. This he calls a "few protein" diet, and proteins are used qualitatively

[1] Trans. Int. Med. Cong., London, 1913.
[2] Tv. Chi. Path Soc., 1916-17, x, 156.
[3] Med. Record, 1913, lxxxiv, 511.

rather than quantitatively. Whether or not this is a correct assumption, it is at least in accord with what little scientific data we have and is certainly worth careful consideration.

Von Noorden[1] insists that there is no reason for leaving meat entirely out of the diet in arteriosclerosis, as we have proved nothing against meat as favoring its production. On the other hand, presumably anything which favors hypertension favors arteriosclerosis and meat certainly, clinically, does increase blood-pressure when a large constituent of the diet. He does lay great stress on restriction of fermentable foods, heavy meals and more than a total of 1½ pints of fluid in the twenty-four hours, which alone he says often reduces the pressure 20 to 40 mm. Hg. (See Relation of Obesity and Reduction Cures to Hypertension.)

Diet in Hypertension.—That which applies to arteriosclerosis applies to hypertensive cases with apparently equal force, therefore it would seem wise to limit the amount of protein intake to the low level compatible with nitrogenous equilibrium, especially the purine bodies, as well as the limitation of quantity, calorically, to meet the needs of the patient as gauged by his various activities. The prevention of indicanurea is apparently of distinct advantage. Eustis[2] observed that all (?) cases of high arterial tension were accompanied by indicanurea, relief of which, by giving a non-nitrogenous diet, was often prompt. The explanation of this is based on Bargers[3] finding parahydroxyphenylethylamine (a pressor substance) in the blood of such patients. This, with Dale and Dixon, he also isolated from the tyrosin of putrefactive meat, another similar substance was produced from leucin from putrid meat.

Cornwall's[4] rules for diet in hypertension probably represent the consensus of medical opinion and might be formulated somewhat as follows:

1. Keep the diet low in protein, 60 to 65 gm. per day, largely purine-free or with low percentage of extractives (soups and meat).

2. Regulate the quantity to secure the minimum of work from the organs with maximum nutrition. The caloric value of which should vary from 1500 to 2000 to 3000 accordingly, as a patient is in bed, leading a sedentary life or working.

3. Restrict the diet so as to meet indications presented by the kidneys, liver, heart and gastro-intestinal tract.

[1] Post Graduate, 1913, xxviii, 426.
[2] Southern Med. Jour., 1912, v, 244.
[3] Trans. Eng. Chem. Soc., 1909, xcv.
[4] New York Med. Jour., 1912, xcvi, 315.

4. The diet should be antiputrefactive, excluding fermentable carbohydrates and should be laxative as well.

The Effect of Various Substances on Blood-pressure.—
1. *Food substances* causing an increase of blood-pressure are principally the purine bodies in meat or meat soups, *i. e.*, the extractives, for the lower the percentage of the latter in meats the less prone are they to increase blood-pressure. For this reason glandular organs are usually more likely to increase blood-pressure than other parts of the animal, and meat that is roasted or broiled has more effect than if boiled or, least of all, if boiled in two waters. Here too, food of almost any kind is much more apt to increase pressure if taken in large amounts, for, as already stated, overeating seems to be one of the chief factors in the production of arteriosclerosis and hypertension. Alcohol in moderate dosage probably has little or no effect on blood-pressure—when taken more liberally it causes a fall in pressure. Excess of fluid in any form tends to increase pressure.

2. Those foods which tend to decrease blood-pressure are the carbohydrate foods; farinaceous foods, vegetables, fruits, fats, and milk preparations, as the latter are purine-free.

Aneurysm.—Aneurysm has also been the subject of special dietary attention, Tufnell prescribing the best-known regimen which is noted for its extreme restriction: Breakfast 2 ounces of bread and butter, 2 ounces of milk or cocoa. Noon, 3 or 4 ounces meat with 2 or 3 ounces of potato or bread and 3 or 4 ounces of water. Night, 2 ounces of bread and butter, 2 ounces of milk or tea. Of course this is an absurd diet and only a strong person could stand it at all; the resulting blood concentration which it is hoped to gain is more than offset by the starvation necessary and would be distinctly bad for weak persons. All blood-pressure-raising foods should be avoided, however, as well as psychical irritation, intestinal fermentation and bodily over-work.[1]

Angina Pectoris.—Both the rules for avoiding the production of arteriosclerosis and hypertension should be made use of, special attention being given to the avoidance of acute attacks of indigestion which often accompany a fatal attack of angina, although many times indigestion is undoubtedly secondary to the claudication rather than the cause of the anginal attacks. The evening meal should be simple and light.

Tobacco in Relation to Cardiac Disease.—While not a food, tobacco is so generally in use that a word as to its place

[1] Hecht Zwit. Fr. Med. Klin., 1912, lxxvi, 87.

in cardiovascular cases is not amiss. Not much is really known about the continued effect of small doses of tobacco and its contained alkaloids, although there are many theories; there is, however, practical unanimity of opinion regarding its large or excessive use and that so used it is of distinct disadvantage. By its blood-pressure-raising qualities, its proneness to disturb digestion in some persons, to cause irritation of the myocardium (extra systoles) it is certainly best left alone in these conditions; whether a very moderate use of tobacco by its soothing and contenting effects may not offset the possible bad effect of continued small amounts is a question to be decided in each case. If a patient becomes susceptible to its effects or if used in large amounts, there is every reason for interdicting the use of this substance.

CHAPTER XX.

FEEDING IN DISEASES OF THE LUNGS.

MUCH of what has been said in regard to the relation of diet to diseases of the circulatory apparatus holds equally true for the pulmonary diseases. In addition, food must be considered in its relation to acute or chronic infections, and from the mechanical stand-point as a possible factor in increasing symptoms by pressure from an overloaded or distended stomach; besides, of course, its nutritional value.

In pneumonia, lobar or lobular, we are dealing for the most part with a self-limited disease of short duration, *i. e.*, as compared with typhoid for example. On this account the food quantities that are given would perhaps not be so important if we could be sure a case would run for not more than seven to ten days. Unfortunately some of the cases run considerably longer or else develop serious complications, such as empyema, in which it is of the utmost importance that the patients should not have lost flesh and strength unnecessarily and so arrive at the late stages of the disease or its complications, in an overweakened condition. On this account the proper dietary treatment may have a very real bearing on the prognosis of the disease.

The routine diet in these cases has usually been feeding of milk, broth, albumin water and gruels with a total nitrogenous content and caloric value far below the body's requirements. Coleman, on the other hand, has applied the principles of the high caloric diet as used in typhoid and apparently with some success, but the need for the prevention of abdominal distension makes the giving of large quantities of food, especially carbohydrates, questionable, and as the majority of cases run but a week it is perhaps wisest to be content with nourishing patients, if not to the full limit of a theoretical capacity, at least sufficiently to prevent undue losses.

The necessity for keeping the excretory organs unhampered by excessive amounts of the products of food metabolism must also be kept in mind, for at times it seems as if we could ask little more than that the organs should remove the disease toxins as rapidly as they are formed. It is nevertheless most important that sufficient food of the right sort should be given in order that the natural antitoxin-producing organs should run at their highest efficiency, under the circumstances, and as well, to prevent a starvation acidosis from further complicating the picture. We know, too, that in pneumonia the percentage of uric acid in the blood is always higher than normal, due to an excessive endogenous uric acid metabolism, and one should therefore avoid as much as possible feeding the purine bodies in the food. These two indications are met by giving a fair but not excessive amount of carbohydrate and fats and a low purine or nearly purine-free diet, during the acute stage of the illness, all in a liquid or semisolid form.

To adults accustomed to their cup of tea or coffee in the morning, this should be continued, but not in large amount, for Mosenthal has shown that the giving of caffeine to an already inflamed and overburdened kidney sometimes brings disaster. The broths and meat extracts and jellies are best left out of the dietary, as they contain only infinitesimal amounts of food and a high percentage of purine bodies. There is one legitimate use of meat extracts or broths in small amounts, namely, when anorexia is present a small cup of well-seasoned broth does more to cheer up a forlorn appetite than anything else. The diets No. 1 and No. 2 as outlined for typhoid fever represents a very good assortment of foods, leaving out the broth where indicated, also omitting some of the lactose if there is any indication of tympanites. A good diet for an average-sized person might be formulated somewhat as follows:

8.00 A. M.   Milk and coffee, each 120 c.c. (4 oz.), 240 c.c. (8 oz.); sugar.

10.00 A. M.   Milk in any form, hot or cold, 240 c.c. (8 oz.).

12.00 M.   Gruel, 120 c.c. (4 oz.), with milk 180 c.c. (6 oz.).

2.00 P. M.   Milk feeding, as at 10.00 A. M., 240 c.c. (8 oz.).

4.00 P. M.   Gruel, 120 c.c. (4 oz.), with milk, 180 c.c. (6 oz.).

6.00 P. M.   Custard with lactose (4 oz.) 1 cup.

8.00 P. M.   Milk feeding, as at 10.00 A. M., 240 c.c. (8 oz.).

10.00 P. M.   Whey, 180 c.c. (6 oz.), with one whole egg and sherry, 15 c.c. ($\frac{1}{2}$ oz.)

12.00 P. M.   Gruel, as at 12.00 o'clock noon.

2.00 A. M.   Milk as at 10.00 A. M.

4.00 A. M.   Whey, 180 c.c. (6 oz.), or hot milk 240 c.c. (8 oz.).

6.00 A, M.   Milk, as at 10.00 A. M.

Approximate values: Protein, 90; fat, 91; carbohydrate, 220 gm.; calories, 1825.

The value of this diet can be considerably increased by adding 500 c.c. (1 pint) of cream if divided between each milk or gruel feeding, which would make the total values, protein 103, fat 180, carbohydrate 235, and calories 2800.

Since sleep is of the utmost importance in pneumonia, a rest from feedings at night of from six to eight hours is advisable if the patients will sleep, but they are to be fed when awake not oftener than every two hours. With the onset of tympanites feedings must be stopped for a few hours so that the beneficial effects of stupes to the abdomen and a hypodermic of pituitary extract, etc., may be obtained. When feedings are resumed it is often better to leave sugar and milk out of the diet unless the latter is fully peptonized (2 hours) or else given in some other form than raw milk. The use of other artificial digestants is often of service.

In this connection it seems worth calling attention to the use of a good Bulgarian bacillus culture given in a little sweetened water three times a day on an empty stomach. The apparent effect of this is often most happy in reducing the distention, as is also indicated in the discussion of typhoid fever.

The feeding of cases of pneumonia complicated by nephritis will depend upon the severity of the latter disease but the aforementioned diet usually serves well, although it is often wise to have it prepared without salt.

Drinks.—In addition to large amounts of plain water (provided the circulatory apparatus is in order), patients are usually grateful for fruit juices with water, such as lemonade, orangeade, grape juice, etc. When the ordinary foods are taken poorly a 5 per cent. solution of gelatin flavored with one of these juices makes it possible to supply a good deal of nourishment, almost without the patients realizing that they are taking anything but flavored water.

When the temperature falls and the symptoms of toxemia are past, a gradual return to a more normal diet may be begun, first by using soft diet, later adding meat and vegetables as convalescence proceeds. A thorough emptying of the intestine by a cathartic, after the temperature is normal, is an invaluable aid to the digestion and helps the appetite to return.

BRONCHITIS.

Acute Bronchitis.—In adults, this is a condition *sui generis*, or a result of infection, possibly also due to sudden climatic changes, although this latter is presumably only predisposing. Then, too, there are the complicating cases of acute bronchitis occurring in the course of almost all the infectious diseases, such as pneumonia, typhoid fever, measles, etc.

In certain elderly people acute bronchitis is a local manifestation of some general diathesis, *e. g.*, gout and nephritis, and in these cases certain dietetic regulations referable to the underlying cause must be taken into consideration and the diet made to harmonize with it. Again in other cases it is a matter of general undernutrition and the bronchitis continues to recur indefinitely until the organism is put in fighting trim by forced feeding and all measures to raise the physical resistance, *e. g.*, fresh air, exercise and general hygiene.

When fever is present the diet should consist of liquid and soft solid foods, milk, cream, cereals, fruit juices, egg, creamed toast. bread, butter, coffee, cocoa, weak tea, mineral water and a large amount of any good drinking water.

The appetite must be consulted and as this is often very poor, the patients for the first day or two frequently wish for nothing but cold liquids of one or another sort. If the intestinal canal has been thoroughly emptied at the outset, the appetite frequently improves, and it is then more easily possible to increase the food. Whenever possible it is always advisable to feed these patients up to the limit of their digestive capacity as it shortens convalescence and Coleman and Shaffer have found in their typhoid diet investigation that even a high degree of body temperature is not incompatible with liberal feeding, as the average patient is able to digest and metabolize food practically as well as in health, provided the proper foods are used.

As soon as the patient wants solid food it may be given, omitting only the well-known indigestibles and much meat.

Chronic Bronchitis.—Chronic bronchitis is frequently a condition accompanying chronic emphysema, and when so present is to be dieted in accordance with the suggestions detailed for that disease. In many cases it is the initial feature of asthma and as such is in need of an etiological diagnosis, when possible, in order to prescribe diet on any satisfactory basis. Thus we may find it a local expression of a general erythema, urticaria or anaphylactic reaction to foreign protein; or a reaction to some form of endogenous toxicosis, gout or uremia; a complication of pulmonary tuberculosis or a reflex from some distant organ. Where any one of these causal condition are found, the diet appropriate for the underlying condition must be made use of. If, however, none of these factors can be found as responsible for the trouble, the only possible method is to proceed on empiric lines and frame the diet with a view to the least disturbance of digestion, both from the direct digestive point of view and the avoidance of mechanical factors which would work adversely in causing precordial pressure and embarrassment of respiration.

Foods to Avoid.—Keeping in mind both these possibilities, we must avoid ordering foods in themselves indigestible, or which are easily fermentable, such as members of the cabbage family; cauliflower, cabbage, Brussels sprouts, and heavy sweets.

Foods Suitable in Chronic Bronchitis.—All simple foods, simply prepared, keeping down the amount of protein food, especially in elderly people; fat foods such as cream, butter, fat meat, etc., enjoy a favorable reputation in all chronic pulmonary affections and should be freely used. Laxative foods, such as fruits, green vegetables and simple salads, should form a considerable element in the diet, as excretion is to be promoted in every direction and a clear colon is of especial importance, for an acute exacerbation of the bronchitis is often traced to an increase in constipation. Water drinking, up to six to eight glasses a day should be insisted on, either as plain water or in the presence of any considerable degree of urinary acidity, partly as mineral alkaline water.

EMPHYSEMA.

Emphysema being for the most part a presenile change and usually accompanied by a general sclerosis of the other organs and bloodvessels, its dietetic treatment resolves itself principally into dietetics of the concomitant conditions, such as bronchitis, chronic nephritis and arteriosclerosis.

The food should be simple, easily digestible and not apt to cause flatulence; the sugars and starches should on the latter account be largely restricted. In fact any embarrassment of the circulation by abdominal distention may easily prove serious, particularly in the presence of marked arterial changes. There is no way of directly influencing the emphysema except by promoting the general health by means of careful attention to the details of eating, not alone in the character of the foods ingested, but the method of eating plays a considerable part in the care that can be given these people.

In the first place great care should be taken not to overeat, not alone on account of the possible mechanical factors but because the waste products of digestion play such a part in the increase of symptoms due to the complicating conditions already enumerated. On the same account elimination should be promoted in every way and often the discomforts of digestive disturbances of all sorts are minimized by this means. It would seem as if Fletcher's principles of eating might afford great relief from the annoying complications, reducing as it does, the protein ration to the low level of physiological economy in nutrition and rendering the methods of forced elimination almost unnecessary, as there is the minimum of waste matter to be gotten rid of (see Fletcherism p. 649). Whether one follows this philosophy or not there is unquestionable virtue in keeping the intake of protein low and rendering combustion and elimination of food products as complete as possible.

ASTHMA.

As asthma is but a symptom of disturbance either primarily in the bronchial tree or remote in other organs, the first step in ordering a diet must be to determine what the underlying pathological condition is. If it is due to a bronchitis, to a toxicosis as in nephritis or from gastro-intestinal disease, relief must be sought in the correction of the abnormal conditions including the diet suitable for each (*q. v.*). Formerly asthma was thought to be due to many nervous influences acting in a reflex manner, and while this may be true in a certain small proportion of the cases, it is by no means proved. A true explanation of many of the hitherto obscure cases is found in the phenomenon of anaphylaxis due to the effect of a foreign protein on an organism already sensitized to that protein. This is seen in hay fever very frequently and from dietary indiscretions where persons with a known idiosyncrasy to egg white, for example, develop an attack of asthma after eating some dish made with egg. Where the cause is known or easily found, the diet may be readily adjusted. But there remains a large number of cases of asthma which cannot easily be etiologically classified—in these persons it is often helpful to test out the skin reaction to different proteins in the food, and where a protein is found to give a positive skin reaction it should be eliminated from the diet. After such a change in diet it is necessary to persist in it for at least ten to fourteen days, until all that particular protein from previous ingestion is eliminated, before it is possible to decide whether the suspected protein is responsible for the attacks of asthma or not. In certain individuals when the anaphylactic reaction is not too marked, it is often possible to overcome this condition by repeated feeding of small amounts of the food in question, gradually increasing the amount.[1]

When it is not possible by any method to come to a definite conclusion as to the cause of the asthma in a particular case, it is necessary to order diet on purely empirical lines, keeping in mind the following points:

1. Indigestion, either gastric or intestinal, should be avoided by ordering only simple food simply prepared.

2. The diet should be laxative as far as possible, as intestinal torpor in all its forms distinctly predisposes to the production of asthmatic attacks.

3. It is probable that in many cases of unknown origin some one or other of the proteins is at fault, most often perhaps an animal protein. On this account it is often useful to curtail the amount of protein ingested, keeping the total daily intake down to the lower limits of physiological economy in nutrition, as suggested by Chittenden. Another reason why this is often helpful is, that, in many of the older or long standing cases, renal excretion is deficient and with nitrogen retention, symptoms of toxemia often develop.

4. Where the asthma is nocturnal, the evening meal should be exceedingly sparing and nothing allowed which by its bulk or from fermentation would add an element of embarrassment to the circulation in the lungs, by pressure upon the thoracic organs.

5 Patients with asthma should take sufficient mild exercise to assist in the complete burning of the food-stuffs, leaving as little residue, either intestinal or systemic, as possible.

6. Most of these patients are helped by drinking a fair amount of water, particularly between meals, and night and morning—six to eight glasses. With these suggestions in mind it should be a simple matter to order foods which meet the necessary conditions so far as it is possible to know them.

Foods to Avoid.—Much sweet food, or heavy sweets of all kinds—syrups, candy, layer cake and preserves. Readily fermentable vegetables, such as cauliflower, cabbage, Brussels sprouts, much onion or potato. Alcohol, except in the most sparing amount and then only for some special indication. Indigestible meats as: goose, duck, veal (unless very tender) and fresh pork. Tobacco should be used sparingly, if at all.

[1] Am. Jour. Elec. Rad., 1917, xxxv, 529.

What has been said in regard to diet in asthma holds equally true for cases of urticaria, which is usually, if not always, an anaphylactic skin reaction.

PLEURISY WITH EFFUSION. HYDROTHORAX.

In both of these conditions there is fluid in the pleural sac. In the case of a pleurisy it comes as a product of inflammation, in hydrothorax it is merely a transudation, principally from stasis, although even this is said by some authorities to be due to a low grade inflammation.

In the early stages of pleurisy if there is fever the patient must be fed as for any fever. When the exudate is established and the patients afebrile an attempt may be made to regulate the diet so as to assist in the removal of the fluid, for although not successful in the case of large exudates, small ones may be absorbed, often without recourse to tapping. To this end the two chief indications are to curtail the water intake to 800 to 1000 c.c. and exclude salt from the diet by the use of one of the salt-poor diets. (See Nephritis.)

It must be remembered in employing these diets that frequently little result, so far as diminishing fluid or edema, occurs during the first few days, then, when the sodium chloride reserve is considerably diminished, the free excretion of the fluids often begins.

The dietetic treatment of hydrothorax depends more or less upon the underlying condition which is the cause of the fluid accumulation, *e. g.*, nephritis and cardiac decompensation. In either condition the same regimen as prescribed for pleuritic effusion is indicated, viz., limitation of fluids and a salt-poor diet, the details of either being dependent on the form of the nephritis or the degree of decompensation.

EMPYEMA.

Empyema whether due to invasion of the pleural sac by one of the ordinary pus organisms or whether the original infection is tuberculous with a secondary infection added, the dietetic indications are the same. The formation of pus, particularly in such great quantities as takes place in empyema, takes a large amount of fat from the body, as the percentage of fat in pus is exceedingly high. On this account it is necessary to feed in large amounts as well as to prevent undue loss of body weight. If the fever is high it will be necessary to modify the usual diet in accordance with the principles of fever requirements both in quantity and quality, but the fact must not be forgotten that if we are to hope for any success in our treatment the chief requisite is a body nourished up to the height of its capacity.

To this end it is essential that a careful record be kept and the caloric value of the food estimated, for it is likely that if the patient's appetite is allowed to dictate the terms of the menu the total energy value of the food will be too low. If the appetite is poor, remember that milk either alone or modified upward by the addition of cream and lactose (see Typhoid Fever) can practically always be digested, even in the absence of appetite, provided too high a formula is not used. If the appetite is fair or good, then one must go ahead and feed liberally all digestible and nourishing foods, making sure that the proportion of fat in the diet is high by giving cream, 250 to 500 c.c., ½ or 1 pint per day, butter up to 250 gm. (¼ pound), or as nearly that amount as will agree with the patient; for the rest the appetite may be trusted largely to determine the choice of foods.

If the case is tuberculous in origin the diets as recommended for tuberculosis will be found useful. In either case great attention should be paid to the digestion to make sure that through light exercise or massage the muscular system is kept in condition.

TUBERCULOSIS, PULMONARY OR GENERAL.

In *none of the infectious diseases* is a proper dietary of so great importance as it is in tuberculosis; one has only to think of its older name "consumption" to realize the truth of this statement; and whether the disease is seen in its acute or chronic form, pulmonary or other distribution, the necessity for a definite feeding plan is paramount. There can be no possible doubt that food, good food, properly chosen, properly prepared and eaten in cheerful surroundings is our sheet-anchor in this disease. So much has been written in all languages in regard to this, that it hardly seems necessary to dwell upon it, but apparently many practitioners either do not appreciate these facts or are too easy going to take them seriously and valuable time is lost, to say nothing of the patient's weight.

Among the earliest symptoms of tuberculosis, the various disturbances of digestion rank a good second in importance, as many of the incipient cases first complain of gastro-intestinal symptoms, such as gas, heaviness after meals and often sour stomach. Jacob[1] who examined the gastric con-

[1] New York Med. Jour., 1913, xcvii, 297.

tents, after test meals, in 50 cases, found hyperacidity or normal acidity the rule in incipient cases, and that the symptoms complained of were often similar to those of organic gastric lesions. He also concluded that the secretion of hydrochloric acid in fever was quite independent of the height of the temperature.

By the older method of stuffing these patients with food, particularly in using large amounts of milk, the patients often developed the symptoms of gastric atony and many cases returned from sanotoria with a well-marked atony, due of course, to the very real weakness of the gastric muscle which was part of the general asthenia, but immensely exaggerated by overfeeding. Fortunately this mistake is now more rarely seen, particularly where any sort of intelligent care has been exercised in the selection of a diet. Toxemic dyspepsia in the tuberculous is also a cause for loss of weight or failure to gain. What then, should be the general principles upon which a suitable diet may be constructed? To this question one will find many answers. Some advocating high protein diets, others high fats and still others a diet high in both of these elements.

First, the question of what should be the object sought in diet, may well be asked. There is now unanimity in the belief that a great gain in weight above the normal for the individual should not be sought and a weight of not over five to ten pounds overweight represents the optimum. Too much weight increases the work of the other organs and hampers the heart and lungs. When this has been gained Brown's[1] advice is certainly founded on experience and common sense, when he advises patients to eat just enough to maintain this increase, avoiding milk. The little flare-ups and upsets in the course of the disease which cause loss of weight will come, and he then advises patients to take milk in addition to their regular diet until this weight is regained, then to drop it. (The use of milk will be further discussed later on.)

The amount of protein proper for the tuberculous to eat has been the subject of much comment and discussion, one set of clinicians insisting that a considerable increase in this should be the rule, particularly as applied to animal protein, and Watson[2] estimates that this diet should be one-third more nutritive for the tuberculous than for the non-tuberculous. This increase he applies to proteins and fats but not to carbohydrates on account of their tendency to fer-

[1] Canada Pract. Rev., 1912, xxxviii, 529.
[2] Practitioner, 1913, xc, 102.

ment. In recommending this increase in animal protein he refers to experiments proving that meat in uncooked form is especially beneficial, the effect being from the juices of the meat rather than the fiber, and that in some way the thyroid is favorably influenced by uncooked meat, eggs and milk. He probably has in mind Cornil and Chautemesse's experiments in which they found that dogs fed on raw meat resisted artificial tuberculous infection better than those fed upon cooked meat. In advocating the meat diet (zomotherapy) in certain cases, Sutherland advises keeping up an exclusive meat diet as long as the patient continues to gain weight, weeks or even months. As they get better, heavier (having been underweight), the meat diet may be relaxed and varied menus given. If gastro-intestinal symptoms develop the meat diet should be stopped, calomel or other cathartic given and the patient put on a milk diet 3 to 4 pints (1500–2000 c.c.) daily, diluted with barley, lime or sodawater. After two or three days the meat diet may be resumed.

Kendall,[1] on the other hand, is against an excessive protein feeding on account of the extra work thrown on the kidneys in excretion, and quotes Bardswell and Chapman who thought that "patients made less satisfactory progress on diets of very large nutritive value than when smaller value and any considerable increase in the amount of protein in the diet produced a disproportionate excretion of nitrogen, an increase in the amount of imperfectly oxidized proteins in the urine, a decrease in the percentage of nitrogen absorbed and an increase in the amount of aromatic sulphates excreted, indicating increased intestinal putrefaction." Certain it is that we wish to keep the patient in at least full nitrogenous equilibrium, and while this can be worked out with scientific accuracy in a fully equipped sanitarium or hospital where nitrogen estimations can be made of intake and output, such a procedure is outside the range of possibility in ordinary practice.

In planning the ideal diet for the tuberculous, one must take into consideration several factors. The question whether the patient has fever or not, whether it is necessary to continue at work or whether freedom from care and work can be assured, for naturally the fever patient or one who is obliged to work needs more food than another, and individual judgment on the part of the physician must be used; but for the ordinary resting case, protein 80 to 100 gm., fats 80 to

[1] Canada Med. Assn. Jour., 1912, p. 670.

100 gm., carbohydrates 300 to 350 gm. would represent a good average, giving a total caloric value of 2500 to 3000 calories. These, as in the case of other diets, can be worked out from the table of 100-calorie portions. Suitable diets for the tuberculous are so much a matter of money that although the patient with means can usually reach a good dietary under supervision—the poorer members of society often have an exceedingly hard time to secure even a maintenance diet. A detailed study of some T. B. Dispensary families' diets for two weeks among Russian Jews, Poles, Italians and Negroes showed[1]

(1) The average Dispensary family obtains about four-fifths the nourishment it should.

(2) Ignorance of food values, poor judgment in buying were largely responsible, besides the poverty.

To offset this condition Chadwick advocates a Caffeteria service for the Tuberculous poor as offering the most for the expenditure.[2]

Diets in Tuberculous.—As an example of the high protein diet we have the following published by Watson[3] which he especially recommends, No. 1 is largely a milk diet, No. 2, largely a meat diet.

No. 1

7.00 A.M.	Milk, ½ pint (250 c.c).
8.30 A.M.	Milk, ½ pint (250 c.c) with casein ½ ounce (15 gm.), flavored with coffee or cocoa; gruel, made with milk and flavored with cream.
11.00 A.M.	Soup, thickened with ¼ pound (120 gm.) raw scraped beef; or soup thickened with an egg.
1.00 P.M.	Chicken essence or veal jelly, strengthened with casein ½ ounce (15 gm.) and milk ½ pint (250 c.c); or raw meat minced ¼ pound, with milk; or raw meat rissoles, with milk or raw meat sandwiches with milk.
3 00 P.M.	Milk with egg on thin custard.
5.00 P.M.	Milk tea, ½ pint (250 c.c) with cream.
7.00 P.M.	Meat juice, *e. g.*, Wyeth's Leube-Rosenthal's meat solutions mixed with port or Burgundy; or soup with raw meat, or beef ex-

[1] 13th Rep. Phipps Inst. 1917.
[2] Mod. Hosp. 1917, 14, 403.
[3] Practitioner, 1913, 4C, 102.

tract with egg and milk forming a custard;
or milk and arrow root, with casein and
cream, ½ pint (250 c.c.); (brandy may be
added).

8.00 P.M. An invalid food made with milk, ½ pint (250
c.c), and casein.

11.00 P.M. Milk and egg or chicken broth and egg.

In severe cases milk may be taken peptonized or fermented
e. g., kumyss, zoolak; buttermilk or ripened milk (Bulgarian
bacillus) may agree better.

No. 2. A diet largely of meat, often helpful when dyspepsia follows large meals.

6.00 A.M. Milk, ½ pint (250 c.c.).

8.00 A.M. Milk, ½ pint, with casein ½ ounce (15 gm.),
flavored with coffee, or cocoa and peptonized; slice of toast with butter; bacon, ham,
eggs, fish, meat rissoles or steak (taking
two things).

11.00 A.M. Glass of hot milk with eggs, or raw meat
soup.

1.00 P.M. *Luncheon*—soup from strong stock, or fish
soup or a helping of fish; mince, lightly
grilled tender steak or chop, or slice of
underdone sirloin of beef, or roasted leg of
mutton; stewed fruit and custard or jelly
with cream; toast, glass of milk.

4.00 P.M. Cup of milk, tea, toast, butter, or biscuit and
butter.

7.00 P.M. *Dinner*—same as luncheon; a little wine.

Prophylaxis for Children of Tuberculous Inheritance.—
When one has to do with children of tuberculous parents or
those who are more or less constantly exposed to this infection, the necessity for a proper feeding plan is self-evident.
Especial attention should be given to following the weight
of the child from month to month so that the first sign of
loss or even of failure to gain may be noted. The food should
be especially nourishing and all other foods eliminated from
the diet as much as possible. Particular hygienic care should
be exercised in the daily routine and everything done in diet,
work, play, sleep and fresh air to promote the greatest degree
of physical efficiency.

Plan of Feeding.—When a patient is able to take ordinary
full diet the best plan is to give only three meals a day, provided of course, the patient can eat sufficient at a meal to
produce the required gain or to maintain an increase already
accomplished. When a patient cannot attain this result on

three meals alone, it is best to try between-meal lunches of reinforced milk, sandwiches, etc. Still other patients, of course, can eat only smaller amounts at a time and here the feedings must be more frequent, but if possible, three or four hours should elapse between them, using the two-hour interval only if necessary and taking care not to overcrowd a gastric muscle which may be already losing its tone.

When the stomach is very irritable, any of the feedings referred to under gastric irritability may be used for this condition, or even gavage if necessary, as this often results in more food being retained than when given by mouth.

Special Foods for the Tuberculous.—Milk.—Milk has from time immemorial, held the first place as an extra in the diet of these cases, but of late years a certain prejudice has arisen, particularly against its large use. The reasons for this have already been intimated in that it takes an excessive amount of milk, if one attempts to feed milk alone, which overdistends the stomach, often resulting in atony, so that many clinicians have discarded its use entirely, while others use it for certain indications in very moderate amounts. The exclusion of milk from the dietary is no more sensible than its excessive use, but the indications for it may be perfectly definite and it then is, of course, most useful, *e. g.*, to add an extra to the diet in cases of failing nutrition; when people are especially fond of milk and in irritable conditions of the gastro-intestinal tract. In the latter, especially for cases with nausea, vomiting, diarrhea or fermentation; buttermilk or artificially ripened milk, keffir, zoolak, etc., may be used to the greatest advantage. A very good way in these cases is to feed one of these prepared milks every two hours and with every other feeding to add some soft solid.

Eggs.—Another form of food long popular in the treatment of tuberculosis, eggs still hold a prominent place in its dietary, but in the light of present-day physiological chemistry, eggs must be used as a very potent albuminous and fat food and enter into calculations of the diet as such, not to be taken indiscriminately in massive daily quantities in addition to regular meals, on the assumption that for the tuberculous patient the more food the better. Incidentally, slightly cooked eggs are better and more completely digested than raw eggs, since often only one third of the raw albuminous portion is digested at all, as shown by examination of the stools.

Fats.—These hold a high place in the diet, for they are non-fermentable and their excretion does not tax the kidneys, being oxidized into water and CO_2. Animal fats being more nearly homologous are probably better than vegetable oils, and the fat from cod livers stands at the head of the list; for certainly this fat furnishes something which is in addition to its hydrocarbon content. Possibly it is its iodine and possibly something belonging to that little-understood class of food-stuffs called vitamines, but at all events clinically it does more for the patient than other fats do. To be sure, this can be taken only in limited quantities and the bulk of the fat in the diet must be made up of meat fat, butter, eggs and cream. The latter should always be taken fresh and not altered by pasteurization or sterilization. This applies to milk as well.

The working standard for a diet in tuberculosis, according to King,[1] must take into consideration the following factors:

"(*a*) Men of the same respective age and weight seem to require a larger diet than do women.

"(*b*) All other conditions being equal, a larger diet is apparently required by persons under thirty years of age than is the case after that period.

"(*c*) The laboring class. *i. e.*, those who earn their living by muscular work, require more food than is the case with those living a more sedentary life, and in a certain measure the dietetic habits necessitated in the first place by occupation persist after occupation distinctions are removed.

"(*d*) The urban dweller consumes a larger relative amount of animal food and therefore derives a larger percentage of his energy from the protein constituent of his diet than is the case with the country dweller. This, of course, applies only to the higher orders of civilization."

King then goes on to say, with these points in view and also keeping in mind individual variations, we may assume the following standards for ambulant cases of comparatively quiescent tuberculosis under sanitarium treatment:

"(1) For young adult men of the 'working class' on very light exercise from 2800 to 3200 calories of which from 110 grams to 125 grams shall be protein.

"(2) For the same class on five or six hours' vigorous exercise (sawing or chopping wood, working with shovels, pickaxes, barrows, etc.), from 3100 to 3600 calories of which 125 grams to 140 grams shall be protein.

"(3) For women of this class 200 calories and approximately 10 grams protein may be deducted in each case.

"(4) For young adult men, whose occupation has been more sedentary—*e. g.*, clerks, bookkeepers, tailors, students,

[1] Med. Rec., 1909, October 16.

etc., on moderate exercise (walking from one to three hours daily)—2600 to 3000 calories, of which not over 115 grams need be protein.

"(5) For women of this class not to exceed 2500 calories and 100 grams protein.

"(6) For older patients, a slight reduction in caloric value and a considerably lower protein constituent are desirable in each case.

"(7) For the country dweller a somewhat larger bulk, without increase in protein value is usually desirable, all other conditions being similar, than is the case with the patient from the city."

King[1] then reports interesting experiences with diets in the Loomis Sanitarium. In 1905 the ration was about as follows: Protein 166 gm. (5½ oz.), fat 214 gm. (7 oz.), carbohydrate 323 gm. (10½ oz.), calories 3955. While on this the patients seemed to thrive and gain, but digestive disturbances were common. The following year the standard diet was changed to protein 131 gm. (4⅓ oz.), fat 113 gm, (3⅔ oz.), carbohydrate 385 gm. (12⅔ oz.), calories 3166. On this diet the gains in weight were equally satisfactory and there were very few digestive disturbances. It was also found that those patients who were able to work consumed more food and had a better digestion than those who did not or could not. The comparison of these diet values with those worked out by Bardswell and Chapman is as follows:

Bardswell and Chapman.	Former Loomis Annex standard.	Later Loomis Annex standard.
Protein . . 150 gm.	Protein . . 166 gm.	Protein . . 130 gm.
Total calories 3200	Total calories 3667	Calories . . 3200

While the caloric value of Bardswell and Chapman is the same as the later Loomis standard, King felt that the lower protein allowance was a distinct advantage on account of (a) economy, (b) increased efficiency, (c) better digestion.

Complications.—In pregnancy, complicated by tuberculosis, the diet should receive special care and on account of a tendency to decalcification, said by some to exist,[2] some form of lime should be freely supplied in milk and gelatin (the calcium content of milk and gelatin being comparatively high), or even as calcium lactate in regular daily amounts. This question of decalcification is still unsettled so far as the biochemists are concerned, but until it is positively determined it would be the wiser error to give calcium to these

[1] Diets in Tuberculosis.
[2] Dreman: Am. Jour. Obstet., 1913, lxxvii, 893.

cases in some form. The diet should also contain more protein than at other times.

Diabetes, from a diatetic point of view, is one of the most difficult complications of tuberculosis to treat. This is not an infrequent association and certainly taxes the ingenuity ot the physician to the utmost. The associated hyperglycemia apparently favors the further development of the tubercle bacillus and yet a marked reduction in carbohydrates is not always easy to obtain. The rules laid down for diabetes must be followed and an attempt made by increasing the proteins and fats to keep the body weight up to normal and of course under these circumstances the kidneys cannot be spared, as they must be called on to excrete the excess nitrogen.

General Rules for Feeding in Tuberculosis.—An epitomized statement for diet in tuberculosis might be put somewhat as follows:

1. Forced feeding is not necessary.

2. Milk and eggs are to be used strictly with respect to their food values

3. A protein content of the food which furnishes a little in excess of ordinary requirements is best.

4. Fats are especially useful.

5. Three meals alone or three meals with three small lunches between and at bedtime offers the best distribution of meals.

6. Avoidance of very bulky or fermentable foods should be insisted on.

7. After normal weight or a weight slightly in excess of normal is reached, as little food should be taken as will maintain this weight.

8. Food should be eaten slowly under the most agreeable circumstances possible.

CHAPTER XXI.

DIET IN DISEASES OF THE STOMACH

THE most important factor in the treatment of diseases of the digestive system is, of course, proper food, as this far outweighs everything else; medicine and mechanical treatment taking an inferior position. The selection of a proper diet for these diseases depends upon a number of things which must be taken strictly into account if one wishes to obtain anything like satisfactory results.

When the trouble is in the esophagus, one has to meet the conditions of stricture, dilatation or ulceration, either singly or combined. In gastric disturbances we have, speaking broadly, conditions of hyperacidity, hypoacidity, disturbed motility, narrowing at the pylorus, dilatation, and inflammatory conditions ranging from the simplest catarrhal inflammation to severe ulceration or cancer.

In the intestinal canal we must reckon with inflammatory conditions, narrowing, dilatation, disturbances of secretion or motility or any combination of these. Besides the elements already enumerated there must be considered the integrity of the accessory digestive glands, such as the liver and pancreas. Hence it can be seen at a glance how many possibilities must be considered in choosing a rational diet for disease in any part of the gastro-intestinal tract.

Among the most important factors that must be taken into account are the influences exerted upon gastric secretion by various agents. In general these may be classed as either excitants to gastric secretion or depressants. Among the former may be included, acids, spices, condiments, water, alcohol, rough foods, proteins with high percentage of extractives, concentrated sugar solutions. Among the depressants, fats (if they are bland) and alkalies are most important. Nervous influences, either reflex or psychic, act either as excitants or depressants to gastric secretion.

In no other class of diseases is the personal factor so great as in digestive disturbances, for foods which may be perfectly digested by a patient in health may not be in illness, so that one is constantly forced to vary the diet, not only for the different phases of these digestive troubles, but for each individual and the individual variations in each patient.

There is however, immense satisfaction in the careful dieting of gastro-intestinal cases, for in no other diseases is the

335

proper diet more salutary than in these, save alone possibly some of the diseases of metabolism, notably diabetes.

INDIGESTION.

The proper digestion of food is such a complex matter that when one speaks of "indigestion" an endless variety of conditions naturally come to mind. Some of these are directly connected with the digestive processes and one may expect to get symptoms of so-called "indigestion" of an acute or chronic nature when any one of the digestive organs are involved in some form of derangement, and as well, the accessory digestive glands. On the other hand, one can have the most violent and persistent forms of indigestion referred to the stomach, whose origin is almost at the other end of the digestive tube; witness the effects on gastric digestion of a chronically diseased appendix, nephrolithiasis, cholelithiasis, adhesions, bands, etc., which may all result in digestive symptoms and which the patient refers to the stomach. It is in many ways unfortunate that the stomach seems to be the mirror for the whole abdominal cavity and almost everything that happens within the abdomen, particularly when of a severe nature, has its gastric reflex, and the stomach, itself to blame for a sufficient amount of trouble has been obliged to carry the opprobrium for digestive troubles which have their origin elsewhere. Then, too, when one uses the word "indigestion" one thinks at once of the gastric and intestinal variety, so that it is necessary, so far as possible, to fix the blame where it belongs and use a term as broad as this with caution, properly hedged with a definite statement as to the organ at fault. Almost every form of pathological, anatomical or functional disturbance affecting the abdominal organs has its gastric or intestinal symptomatology. As an example of this one has only to mention any one of the chronic catarrhal conditions affecting stomach or intestine to bring to mind certain so-called symptoms of indigestion and to this must be added various abnormal states of pancreas, liver, kidneys, etc., with gastrointestinal symptoms in order to realize what a loose generalization the term "indigestion" denotes.

Given however, a normal gastro-intestinal canal and accessory glands there are certain conditions and substances which can produce symptoms which pass under this general name; various individuals differing in their reaction to different forms of irritation which may be mechanical, chemical or thermal in origin. What suits one individual's digestive apparatus may have an entirely different effect on another's and one has only to mention such substances as lobster, deviled crabs, hot breads, certain heavy sweets or fats with a high melting point in order to realize that some people cannot take these articles of food without a digestive upset, whether from anaphylactic action or a difference in digestive juices or motor function, while still others can take them with impunity. Foods, such as those undergoing putrefaction or fermentation, almost universally cause a more or less serious disturbance because very few possess the ability to detoxify these materials. Then, too, faulty mastication either from bad teeth, or lack of them, is very apt to result in disturbances which may be only functional, but are usually in the long-standing or chronic cases due to actual pathological lesions of the gastro-intestinal tract. Rapid eating acts in the same way, also improperly prepared food, to say nothing of vegetable substances which are unripe. Experience has shown that certain foods are always better borne when cooked than if eaten raw, and there is no doubt but that individual racial differences and habits cause the digestive apparatus to adjust itself to conditions which would spell "disaster" for people not accustomed to such a dietary. Could we eat the food of our ancestors of the stone age without disaster to our digestions? and the diet of our Eskimo brothers would, if eaten by us, cause many a troubled dream. Hence we see that the variety of differences in different peoples and different individuals of the same people is infinite, not only in face and form, but in their reaction to different foods, and it is a wise man who early learns his own dietary impossibilities and has the strength of mind to avoid them. Still another factor enters into the question of the digestibility of foods, such as for example, the physic effect of anger, fear, etc., which inhibits the action of the secretory glands or causes motor irregularities of the stomach and intestine. Great stress is laid by Hayden[1] on treating cases of chronic indigestion by advanced suggestion (neuro-induction) after first finding out about physiological possiblities. Among the cases successfully treated are those who have been unable to take certain foods since childhood (excepting of course from anaphylaxis). These are often cured in one treatment. Again the effect of overwork, muscular or mental, is often to inhibit the digestive processes with the well-known sequelæ of digestive disturbance; and everyone knows that some foods which may

[1] Med. Press and Circl., 1918, n. s., cv, 146.

22

be eaten at one time without difficulty prove a veritable source of sorrow when taken under other circumstances. One might go on indefinitely multiplying the factors which modify the digestibility of foodstuffs, but enough has been said to make the fact evident that there are individual differences in people, in foods, and in the circumstances under which they are eaten, that play an enormous role in the production of digestive unrest and result in what is generally spoken of as "indigestion" in some one of its forms. One must, on the other hand, always seek for the underlying cause whether it be a condition of true pathology, functional derangement or individual idiosyncrasy, else one easily falls into the habit of thinking of "indigestion" as an indefinite, but comfortably large scrap-basket into which may be tossed a digestive symptom-complex, without taking the trouble to really get at its true significance.

Diet in Irritable Stomach[1] (With Vomiting).—An irritable stomach with nausea or vomiting is often a difficult problem in feeding.

From whatever cause (after all that is possible has been done to find and remove it) it is usually best to give a stomach absolute rest. The length of time this is necessary will depend on many factors, but, generally a rest of from four to eight, twelve or twenty-four hours is enough, after which we may begin feeding somewhat on the following plan.

Chloroform water (perfectly fresh) dram 1 (4 c.c.). Peptonized milk (given five minutes later) oz. ½ (15 c.c.). Repeat every hour, four doses. If there is no vomiting give chloroform water, dram 1 (4 c.c.). Peptonized milk (given five minutes later) oz. 1 (30 c.c.). Repeat every hour for four doses. If no vomiting advance to peptonized milk oz. 2 (60 c.c.).

GASTRIC HYPERACIDITY, HYPERCHLORHYDRIA.

Acid dyspepsia is a very common diagnosis and it is probably true that more than half of the patients who consult a physician for gastric troubles are found on examination to have a hyperacidity due to an excess of free HCl. The time has gone by, however, when one can rest content with such a diagnosis, for hyperchlorhydria is in almost every, if not in every instance, merely a symptom and not a disease entity. One must therefore seek for the underlying cause which with care can almost always be successfully done. *Kauffman's*[2] *classification* covers the etiology satisfactorily and divides the cases into:

[1] Allen Whipple.
[2] Kauffman, in Forchheimer, iii, 75.

1. Those with an inborn disposition toward acidity.
2. Due to faulty habits.
3. Chronic intoxications.
4. Reflex from disturbances in other organs (or in the stomach itself).

1. Little is known about the first class except that one occasionally does find people who have always had a hyperacid stomach extending from childhood, without evidence of a pathological basis. In these cases at the same time, must be borne in mind possible, but hidden, reflex causes, such as chronic appendicitis.

2. Faulty habits account for a certain number of cases, of which may be mentioned, rapid eating, highly spiced foods, a great amount of acid food, or very sweet food and mental overwork. Students are very prone to have an exacerbation of hyperacidity during examination times, whether they have a real pathological lesion or not.

3. Too free use of tobacco in any form accounts for certain cases, and for some this means any use whatever of the weed. Some patients can smoke cigarettes or cigars in moderation without symptoms, while others have been known to precipitate an attack of hyperacidity by a few days of pipe smoking so regularly that the pipe has been given up.

Alcohol, particularly when taken strong on an empty stomach, in the form of cocktails or neat spirits frequently leads to a hyperacidity, and of course an actual catarrh later on if persisted in. Some patients cannot take coffee without increasing considerably the hyperacidity.

4. The reflex conditions which may produce a hyperacidity are legion and one has but to mention chronic appendicitis, cholelithiasis, nephrolithiasis and peptic ulcer, to bring to mind numberless cases falling into this class.

Given a case of hyperchlorhydria, if the cause can be found, of course treatment and diet must be directed along lines suitable for the particular condition at fault, but nevertheless a certain number of cases remain which are evidently hyperacidity with the symptoms of pyrosis, eructations, often very acid, and some discomfort or burning in the epigastric region at the height of digestion. When there is actual pain, repeated daily, usually one to three hours after meals, there is almost always an organic lesion at fault, but if this can be reasonably ruled out, we must take dietetic measures to reduce the hyperacidity to a minimum. A diagnosis of hyperacidity can only be made satisfactorily by means of a test meal and, in fairness to the patient, this precaution should never be omitted.

The Reduction of Gastric Hyperacidity by Diet.—This is done first by the avoidance of certain foods which are sure to induce a certain amount of physiological increase in acidity and secondarily to give such foods as will render the excess of acid as innocuous as possible. To these ends one must avoid taking all acids, spices, condiments, salt meat or salt fish, and the use of salt on the food should be reduced to the minimum. It has been shown possible, in dogs, to feed meat boiled in distilled water until the salt intake is reduced almost to zero, when this is done the free hydrochloric acid production is actually controlled. This cannot be continued indefinitely in human beings, as sodium chloride in a certain minimal amount (1 or 2 gm. per day) is necessary to health, but all excess can be obviated with some resulting diminution in acid values in their gastric secretion. All foods must be avoided, which by their tough consistency would remain in the stomach a long time, such as very coarse vegetables, seeds, fruit skins or fats with a high melting-point, as mutton fat. Very hot or cold drinks or foods act in much the same way and must be left alone. Alcohol is especially bad in all forms. Meat soups are stimulating and are best omitted from the diet as are all hors d'oeuvre, such as caviare, olives and pickles, etc. Very sweet food has much the same effect, so all candy, rich cake, heavy preserves, sweet jellies must be left out of the diet.

When one comes to construct a diet suitable for these cases one meets at once theoretical objections to many forms of food, and authority can be found for barring carbohydrate or protein food, especially meats in all forms, for although they have a high combining power for the free HCl, they in turn are gastric excitants and would thereby defeat their own object. Diets based on this view are constructed largely of carbohydrates and theoretically these should be well tolerated, but as a matter of fact for one reason or another they do not seem to act practically as we should expect, probably because although they call out a smaller acid secretion, they have little to offer to combine with the free HCl, which, once it accumulates in any quantity, causes the symptoms for which we are attempting to find the ideal diet. Fats do actually depress the acid secretions and when of a low melting-point, such as sweet butter, or when bland and liquid, as olive, peanut or cotton-seed oil, they are very valuable foods in hyperacid conditions for this quality, as well as for their high nutritive and caloric value.

But one cannot live on fats, so that to a certain extent a mixed diet must be used. Experience has shown that although milk·is more or less a gastric stimulant, it offers such a high percentage of protein for binding the free HCl, that it is of great value, and a few days of a milk-and-cream diet is often most useful in quieting an overproductive gastric secretion. Eggs are good for the same reason although some authorities think that as the fat is in emulsion it is more stimulating than should be used; this is not, in the view of most clinicians, of sufficient weight to prevent their free use to advantage. The fine cereal preparations, such as farina, cream of wheat, malted breakfast food, wheatena, are all usable and are better than oatmeal. Bread is at times a marked gastric stimulant and Kauffman refers to hyperchlorhydria in vegetarians for which he largely blames the excessive use of bread. Stale bread, toast, zweiback or crust of roll may be taken by these cases in moderation.

Diet in Hyperacidity.—The diet in hyperacidity may be advantageously made up of the following articles, using considerable quantities of the less stimulating proteins:

—*Raw oysters* with a very little salt or a few drops of lemon juice.

—*Soups:* Cream or purée (except tomato) and made without meat stock.

Fish: All white-meated, non-fatty fish, such as fresh cod, halibut, bass, white fish, boiled and served with egg sauce, or broiled (never fried).

Meat: In marked hyperacidity meat is best let alone, except occasionally boiled or roasted and chicken or turkey. In less severe cases, minced lamb, without fat, guinea-hen, well-done beef without gristle, fat or gravy, in small amounts and never more than once a day, may be allowed.

—*Vegetables:* The soft green vegetables, such as young peas, string beans, spinach with egg, beet tops, celery, squash, vegetable marrow, rice, all boiled. Baked Hubbard squash, baked white potato, spaghetti. (No cabbage, Brussels sprouts, cauliflower or onions to be used on account of their tendency to ferment and cause flatulence.)

Cheese: Cream, Neufchatel, Swiss.

Desserts: All cream desserts, those made of egg and milk, such as custards, blanc mange, floating island, junket, soft rice, farina or bread puddings without rich sauces and best eaten with cream. Gelatin desserts if not highly flavored, all made with the minimum amount of sugar.

Fruit: None at all in severe cases. In milder cases when constipation is marked, soft, subacid, stewed friuts may be taken in fair amount, but no fruits with seeds or those with tough skins should be used, such as figs, raspberries, blackberries, gooseberries and prunes.   Fruit should be stewed or baked with very little sugar.

Bread: Toast, dry roll, zweiback, toasted crackers.

Butter: Either fresh butter, or salted butter, if used, should be worked over in fresh water to take out as much of the salt as possible.

Drinks: Weak tea, cocoa made with milk, cream, water, Vichy not too cold and never sparkling.

Cereals: All fine well-boiled cereals.

Eggs: In any form but fried or hard-boiled and not made into fancy entrees.

Cake: A little cup cake, dry cookies and sponge cake.

Foods to Avoid: All highly spiced, sour, salty foods, condiments, pickles, jellies, salted nuts, olives, raw vegetables as celery, salads, radishes, etc.   Very cold or hot foods or drinks, or if taken in small amount they should be kept in the mouth long enough to bring their temperature to about body heat.   Uncooked vegetables of all sorts and hard substances as corn.   Coffee, wines, beer, liquors, cordials, ale, ginger ale and cold soft drinks.   Pies, syrups, pancakes, hot biscuits, cake other than those already mentioned.

GASTRIC HYPERSECRETION.

Since hypersecretion whether intermittent or continuous is a symptom of disease and not a disease itself, it is necessary, in order to prescribe a rational diet, to know if possible what the underlying cause may be.   In the intermittent variety we may be dealing with merely a part of a general neurosis or it may be a gastric manifestation of a lesion of the central nervous system, such as tabes or lateral sclerosis, where it is regularly an accompanying feature of the gastric crisis.   It may also follow the excessive ingestion of alcohol or gastric irritants or accompany acute gastric dilatation (*q. v.*).

In the intermittent variety the diet should be arranged so far as possible in accord with the etiological factor.   Since hypersecretion is practically always accompanied by a definite hyperchlorhydria the diet should be chosen on the basis of the foods recommended for this condition.   A few days or a week or more of a milk diet with or without the addition of very soft-boiled eggs, gives relief to most of the cases, regardless of the etiology, excepting only those cases due to a lesion of the central nervous system, as tabes.   The relief is, however, often only symptomatic and a test meal will still show hypersecretion and hyperacidity unless in case of ulcer there had been actual healing.

Continuous Hypersecretion is for the most part a symptom of gastric or duodenal ulcer and unless this can in some way be excluded, as by *x*-ray examination, it is fair to assume such a relationship, particularly in the presence of ulcer symptoms, and institute an ulcer cure.

The pain which so often accompanies hypersecretion may be ascribed probably to pylorospasm or possibly to an irritated ulcer and, while a milk diet will also bring relief to this symptom it will do so permanently only so far as the diet is successful in curing the underlying ulcer.

While usually a high protein diet is advocated for hypersecretion, it will be seen from what has been said that this is rather a shot in the dark and that if one wishes to use foods intelligently it is absolutely necessary to first make an etiological diagnosis.

In general it may be said that the protein of milk and egg is the best for all cases of hypersecretion, whereas, meat or meat products are distinctly stimulating to gastric secretion and should be omitted from the diet at first, and later allowed only in small amount and in the more easily digested forms, *e. g.*, chicken, mutton and sweetbreads. Soft farinaceous puddings and cereals are allowed in moderation and purée of vegetables, as in hyperchlorhydria (*q. v.*). Especial importance is attached to the avoidance of condiments, acid food and drink, rough foods, skins, seeds, corn, etc., all of which remain a long time in the stomach and produce thereby irritation, and in addition the thermal irritants, such as very hot or very cold foods, are to be avoided.

GASTRIC HYPOACIDITY AND ACHYLIA GASTRICA.

Diminution or absence of gastric acid and ferments, as its name implies, is the direct opposite of hyperchlorhydria and may be due to a variety of causes, either organic or functional. Of the organic causes any long-standing catarrh of the stomach will lead to it and it is found as a frequent complication of catarrhal gastritis and gastric carcinoma, pernicious anemia, severe infectious diseases at times and in many elderly people. In any event permanent achylia is accompanied by atrophy of the mucous membrane of the stomach and its secreting glands.

Of the functional causes, many cases are due to profound neurasthenic conditions and as a reflex from organic disease

in some of the other abdominal organs, *e. g.*, chronic appendicitis or cholelithiasis.   There is still another class of case
in whom the achylia gives rise to no symptoms and is only
found by accident in the course of a routine examination.
The cause of this variety is far from clear.

The degree of the hypoacidity varies within wide limits and
runs from a slight reduction in the free HCl and total acid
values and without change in the pepsin-rennin secretion,
all the way to complete achylia with total absence of acids
and ferments.   In passing, it might be remarked that the
acids are diminished more frequently and in greater proportion than the ferments.   In the cases in which the hypoacidity is dependent on a definite lesion, as for example
gastritis, the return of the acid is greatly dependent on the
outcome of the underlying cause, which if cleared up may
result in a return of the secretions.   Other cases are found
without definite cause as already stated and remain achlyia
to the end of the chapter, apparently with little effect on the
general health,

The diet problem in hypoacidity is in many respects a
much more simple matter than in most cases of marked
hyperacidity and within certain limits the foods which are
inadvisable in hyperchlorhydria on account of their tending
to excite gastric secretion, are the ones which we may often
freely use in this opposite condition.

Mention has already been made of the diet best for these
cases in connection with chronic gastritis with hypoacidity
(p. 348), but it is necessary to go more into detail.   Where
there is a definite organic cause or accompanying condition
to the hypoacidity or achylia the diet must be in accordance
with this complicating feature and all foods which are in any
way irritating must be avoided, such as condiments, strong
acids, very rough or hard foods, skins, seeds, etc., as the
mucous membrane in many of these cases is exceedingly vul-
nerable and bleeds easily, even on the introduction of the
stomach-tube.   Very hot foods or large quantities of acid
food or drinks must be avoided.

Theoretically very limited protein should be given, as in
the absence of the normal HCl and pepsin, gastric digestion
is at a minimum or entirely absent.   Within certain limits
this objection holds good, namely for all protein foods difficult of digestion, *e. g.*, veal, tough meats of all sorts, connective tissue (which latter is only digested in the presence
of free HCl and pepsin) and tough clams, lobster, etc.   On
the other hand, the patients must receive their full daily
allowance of protein and will be able to digest the proper

kinds in the course of pancreatic and intestinal digestion. Of these, milk, eggs, tender meats and fowl cut very fine without gristle or connective tissue, mild cheeses tender white-meated fish and vegetable protein of all sorts must form the bulk of the protein ration, but given preferably in only moderate amount say from 70 to 90 grams per diem, and not to the high limit allowable in a normal person. While a moderate amount of these protein foods can be entirely digested in the intestines, any excess will throw too much work on these accessory digestive processes which may easily go out of commission on this account, with the result that the proteins in excess undergo putrefaction in the intestine, giving rise to many uncomfortable symptoms of toxemia. This is the more prone to happen as the normal gastric juice is a strong antiseptic for all foods brought to the stomach and it is a hardy germ that can live through the acid immersion it receives there. On this account the normal chyme is comparatively free from bacteria; a fortunate provision of nature when one considers the quantity of poor gastric surgery that is done, much of which would be followed by greater disaster were it not for this fact.

Since the natural barrier to the entrance of pathological bacteria is largely or entirely missing in these cases of hypoacidity, it is of *the greatest importance that the food taken be all thoroughly cooked to render it sterile.* Fruit with skins may be an exception to this rule, as they are really practically sterile within their skins. For the same reason great care should be taken of the mouth and its toilet made before and after meals, using toothpick, dental floss, tooth brush and a good mouth wash. This seems excessive care, but many cases of diarrhea and chronic intestinal infection are started by reason of carelessness in these respects.

Clear soups are good for their appetizing and stimulating effects on the gastric glands that are still capable of stimulation and other protein foods as already indicated, may be eaten. All vegetables that are soft and non-irritating, fats, particularly butter and oils and cream. All carbohydrate foods are easily digested as the gastric ptyalin digestion proceeds uninterruptedly in the absence of gastric acidity. At the same time excessive use of sweets should be avoided as likely to disturb digestion. All simple desserts may be used to advantage.

There is still another condition which must be reckoned with in these patients, namely, that while the gastric motility is usually well preserved in all but cancer cases, there may be the opposite condition of gastric atony. In this latter complication one may use the same class of foods as recommended for the cases with good motility, but they should be given in smaller amounts and at more frequent intervals, following generally the dietetic rules laid down for atony, particularly with reference to restricted fluids at meals.

Many of these cases of achylia are complicated by diarrhea probably of pancreatic origin, at all events there are few more brilliant results in medicine than those obtained in most of these cases of achylia diarrhea by the giving of dilute HCl, either alone or with pepsin; and all cases of unexplained and long-standing diarrhea should have determined, by a gastric test meal, the presence or absence of HCl.

The addition of this dilute acid to the dietary in all cases of achylia is of distinct advantage, although it must not be given in too large doses and later when digestion is regulated it may be possible to omit the acid altogether.

GASTRITIS.

Acute Gastritis.—Acute gastritis, except that caused by a toxicosis, must be considered a rare disease, in spite of the frequency of the diagnosis. When the toxicosis is constitutional of course the dietary treatment is along lines laid down for the particular disease at fault, *e. g.*, renal insufficiency, etc. There are however, a fair number of cases caused by the direct effect of irritating substances such as strong acids, alkalies and abuse of condiments, but most frequent of all, the excessive use of alcohol; and it is after a drinking bout that this is most frequently met with. In any case, the cause being what it may, the dietary treatment is practically the same.

The first step is starvation, nothing whatever should be given by mouth and the fluids which the system craves in severe cases accompanied by much nausea and vomiting, may be supplied by the rectum, either in the form of a Murphy drip or by giving from six to eight ounces of warm saline by rectum, every two, three or four hours. After twelve 'to twenty-four hours, or when the vomiting has ceased, one may begin to feed small amounts of cold peptonized milk, or koumyss, buttermilk, white of egg in dilute orange juice beaten up and strained; milk; Vichy or Delafield's mixture:[1] beginning all in very small amounts (a teaspoonful every twenty to thirty minutes) and increasing the amount and

---

[1] Delafield's mixture: Cream, 120 c. c. (oz. 4); milk, 120 c. c. (oz. 4); Vichy, 120 c. c. (oz. 4); soda bicaronate, gm. $\frac{2}{3}$ (gr. 20); cerium oxalate, gm. $\frac{1}{3}$ (gr. 10).

lengthening the interval. In certain cases, small amounts of iced champagne or ice-cold ginger ale are well borne and may even be of assistance in controlling the vomiting.

In acute gastritis or esophagitis, due to taking a corrosive poison, demulcent drinks are of especial value in not only supplying some nourishment, but in quieting an inflamed mucous membrane. Of these drinks a thin solution of gum arabic (2 to 5 per cent.) flavored with a little orange juice is acceptable. Also a solution of Iceland moss made in the same way. After the acute stage is past one begins with gruels, fine cereals, milk, plain or diluted; then soft solids and so on up the scale until the full diet is reached. All rough, highly spiced and peppery, very hot or very cold foods and drinks should be avoided for some time.

Chronic Gastritis.—In contradistinction to the acute variety, chronic gastritis is fairly frequently seen and is practically always secondary to a chronic disease with poor elimination, to chronic congestion, as in hepatic cirrhosis or cardiac decompensation or a chronic form of irritation of which latter, of course, alcohol is the chief example. During an acute exacerbation the diet should be the same as that detailed for acute gastritis. When the disease is found in its later stages many digestive symptoms are traceable to its presence. In arranging the diet for such cases it is almost absolutely essential to have an analysis of a gastric test meal for diagnosis, as many digestive symptoms referred to the stomach and lumped as chronic gastritis are nothing of the sort. They are quite as likely due to secretory or motor disturbances, often secondary to other conditions such as peptic ulcer, chronic appendicitis or gall-bladder disease, and have nothing to do with an increased production of mucus, which is a *sine qui non* of true gastritis.

Then too, some cases of chronic gastritis are accompanied by hyperacidity, others by normal or hypoacidity running even into an achylia gastrica, the certain knowledge of which will be of great assistance in selecting a proper dietary.

In general it may be said that after removal of the cause, whenever that is possible, a certain amount of rest and the entire absence of all irritating food should be insisted upon.

Diet.—When the gastritis is accompanied by hyperacidity, the following articles of food should be forbidden:

Salt foods, spiced foods, acid foods, rough or mechanically irritating foods, fermented foods, *e. g.*, wines, beers and ales. Of course, no case of gastritis should take alcohol in any form except possibly when the patient has been long accustomed to its use, a little whiskey or red wine, both diluted

with Vichy, may be allowed for a short time.   Nothing very
hot or very cold is allowed.   On the other hand, as there is
usually good digestive power to the secretions, a fairly high
protein allowance of a non-stimulating sort may be allowed.
In a general way the diet may be advised as follows:

Early morning on awakening a half-glass of warm Hôpital
or Celestin Vichy, or water with half a teaspoonful of artificial Vichy salts.   This taken at least one-half hour before
breakfast, acts as does a gastric lavage.   If the bowels are
constipated an occasional small dose of some of the laxative
soda salts may be given, phosphate or sulphate of soda.

> *Breakfast:* Cocoa, made with milk, or weak tea; fine
> cereal—farina, cream of wheat, wheatena with
> cream, and very little sugar; soft toast or soft part
> of stale bread, well chewed; eggs in any simple
> form.   Later, apple sauce or baked sweet apple.
>
> *Luncheon, Dinner or Supper:* Cream or purée soup (no
> meat stock).   Simple egg entrée.   A little boiled
> chicken or young lamb, scraped or finely cut beef,
> all without rich gravies or sauces; purée of soft,
> green vegetables, put through a colander, without
> seeds or rough cellulose or skins; cauliflower, cab-
> bage or tomatoes are not allowed, desserts, soft
> custards, puddings, gelatin desserts with cream,
> cream desserts; ice-cream occasionally.   Later soft
> stewed fruits, not acid, and cooked with little sugar;
> junket.
>
> *Beverages:* Alkaline waters, Vichy, High Rock, plain
> water; cocoa or weak tea; milk.

Milk food should be reduced to a minimum in the presence
of gastric atony.   The quantity of food given at each feeding and the length of the feeding interval will depend on the
condition of gastric motility.   When this is good, three
normal-sized meals may be given, when impaired, frequent,
small, dry feedings are better.   This is of course, true of
gastritis by whatever degree of acidity it is accompanied.
(See Diet in Gastric Atony.)   It is advisable to eat a meal
which is easily digested and passed into the intestine as
rapidly as possible, so giving the maximum degree of rest
to the stomach.

**Diet when Gastritis is Accompanied by Hypoacidity or
Achylia.**—Early morning alkaline waters as for hyperacid
cases, except that to them, may be added a little sodium
chloride; or Carlsbad water or sodium salts may be allowed
when constipation is present, or plain water, six ounces
(180 c.c.) with salt gr. v (½ gm.), soda bicarbonate gr. xv

(1 gm.). The chief difference in the diet from that given for hyperacid cases is that less meat protein is allowed. Stewed fruits may be used earlier than in hyperacid cases and stock soups are permitted largely for their appetizing qualities. With impaired motility, however, soup of all kinds is best omitted, as fluids then leave the stomach slowly. Water should be taken in only small amounts with meals and it is well to order patients to drink water about an hour before meals, between meals and at bedtime.

PEPTIC ULCER (GASTRIC AND DUODENAL).

In the acute and so-called medical ulcer of the stomach or duodenum or in the acute exacerbation of a chronic ulcer, the management and dietary are the chief essentials, excepting, of course, those cases which on account of some complication demand surgical intervention. In response to this need, there have sprung up a number of different forms of treatment, some advocates of all of them being found in each community. The fact that the acute medical ulcer has a tendency to heal spontaneously, if given a fair chance, probably accounts for the claims of one or another of the different methods in vogue. With the acute exacerbation of a chronic ulcer it is somewhat different and although the acute symptoms may promptly subside when treated as an acute simple ulcer, the ultimate end sought, namely cicatrization of the old ulcer is a most uncertain chance, although it does take place in perhaps a larger proportion of cases than the surgeons would have us believe, as proved by autopsy findings. The gastric and duodenal ulcers are dealt with together, as their dietary treatment is identical.

The Chief Methods of Dietary Treatment for ulcer may be classed as:

1. Absolute physiological rest to the upper digestive tract, with later mouth feedings either with or without rectal alimentation in addition.

2. Almost continuous, but reduced, physiological activity of the stomach but with food that is in small amounts, principally protein and which has the quality of quickly binding the free hydrochloric acid, turning the albumin into the comparatively unirritating syntonin, and of leaving the stomach quite promptly.

3. Transgastric or duodenal feedings.

4. An essential feature of still another form of treatment is the use of alkalies to reduce the exaggerated acidity, usually present in these cases, together with the feeding of small

quantities at frequent intervals of highly albuminous foods. The use of alkalies may, of course be combined with any one of the forms of treatment and has many advocates.

The first plan has the disadvantage, if carried out to the letter, of almost complete starvation during the time of digestive rest. Where this has been modified by attempts at rectal feeding or water is introduced by rectum, physiology has shown that at once peristaltic unrest is set up throughout the entire gastro-intestinal tract and it also gives rise to gastric secretion, although this is denied by some authorities.

Von Leube Diet in Ulcer.—In the first type of diet as exemplified by the von Leube cure and modified most satisfactorily by G. R. Lockwood, absolute rest is given for three days and not even water is allowed, but the mouth is kept moist by mouth washes. If after twenty-four to forty-eight hours the thirst becomes too excessive, the Murphy drip is instituted whereby from twenty to fifty drops of normal saline solution are allowed to flow into the rectum each minute, depending on the patient's rectal tolerance. To this Murphy drip there may be added sufficient glucose to make a 2 per cent. solution. It also helps to make the patient relaxed, and comfortable to add 50 grains (3.5 gm.) strontium bromide to the day's allowance. If given continuously about three pints of fluid may be introduced into the system preventing absolutely the thirst which is so trying. In patients who are old, feeble or desiccated by vomiting and insufficient food before hand, the first period of starvation is limited to twenty-four hours.

On the second day in these cases, and the third day in sthenic cases, 2 ounces of Celestin or Hôpital Vichy is given every two hours and the following day this is alternated with 2 ounces of albumin water, so that liquids are therefore given every hour. Von Leube also recommends very strongly the continuous use of local heat over the upper abdomen either as hot compresses or the use of the electric pad over a moist compress, except in cases of recent hemorrhage. On the next day fully peptonized milk, 2 ounces at each feeding, every two hours is alternated with the Vichy so that the patient gets one or the other every hour. During the first few days of this diet, if the thirst is troublesome, either the Murphy drip can be continued or from 4 to 6 ounces of warm saline may be given by rectum every three or four hours. Each day the peptonized milk is increased 1 ounce, until 8 ounces are being taken. The Vichy is increased 1 ounce daily until 4 ounces are given at a time. Both

Vichy and fully peptonized milk[1] have been shown by Cannon to leave the stomach very rapidly. The bowels are kept regular by enemeta and if there is troublesome gastric acidity, alkaline powders are given. About the tenth day soft milk toast, junket or fine cereal may be added. It is well to add these to one of the peptonized milk feedings, then to two, three or until with every other milk feeding the patient gets a soft solid. When a soft solid is given it is better not to give over 4 oz. (120 c.c.) of the peptonized milk. In the third week, the quantities may be increased and creamed mashed potato, fresh creamed halibut or cod fish, macaroni, purée soups made without meat stock are added, also purée of vegetables, such as purée of peas. Farinaceous desserts can then be added, such as cornstarch, farina, blanc mange and custard. During these three weeks the patient remains in bed, still continuing the hot applications. During the fourth week they may be allowed up in a chair and put gradually on any soft food, leaving out fruit, coffee, acids, irritants of all kinds, whether mechanical, thermal or chemical.

This dietary cure takes time and cannot be hurried if one wishes to give the patient the best chance of recovery. When the mouth feedings have begun some clinicians prefer to use nutrient enemata as an additional supply of fluid and some nourishment. The best food for this purpose is undoubtedly fully peptonized milk, the same as that given by mouth with or without the addition of glucose sufficient to make a 2 to 4 per cent. solution. Often the milk alone is better borne in varying quantities, some patients taking as much as 1 pint every six hours, others a less amount at more frequent intervals, all of which must be determined for each case individually. (For details see Rectal Feeding.)

Those who prefer to use the von Leube diet as originally outlined by him, will find the following plan useful.

Von Leube's Diet[2] (*Original*):

First Three Days:

    7 A.M.   150 c.c. of milk (5 oz.).

    8 A.M.   150 c.c. of milk (5 oz.).

    10 A.M.   150 c.c. of milk (5 oz.) with strained barley water.

[1] For complete peptonization of milk, Lockwood's directions are most satisfactory. Divide a quart of milk in half, bring one-half (1 pt.) to boiling and add the other cold pint. This produces the correct temperature. To this add two tubes of Fairchild's peptonizing powder rubbed up in 4 ounces of water. Put the milk in scalded bottles and stand in a pail of water at 105° F. and keep there with occasional shaking for two hours. Then scald and put on ice.

[2] Smith: What to Eat and Why, p. 193.

11 A.M.   150 c.c. of milk (5 oz.).

1 P.M.   150 c.c. bouillon with peptone preparation.

Fourth to Eleventh Day:

7 to 9 A.M.   300 c.c. of milk (10 oz.).

11 A.M.   300 c.c. of milk with barley, rice or oatmeal water.

1 P.M.   One cup of bouillon (200 c.c.) with a beaten egg.

3 to 5 P.M.   300 c.c of milk (10 oz.).

7 P.M.   Milk with barley water.

9 P.M.   300 c.c. of milk (10 oz.).

Eleventh to Fourteenth Day:

7 to 9 A.M.   300 c.c. of milk (10 oz.) and two crackers, softened with barley water.

11 A.M.   300 c.c. of milk (10 oz.).

1 P.M.   200 c.c. bouillon (6⅓ oz.,), one egg, two crackers.

3 P.M.   300 c.c. of milk (10 oz.), one egg.

5 P.M.   300 c.c. of milk (10 oz.), two crackers.

7 P.M.   Milk with barley water.

9 P.M.   300 c.c. of milk (10 oz.).

Fourteenth to Seventeenth Day:

7 to 9 to 11 A.M.   As above.

1 P.M.   Scraped meat 50 gm. (1⅔ oz.), two crackers, one cup of bullion, 200 c.c. (6⅓ oz.).

3 P.M.   300 c.c. of milk (10 oz.).

5 P.M.   300 c.c. of milk (10 oz.), one soft-boiled egg, two crackers.

7 P.M.   300 c.c. of milk (10 oz.) with farina.

9 P.M.   300 c.c. of milk (10 oz.).

Seventeenth to Twenty-fourth Day:

7 A.M.   Two soft-boiled eggs, butter (1 gm.), toasted bread 50 gm. (1⅔ oz.), 300 c.c. of milk (10 oz.).

10 A.M.   300 c.c. of milk (10 oz.), crackers 50 gm. (1⅔ oz.).

1 P.M.   Broiled lamb chop 50 gm. (1⅔ oz.), mashed potato 50 gm. (1⅔ oz.), butter 10 gm. (⅓ oz.), cup of bouillon 200 c.c. (6⅓ oz.).

4 P.M.   Same as 10 A.M.

6.30 P.M.   300 c.c. (10 oz.), of milk with farina, crackers 50 gm. (1⅔ oz.), butter 20 gm. (⅔ oz.).

9 P.M.   300 c.c. milk (10 oz.).

Of the second method of feeding these cases, viz., that of continued physiological activity with small amounts of bland and highly albuminous food, the Lenhartz diet is the best known and most generally used. One great object of this diet is to do away with any period of actual starvation, on the principle that the better nourished a patient can be kept the greater chance for healing. In addition, what has already been said, in regard to the favorable influence of the rapid combining of the free hydrochloric acid with the albumin in the diet, of which there is great abundance, holds true.

General Directions for Lenhartz's Diet..—Patients must be in bed and kept there the entire time not even allowed up for use of the commode; naturally the best and sunniest room available should be chosen for all of these cases, regardless of the form of diet.

The eggs used in each day's feedings should be beaten up raw and divided equally into seven feedings, putting the feedings into seven medicine or small glasses for accuracy and keeping them all in the ice-box until used. The milk used for the day should be put on ice and the feeding spoon kept on ice. All feedings should be very slowly given by spoonfuls. A very little salt may be allowed on the egg feedings, otherwise none. As will be seen from the schedule of feedings, they are given every hour from 7.00 A.M. to 7.00 P.M., or 8.00 A.M. to 8.00 P.M. if more convenient, leaving a full twelve-hour rest. The following are the details of each day's diet.

FIRST DAY

7.00 A.M.	Egg.
8.00 A.M.	Milk, 20 c.c. (⅔ oz.).
9.00 A.M.	Egg.
10.00 A.M.	Milk, 20 c.c. (⅔ oz.).
11.00 A.M.	Egg.
12.00 NOON	Milk, 15 c.c. (½ oz.).
1.00 P.M.	Egg.
2.00 P.M.	Milk, 15 c.c. (½ oz.).
3.00 P.M.	Egg.
4.00 P.M.	Milk, 15 c.c. (½ oz.).
5.00 P.M.	Egg.
6.00 P.M.	Milk, 15 c.c. (½ oz.).
7.00 P.M.	Egg.

Total, first day, eggs (raw), 2; milk, 100 c.c. (3⅓ oz.); calories, 280.

SECOND DAY

7.00 A.M.	Egg.
8.00 A.M.	Milk, 35 c.c. (1 oz.).
9.00 A.M.	Egg.
10.00 A.M.	Milk, 35 c.c. (1 oz.).
11.00 A.M.	Egg.
12.00 NOON	Milk, 35 c.c. (1 oz.).
1.00 P.M.	Egg.

23

2.00 P.M.	Milk, 35 c.c. (1 oz.).
3.00 P.M.	Egg.
4.00 P.M.	Milk, 35 c.c. (1 oz.).
5.00 P.M.	Egg.
6.00 P.M.	Milk, 30 c.c. (1 oz.).
7.00 P.M.	Egg.

Total second day, eggs (raw), 3; milk, 200 c.c. (6⅔ oz.); calories, 470.

THIRD DAY

7.00 A.M.	Egg; sugar, 2 gm. (½ dr.).
8.00 A.M.	Milk, 50 c.c. (1⅔ oz.).
9.00 A.M.	Egg; sugar, 3 gm. (¾ dr.).
10.00 A.M.	Milk, 50 c.c. (1⅔ oz.).
11.00 A.M.	Egg; sugar, 3 gm. (¾ dr.).
12.00 NOON	Milk, 50 c.c. (1⅔ oz.).
1.00 P.M.	Egg; sugar, 3 gm. (¾ dr.).
2.00 P.M.	Milk, 50 c.c. (1⅔ oz.).
3.00 P.M.	Egg; sugar, 3 gm. (¾ dr.).
4.00 P.M.	Milk, 50 c.c. (1⅔ oz.).
5.00 P.M.	Egg; sugar, 3 gm. (¾ dr.).
6.00 P.M.	Milk, 50 c.c. (1⅔ oz.).
7.00 P.M.	Egg; sugar, 3 gm. (¾ dr.).

Total, third day, eggs (raw), 4; milk, 300 c.c. (10 oz.); sugar, 20 gm. (5 dr.); calories, 637.

FOURTH DAY.

7.00 A.M.	Egg; sugar, 2 gm. (½ dr.).
8.00 A.M.	Milk, 70 c.c. (2⅓ oz.).
9.00 A.M.	Egg; sugar, 3 gm. (¾ dr.).
10.00 A.M.	Milk, 70 c.c. (2⅓ oz.).
11.00 A.M.	Egg; sugar, 3 gm. (¾ dr.).
12.00 NOON	Milk, 65 c.c. (2 oz.).
1.00 P.M.	Egg; sugar, 3 gm. (¾ dr.).
2.00 P.M.	Milk, 65 c.c. (2 oz.).
3.00 P.M.	Egg; sugar, 3 gm. (¾ dr.).
4.00 P.M.	Milk, 65 c.c. (2 oz.).
5.00 P.M.	Egg; sugar, 3 gm. (¾ dr.).
6.00 P.M.	Milk, 65 c.c. (2 oz.).
7.00 P.M.	Egg; sugar, 3 gm. (¾ dr.).

Total fourth day, eggs (raw), 5; milk, 400 c.c. (13⅓ oz.); sugar, 20 gm. (5 dr.); calories, 777.

FIFTH DAY

7.00 A.M.	Egg; sugar, 4 gm. (1 dr.).
8.00 A.M.	Milk, 80 c.c. (2⅔ oz.).
9.00 A.M.	Egg, sugar, 4 gm. (1 dr.).

10.00 A.M.	Milk, 80 c.c. (2⅔ oz.).
11.00 A.M.	Egg; sugar, 4 gm. (1 dr.).
12.00 NOON	Milk, 80 c.c. (2⅔ oz.).
1.00 P.M.	Egg; sugar, 4½ gm. (1 dr.).
2.00 P.M.	Milk, 80 c.c. (2⅔ oz.).
3.00 P.M.	Egg; sugar, 4½ gm. (1 dr.).
4.00 P.M.	Milk, 80 c.c. (2⅔ oz.).
5.00 P.M.	Egg; sugar, 4½ gm. (1 dr.)
6.00 P.M.	Milk, 90 c.c. (3 oz.).
7.00 P.M.	Egg; sugar, 4½ gm. (1 dr.).

Total, fifth day, eggs (raw), 6; milk, 500 c.c. (16⅔ oz.); sugar, 30 gm. (1 oz.); calories, 966.

Sixth Day

7.00 A.M.	Egg; sugar, 4 gm. (1 dr.).
8.00 A.M.	Milk, 100 c.c. (3⅓ oz.).
9.00 A.M.	Egg; sugar, 4½ gm. (1 dr.); scraped beef, 12 gm. (3 dr.).
10.00 A.M.	Milk, 100 c.c. (3⅓ oz.).
11.00 A.M.	Egg; sugar, 4½ gm. (1 dr.).
12.00 NOON	Milk, 100 c.c. (3⅓ oz.).
1.00 P.M.	Egg; sugar, 4½ gm. (1 dr.); scraped beef, 12 gm. (3 dr.).
2.00 P.M.	Milk, 100 c.c. (3⅓ oz.).
3.00 P.M.	Egg; sugar, 4½ gm. (1 dr.).
4.00 P.M.	Milk, 100 c.c. (3⅓ oz.).
5.00 P.M.	Egg; sugar, 4 gm. (1 dr.); scraped beef, 12 gm. (3 dr.).
6.00 P.M.	Milk, 100 c.c. (3⅓ oz.).
7.00 P.M.	Egg; sugar, 4½ gm. (1 dr.).

Total, sixth day, eggs (raw), 7; milk, 600 c.c. (20 oz.); sugar, 30 gm. (1 oz.; scraped beef, 36 gm. (9 dr.); calories 1135.

Seventh Day

7.00 A.M.	1 soft-boiled egg.
8.00 A.M.	Milk, 100 c.c. (3⅓ oz.).
9.00 A.M.	Egg; sugar, 13 gm. (3 dr.).
10.00 A.M.	Milk, 100 c.c. (3⅓ oz.); scraped beef, 23 gm. (6 dr.); boiled rice, 33 gm. (1 oz.).
11.00 A.M.	1 soft-boiled egg.
12.00 NOON	Milk, 125 c.c. (4 oz.).
1.00 P.M.	Egg; sugar, 13 gm. (3 dr.).
2.00 P.M.	Milk, 125 c.c. (4 oz.); scraped beef, 23 gm. (6 dr.); boiled rice, 33 gm. (1 oz.).
3.00 P.M.	1 soft-boiled egg.

4.00 P.M.	Milk, 125 c.c. (4 oz.).
5.00 P.M.	Egg; sugar, 14 gm. (3⅓ dr.).
6.00 P.M.	Milk, 125 c.c. (4 oz.); scraped beef, 24 gm. (6 dr.); boiled rice, 34 gm. (1 oz.).
7.00 P.M.	1 soft-boiled egg.

Total, seventh day, eggs (raw), 4; soft-boiled, 4; milk, 700 c.c. (23⅓ oz.); sugar, 40 gm. (1⅓ oz.); sraped beef, 70 gm. (2⅓ oz.); boiled rice, 100 gm. (3⅓ oz.), with beef juice; calories, 1580.

EIGHTH DAY

The diet changes on the eighth day, requiring only four raw eggs, which may be divided into three feedings. The other four eggs are to be soft-boiled and given as directed by diet.

7.00 A.M.	1 soft-boiled egg.
8.00 A.M.	Milk, 135 c.c. (4½ oz.).
9.00 A.M.	Egg; sugar, 13 gm. (3 dr.).
10.00 A.M.	Milk, 133 c.c. (4½ oz.); scraped beef, 23 gm. (6 dr.); boiled rice, 33 gm. (1 oz.).
11.00 A.M.	1 soft-boiled egg; zweiback, 10 gm. (2½ dr.).
12.00 NOON	Milk, 133 c.c. (4½ oz.).
1.00 P.M.	Egg; sugar, 13 gm. (3 dr.).
2.00 P.M.	Milk, 133 c.c. (4½ oz.); scraped beef, 23 gm. (6 dr.); boiled rice, 33 gm. (1 oz.).
3.00 P.M.	1 soft-boiled egg.
4.00 P.M.	Milk, 133 c.c. (4½ oz.).
5.00 P.M.	Egg; sugar, 14 gm. (3½ dr.); zweiback, 10 gm. (2½ dr.).
6.00 P.M.	Milk, 133 c.c. (4½ oz.); scraped beef, 24 gm. (6 dr.); boiled rice, 34 gm. (1 oz.).
7.00 P.M.	1 soft-boiled egg.

Total eighth day, eggs (raw), 4; soft-boiled, 4; milk, 800 c.c. (26⅔ oz.); scraped beef, 70 gm. (2⅓ oz.); boiled rice, 100 gm. (3⅓ oz.); zweiback, 20 gm. (5 dr.); sugar, 40 gm. (1⅓ oz.); calories, 1720.

NINTH DAY

7.00 A.M.	1 soft-boiled egg.
8.00 A.M.	Milk, 150 c.c. (5 oz.).
9.00 A.M.	Egg; sugar, 13 gm. (3 dr.).
10.00 A.M.	Milk, 150 c.c. (5 oz.); scraped beef, 23 gm. (6 dr.); boiled rice, 66 gm. (2 oz.).
11.00 A.M.	1 soft-boiled egg; zweiback, 20 gm. (5 dr.).
12.00 NOON	Milk, 150 c.c. (5 oz.).
1.00 P.M.	Egg; sugar, 13 gm. (3 dr.).

2.00 P.M.	Milk, 150 c.c. (5 oz.); scraped beef, 23 gm. (6 dr.); boiled rice, 67 gm. (2 oz.).
3.00 P.M.	1 soft-boiled egg; zweiback, 20 gm. (5 dr.).
4.00 P.M.	Milk, 150 c.c. (5 oz.).
5.00 P.M.	Egg; sugar, 14 gm. (3½ dr.)
6.00 P.M.	Milk, 150 c.c. (5 oz.); scraped beef, 24 gm. (6 dr.); boiled rice, 67 gm. (2 oz.).
7.00 P.M.	1 soft-boiled egg.

Total, ninth day, eggs (raw), 4; cooked, 4; milk, 900 c.c. (**30 oz.**); sugar, 40 gm. (1⅓ oz.); scraped beef, 70 gm. (2⅓ **oz.**); **rice,** 200 gm. (6⅔ oz.); zweiback, 40 gm. (1⅓ oz.) or **toast,** 20 gm. (dr.); calories, 2138.

TENTH DAY

7.00 A.M.	1 soft-boiled egg.
8.00 A.M.	Milk, 166 c.c. (5½ oz.).
9.00 A.M.	Egg; sugar, 13 gm. (3 dr.).
10.00 A.M.	Milk, 168 c.c. (5½ oz.); scraped beef, 23 gm. (6 dr.); boiled rice, 66 gm. (2 oz.).
11.00 A.M.	1 soft-boiled egg; zwieback, 20 gm. (5 dr.); butter, 4 gm. (1 dr.).
12.00 NOON	Cooked chopped chicken, 25 gm. (6 dr.); milk, 166 c.c. (5½ oz.).
1.00 P.M.	Egg; sugar, 13 gm. (3 dr.).
2.00 P.M.	Milk, 166 c.c. (5½ oz.); scraped beef, 23 gm. (6 dr.); boiled rice, 66 gm. (2 oz.); butter, 4 gm. (1 dr.).
3.00 P.M.	1 soft-boiled egg; zwieback, 20 gm. (5 dr.); butter, 4 gm. (1 dr.).
4.00 P.M.	Cooked chopped chicken, 25 gm. (6 dr.).
5.00 P.M.	Egg; sugar, 14 gm. (3½ dr.).
6.00 P.M.	Milk, 166 c.c. (5½ oz.); scraped beef, 24 gm. (6 dr.); boiled rice, 67 gm. (2 oz.); butter, 4 gm. (1 dr.).
7.00 P.M.	1 soft-boiled egg.

Total, tenth day, eggs (raw), 4; cooked, 4; milk, 1000 c.c. (33⅓ oz.); sugar, 40 gm. (1⅓ oz.); scraped beef, 70 gm. gm. (2⅓ oz.); boiled rice, 200 gm. (6⅔ oz.); zwieback, 40 gm. (1⅓ oz.), or toast, 20 gm. (5 dr.); chicken, 50 gm. (1⅔ oz.); butter, 20 gm. (5 dr.); calories, 2478.

ELEVENTH DAY

7.00 A.M.	1 soft-boiled egg; milk, 250 c.c. (8⅓ oz.); zwieback, 10 gm. (2½ dr.); butter, 4 gm. (1 dr.).
8.00 A.M.	Egg; sugar, 13 gm. (3 dr.); scraped beef, 20 gm. (5 dr.); boiled rice, 75 gm. (2½ oz.); zwieback, 10 gm. (2½ dr.); butter, 6 gm. (1½ dr.).

11.00 P.M.	1 soft-boiled egg; milk 250 c.c. (8⅓ oz.); butter, 6 gm. 1½ dr.); zwieback, 10 gm. (2½ dr.).
1.00 P.M.	Egg; sugar, 13 gm. (3 dr.); cooked chopped chicken, 25 gm. (6 dr.); boiled rice, 75 gm. (2½ oz.).
3.00 P.M.	1 soft-boiled egg; milk, 250 c.c. (8⅓ oz.); scraped beef, 20 gm. (5 dr.); boiled rice, 75 gm. (2½ oz.); zwieback, 10 gm. (2½ dr.); butter, 6 gm. (1½ dr.).
5.00 P.M.	Egg; sugar, 14 gm. (3½ dr.); cooked chopped chicken, 25 gm. (6 dr.); boiled rice, 75 gm. (2½ oz.); butter, 6 gm. (1½ dr.).
7.00 P.M.	1 soft-boiled egg; milk, 250 c.c. (8⅓ oz.); zwieback, 10 gm. (2½ dr.); butter, 6 gm. (1½ dr.); scraped beef, 30 gm. (1 oz.)

Total, eleventh day, eggs (raw), 4; cooked, 4; milk, 1000 c.c. (33⅓ oz.); butter, 40 gm. (1⅓ oz.); sugar, 40 gm. (1⅓ oz.); scraped beef, 70 gm. (2⅓ oz.); boiled rice, 300 gm. (10 oz.); zwieback, 60 gm. (2 oz.); chicken, 50 gm. (1⅔ oz.); calories, 2941.

TWELFTH DAY

7.00 A.M.	1 soft-boiled egg; milk, 250 c.c. (8⅓ oz.); zwieback, 10 gm. (2½ dr.); butter, 4 gm. (1 dr.).
9.00 A.M.	Egg; sugar, 13 gm. (3 dr.); scraped beef, 35 gm. (1 oz.); boiled rice, 75 gm. (2½ oz.); zwieback, 10 gm. (2½ dr.); butter, 6 gm. (1½ dr.).
11.00 A.M.	1 soft-boiled egg; milk, 250 c.c. (8⅓ oz.); zwieback, 20 gm. (5 dr.); butter, 6 gm. 1½ dr.).
1.00 P.M.	Egg; sugar, 13 gm. (3 dr.); cooked chopped chicken, 25 gm. (6 dr.); boiled rice, 75 gm. (2½ oz.); zwieback, 10 gm. (2½ dr.); butter, 6 gm. (1½ dr.).
3.00 P.M.	1 soft-boiled egg; milk, 250 c.c. (8⅓ oz.); scraped beef, 35 gm. (1 oz.); boiled rice, 50 gm. (1⅔ oz.); zwieback, 10 gm. (2½ dr.); butter, 6 gm. (1½ dr.).
5.00 P.M.	Egg; sugar, 14 gm. (3½ dr.); cooked chopped chicken, 25 gm. (6 dr.); boiled rice, 75 gm. (2½ oz.); zwieback, 10 gm. (2½ dr.); butter, 6 gm. (1½ dr.).

7.00 P.M.   1 soft-boiled egg; milk, 250 c.c. (8⅓ oz.); zwieback, 10 gm. (2½ dr.); butter, 6 gm. (1½ dr.).

Total, twelfth day, eggs (raw), 4; cooked, 4; milk, 1000 c.c. (33⅓ oz.); sugar, 40 gm. (1⅓ oz.); scraped beef, 70 gm. (2⅓ oz.); boiled rice, 300 gm. (10 oz.); zwieback, 80 gm. (2⅔ oz.); chicken, 50 gm. (1⅔ oz.); butter, 40 gm. (1½ oz.); calories, 2941.

THIRTEENTH DAY

7.00 A.M.   1 soft-boiled egg; milk, 142 c.c. (4⅔ oz.); zwieback, 10 gm. (2½ dr.); butter, 4 gm. (1 dr.).

9.00 A.M.   Egg; sugar, 13 gm. (3 dr.); milk, 142 c.c. (4⅔ oz.); scraped beef, 20 gm. (5 dr.); boiled rice, 75 gm. (2½ oz.); zwieback, 20 gm. (5 dr.); butter, 6 gm. (1½ dr.).

11.00 A.M.   1 soft-boiled egg; milk, 144 c.c. (5 oz.); zwieback, 10 gm. (2½ dr.); butter, 6 gm. (1½ dr.).

1.00 P.M.   Egg; sugar, 13 gm. (3 dr.); milk, 142 c.c. (4⅔ oz.); cooked chopped chicken, 25 gm. (6 dr.); boiled rice, 75 gm. (2½ oz.); zwieback, 10 gm. (2½ dr.); butter, 6 gm. (1½ dr.).

3.00 P.M.   1 soft-boiled egg; milk, 144 c.c. (5 oz.); scraped beef, 20 gm. (5 dr.); boiled rice, 75 gm. (2½ oz.); zwieback, 10 gm. (2½ dr.); butter, 6 gm. (1½ dr.).

5.00 P.M.   Egg; sugar, 14 gm. (3½ dr.); milk, 142 c.c. (5 oz.); cooked chopped chicken, 25 gm. (6 dr.); boiled rice, 75 gm. (2½ oz.); zwieback, 10 gm. (2½ dr.); butter, 6 gm. (1½ dr.).

7.00 P.M.   1 soft-boiled egg; milk, 144 c.c. (5 oz.); zwieback, 10 gm. (2½ dr.); butter, 6 gm. (1½ dr.).

Total, thirteenth day, eggs (raw), 4; cooked, 4; milk, 1000 c.c. (33⅓ oz.); sugar, 40 gm. (1⅓ oz.); scraped beef, 70 gm. (2⅓ oz.); boiled rice, 300 gm. (10 oz.); zwieback, 80 gm. (2⅓ oz.); chicken, 50 gm. (1⅔ oz.); butter, 40 gm. (1⅓ oz.); calories, 3007.

FOURTEENTH DAY

7.00 A.M.   1 soft-boiled egg; minced chop; buttered toast; milk, 142 c.c. (4⅔ oz.).

9.00 A.M.	Boiled rice; buttered zwieback; custard; milk, 142 c.c. (4⅔ oz.).
11.00 A.M. ‡	1 soft-boiled egg; buttered zwieback; junket; milk, 144 c.c. (5 oz.).
1.00 P.M.	Minced chicken; boiled rice; buttered zwieback; custard; milk, 142 c.c. (4⅔ oz.).
3.00 P.M.	1 soft-boiled egg; cooked scraped beef; boiled rice; buttered toast; milk, 144 c.c. (5 oz.).
5.00 P.M.	Minced chicken; boiled rice; buttered zwieback; custard; milk, 142 c.c. (4⅔ oz.).
7.00 P.M.	1 soft-boiled egg; buttered toast; milk, 144 c.c. (5 oz.).

Total, fourteenth day, eggs (raw), 4; cooked, 4; milk, 1000 c.c. (33⅓ oz.); sugar, 40 gm. (1⅓ oz.); scraped beef, 70 gm. (2⅓ oz.); boiled rice, 300 gm. (10 oz.); zwieback, 100 gm. (3⅓ oz.); butter, 40 gm. (1⅓ oz.); chicken, 50 gm. (1⅔ oz.); calories, 3007.

Many patients are unable to take the full amount of food ordered after the sixth day, particularly women who may have long been small eaters. If pushed, the feedings may result in an acute gastric upset, anorexia, nausea, vomiting; in fact this has been very frequent in the writer's experience, often making it necessary to stop all feedings for twenty-four hours or at least, after the sixth day only advancing the diet every other day, thus giving a little more time to become adjusted to the quantity of food. In fact this is the writer's custom whenever this form of diet seems indicated. Whenever any hard substance like zwieback is called for, it is wiser to substitute a little softened toast or even the zwieback softened with hot water.

The usefulness of the Lenhartz diet is confined almost entirely to the treatment of acute ulcer cases and even in these the amount of food given after the first few days is too large for most patients, nausea and vomiting being, not infrequently, the result.

In chronic ulcer it is distinctly less valuable for the same reason and also because meat is added too early to the diet.

Diet Combined with Alkaline Treatment.—There have been advanced many forms of the alkaline treatment combined with proper diet for cases of gastric and duodenal ulcer, but apparently the one most specifically and carefully worked out for this is the treatment arranged and practised by B. W. Sippy[1] of Chicago. By this method he feels that an operative procedure is scarcely ever necessary, as the

[1] Sippy, in Musser and Kelly: Jour. Am. Med. Assn, 1915, lxiv, 20, 1625.

TABLE OF LENHARTZ'S DIET.

Day.	Calories.	Eggs.	Milk, c.c.	Sugar, gm.	Scraped beef, gm.	Boiled rice, gm.	Zwieback, gm.	Butter, gm.	Chicken, gm.
1	280	Raw 2	100 (3⅓ oz.)						
2	470	Raw 3	200 (6⅔ oz.)						
3	637	Raw 4	300 (10 oz.)	20 (5 dr.)					
4	777	Raw 5	400 (13⅓ oz.)	20 (5 dr.)					
5	966	Raw 6	500 (16⅔ oz.)	30 (1 oz.)					
6	1135	Raw 7	600 (20 oz.)	30 (1 oz.)	36 (9 dr.)				
7	1580	Raw 4, soft 4	700 (23⅓ oz.)	40 (1⅓ oz.)	70 (2⅓ oz.)	100 (3⅓ oz.)			
8	1720	Raw 4 soft 4	800 (26⅔ oz.)	40 (1⅓ oz.)	70 (2⅓ oz.)	100 (3⅓ oz.)	20 (⅔ oz.)		
9	2138	Raw 4 soft 4	900 (30 oz.)	40 (1⅓ oz.)	70 (2⅓ oz.)	200 (6⅔ oz.)	40 (1⅓ oz.) or toast, 20 (⅔ oz.)		
10	2478	Raw 4, soft 4	1000 (33⅓ oz.)	40 (1⅓ oz.)	70 (2⅓ oz.)	200 (6⅔ oz.)	40 (1⅓ oz.) or toast, 20 (⅔ oz.)	20 (⅔ oz.)	50 (1⅔ oz.)
11	2941	Raw 4, soft 4	1000 (33⅓ oz.)	40 (1⅓ oz.)	70 (2⅓ oz.)	300 (10 oz.)	60 (2 oz.)	40 (1⅓ oz.)	50 (1⅔ oz.)
12	2941	Raw 4, soft 4	1000 (33⅓ oz.)	40 (1⅓ oz.)	70 (2⅓ oz.)	300 (10 oz.)	80 (2⅔ oz.)	40 (1⅓ oz.)	50 (1⅔ oz.)
13	3007	Raw 4, soft 4	1000 (33⅓ oz.)	40 (1⅓ oz.)	70 (2⅓ oz.)	300 (10 oz.)	80 (2⅔ oz.)	40 (1⅓ oz.)	50 (1⅔ oz.)
14	3007	Same as the thirteenth day.							

cases are so regularly cured by medical means, and he even includes all cases of pyloric stenosis, except those of extreme narrowing, due to definite cicatricial contraction following a healed ulcer. He says that after three, four or more weeks of this treatment the spasm is relieved, the round-celled infiltration disappears as well as the edema of the inflammatory tissues, and the lumen is again established so that in practically every case a motor meal, consisting of meat and vegetables, leaves the stomach within the normal limits of six or seven hours. This is of course, quite radical and might be considered an extreme statement; Sippy, however, is most definite in his statements as to methods, what is to be expected and the results obtained, and since they are made on such responsible authority they warrant a respectful hearing and a very thorough trial in practice. He limits surgical interference in ulcer cases to the following conditions and complications.

1. Perforation.
2. Perigastric abscess.
3. Secondary carcinoma.
4. Hour-glass or other deformity.
5. Hemorrhage of a serious nature under certain conditions.
6. Pyloric obstruction of high grade not influenced by medical treatment.

The underlying principles on which the diet and treatment are founded may be stated as follows: Peptic ulcers would tend to heal spontaneously, as ulcers situated elsewhere, were it not for the fact that they are constantly subjected to the corrosive action of the gastric juice and that if this can be neutralized continuously during the period of gastric and upper intestinal digestion by proper diet and alkalies and the removal at night of any product of continuous hypersecretion, the ulcer will heal without difficulty. With this as a basis, Sippy treats and diets these cases as follows:

"Patients are put to bed from three to four weeks, at the end of which time they are gradually allowed up and out as one would after any illness of a corresponding length, but no real work should be attempted for a period of seven or eight weeks at least. As originally outlined the initial treatment consists of a period of five days in which no food or drink was given by mouth, but about twelve ounces, more or less, of saline was given by rectum four times a day. Subsequently, this period of starvation was abandoned, and presumably, except in the case of severe hemorrhage, the feedings were begun at once. Each morning one-half hour before the first feeding a dram of subnitrate of bismuth is given in a little water. Feedings are given every hour from 7 A.M. to 7 P.M., consisting of equal parts of milk and cream in amounts of a total of 1 to 3 ounces. Although acidity is more easily controlled by hourly feedings, some cases do well on two, three or four hourly feedings. Half-way between each feeding a powder consisting of 10 grains each of calcined magnesia and sodium bicarbonate is given, alternating with another powder of 10 grains of bismuth and 20 to 30 grains of soda bicarbonate. It is best to give the powder containing magnesia as often as possible as the magnesia has four times the power of neutralizing the free hydrochloric acid as compared with the soda; diarrhea, however, is apt to follow its free use, so that one must alternate these powders according to this condition. •After two or three days, soft eggs and well-cooked (fine) cereals are added so that at the end of about ten days the patients are receiving the 3 ounces of milk and cream mixture every hour from 7 A.M. to 7 P.M., 3 soft-boiled eggs, one at a time, and 9 ounces of cereal, 3 ounces given at each of three feedings. These extras are added one at a time until the six extra feedings of eggs and cereals are given evenly spaced throughout the day. The bulk of each feeding should not exceed a total of 6 ounces. In order that the treatment should be successful, an accurate control of the acidity must be maintained throughout the twenty-four hours. This is accomplished by testing the gastric contents from time to time, early in the treatment, by the stomach-tube (or Einhorn's duodenal tube may be used to advantage, as very easy of application). Sippy's method for accurate control of the free hydrochloric acidity is somewhat as follows: the first day or two the tube is passed occasionally to check up the presence of free HCl; if present in the stomach contents the alkali powders must be increased as the treatment aim absolutely to keep the free HCl down to zero. After a day or two this is done as a routine two or three times a week, as practically that is all that is necessary to insure the absence of the hydrochloric acid.

"The amount of alkali can be varied as determined by the examination of the stomach contents. It is particularly necessary to be sure that the stomach does not contain free acid during the night and it may be necessary to give two or three alkali powders between 7 and 10 P.M. to insure this. At 10 o'clock the tube should be passed and all acid hypersecetion removed. If there is a considerable amount of this, the tube should be passed again during the night two or three times. After the first few day's treatment this is rarely necessary as the hypersecretion is usually well controlled and at 10 P.M. nothing but a very few ç.c. of gastric contents are found, which are unimportant.

"In the diet cream soups, vegetable purées or other soft foods may be added or substituted, such as jellies, custards, creams; keeping, however, the milk, cream, eggs and cereal as the basis of the diet.   The best cereals are farina, cream of wheat, rice cooked to a soft pulp.   With this diet it is quite regularly that the cases, according to Sippy, show a gain of from 1 to 4 pounds a week.

"During the third week, soft toast or crackers, purée of potato, cream soups may be added.   In the fourth week the milk and cream may be made 2½ ounces each at each feeding and the period between feedings lengthened to two hours. After two or three weeks more, three-hour feedings may be given, but if the ulcer is of some month's duration it is best not to increase the periods too rapidly and for several months it is wise not to have the patients take less than five feedings a day.   The morning bismuth should be taken for from six to eight weeks and then stopped and the alkaline powders should be continued between feedings for several months.

"During a period of a year or more, milk, cream, eggs, vegetables, purées, cereal, bread and butter and meats should form the basis of the diet."   In cases that for one reason or another milk is distasteful, it often can be given if flavored with tea, cocoa, etc., frozen balls of butter may be substituted for cream and a small quantity of cereal gruel may be given each hour.

Modified Diet for Peptic Ulcer.—In this the essential features of both the Sippy and von Leube methods are combined and fully peptonized milk (two hour peptonization) is used instead of the milk and cream mixture of Sippy. This modified method reproduces medically the conditions that are sought by operation, viz., a continued greatly reduced gastric acidity and even a real alkalinity of the stomach contents, as well as a rapid emptying time, for Canon has shown that fully peptonized milk leaves the stomach with great rapidity.

The following are the details of the method.

The patient is kept in bed for three weeks and the hot pad kept continuously on the epigastrium as in the von Leube routine.   The continuous Murphy drip of 2 per cent. glucose solution is started at once to which is added 50 grains (3 gm.) strontium bromide for the daily allowance. Nothing by mouth is allowed for three days.   Mouth washes are used several times a day.   Mouth feeding is begun on the fourth day, consisting of 2 oz. (60 c.c.) fully peptonized milk, every hour from 7 A.M. to 7 P.M. Half way between feedings the alkaline powders, as recommended in the Sippy routine, are given in two ounces of water (60 c.c.). Each day the milk is increased one ounce (30 c.c.) until four ounces (120 c.c.) are taken every hour, (or eight ounces (240 c.c.) every two hours in some cases). The water allowance is not increased to over three or four ounces (90 to 120 c.c.) with the alkalie. After eight or ten days of feeding, a tablespoonful of well cooked farina is allowed, first twice a day with two milk feedings which are kept up continuously. The tenth day farina, cream of wheat or wheatena are allowed with three of the milk feedings. The twelfth day one may increase the cereal to two tablespoonfuls and a small sprinkling of powdered sugar is allowed. The fifteenth day four soft feedings are given evenly spaced throughout the day, still continuing the peptonized milk feedings; of these soft feedings one may be, one slice of milk toast. The seventeenth day a soft egg is allowed or custard and the milk feedings may be reduced to 2 oz. (60 c.c.). After the twenty-first day, the feedings are arranged so as to give three soft meals at eight, one at six-thirty with a mid-feeding at eleven A.M. and four P.M. of milk, custard, junket or cream cheese sandwich. In the fourth week creamed fresh cod or halibut are added, cream or purée soups, mashed potatoes and well cooked rice.

From the end of the third week the peptonization of the milk is reduced fifteen minutes a day until plain milk is taken but always scalded. During the entire treatment the alkaline mixtures are given in sufficient amount at first to maintain as nearly as possible a continuously alkaline reaction to the gastric contents and when soft feedings are added sufficient to prevent the formation of free HCl at least. The stomach contents must be tested by passing a stomach or duodenal tube and emptying the stomach at bed time and during the night if necessary, as recommended in the Sippy routine.

Ambulatory Diet Cure for Peptic Ulcer.—There are always a certain number of cases that are seen in whom the symptoms are very suggestive of chronic ulcer, but in whom the diagnosis is not sufficiently certain or for one reason or another the patients will not or cannot give the time for a regular course of treatment in bed. In these cases it is advisable to put them on a bland diet which has sufficient food value to keep up the patient's strength, and combine well with the usual large excess of free hydrochloric acid and. be obtainable almost any and everywhere. In this day of the "dairy lunch," it is very easy to obtain this diet anywhere about a city. If the case is actually one of gastric or duodenal ulcer the chances are very great that at least there will be decided temporary relief, sometimes for a year or more and in a few cases, particularly if persisted in for three or four weeks, the writer has seen clinical cures. The diet is also of considerable diagnostic value, as the case which is clinically ulcer but does not get very great or complete temporary relief for weeks or longer, is very probably not ulcer but chronic appendicitis, gall-bladder disease or something else which simulates ulcer.

The diet for these ambulatory cases is planned as follows: For two (or more) full weeks, they take at 8 A.M., 1 and 7 P.M., 2 glasses of milk (¼ cream) and 2 soft-boiled eggs (1 minute), without salt at first. At 11 A.M. and 4 P.M. 1½ glasses of milk (1680 c.c.).

This gives milk 56 oz.

Cream 13 oz. (390 c.c.) 6 eggs.

Protein 105 gm. (3½ oz.); fat 177 gm. (6 oz.).

Carbohydrate 85 gm. (3 oz.) calories 2400.

Before breakfast a dram (4 gm.) of bismuth subnitrate is given in an ounce of water. One half hour after the three principal meals, ½ to 1 dram (2 to 4 gm.) of the following powder; equal parts of bismuth, soda bicarbonate and calcined magnesia, is given in four ounces (120 c.c., of water. The magnesia may be reduced and an equal amount of soda added if the bowels are made too active by the magnesia. One half hour after the 11 A.M. and 4 P.M. feedings one teaspoonful of soda is given in ½ glass of water. At night after the seven o'clock feeding the magnesia mixture is given at 7.45 and a teaspoonful of soda at 8.45 P.M. and 9.45 P.M., each in ½ to ⅔ glass of water.

If possible it is well for the patient to empty his stomach by the tube at 10.30. P.M.

In all these forms of ulcer treatment, except when there has been a recent hemorrhage, if pain persists relief is often obtained by an early morning lavage of the stomach with a silver nitrate solution 1 : 4000 increasing to 1 : 2000 followed after the stomach is left clean by plain water lavage by the bismuth.

After the two weeks are up, or longer in severe cases, fine well-cooked cereals, custards, gruels, cream soups, soft toast; later boiled fish, etc., can be added as in the third and fourth weeks of the von Leube diet.

One does not expect to get the best results with this diet and it should not be advised unless the patient refuses for one reason or another to take a full course of diet with rest in bed. Vichy is the best form in which to take water between feedings or if more alkali is indicated by much acidity. Alkali powders may be given an hour to an hour and a half after the principal feedings. If the milk mixture does not seem to agree, some of the alkali may be added directly, to each feeding.[1] An occasional case has to omit the cream on account of increased gastric acidity.

Transgastric or Duodenal Feeding.[2]—This method of feeding has been devised by Einhorn and is recommended by him in gastric or duodenal ulcer cases or chronic gastric dilatation, to prevent weight on the gastric walls and to allow them to contract down to more nearly their normal size, this of course provided there is no organic obstruction. Also in extreme atony, whether there is pylorospasm or not; in cases where nutrition is difficult on account of asthenia, absolute anorexia and nervous vomiting. Einhorn also recommends it in severe liver diseases to reduce the physiological congestion of that organ and also in inoperable carcinoma of the stomach where the taking of food is painful.

In gastric or duodenal ulcer with which we are particularly concerned here, its usefulness is claimed to lie in the rest, both secretory and muscular,which it gives to the stomach and possibly to a less extent to the duodenum.

The duodenal tube is introduced as follows: The tube is put in the patient's mouth and he is given a swallow or more of water, to wash it down, taking care only that it is not swallowed too quickly, so that it does not rotate on itself, but will go straight into the stomach. The patient then lies on the right side to facilitate the passage of the tube into the duodenum by gravity. This takes a varying amount of time, depending on the acidity present, the motor power of the stomach muscle and the presence or absence of pylorospasm, entering the duodenum quickest in hypoacidity or achylia when accompanied, as it usually is, by good muscular action and no spasm of the pylorus; the time varying from ten to twenty minutes under the latter conditions, to two or three hours for normal individuals and even up to thirty-six hours at the longest. When the tube is beyond the pylorus it is difficult to obtain fluid and what little can be obtained is alkaline and usually contains bile. If still in the stomach the fluid aspirated by the syringe is of course

[1] A very good form of alkaline powder to use is equal parts of soda bicarbonate, heavy burned magnesia and subnitrate of bismuth. Bismuth subnitrate in dram doses is useful to control pain when given on an empty stomach early in the morning.

[2] Einhorn: Post Graduate, 1913.

acid and is in greater quantity. If there is achylia and consequently no acid to test for, we can give a little milk or colored fluid by mouth and immediately aspirate: if the tube is beyond the pylorus no milk will be aspirated. After the tube is once in the duodenum it is left there throughout the period of feeding, twelve to fifteen days, and the mouth kept clean by frequent use of mouth washes.

The regular feedings recommended by Einhorn consist of milk, 7 or 8 ounces, (210 to 240 c.c.) one egg and a tablespoonful of lactose. If diarrhea develops the lactose is omitted. Where it is necessary to prevent loss of weight or to increase weight, 1 or 2 drams(2 to 4 gm.) of butter to each feeding may be added. Where patients for one reason or another cannot take milk, gruels may be substituted but always being sure that the feedings are all free from lumps. The number of feedings is eight a day at two-hour intervals and must be given slowly, taking at least twenty minutes to each; for if given rapidly they cause overdistention of the duodenum and great discomfort. The best way to introduce the food is by means of a syringe with a three-way stopcock so that it need not be disconnected each time.

The food should all be strained and given at body temperature and the thinner the tube the more comfortable for the patient, although the smaller tubes necessitate slower feeding. A very important rule is, that after the food has been given, a little water, then a little air should be passed through the tube to be sure the tube is clean and empty; otherwise the tube is apt to be blocked in a day or two, necessitating its removal for cleaning. Besides the feedings at least a pint of warm normal saline should be given once a day, or this may be given by rectum. After the period of transgastric feedings is finished one begins mouth feedings with fully peptonized milk, then soft thin cereals and gradually increases the feeding as recommended in the von Leube cure, only one need not begin with such small feedings, but the feeding recommended for the eighth feeding day may be used at the start and increased as indicated for that regimen.

DUODENAL FEEDING DIET.   (Einhorn.)

7.30 A.M.	Oatmeal gruel	180 c.c. (6 oz.)
	One egg	
	Butter	15 gm. (½ oz.)
	Lactose	15 gm. (½ oz.)
9.30 A.M.	Pea soup	180 c.c. (6 oz.)
	One egg	
	Butter	15 gm. (½ oz.)
	Lactose	15 gm. (½ oz.)
11.30 A.M.	Same as at 9.30 A.M.	
1.30 P.M.	Bouillon	180 c.c. (6 oz.)
	One egg	

3.30 P.M.	Oatmeal gruel	180 c.c. (6 oz.)		
	Butter	15 gm. (½ oz.)		
	One egg			
	Lactose	15 gm. (½ oz.)		
5.30 P.M.	Same as at 9.30 A.M.			
9.30 P.M.	Bouillon	180 c.c. (6 oz.)		
	One egg			

Total amount: Calories.

Oatmeal gruel	360 c.c. (13 oz.)	=	1476
Eggs	8	=	1352
Pea soup	720 c.c. (26 oz.)	=	384
Lactose	90 gm. (3 oz.)	=	369
Bouillon	360 c.c. (13 oz.)	=	39
Butter	90 gm. (3 oz.)	=	715

                                                  4335

DIET AFTER HEMORRHAGE FROM STOMACH OR DUODENUM.

At the first evidence of hemorrhage the patient is to be kept absolutely at rest and quiet in bed. If the hemorrhage is severe so that life is threatened either from exsanguination or cerebral anemia, the foot of the bed should be elevated on shock blocks and the patient's limbs tied off with broad bandages to keep as much blood in the trunk and head as possible. Each limb should be left tied off not longer than ten minutes at a time, they can be used thus in rotation, one or two at a time. Absolutely nothing should be given by mouth, not even cracked ice, but if there has been great loss of blood, saline may be given by rectum either in 4- to 6-ounce amounts, every three or four hours or by continuous Murphy drip. If the hemorrhage is extreme a saline infusion may be given or better still a blood transfusion from a suitable donor. If the hemorrhage is recurring and too excessive, the question of immediate laparotomy must be considered.

After hemorrhage, it is best, if possible, not to use rectal saline or feeding for at least twenty-four to forty-eight hours unless the thirst becomes too excessive. The chief reason is, that anything put into the rectum starts antiperistalsis which may reach the stomach, and also that it is capable of starting gastric secretion. After this period is past one may begin on one or two lines of treatment.

1. Feeding by rectum entirely, for from two to five days, or even longer, and then begin on the Lenhartz or von Leube diets.

2. By beginning at once with a Lenhartz or von Leube diet, as already explained. In the author's opinion the Lenhartz is better suited to acute ulcerative conditions than to

24

chronic, while the von Leube, particularly as modified by Lockwood, is better for either condition, acute or chronic.

From this point the diet is arranged in accordance with the details of the diet selected. Practically all clinicians of experience favor at least a period of twenty-four to forty-eight hours' absoute rest to the stomach before food or even water is given by mouth.

GASTRIC ATONY.

(Impaired Gastric Motor Function or Myasthenia Gastrica.)

Enough has been said of this condition of atony when complicating chronic gastritis to indicate quite fully the principles involved in prescribing a dietary for the use of patients suffering from motor insufficiency of the stomach.

Since the condition is almost always secondary to a general muscular and nervous debility often found in patients after exhausting or long-continued disease, and in those of enteroptotic habitus, the greatest care must be exercised in choosing a diet in order to overnourish these patients, if possible, so that they can gain in general ways, while at the same time preventing gastric overdistention and the introduction of foods which leave the stomach slowly or with difficulty, such as all coarse or tough foods, heavy fats, etc.

Many patients with motor insufficiency of the stomach get fixed ideas as to what they can or cannot eat and since it is usually the latter, they very quickly add to their troubles marked malnutrition and eventually settling down to a dietary which is hopelessly inadequate to nourish them, with the result that their stomach musculature becomes still further weakened.

Motor insufficiency has been termed by some authorities as "an indigestion of liquids" which simply means that liquids remain in the stomach longer than solids in this condition, so giving rise to fulness, splashing and regurgitation for a longer or shorter time after the stomach should be normally empty. It must also be kept in mind that many if not most of these patients show general improvement, when on a proper diet, a considerable time before the gastric muscle regains its tone and they are constantly tempted to break rules and eat or drink as they choose because they feel so much better and stronger; only a firm adherence to diet and general hygiene with graduated exercises will bring the desired result with a return to normal of the gastric functions. Associated with the myasthenia one finds very frequently a condition of gastric hyperacidity which must also be taken into consideration in the diet planned for these individuals, also many persons with congenital or acquired ptosis of the stomach show the same combination of pathological conditions, namely, myasthenia and hyperacidity, either separately or combined.

General Directions in Gastric Atony.—Before touching directly on the foods best suited to these cases it would be worth while to formulate certain rules for these patients to follow, which will aid the stomach in performing its motor functions with the greatest efficiency under the individual circumstances.

1. Patients should always have a period of absolute rest before meals, reclining for fifteen to thirty minutes. It is astonishing how much this rest will improve the appetite and muscular tone, it means that they eat when rested and do not hurry in to a meal from some occupation; this is one of the greatest aids to good digestion in any abnormal condition of the gastro-intestinal tract.

2. Meals should be small, well-cooked and of easily digested materials, rather dry and of concentrated caloric value, without skins of fruit and vegetable seeds, gristle or fat which does not melt at body temperature, *e. g.*, mutton fat.

3. The interval for feeding in severe cases should be every three hours; 3 or 4 ounces or more of water should be given three-quarters of an hour before meals, best at room temperature or warm, never cold.

4. At meals it is best to take no liquids or at most not over 3 ounces and then only in the less severe cases.

5. It should be remembered that milk often fails to agree with these patients, increasing flatulence.

6. After meals when possible (and always in severe cases), patients should lie for half an hour to an hour on their right side in order to facilitate evacuation of the stomach by gravity.

7. Many cases, particularly those complicated by gastroptosis will get great digestive benefit by wearing a proper corset or belt. This helps to fix a usually flabby abdominal wall and improves the splanchnic circulation, often resulting in a general increase of the systolic blood-pressure; such patients often having an abnormally low arterial tension, 85 to 100 mm. Hg.

8. Other hygienic measures useful in this condition will be found in books dealing with this particular subject, *e. g.*, exercises, bathing, sleep and rest.

Keeping in mind the foregoing rules it would hardly seem necessary to give a specimen dietary for such a case, but many are too busy or lack enthusiasm for these details, hence the following sample diets are given with the caution that such conditions as hyperacidity or hypoacidity, fermentation, pyloric spasm, etc., must be recognized if present and due allowance made in the selection of a diet (see Special Rules for Diet in Hyper- and Hypoacid Gastric Conditions).

Diets for Atony: (Rather liberal).

7 A.M.   2 tablespoonfuls of any well-cooked cereal with butter and sugar (heavy cream if it agrees). Bread or toast and butter, two slices; 1 soft-boiled egg.

10 A.M.   Custard (unsweetened) with cream, 2 or 3 toasted saltines.

1 P.M.   Chopped meat or chicken or fish; bread and butter; rice, cooked to a pulp, with butter and salt, or beef juice or baked potato. Later a small portion of baked hubbard squash, stewed celery, or rice or bread pudding, but both dessert and vegetables should not be taken at the same meal.

4 P.M.   Cream cheese with toasted and buttered saltine biscuits, as a sandwich, one or two of these.

7 P.M.   Fish or eggs (except fried), bread and butter, rice with butter and cream, a simple dessert such as custard, blanc mange, Spanish cream, etc.

10 P.M.   Same as 10 A.M. or 4 P.M., feedings or a plain sandwich made of beef, chicken or mutton; Swiss cheese, bread and butter.

For those who can take milk, it may be used in various ways, plain, buttermilk or junket, etc. Many of these cases of myasthenia being merely a part of a general neurasthenia with malnutrition, do well on the Wier-Mitchell rest cure routine, care only being taken that large quantities of food shall not be taken at one time. In the severe cases it is often best to feed every two hours instead of every three, using small feedings of concentrated nourishment, then gradually increasing, the intervals of feeding and the quantity of food at each feeding.

Diet for Severe Atony:

8 A.M.   Junket, 240 c.c. (8 oz.), with cream, 60 c.c. (2 oz.).

11 A.M.   4 saltines, with cream and cheese.

1 P.M.   Sandwich of bread and beef.

4 P.M.   Cocoa, junket, 360 c.c. (12 oz.).

7 P.M.   Custard, baked or boiled, 180 gm. (6 oz.).

9 P.M.   Sandwich, with chicken and bread.

Wegele's Diet for Atony of the Stomach:

Morning.—Dry toast, 30 gm. (1 oz.); a cupful of cocoa made of leguminose cocoa and 60 gm. (2 oz.) of cream.

Forenoon.—An egg (poached or soft-boiled) and 30 gm. (1 oz.) of toast.

Midday.—Scraped meat, 100 gm. (3½ oz.); mashed potato, 7 oz. (210 gm.); toast, 30 gm. (1 oz.); followed by 30 gm. (1 oz.) of extract of malt. .

Afternoon.—A cupful of cocoa with 60 c.c. (2 oz.) cream,

Evening.—Tapioca cooked to a pulp, 300 gm. (10 oz.). Followed by 20 c.c. (¾ oz.) of malt extract.

10 P.M.—A tumblerful of milk with a dessertspoonful of cognac brandy.

Tibbles,[1] on the other hand, recommends only three meals at 8 A.M., 2 P.M. and 8 P.M., two of them mainly protein, giving most of the carbohydrate at midday, as follows:

Breakfast, 8 A.M.—Fish (sole, haddock, weakfish, seabass, halibut), with a little lemon juice; 1 or 2 eggs poached or lightly boiled. A small amount of crisp dry toast or stale bread, and a cupful of coffee with cream and one piece of sugar (if it agrees).

Midday.—2 P.M. (No meat.) Boiled macaroni with a trace of grated cheese or boiled rice with tomato, purée of cabbage, savory or potato with gravy or extract of meat; boiled spinach, vegetable marrow or squash, string or snap kidney beans. Any milk pudding which has been cooked slowly (four or five hours). Jellies or creams made with gelatin, or fruit jelly or cooked apples, plums, prunes and raw fruit rubbed through a sieve (raspberries, strawberries, blackberries or currants). At the end of the meal 4 or 5 ounces of water, diluted spirit, Burgundy or Bordeaux.

Evening.—8 P.M. Soup about 90 c.c. (3 oz.); fish (same as at breakfast), tender lean beef or mutton, poultry, venison, pheasant or other game (except hare); 30 gm. (1 oz.) of potato purée or boiled rice or toast or stalebread; no pudding or dessert. At the end of meal 2 glasses of wine or 30 c.c. (1 oz.) of whiskey in 120 c.c. (4 oz.) of water. The food has a heat value of 2150 calories and contains:

Protein.	Fat.	Carbohydrates.	Alcohol.
209.6 gm.	58.7 gm.	142.5 gm.	35 c.c.

[1] Dietetics, Lea & Febiger, p. 295.

Diet for Mild Atony:[1]

8 A.M.   Cup of coffee or cocoa, with cream, sugar, fine cereal.

11 A.M.   Egg shake, Russell's emulsion or koumyss.

1 P.M.   Steak or chop, one vegetable, rice pudding, bread and butter.

4 P.M.   Chicken sandwich and a glass of hot milk.

7 P.M.   Fish or chicken, two green vegetables, tapioca pudding.

For advanced atony, still smaller meals are best, *e. g.,*:

8 A.M.   Cup of coffee or cocoa with cream, sugar; soft-boiled egg, bread and butter.

11 A.M.   Baked custard.

1 P.M.   Minced chicken on toast, cornstarch pudding.

4 P.M.   Scraped beef sandwiches.

7 P.M.   Small broiled chop, creamed spaghetti.

10 P.M.   Cup of malted milk.

The same rules in regard to drinking as before outlined. Meals should be dry, never more than one glassful of fluid and better less, half a glassful between meals once or twice.

ORGANIC GASTRIC ACIDITY.

This may be of two sorts, one due to the ingestion of organic acids in foods, such as acetic acid in pickles, cider, vinegar or acid-wine preparations; butyric acid from butter, lactic acid from buttermilk or other fermented or ripened milks. The other form of organic acidity is that due to the development of acids arising in the process of gastric fermentation, thus lactic acid from bacterial action on carbohydrates, butyric acid from dextrose and in fact any sugar, also from lactic acid. When gastric hydrochloric acidity is normal, bacterial activity is checked and organic acids are not found in the gastric contents unless they are ingested except in minimal amounts.

The dietary treatment of organic acidity depends, of course, first on the prevention of the ingestion of the acids and then upon the omission from the diet of acid-forming bodies, such as wines, butter, sugar and starches. At times it is best to put the patient on a milk diet for two or three days, then to add eggs, meat, fish, green vegetables and fruits, but omitting all farinaceous foods for a time. When all symptoms have subsided, well-toasted bread or cereal food may be allowed once a day, then twice a day and later three times a day and so on until the patient is back to a full mixed dietary.

[1]Lockwood: Diseases of the Stomach, p. 327.

CARCINOMA OF THE STOMACH.

The presence of a cancerous growth anywhere in the body is a guarantee that sooner or later the patient's nutrition will suffer and in spite of a sufficient intake these people lose weight out of apparent proportion to the size of the growth or indeed its location. To this rule there are numerous exceptions and all clinicians are familiar with the latent type of carcinoma that develops silently without giving the usual outward signs of nutritional disturbance until toward the end of the course of the disease. Some of these cases maintain a remarkable degree of nutrition up to the end, but of course, most of them lose very rapidly as the disease progresses and the emaciation in long-standing cases, particularly where the digestive tube is involved, is often extreme. The toxic destruction of tissue protein keeps a negative nitrogen balance in spite of a high protein intake and when the amount taken is below the average normal, the emaciation is especially rapid.

The partial or complete failure of free hydrochloric acid in the gastric secretion is an usual accompaniment of gastric carcinoma at some time in the course of its development, although it may not be evident in the earlier stages, but what is often lost sight of, is the fact that this same hypoacidity may be present, when carcinoma is present at some point remote from the stomach. This fact has in all probability much to do with the disturbances in digestion, as the lack of normal gastric secretion results not only in the lessening of gastric digestion but the normal stimulus for the pancreas and intestine is diminished or wanting and so the normal preparation of food-stuffs for absorption is interfered with, the results of which soon become evident.

Diet in Carcinoma of the Stomach.—The diet suitable for this disease depends principally upon the complications which may be present, and there are some fundamental facts which must be kept in mind.

1. These cases of carcinoma on account of the hypoacidity should be given only moderate amounts of meat products, unless there are other further contra-indications.

2. The gastric motility is apt to be disturbed with delayed emptying of the stomach, particularly in the later stages when this is present, it is necessary to diet according to the rules laid down for myasthenia gastrica (atony).

3. When ulceration is evident one must be governed somewhat by the principles advised for a peptic ulcer diet, in that the foods should be soft and non-irritating. It is not

necessary to reduce the quantity except in the presence of rather extreme ulceration, for there is no chance of healing a carcinomatous ulcer by diet, and it is most important to keep up the patient's nutrition to as high degree as possible, so these patients should be fed to the limit of their capacity with suitable liquids, semiliquids and soft foods.

4. Where ulceration is extreme or the anorexia so severe that nutrition is interfered with out of proportion to the development of the growth, good results may be obtained by duodenal feedings, using liquid foods of high caloric value, as suggested under the chapter on Duodenal Feeding (p. 368). A fair amount can be done in this way to maintain the patient's weight and strength.

The use of an early morning saline drink is especially good both for the cleansing effect on the gastric mucous membrane and for a laxative effect when this is necessary. Those waters with sodium chloride are good for their cleansing effect, particularly as there is usually an absence of chlorides in the stomach. Weisbaden or Carlsbad sprudel represent the two types, Weisbaden that without laxative effect and the Carlsbad when a laxative effect is needed. For most cases Vichy, either French or artificial, 4 ounces, does very well, or failing this, the use of 20 grains of soda bicarbonate and 10 grains of common salt in 6 ounces of water answers every purpose, with the addition of sodium sulphate or phosphate when additional laxative effect is desired.

Most of these patients crave food more highly seasoned than usual and there is no objection to this within reason.

In the apparent absence of ulceration alcohol should be taken only sparingly on account of its tendency to disturb digestion. As an appetizer with meals, a little diluted wine or whiskey finds no contra-indication in fact unless, again ulceration is present. Foods that irritate or ferment readily should not be taken and are hardly likely to be, as anorexia is often a prominent symptom.

When the growth involves either the cardia or pylorus, after a time only liquid food will pass a stricture. This food should be chosen with a view to its concentration as well as its fluid consistency and to this end milk, cream and lactose mixtures, with gruels made from cereals, pea soup with considerable amounts of butter, or purée soups in which cream is a large ingredient, and with ice-cream, made with eggs and liberally sweetened with lactose must form the bulk of the diet. In the preparation of milk to be used in the presence of pyloric stenosis, it is well to boil it first then flavor it with cocoa, coffee, tea, etc., as boiling causes the curd to be fine and soft and to offer less difficulty in passing the pylorus. This is a necessary precaution, as even in the absence of normal gastric digestion whole milk will curd from what little acid there may be present, but the further chymification is interfered with on account of the diminished hydrochloric acid and pepsin, so that the thick curd may remain in the stomach an indefinite length of time. Adding 1 or 2 grains of sodium citrate to each ounce of milk has the effect also of preventing the formation of any but light flocculent curds.

The liquid beef preparations are good as appetizers and for their stimulant effect, but their food value is so small that one must not be deceived by their bulk in thinking that anything of great food value is being given. The malted milk or dried-milk preparations are good to use for the sake of variety, but after all, the more normal the constituents of the diet can be kept the better the appetite and nutrition will be preserved. Any one of the predigested proteins is good to use.

In the presence of hemorrhage, unless excessive, it is not wise to stop food for more than a few hours, although the quality and quantity of food taken afterward might better conform for a time to one of the peptic-ulcer diets, but as already stated, in connection with severe ulceration, the quantity must be rapidly advanced after a day or two of semistarvation, otherwise the loss of flesh and strength will be out of proportion to the uncertain improvement in the pathological condition present.

When the pain from ulceration is so great as to cause great distress on the ingestion of food, it is well to give the patient a 5-grain orthoform tablet to dissolve in the mouth before meals or a small amount of cocaine in solution may be given, ½ or 1 grain, but this should not be done regularly. Anesthesin, 2 per cent., in olive oil may be given in ½-dram doses before meals, or bits of cracked ice with or without a little elixir of menthol[1] may add greatly to the patient's comfort if given before feedings. When the cancerous condition reaches this stage it is of course best to keep up a certain amount of morphine regularly, and the question of gastrostomy or gastroenterostomy must be considered as a temporizing measure.

The relief to certain cases from these operations is, at times, exceedingly great, depending on the anatomical condition present, often permitting the patients to gain weight

[1] Elixir of menthol; Menthol 1.0, Spts, Vin. 25.0, Aq. destil. and Syr. simpl. āā 12.0.

and a certain amount of well-being which may last several months before they finally succumb to the disease. When all else fails resort may be had to rectal feeding, but this, as already pointed out in the chapter on artificial modes of feeding, is inadequate in furnishing sufficient food to maintain life for any considerable length of time, except at a low ebb, and acts as little more than a placebo, although sufficient fluid can be given to prevent great thirst and desiccation.

GASTRIC DILATATION.

In considering the question of gastric dilatation one naturally divides the condition into an obstructive and non-obstructive variety and again into an acute and chronic type.

In the acute form whether from obstruction, such as an arteriomesenteric constriction, in very thin individuals, or obstruction due to acute kinking of the duodenum, or that due to paralytic causes, either central or peripheral, of which postoperative or postanesthetic, overdistention or toxic are the chief varieties,[1] the treatment is identical and so far as diet goes is quickly written. Give nothing whatever by mouth, neither food nor water. The former is not needed for a time and the latter may be supplied by rectal salines, or if necessary by hypodermoclysis. Lavage every two or three hours to remove the accumulated fluid with proper postural treatment with the patient lying well over on the right side or on the stomach are the forms of treatment needed. After it is seen that the dilatation has subsided and one no longer gets the characteristic brownish fluid by the stomach-tube, one can begin to feed small amounts of peptonized milk or gruel, gradually increasing the amount of food and the quality from fluid to semisolid and then to soft until after a period of three or four days to a week one can return to soft solid food, provided the general condition of the patient warrants it.

In the chronic forms of dilatation, if this is due to obstruction at the gastric outlet, one usually finds a good gastric muscle tonus, in fact it is often hypertonic, as the visible peristaltic waves testify; but the difficulty is that the outlet is more or less narrowed so that first, heavy coarse articles of food fail to pass the obstruction, then later ordinary mixed or soft foods cannot leave the stomach completely and stagnate, until finally, in the more advanced stage, even liquids cannot pass the pylorus. Of course before one considers

[1] Lockwood: Diseases of the Stomach, p. 335.

dietetic treatment an accurate diagnosis is necessary for any intelligent mode of action. Having determined the degree of stenosis one gives a diet suitable for the underlying cause whether it be ulcer or simple cicatricial stenosis of varying degree. In the latter, if moderate, only soft diet finely divided, milk citrated to prevent a heavy curd (1 grain sodium citrate to the ounce of milk) or boiled to the same end, may be given, with lavage at bedtime to prevent stagnation. In the more advanced cases when only fluids will pass one can use fully peptonized milk, purée soups, cream soups with butter and meat extract or meat jelly. Of course in such an instance of extreme stenosis, operative procedure must be contemplated and decided upon before the patient loses vitality and strength. If Sippy's claims are substantiated most of the cases due to ulcer and round-celled inflammatory exudate recover without operation on the diet as outlined by him (see p. 360). Where the chronic dilatation is secondary to a general or gastric myasthenia the diet must be in accordance with that laid down for the dietetic treatment of atony (p. 372), and the principles of small dry meals with total reduction of fluid during the twenty-four hours to one quart, or at times less, must be adhered to. Certain authors recommend in this condition small feedings of concentrated soups frequently repeated, and this plan may be followed if that already referred to does not succeed.

The acute form of dilatation is most satisfactory to treat if recognized early, the chronic form most unsatisfactory as a rule, for if the dilatation is due to an actual obstruction, although the diet may be modified as already explained to meet varying degrees of stenosis, the time eventually comes in practically all cases when the case becomes a surgical condition (if indeed it is not from the beginning), and an operation imperative.

GASTRIC NEUROSES.

The forms which gastric neuroses can take are many, but they group themselves naturally about disturbances in— I, secretion; II, sensation, and III, motility.

The neuroses play a much smaller role in diagnosis than they formerly did, since we have come to know that many conditions previously considered neuroses have a definite pathological basis, that, for example, Reichman's disease or continuous gastric secretion can no longer be placed with the neuroses but is due to some form of chronic irritation along the gastro-intestinal canal, and is perhaps most frequently associated with chronic gastric or duodenal ulcer. So too, if one considers the so-called neuroses of sensation we find it necessary to recast most of these diagnoses and the persistent gastralgia formerly classed as a neurosis is now known to betoken real trouble in practically every instance, due to chronic ulcer, appendicitis or gall-bladder disease in most instances. So it goes throughout the entire list; nevertheless there are some real digestive neuroses left belonging to all three classes which require attention, medically and dietetically.

Secretory Neuroses.—By far the greatest number of these cases have an excess of secretion, particularly of hydrochloric acid. This gives rise to nervous hyperchlorhydria with its attendant symptoms of acid eructation, belching, constipation, etc., all coming on at times of stress when the nervous system is overirritated, as for example in students preparing for examination, young speakers and actors. Even in these cases if there is continued repetition of the symptoms one must be on the lookout for a pathological basis. The diet here should be that described for hyperchlorhydria, avoidance of all irritants must be insisted upon, such as: chemical, *e. g.*, acids, alcohol and condiments; mechanical, *e. g.*, seeds or hard substances; thermal, *e. g.*, hot or iced drinks or foods; and as well, food should be simply prepared, eaten slowly at regular intervals and with full attention to proper methods of eating. The general hygiene of the nervous system should also receive attention (see Hyperchlorhydria). Excessive secretion may at times be purely nervous, but continuous secretion is usually of pathological significance.

In other cases the neurosis takes the form of a hypoacidity even to an achylia gastrica which has been supposed at times to be of nervous origin, although probably even in many of these an anatomical basis may be found. The diet for this should be that advised for hyposecretion or achylia gastrica (see p. 343) and in general should be stimulating but not irritating.

Neuroses of Sensation.—All sorts of morbid gastric sensations may be felt by the neurasthenic, ranging from merely a sense of uneasiness or fulness to actual pain, the latter, however, as already stated if persistent or recurring is almost always due to some pathological state of the digestive tube itself and is not a neurosis. The treatment here should be of course, largely along neurological lines, the diet must be full, simple and nutritious and if the symptoms occur in patients (especially women) who are thin, and so to speak "on wires" nervously, they should be put to bed and given the rest cure regimen, such as that devised by Wier Mitchell or some modification of it. The digestive symptoms usually disappear within the first week of this routine.

Motor Neuroses.—Many of the abnormal sensations included under this last group are due to a nervously disturbed gastro-intestinal musculature, giving rise to peristaltic unrest which in a normal state passes unnoticed, but which loom large to the nervous person. Another and familiar form of motor disturbance is seen in nervous vomiting which is often so difficult to control. All these forms of motor neuroses must be treated first from a general hygienic and neurological point of view by hydrotherapy, suggestion, etc., diet may often be ignored and in many instances if we can gain the patient's confidence they can often be told to eat anything they want and it will many times be found that such seeming indulgence works wonderfully well, anything within reason being digested. At other times one must treat these cases as one does a stomach which is irritable from some pathological cause, for often a digestive organ that has been misbehaving for a long time develops a secondary irritation which is real and must be definitely treated by a diet that is useful in any irritable stomach, e. g., fluids, as milk and Vichy or buttermilk and Vichy, egg albumen in cracked ice and water, iced bouillon, iced malted milk, gruels, thin soft solids, cereals, custards, blanc mange, soft eggs, cream toast, back to solids with white meat of chicken, baked farina, vermicelli, noodles and by degrees to a normal dietary.

GASTRIC TEST MEALS.

Ewald-Boas Test Breakfast.—Water, 400 c.c. (13 oz.); bread or roll, 40 gm. (1⅓ oz.). Given on an empty stomach. Expressed by aspiration one hour later.

Ewald Test Dinner.—Chopped meat 165 gm. (6 oz.); stale bread, 35 gm. (1 oz.); butter. Aspirate three hours afterward.

Test Meal of Germain, See.—Chopped meat, 100 to 150 gm. (3 ⅓ to 5 oz.); white bread, 60 to 80 gm. (2 to 2⅔ oz.); water, 300 c.c. (10 oz.). Examine contents two hours later.

Reigel's Test Dinner.—Meat broth, 400 c.c. (13 oz.); beefsteak, 150 to 200 gm. (5 to 7 oz.); mashed potato, 50 gm. (1⅔ oz.); roll, 35 gm. (1 oz.). Should be aspirated four hours later.

Klemperer's Test Meal.—Milk, 500 c.c. (1 pt.); 2 rolls (70 gm.). Give on empty stomach and aspirate two hours later.

Boas (*Non-lactic Acid-containing*) *Test Meal.*—One oz. (30 gm.) rolled oats boiled in 1 pt. (500 c.c.) water; salt q. s., or 2 shredded wheat biscuits with 300 c.c. (10 oz.) water. To use when testing for lactic acid the stomach should be washed out the night before.

Salzer's Double Test Meal.—Beef, 40 gm. (1⅓ oz.), scraped and broiled; milk, 250 c.c. (8 oz.); boiled rice, 50 gm. (1⅔ oz.); 1 soft-boiled egg. Four hours later give Ewald-Boas test meal and remove one hour afterward.

The Ewald meal may be used or one pint of gruel made of strained oatmeal or any cereal just thin enough to be aspirated through the small tube ordinarily used. A sample of the gastric contents is aspirated and tested chemically ½, 1, 1½, 2 and 2½ hours after taking the meal.

GASTRIC MOTOR MEALS.

Von Luebe.—Soup, 400 c.c. (13 oz.); beef, 200 gm. (6⅔ oz.); bread, 50 gm. (1⅔ oz.); water, 200 c.c. (6⅔ oz.). If at the end of six hours gastric lavage fails to show a residue, the motor power of the stomach is normal.

Boas.—If two hours after an Ewald-Boas test meal the stomach is empty by lavage, there is normal motor power.

Hausman's Stagnation Test Meal.—Four tablespoonfuls of boiled rice and a glass of water are given at 9 P. M. (a little sugar and milk may be taken on the rice). If at 9 A. M. next morning fasting, lavage fails to show macroscopic or microscopic rice residue, there is no stagnation. (A drop of Lugol's solution stains any starch granules blue so that they are easily seen.)

Test Supper.—For supper, meat, bread, butter and water or two cups of tea. Lavage in the morning following should fail to show any residue in a normal stomach.

Water Test for Acidity.[1]—Carlson, Orr, Hanke, Brackman and Rehfuss all observed that the taking of water stimulated gastric secretion, producing an acidity that was about 100 in less than twenty minutes after stimulation. They found that in ten to twenty minutes 500 c.c. (10 oz.) of water would leave the stomach (? Ed.) and also that after drinking 50 c.c. (1⅔ oz.) of water as much as 225 c.c. (7 oz.) of gastric juice could be obtained.

Austin's meal directions are as follows, partially based on the foregoing: Previous evening the patient takes a meal of meat, potato, bread, butter, rice and raisins and presents himself the next morning for examination, fasting. Then

[1] Austin: Boston Med. and Surg. Jour., 1915, clxxii, 857.

350 c.c. (12 oz.) of water are given and removed by the stomach-tube in twenty minutes. Austin found the total acid values much lower than those already quoted, varying from 19 to 31.

Intestinal Motor Meal (Schmidt-Strassburger).—With the meal two capsules, each containing 0.5 gm. (7½ gr.) of charcoal are given to mark the meal, then the following: finely cut meat, 80 gm. (2⅔ oz.); mashed potato, 200 gm. (6⅔ oz.); eggs (2); butter, 40 gm. (1⅓ oz.); oatmeal gruel made with milk, 1500 c.c. (3 pt.); clear soup, 250 c.c. (8 oz.;) very dry toast or zweiback, 100 gm. (3⅓ oz.). In health it is said this should pass through the intestine in fifteen to twenty-five hours. In diarrhea due to colitis, in ten to fifteen hours. In enterocolitis with diarrhea, in three to five hours (Strauss).

For further intestinal test diet see Schmidt, Intestinal Diet (p. 387).

CHAPTER XXI.

DIET IN DISEASES OF THE INTESTINES.

In diseases of the intestines, no less than in gastric disturbances, diet plays a most important role, not alone from the therapeutic standpoint but from that of prevention as well. Another interesting development of more recent years is the effect of various foods on the intestinal flora and the possibility of changing this at will by the institution of a definite diet.

One group of bacteria designated as putrefactive thrive particularly in the large intestine.[1] A second group, the fermentation bacteria, may also thrive and where they do acid conditions are likely to arise which inhibit the growth of the putrefactive organisms. According to Hester and Kendall[2] the absence of carbohydrate in the diet allows the proteolytic bacteria to predominate,—this is told by the fecal discharges, as well as the finding of indican and its congeners in the urine.

Torry[3] found in typhoid cases fed with an unusual quantity of lactose that the ordinary type of flora was changed to one largely cominated by the bacillus acidophilus. Lactose and dextrine added to a meat and rice diet caused a marked development of aciduric bacteria of the bacillus acodophilus type almost to the suppression of the proteolytic type. Glucose did not have this effect. Starchy food also had the tendency to eliminate the putrefactive bacteria. Protein foods failed to produce a stereotyped change. Milk for example was less likely to give rise to putrefaction than did meat. Torrey also found that vegetable protein was less likely to encourage the putrefactive bacteria than animal protein. Fats seemed to lack a determining influence.

From all this it can be readily seen that the dieting of some cases of chronic intestinal disturbances must be founded on carefully collected data in which the examination of the stools, not only for gross and chemical changes but for bacterial divergences from the normal is made.

Then too, certain cases of diarrhea originate from abnormalities in the gastric or pancreatic secretions, which must be tested if one is to come to a rational etiological diagnosis. Thus one sees cases diagnosed as chronic enteritis

[1] Ed. Jour. Am. Men. Assn. May 10, 1919, page 1370.
[2] Jour. Biol. Chem, 1910, vii, 203.
[3] Jour. Inf. Dis., 1915, xvi, 72.

in which the intestine is practically normal except for slight secondary inflammatory changes and the diarrhea is caused by a failure of gastric secretion, the so-called gastrogenic diarrhea already referred to. In the intestine too, we have the most marked examples of functional neurosis, due to lack of nervous stability, resulting in diarrhea of various types, as well as constipation.

ACUTE ENTERITIS.

Enteritis, or inflammation of the small intestine, is of frequent occurrence and one has only to glance over the etiological factors to realize how many conditions there are that may give rise to it. Among these causes may be mentioned dietary indiscretions, unhygienic surroundings, frequent exposure to sudden atmospheric changes, irritants, as some acids, mercury, arsenic, cantharides, copper, tartar emetic, garlic, alcohol. Blood irritants, seen in uremic conditions; mechanical irritants; bacillary infections of the intestinal tract; parasites; the exanthemata; chronic constipation; intestinal obstruction; disturbances of circulation; drinking ice-water to excess,[1] etc.

The inflammation may affect any part of the small bowel, so that we may have a duodenitis (distinguishable from the other locations on account of the frequency of a complicaing jaundice); jejunitis and ileitis. Aside from the duodenitis, of course it is impossible clinically to distinguish which part of the bowel is involved.

Conheim[2] *divides* enteritis into:

1. Mild enteritis without diarrhea, but with numerous symptoms, such as meteorism, abdominal pains, flatulence and loss of strength.

2. Moderately severe enteritis with much intestinal fermentation and frequent diarrhea.

3. Severe cases with persistent diarrhea.

The dietetic treatment of the acute cases resolves itself into a negative and positive phase. Under the former we are content during the acute onset to withhold all food for twenty-four hours or possibly longer, giving only water and a good cathartic to relieve the bowels of any offending matter; for in spite of the diarrhea which is present in the moderate or severe cases, nature usually needs assistance in this.

This is particularly true in the severe acute type, ordinarily known as cholera morbus. After the preliminary period of

[1] Gant: Diarrhea Inflammation and Parasitic Intestinal Diseases, p. 176.
[2] Forchheimer: Therapeutics, iii, 197.

25

starvation one may begin feeding thin gruels, albumin water, rice, or toast, water and weak tea. Milk is best left out of the diet at the outset, for it is seldom properly digested while peristalsis is so active and even in the late stages it fails to agree as well as some of the carbohydrate or other protein foods. Some cases, however, do well on boiled milk, for the boiling causes it to respond to the gastric enzymes in a fine flocculent curd; in still others it can be given advantageously raw and over long periods. When the disease reaches the subacute stage in mild cases, one may feed most of the soft foods, such as eggs, soft meats, sweetbreads, stewed or boiled chicken, creamed fresh cod, halibut and whitefish. If there is not much flatulence one may give the fine cereals well cooked, farina, cream of wheat, rice, wheatena, malted breakfast food with a little butter and salt. These cereals are not good when there is a tendency to or actual excessive carbohydrate fermentation in the intestine, as shown by explosive acid stools and an active formation of CO_2 in the fermentation tube. Later on soft-cooked or purée vegetables put through a colander are allowable, such as spinach, peas, potatoes, carrots and celery, but as a rule vegetables should be left out of the diet on account of their laxative effect. Soft custards, blanc mange, farina or rice pudding and gelatin desserts are allowable in the mild or subacute cases.

There are very definite foods which should not be eaten at any time in any type of this trouble, such as coarse or irritating foods, those which ferment easily or putrify readily, and all the foods given must be soft and free from indigestible particles. Not much sugar should be given. Wines, beer or champagne are not allowed with the exception that in the later stages a little diluted claret or sherry may be permitted.

Among the vegetables under the ban are cauliflower, turnips, cabbage, radishes, onions, tomatoes, celery root, oyster plant and Brussels sprouts. No fruit may be taken, nor cake, rich jellies or other sweets. Rich cheese, high meat or game are also forbidden.

In general the milder the case, the less strict need the diet be and *vice versa*.

CHRONIC ENTERITIS.

This may be chronic from the start or may be the remains of an acute attack, the etiology being the same as that of the acute cases, but acting more slowly, or it may be an accompaniment of other diseases of the bowels as, *e. g.*, carcinoma, intestinal obstruction, fecal impaction, etc.[1] In the chronic forms of enteritis, it is particularly satisfactory to make a

[1] Stengel, in Osler's Mod. Med., 1914, 2d ed.

definite test of the patient's digestion as affecting the proteins, fats and carbohydrates, after which it is possible to plan a rational diet suited to that individual's needs.

This is arrived at most certainly by placing the patient on a Schmidt test diet, which is as follows:

Schmidt Test Diet.—*In the morning*, 0.5 liter (16 oz.) milk, or, if milk does not agree, 0.5 liter (16 oz.) cocoa, prepared from 20 gm. (⅔ oz.) cocoa powder, 10 gm. (⅓ oz.); sugar, 400 c.c. (13 oz.) water and 100 c.c. (3⅓ oz.) milk.

In the forenoon. 0.5 liter (16 oz.) oatmeal gruel, made from 40 gm. (1⅓ oz.) oatmeal, 10 gm. (⅓ oz.) butter, 200 c.c. (6½ oz.) milk, 300 c.c. (10 oz.) water; 1 egg strained.

At noon, 125 gm. (4 oz.) chopped beef (raw weight), broiled rare with 20 gm. (⅔ oz.) of butter, so that the interior will still remain raw. To this add 250 gm. (8 oz.) potato broth, made of 190 gm. (6⅓ oz.) mashed potatoes, 100 c.c. (3⅓ oz.) milk, and 10 gm. (⅓ oz.) butter.

In the *afternoon* as in the morning.

In the *evening* as in the forenoon.

This diet consists of:

Milk	1.5 liters (1½ qt.)
Zwieback	100.0 gm. (3½ oz.)
Eggs	2.0
Butter	50.0 gm. (1 [")
Beef	125.0 gm. (4 ")
Potatoes	190.0 gm. (6½ ")
Oatmeal (gruel)	80.0 gm. (2⅔ ")

This contains protein, 102 gm. (3⅓ oz.); fat, 111 gm. (4 oz.); carbohydrates, 191 gm. (6⅓ oz.); calories, 2234.

In order to carry this diet out most satisfactorily it is best to give it for a couple of days and then give two capsules each containing 10 grains of charcoal. This is given again at the end of the test period of two, three or four days as may have been decided and the stools and urine saved accurately for the period which is marked at its beginning and end by the charcoal.

The result of the examination of the feces will show whether the stools contain undigested food, meat fibers connective tissue, free starch, fat drops, fatty acid crystals, soaps or parasites. At the same time the pancreatic ferments may be tested for and the presence of carbohydrate and protein fermentation disclosed if it is present. Also the prevailing bacterial growth whether Gram-negative (normal) or Gram-positive.

It will be found that a good many patients, particularly women and especially so if both their stomach and intestinal digestion are poor, cannot take the full Schmidt diet, the quantity is too great. In such instances the test diet as modified by the author will be found very serviceable as containing the proper proportions of food elements and of sufficient caloric value.

MODIFIED SCHMIDT DIET.

			Protein.	Fat.	Carbohydrate.	Calories.
Oatmeal .	. 165 gm.	(5½ oz.)	4.4	0.8	18.2	100
Rice .	. . 90 "	(3 ")	2.4	0.8	21.0	100
Milk .	. . 1500 c.c.	(50 ")	49.5	60.0	67.5	1080
Butter .	. 40 gm.	(1⅓ ")	0.6	34.0	..	318
Bread .	. 120 gm.	(4 ")	13.1	2.4	80.0	400
Chopped meat	65 gm.	(2 ")	17.1	4.7	..	100
			87.1 gm.	102.7 gm.	186.7 gm.	2088

Breakfast.	Dinner.	Supper.
Oatmeal, 165 gm. (5½ oz.)	Meat, 65 gm. (1 oz.)	Rice, 90 gm. (3 oz.)
Milk, 250 c.c. (3 ")	Bread, 40 " (1⅓ ")	Bread, 40 " (1⅓ ")
Bread 40 gm. (1⅓ ")	Milk, 250 c.c. (8 ")	Butter, 15 " (½ ")
Butter, 15 " (½ ")	Butter, 10 gm. (⅓ ")	Milk, 250 c.c. (8 ")
At 10, 3, and 9 o'clock, 250 c.c. milk.		

Having determined the digestive capacity of the pancreatic or intestinal enzymes by the use of the Schmidt diet, the task still remains of constructing a suitable diet for these patients. Chronic enteritis is not a condition that shows rapid improvement and weeks and months must often elapse before anything like satisfactory progress can be expected. On this account patients must be warned and told to expect slow changes, as otherwise they are quite sure to become discouraged and blame their medical attendant for failure to improve rapidly. When the stools show undigested food, whether diarrhea is present or not, the diet is not what it should be and the first constant aim must be to get a diet that can be digested, showing a normally smooth stool, even though its consistence may be too soft or fluid. This, of course, can only be done by painstaking changes with constant stool inspection to check up the condition of digestion.

It is usually a good plan in starting the dietary treatment of these cases to begin with a liquid or semiliquid diet. Just which combination of foods will fit the individual case can only be determined by trial, but an ordinarily successful plan is to feed them every two hours with gruel, malted milk, cocoa and soft egg alternately. Some cases digest boiled milk well and it is often deserving of a trial. If it is not digested as shown by curds and more active diarrhea then it should be omitted, even in the cocoa which should then be made with water. After a few days of this rigid diet, one may begin to add one extra at a time, preferably with every other feeding. *i. e.*, every four hours. These extras may be in the form of fine cereal, farina, cream of wheat, wheatena, eaten with a little butter and salt or with a little malted milk over them. Then dry toast with or without butter is added. After which one may keep on gradually increasing the foods to boiled rice, macaroni, dry cheese, cream cheese, toasted crackers. By this time, it is well to lengthen the feeding interval to three or four hours. The character of the diet can be changed as rapidly as improvement in symptoms comes, adding next finely minced chicken and sweetbreads, lamb, boiled fresh white-meated fish. Desserts made of gelatin, egg or farinaceous puddings, later cream desserts, all made with the minimum amount of sugar. All vegetables should be left out of the diet for a long time, but when taken they should be thoroughly cooked, soft, and put through a colander, or in the form of a purée. Fruits should be added last and then only well-cooked, soft fruits, such as baked apple (without the skin), apple sauce, etc. Of course, fruit should not be given until the stools are of normal consistence and well digested and it will be probably weeks or months after starting treatment before it can be given.

ACUTE COLITIS OR ACUTE DYSENTERY.

Acute dysentery is caused by a variety of factors, bacillary, protozoon and constitutional, and results in an acutely inflamed colon mucous membrane which may or may not go on to ulceration, depending on the form and severity of the exciting cause. It is often found as a part of an infection involving the small intestine as an enterocolitis, or it occurs alone.

When it occurs as part of an infection higher up, the dietary treatment is in accordance with the needs of the small intestine, when it occurs alone it is often very sudden and severe in its onset and requires great care in treatment. After a complete emptying of the bowel by catharsis, it is a good plan to withhold food for twenty-four hours in order to quiet the peristalsis, using opium or other antiperistaltic agent. When feedings are begun they should be liquid and at first largely protein, as whey, albumin water and clear soups, then gruel made of oatmeal, farina or wheat cereals or koumyss: sweet milk should not be given, as it tends to increase the diarrhea, although this is less marked if the milk is boiled. Later scraped meat, dry toast, well cooked, fine cereals, soft-boiled or poached eggs, macaroni, well-boiled rice, weak tea or a little dilute whiskey or claret form the bulk of the diet. When the acute symptoms subside the patients are either well or the disease goes on into the chronic stage. In the acute stage fruit and vegetables are to be avoided. In the severe forms, withholding food for several days is often a good plan.

CHRONIC COLITIS.

Whatever the origin of the colitis or whatever pathological form it takes, there are certain dietary conditions which must be taken into consideration and met in all cases.

1. That the diet must be made up of easily digestible foods.

2. That the foods must not be stimulating to peristalsis.

3. That all food must be finely subdivided, soft and with as little digestive residue as possible.

4 The quantity of food must be sufficient for complete nutrition in nitrogen and caloric content.

As to the first point the foods particularly suitable are:—clear, cream or purée soups, white-meated fish; (other richer forms later if they agree wth gastric digestion); soft part of oysters, beef, mutton, chicken, sweetbreads, eggs, fine cereals, farina, cream of wheat, malted breakfast food, wheatena, tea, coffee, cocoa made with water, butter, toast, stale bread, roll, purée of vegetables such as potato, lima beans, peas, spinach, stewed celery, baked Hubbard squash. (In many cases no green vegetables can be taken at all on account of increased peristalsis.) Farinaceous puddings, gelatin desserts, egg desserts. (For food stimulating to peristalsis see Section on Diarrhea.) In general it may be said that fruits, coarse vegetables (in some cases any vegetables), very sweet foods, much fat food, are all stimulating and must be avoided. Milk is also in this class for most patients, although occasionally a patient can take it boiled or diluted with gruels. Sometimes koumyss will be better digested than plain milk. White wine, beer, ale and champagne are contra-indicated.

That patients should receive sufficient food for nutritional uses is self-evident, but it is not by any means easy to nourish many of these patients completely, as there is often much anorexia, and if pain is also present, it is still more difficult to feed them.

In the long-standing cases, particularly those due to ulcerative colitis, malnutrition is more or less the rule and some patients lose as much as half their body weight, it being impossible to get them to take a sufficient supply, and the ingenuity of the physician is put to a severe test. In these long-standing and severe cases the use of artificial food materials is often useful (see Artificial Foods) to fortify soups and gruels.

MEMBRANOUS COLITIS, MUCOUS COLIC OR CHRONIC MUCOUS COLITIS.

It was formerly thought that these cases were in the last analysis of a neurotic origin, occurring only in nervous persons; and while many of the patients were nervous it was also observed that the disease occurred in those who were not at all so. Nothnagle was largely responsible for this general belief, but time has proven it untenable when applied to the cases as a class. The characteristic feature of the disease is the passage of mucous strips, bits, ribbons or even entire casts of parts of the colon and accompanied by more or less abdominal pain. There are two groups[1] ordinarily distinguished.

1. Those with pain along the colon and a tendency to diarrhea, *i. e.*, chronic mucous colitis.

2. Those occurring in nervous persons who have chronic constipation and attacks of "membranous colitis" or "mucous colic."

The diet in the first group is so constructed as to spare the bowel as much irritation as possible and consists largely of albuminous foods together with farinaceous gruels, all coarse foods are excluded as well as vegetables and fruits, the rest of the feedings are as already described in the section on Enteritis or Chronic Colitis. In the second group there is really a catarrh of the bowel and in addition chronic constipation. Von Noorden fastened upon the chronic constipation as the essential feature of the disease and by combating this was able to clear up the mucous stools. In order to accomplish this he prescribed a diet with much cellulose, indigestible residue in skins and seeds, coarse black or rye bread, crude vegetables, raw or cooked, but the rougher the better, cabbage, tomatoes, turnips, carrots, celery, cauliflower, Brussels sprouts, corn, etc., also large amounts of fats in the form of cream, butter, fat meats and oils. Cider and buttermilk are both good for this purpose.

The following diet devised by Butman is recommended and is also good for chronic constipation generally.

On rising a glass of cold water.

> *Breakfast:* Oatmeal, whole wheat or graham bread (or bran bread), butter, coffee, raw or cooked fruit. Marmalade (honey).

[1] Forchheimer, vol. iii.

Midmorning: A glass of buttermilk or cider, or water, dried fruit, figs, dates or prunes.

Luncheon: A small amount of meat, fish or other seafood, two or more green vegetables, coarse bread, butter. Fruit.

Midafternoon: A glass of buttermilk or cider, etc.

Dinner: Fruit, meat or fish, two or more green vegetables, coarse bread, butter (bran bread or biscuits), salad, dessert, preferably a fruit dessert.

Bedtime: Same as midmorning.

Or the diet recommended under Chronic Constipation.

ULCERATION OF THE SMALL OR LARGE INTESTINE.

Ulceration of the small or large bowel occurs in a variety of conditions, *e. g.*, simple ulceration as in duodenal ulcer or as the result of typhoid fever, tuberculosis or other bacterial or protozoan diseases.

In simple or typhoid ulceration the diet has already been described under these headings. In tuberculous ulceration and that due to other bacteria, as in chronic dysentery or amebic dysentery, the dietary regulations are practically alike. The diet should be free of irritating foods, seeds, skins, raw vegetables or those with a rough residue, as corn, bran, etc. Everything should be exceedingly soft and of moderate bulk. When diarrhea is present one must be governed in the selection of food by a knowledge of what foods are naturally laxative and avoid them, using on the contrary the classes of foods which have been described under Enteritis and Diarrheal Diseases in general.

Laxative foods include fruit, vegetables, indigestible fats, sugars, game, "high" meat, malt liquors, rough substances, such as bran.

INTESTINAL HEMORRHAGE.

The diet in intestinal hemorrhage, if at all severe, should be regulated much as has already been described under Hemorrhage in Typhoid. All food by mouth should be stopped at once. If the hemorrhage is from a point high up in the intestine, as that from duodenal ulceration, not even water should be given for from forty-eight to seventy-two hours. (See Duodenal Ulcer, p. 349.) If the patient is desiccated it will be necessary to give warm saline by the rectal route within six hours of the hemorrhage, either as a continuous Murphy drip, or in repeated amounts of 4 to 6 ounces every two, three or four hours. If the hemorrhage is from lower down, as from the ilium in typhoid, water may be begun within six hours, and within twelve to twenty-four hours one may again begin mouth feedings with broth, albumin water, malted milk or diluted citrated milk (1 grain of sodium citrate to the ounce). After another six to twelve hours the feedings may be gradually and steadily increased again until full fluids are being taken. It is not necessary to interdict water in these cases and this may be given in small amounts, frequently repeated two or three hours after the hemorrhage. Large or very hot enemata of water should not be given on account of their tendency to dilate the abdominal vessels, which of course, increases the danger of hemorrhage. When the hemorrhage is from the colon, it is scarcely ever severe enough to cause anxiety and only in exceptionally large hemorrhages need one hesitate to continue giving fluids by mouth. Of course, under this circumstance no fluid should be given by rectum.

DIARRHEA.

As diarrhea is merely a symptom, a classification of its etiology would include a discussion of every condition which may give rise to this symptom, the treatment being often quite as various as the etiology.

The Causes of Diarrhea.—In general the causes of diarrhea may be enumerated as follows:

Gastrogenic.—When achylia gastrica is present this in some way predisposes to diarrhea, probably the lack of acid secretion fails to call out the pancreatic enzymes sufficiently to properly digest the food, and diarrhea results.

Toxic.—In cases of chronic Bright's, diarrhea is often present and represents the attempt of nature to eliminate water, chlorides, toxic material and probably nitrogen by way of the intestinal mucosa, being therefore a vicarious diarrhea. Other varieties of toxic origin are seen in the acute bacterial intestinal diseases, typhoid, cholera and cholera morbus; ptomaine toxemia including all forms of food poisoning, which are almost invariably accompanied by diarrhea. The toxic effect of the inorganic salts must also be included, principally arsenic, mercury and antimony, and to the milder toxic infections, such as intestinal catarrh, acute and chronic.

Irritative Diarrhea, which may be toxic or merely mechanical, as the eating of quantities of indigestible food such as corn, fruit in excess, etc., excess of gastric HCl.

Drug Diarrhea, due to ingestion of laxative drugs which if taken in excessive amount or over long periods, often continue the diarrhea after the complete elimination of the drug which is then probably due to a catarrhal inflammation. Ulcerative conditions of the gastro-intestinal tract—peptic, tuberculous and simple ulcer or the numerous forms of diarrhea due to a diseased colon.

Nervous Diarrhea.—Many people have this difficulty in the face of some unusual excitement, soldiers, musicians, and in hysteria and are all due to vasomotor dilatation in an unstable nervous system, causing the so-called "sweating" of the intestine. Under this heading the diarrhea of hyperthyroidism may belong, although this is quite as likely to be due to the general toxemia seen in these cases. Reflex diarrhea is also of nervous origin.

Habit Diarrhea.—Some persons normally have several more or less watery stools a day or they may have a morning diarrhea, often due to catarrh, however.

Diarrhea due to Food Idiosyncrasy.—In these cases some one article of food may habitually excite a diarrhea quite apart from any known toxic or mechanical effect, although it is probably of toxic origin in the last analysis.

Diarrhea of Pancreatic Origin.—Where the ferments are deficient, as the well-known fatty diarrhea.

Diarrhea occurring as secondary to periods of fecal impaction with a tunneling of the fecal mass, or alternating with severe constipation.

With all these forms of diarrhea the etiology gives the clue to the dietetic treatment and an accurate diagnosis is always essential to a satisfactory and intelligent ordering of foods.

It is unfortunately not possible to find in every cases the actual cause, so that the clinician is not infrequently called upon to prescribe a diet for diarrhea in which the etiology is obscure and eludes the most painstaking investigation. The underlying principles are much the same in ordering diets for almost all the forms of diarrhea and may be described as follows:

Dietary Regulations.—The diet should be non-irritating, easily digested, not a stimulant of peristalsis, free from taint of putrefaction, finely comminuted and should include as many articles of food that are naturally astringent as possible, and not apt to ferment.

In acute diarrhea from any cause a period of starvation following an intestinal purge is the best dietetic routine, allowing fresh but not cold water in abundance. When the appetite begins to demand food, clear broth, beef tea, cereal gruels, dry toast and tea are best for a day or two, gradually extending the list from foods which are allowed in chronic diarrhea.

Foods to Avoid in Chronic Diarrhea.—Very fatty foods, except a moderate amount of butter. Raw milk and cream. Green vegetables of all sorts. Boiled potato. Corn is especially irritant. Fruit in all forms is forbidden, whether stewed or fresh. Salads, nuts, pickles, condiments. Salt meat or salt fish. Smoked meats or fish. Goose, duck, pork as too fat. Sweets, cake, pie, candy, and preserves. Cream or milk desserts. Sweet wine, beer and ale.

Foods Recommended in Diarrhea.—Clear soups, white-meated fish (not fatty), *e. g.*, cod, halibut, bass. Chicken, mutton or lamb, scraped beef, soft part of oysters. Guinea hen. Soft eggs. Rice, macaroni, noodles. Baked potato may agree. Cereals except oatmeal or Pettijohn. Stale bread or dry toast, crust of roll. Toasted crackers. Cream, Edam, Canadian cheese. Farinaceous puddings made with little sugar, preferably baked. Calf's foot or wine jelly. Tea, clear coffee (in some cases this is laxative), water, claret, Burgundy. A little diluted whiskey or brandy. In some instances malted milk is well tolerated, while in others it is laxative. In a few cases it is possible to give boiled milk, but for the most part milk in any form is very badly tolerated causing an increase in the diarrhea with the passage of undigested curds.

Foods Allowed in Certain Cases.—The use of malted milk or cereal is useful unless it proves laxative. Crisp bacon, turkey, koumyss, zoolak, buttermilk. Thoroughly stewed celery, baked Hubbard squash, creamed spinach, tender boiled peas or lima beans mashed through a colander, removing the skins.

Chronic Diarrhea—Cohnheim's Diet List (American Modification).

7.00 A.M.　Mineral water, 75 to 150 c.c. (2½ to 5 oz.), taken hot on rising. The choice of water will depend on gastric secretions, with hypo-acidity or achylia, sodium chloride and alkaline waters are best. At home 10 grains of salt and 10 of bicarbonate of soda may be added to the allowance of hot water.

7.30 A.M.　Philip's digestible cocoa (2 teaspoonfuls to a cup) made with water. Toasted white bread and butter.

10.30 A.M.　Fine cereal, cream of wheat or farina or malted breakfast food, one soft-boiled egg or scraped meat or lamb chop cut fine.

1.00 P.M.   Broth with macaroni, vermicelli or noodles. In mild cases vegetable purées. One glass of claret.

4.00 P.M.   Same as 7.30 A.M.

6.00 P.M.   Mineral water as in early morning.

7.00 to 8.00 P.M.   Tea with claret. Toast, butter and a little cold chicken.

9.00 to 10.00 P.M.   A cup of hot peppermint tea or chamomile tea. If the case is mild and the stools soft rather than liquid, some soft carrots, fillet of sole or baked fish is allowed.

Absolutely Forbidden Articles.—Cold drinks, all rough or coarse vegetables, such as cabbage, potatoes, cheese, sweets, coffee. All legumes unless served in soups; goose, duck, fat fish as salmon, mackerel, blue fish, meat fats, gravies, raw fruits.

INTESTINAL NEUROSES.

These follow much the same classification as the gastric neuroses except that the intestinal pain of a purely nervous origin is rare and as a diagnosis should only be made after a careful process of exclusion and even then with reservation. The diet in these intestinal cases is much on the same lines as that recommended for definite intestinal pathological states which symptomatically they often so closely simulate, *e. g.*, in nervous constipation. Besides the general tonic treatment of the nervous system, the diet should be that recommended for chronic constipation with a large percentage of roughage in the form of fruits, vegetables and bran. With the opposite condition, namely, that of a nervous diarrhea, a diet such as that advised for chronic diarrhea is advisable (p. 394). On the other hand, one sees not a few cases of a type of nervous diarrhea which present a characteristic picture of an undernourished, anemic, worried, irritable individual, man or woman, who gives a history of a diarrhea of month's or years' standing, from whom the history is obtained that little by little they have curtailed their diet with the idea that first one thing, then another disagrees and causes the diarrhea, until they are living on perhaps only three or four articles of food with an entirely inadequate number of calories. The stools are more or less numerous, liquid or semiliquid which on analysis show no other abnormal characteristic than possibly some little mucus and a few leukocytes. If one is sure of one's ground in dealing with these people and can reassure them and gain their confidence it is usually possible to begin feeding them liberally at once and a good meal of finely cut tenderloin, baked potato or rice, green peas and a simple dessert will do more to restore confidence than anything else. The character of the stool may not change at once, but will usually return to normal within a few days and the diet can then be rapidly increased to a general mixed one with full confidence that it will be satisfactorily digested.

The anemia should also be treated and a general course of sensible hygiene insisted upon.

CHRONIC CONSTIPATION.

If an aboriginal text-book on medicine should be found, it would probably be noted that there was no chapter on chronic constipation, this being a disease of modern life, a product of inactivity and a non-stimulating diet. The causes of constipation are numerous, some predisposing, some direct. Faulty habits of eating are most largely responsible and a diet with little residue from cellulose will be very apt to result in constipation. Any condition which tends to the weakening of the voluntary or involuntary muscles will also tend to produce or exaggerate a tendency to constipation, such as illnesses of all kinds, lazy habits of exercise and irregularity in attempted evacuation, all have much to do with it. Chronic constitutional diseases producing a congestion of the abdominal organs will result in constipation.

Varieties of Constipation.—The cases divide themselves into:

1. Functional, either (*a*) atonic or (*b*) spastic.

2. Organic from mechanical obstruction of the lumen of the gut, from within or without.

Of all forms, the atonic comprises most of the cases, possibly 90 per cent., and is due to a lazy or inactive bowel. The spastic variety is the direct opposite of this, in that it occurs as a product of overstimulation of the intestinal nerve-endings, giving rise to spastic contraction of the bowel and pain. The form of constipation due to mechanical obstruction speaks for itself and is of only minor interest from a dietetic point of view.

In the atonic constipation, every means possible must be used to awaken the bowel by mechanical stimulation, as by massage, exercise of the abdominal muscles and general body exercise, calisthenics or out-of-door work.

In the selection of a diet the two important facts to be remembered are that the food must be as coarse and rough as possible, and that all sorts of fats are very valuable in promoting ease of evacuation. In many or most of the patients suffering from chronic constipation, the stools are of small bulk and the more severe the constipation the smaller the bulk of the stool, as the sluggishness gives an extra amount of time for the further and more complete disintegration and absorption of the foods. In other words, digestion and absorption are often at their highest in chronic constipation, and if there was not sometimes absorption of other things besides the food, such as various digestive by-products and the products of bacterial putrefaction, chronic constipation would not be so undesirable. As it is, the condition is not ordinarily a favorable one for health or well-being; although there are many cases who do not have a movement of the bowels more often than once or twice a week, yet who seem to keep in perfect health and vigor.

Taking food into the stomach at once excites not only peristalsis of the stomach but also of the bowels and particularly of the caput coli, so that there is good physiological reason for the desire to defecate shortly after a meal and particularly after breakfast, which should be the preferable time for evacuation. Peristalsis is especially "stimulated by indigestible meat residue, vegetable fiber, cellulose, sugar and organic acids. Peptones stimulate it feebly, oils more strongly, and gases in especially CH₄ and SH₂ even more powerfully."[1]

Atonic Constipation.—Since in this condition the bowel needs stimulation one must give a coarse diet with a large residue much as has been recommended for "membranous colitis," following von Noorden's suggestion and copying artificially, so far as one can, the diet that is eaten by semi-civilized or wholly barbarous people. This should include much uncooked food in the form of vegetables, nuts and fruits of all sorts. The bread eaten should be whole wheat, rye, gluten or bran bread, to which nuts and raisins can be added.

Vegetables.—All vegetables are good, raw celery and cold-slaw or cooked cauliflower, turnips, asparagus, carrots, parsnips, salsify or oyster plant are especially good. Jerusalem artichokes, raw or cooked celery, squash, either the summer variety or Hubbard squash, the latter preferably baked; all beans and all vegetable and fruit salads. A good rule for these patients is to help themselves to a double portion of vegetables.

[1] Tibbles: Food in Health and Disease, p. 349.

Meat.—Fat meats are best, unless it is important to keep down the weight.

Eggs and *fish* are also allowed.

Cheese, except cream cheese, is forbidden.

Fruits, especially those with much residue, pears, melons, apple (a raw apple at bedtime often being very serviceable). Oranges and grapefruit, if the section divisions are also eaten, particularly in oranges. All berries except blackberries, which are rather constipating. Dried fruit of all sorts, figs, pulled or stewed, dates and raisins and all nuts.

Desserts.—Fruit desserts or puddings, blanc mange, made with prunes, figs, raisins or fresh fruits. Other desserts are allowed, but are less stimulating.

Salad.—All kinds. The coarser, the better. Those made of fruit and vegetables are particularly good, as apples and celery, alligator pear or any other fruit salad with lettuce.

Fats.—Fats of all sorts, animal, vegetable and mineral are useful. The mineral oils introduced by Lane for intestinal stasis are often very beneficial.

Each case of atonic constipation must be considered individually in prescribing a diet, as for example it would be actually wrong to order a diet with high fats for a person already overweight, or a diet principally vegetable and fruit for a person suffering from inanition.

Chronic Constipation.—The following diet will be found generally useful, having due regard for the foregoing factors.

On rising drink a glass of water, one third to one-half grape juice or two glasses of plain water.

Breakfast: Stewed fruit or fresh fruit. Oatmeal or pettijohn breakfast food (25 per cent. bran), with cream and sugar, white or brown; or cornmeal mush with molasses, golden drip or maple sugar; eggs or bacon, whole-wheat bread or bran bread or Grant's health crackers (bran) with fresh butter, if it is obtainable (one eats more butter when it is fresh than when salted), or cooked bran may be mixed with the morning dish of cereal.

Midmorning: Drink a glass of water or eat some dried fruit, figs, dates or Bordeaux prunes, or fresh fruit in season.

Luncheon or Supper: Small piece of meat or fish, two green vegetables from the list, whole-wheat bread and fresh butter, bran bread or crackers. Fruit fresh or stewed. Prune or fig pudding, or salad with oil dressing.

Dinner: Grapefruit, vegetable soup. Entrée of fish or egg with caper sauce or plain. Small piece of fowl or red meat with fat. Two or more green vegetables from list, taken in double quantity, and cooked with butter or oil, unless it is necessary to keep the weight down. Salad of celery and fruit or lettuce and other vegetable with ship biscuit or bran cracker. Cold slaw. Olives, radishes. Dessert—a fruit pudding, fresh fruit, stewed fruit, figs, nuts, raisins.

Bedtime. Two figs, prunes or several dates.

Of course one is not supposed to eat all the articles mentioned at one meal, but a choice made for each, varying it as to fats or vegetables, as necessity requires.

Drinks.—Coffee, buttermilk, cider, water, Vichy, grape juice, raspberry vinegar or some sweet wine, if one must have alcohol.

The use of agar-agar preparations is sometimes recommended in these cases to give bulk to the feces owing to their power of taking up water. But much the same result can be obtained by the use of good amounts of vegetables and fruit.

Spastic Constipation.—In this form of constipation it is necessary to furnish considerable bulk to the feces, but keeping all the foods soft and non-irritating, also include a large percentage of fats and oils, making an especial point of this latter feature. It is here that the mineral oils may have their best effect and should be tried freely and thoroughly and as well, the injecting of 2 to 4 ounces of some bland oil into the rectum at bedtime. For this purpose one may use olive, cottonseed, peanut or sweet oil. Larger quantities are often recommended, but serve no more useful purpose than the small amount. In this diet the fruits should be freely used, but not those with seeds or skins; and raw, rough or uncooked vegetables must be left out of the diet.

Potatoes, spaghetti and all cereal foods are good, except oatmeal or bran preparations and, of course, fish, eggs and a moderate amount of meat, free of connective tissue, are all allowable.

If one will keep in mind the facts already stated, that the diet must contain a greatly increased bulk of soft vegetables and fruit and as large an amount of oils and fats as one can digest readily, the diet may be easily constructed. It is often better to take all the vegetables as a purée or after being passed through a colander.

Obstructive Constipation.—The texture of the diet in this condition will depend largely upon the degree of obstruction; if slight, it will be only necessary to exclude all coarse food from the diet which will leave us much the same diet as has been recommended for spastic constipation. When the obstruction is more marked or severe, it will be necessary to confine the foods to those which leave the stomach largely in fluid or semifluid form, such as malted milk, citrated milk (1 grain of sodium citrate to the ounce of milk), cream and purée soups, cream, meat cut very fine or scraped. Soft eggs. Mashed potato, oils, butter, fine cereal gruels, ice-cream and syrups. Of course when an obstruction reaches this point it becomes a surgical condition and should be so treated. The only cases of severe obstruction in which it is necessary to consider the diet for any but a few days, are those cases, which, for one reason or another are inoperable.

The Use of Mineral Oil in Chronic Constipation.—This oil comes in various grades, heavy and light, made here and abroad, formerly in Russia, hence the common name "Russian mineral oil." Many cases of chronic constipation are greatly helped by varying doses, from a tablespoonful morning and night to double that dosage or more. Still others find that a tablespoonful at bedtime is amply sufficient, in short, each patient has to find the individual dose suited to the needs of their case. Many patients cannot take this oil at all, for although it is not absorbed, the entire amount ingested being recoverable in the feces, it not infrequently interferes with the normal digestive processes giving rise especially to intestinal indigestion, characterized by the symptoms of a mild enteritis accompanied by loss of appetite. Whether this acts partly on account of the depressing effect of oils on gastric secretion or possibly on account of the same effect on the intestinal enzymes or again by mechanically preventing the digestive juices from attacking the foods is not definitely known. The essential thing, however, to remember is that it does not agree with all patients by any means and its effect on digestion must be watched. After considerable investigation in regard to the different mineral oils and the different methods of giving it, Bastedo[1] came to the following conclusions, which are borne out by clinical experience.

Dosage.—Half an ounce to three ounces a day. In the same patient, the same amount of each of the oils was required, *i. e.*, heavy and light oil.

Frequency of Dose.—The same amount daily seemed as efficient when given in one dose as when given in divided doses two or three times a day.

Number of Stools.—To produce one or two copious stools a day the dose required varied considerably, but there was no

[1] Jour. Am. Med. Assn., 1914, lxiv, 808.

difference noted on account of difference in the specific gravity or character of the oils.

So far as therapeutic results are concerned the differences in the action of the three varieties of liquid petroleum, namely, light Russian liquid petrolatum, heavy Russian liquid petrolatum and American liquid petrolatum, are too slight to be of importance.

Character of Stools.—The stools were soft, usually formed, sometimes mushy, obviously greasy. They had a peculiar odor described as sour. Their consistency varied with the dose, but was the same for the different kinds of oil.

Admixture of Oil with Other Ingredients of Stools.—Generally well mixed, but from time to time a patient would have a stool of free oil. This occurred with all varieties of oil. (It necessitated reduction of the dose, and if then the bowels were not active enough, the administration in addition of cascara, aloin, etc.)

The increase in the quantity of oil used in America has stimulated production on this side of the water until now all grades of mineral oil may be had of native manufacture which are in every way as good as the imported brands.

INTESTINAL ATONY.

This condition affects chiefly the muscular coat of the large bowel and results in constipation, in fact a large majority of cases of chronic constipation are the result of an atonic colon.

The diet to combat intestinal atony should be much the same as that recommended for chronic constipation and contains as large a percentage of cellulose and fats as possible. Suitable foods are: the breads which should be those made with whole-wheat flour, rye flour or bran; vegetables; the best varieties of which are those having the largest residue, such as the cabbage family, spinach, string beans or dried beans, peas, parsnips, sweet potatoes, beet tops, etc.; the rough cereals as oatmeal (Irish) or Pettijohn (which is 25 per cent. bran) or Kellogg's cooked bran, which can be eaten alone or mixed with other cereals. All fruits, fresh stewed or dried are useful and should be taken in some form at least three times a day. Molasses, honey, marmalade and maple syrup are all stimulating to the intestine. The best fats are cream, olive oil, butter and fat meats—as bacon. Protein foods may be unrestricted in kind but should be somewhat limited quantitatively, for when taken in large amounts they tend to spoil the appetite for the more bulky and necessary vegetables and fruits.

As additional measures, massage of the colon and electricity (given with one electrode in the rectum) assist in waking up a sluggish bowel, and general hygiene.

APPENDICITIS.

Acute Appendicitis.—Acute appendicitis whether catarrhal, suppurative, gangrenous or perforative, is essentially a surgical disease and should be so considered from the onset. There are certain conditions, however, under which acute appendicitis may arise, which, for one reason or another make an operation either impossible or inadvisable, as for example, if the patient absolutely refuses surgical aid, in spite of knowing the dangers of that course; when surgical aid is not to be had or only a very poor variety; in people of great age where it is feared the shock of any operative interference would be fatal and last but not least important, in those cases which have been neglected until general peritonitis is present with distention and an almost moribund condition, when operation is considered as a last hope. These last-named cases almost invariably die if operated upon and are likely to die if they are not, but a few may survive careful medical treatment. Of course, it is a matter of very fine distinction and surgical judgment when this point is reached and rejection of surgery should not be encouraged except after mature deliberation and full consultation.

In all these conditions it will be necessary at times to turn to general medical care without operation and the dietary and general routine care of such patients are of the utmost importance. Formerly in these conditions reliance was placed on opium in full doses, and many cases were successfully carried through with its aid. The effectiveness of opium depended on the fact that it quieted the bowel, tending to stop peristalsis and the consequent transference from the iliac fossa of the septic material all over the abdominal cavity, an easy matter when peristalsis is active; and no doubt also to the fact that it helped to destroy the appetite, and so limit distention from fermentation of ingested food. Of late years this method has fallen into disrepute because of the fact that opium so completely masks the symptoms in the early stages that one cannot tell of the progress of the disease and one is apt to miss the true significance of the patient's condition.

Ochsner's Treatment for Appendicitis.[1]—In the early nineties, Ochsner devised the treatment which goes by his

[1] Handbook of Appendicitis, 1906, p. 132.

name and although it has been the storm center of many arguments, under the conditions mentioned, where operation is impossible or inadvisable, it remains today the best method we have and often gives surprisingly good results. In a word it consists of withholding everything by mouth, forbids catharsis and insists upon gastric lavage when there is nausea or vomiting and depends upon rectal absorption of small amounts of predigested food and salines.

Ochsner bases his recommendation of this method founded on experience on these two cardinal facts.

1. "The anatomical location of the appendix m. kes it easy to be shut off from the general abdominal cavity, *if the surrounding structures remain at rest for a time.*"

2. "If at rest, the cecum, omentum and small int*estine* surround the diseased appendix, no matter what its pathological condition—so shutting it off from the general cavity.

The effect of taking food is to excite peristalsis and no matter how light the food, it may, by exciting peristalsis, carry septic material all over the peritoneum and the gas produced by food passing down disturbs an inflamed appendix. He therefore forbids absolutely everything by mouth. This does not mean that a little broth or water or milk may be given, but means that at first *nothing is to pass the lips.* Ochsner further states "no matter whether the patient has a catarrhal appendicitis with or without a foreign body in the appendix or whether the appendix is gangrenous or perforated he will almost invariably recover, if from the beginning of the disease absolutely no food is given by mouth."

He also insists on gastric lavage if there is nausea or vomiting or if the patient begins his appendiceal symptoms shortly after a meal. This removes material that excites peristalsis and will later surely ferment and form gas if it be not promptly removed. The lavage is to be repeated at least once if the nausea and vomiting recur; usually after the first twenty-four hours water may be given by mouth in small amounts, but if peristalsis is thereby excited it must be given only by rectum.

The last feature of Ochsner's treatment is to give nutrient enemata every three to six hours not to exceed 4 ounces at a time, made up of ½ or 1 ounce of some predigested commercial food in 3 or 4 ounces of normal saline solution and given by a small tube after adding twenty drops of tincture opii deodorata, for an adult, to the first feeding, and one-half that amount to the other feedings (children in proportion), unless the patient is entirely free of pain or restlessness. These directions are to be followed until the patient is well along toward recovery and in very severe cases he continues the rectal feeding for ten days or even longer. Theoretically there is objection to giving anything by rectum, as peristalsis is at once excited in the entire length of the large intestine, as it is so clearly shown by the fluoroscope when bismuth or barium are mixed with the enema. Practically, however, this objection does not seem to invalidate the treatment, probably because the peristalsis is along definite and fairly fixed lines, unlike the movement of the small intestine.

Of course, as shown in the chapter on Rectal Feeding, these enemata furnish little besides fluid, although some protein in the form of amino-acids and some of the sugars are absorbed in solution. Probably completely pancreatized ("peptonized") milk (two hours) after being sterilized is quite as efficient as the commercial predigested foods.

Ochsner himself is a strong advocate of surgical intervention in appendicitis and only recommends the foregoing when an operation is either impossible or inadvisable, as already explained.

Chronic or Larval Appendicitis.—In chronic appendicitis or larval appendicitis, conditions are quite different from the acute variety and while operation is advisable when a diagnosis is made, it may for one or another reason, be necessary to postpone it until some later time. Then too, when not acutely ill it is not always so easy to persuade one's patients to undergo the operation, although they should be warned that an acute exacerbation is possible at any moment which may make an operation imperative. If, on the other hand, it is necessary to tide these patients along for one or another reason, dietary regulations will help in reducing the symptoms in many cases, until an operation can be done.

In very many of these patients there is an accompanying constipation which is more or less marked and in them the diet as advised for chronic constipation will be of distinct value, for by facilitating the constant removal of fecal masses from the colon the congestion of the caput coli and appendix region will be considerably reduced, so lessening at all events the pain and many of the symptoms of chronic indigestion which these patients have, also any pressure on the appendix from impinging fecal masses will be relieved. In these patients it is advisable to give a morning dose of some one of the saline cathartics, at least until the bowels act regularly themselves. The following mixture as recommended to the author by R. Freeman, has proven its value many times. Sodium salicylate ʒi (4 gm.), sodium phosphate ʒss (16 gm.), sodium sulphate ʒiss (45 gm.), giving a teaspoonful of this combination (more or less as required), in the early morning, at least one-half or three-quarters of an hour before breakfast. It should be dissolved in a little hot water and the glass filled at least three-quarters full with cool, but not cold water. The addition of the salicylate salt helps to reduce fermentation and consequent distention. The chronic cases with constipation have the latter feature lessened by the use of some preparation of mineral oil, provided it does not disagree (see Chronic Constipation).

When constipation is not a feature of the condition a diet containing the minimum amount of fermentable vegetables is advisable. *i. e.*, leaving out potatoes, onions, cauliflower, cabbage, Brussels sprouts, sweets, fresh breads or uncooked starches, pies, cakes, syrups, fried foods or foods that are famously indigestible (see Section on Indigestion). Here, too it is advisable to give a smaller dose of the saline or the above-mentioned salts which help to drain the appendix and reduce congestion about it. Rest before and after meals is advisable and it is especially desirable that these patients should eat without haste and thoroughly masticate their food.

The author has seen many cases in which this plan of treatment has reduced the symptoms to a minimum and in a number relieved the patients entirely, although, of course, it is presumable that further trouble will recur at a later time, particularly if the appendicitis is of the chronic involuting variety.

CHRONIC TYPHLITIS AND PERITYPHLITIS.

The dietary routine for these conditions is much the same as that given for chronic appendicitis, although here oil and fat foods play a more prominent part and the injection of two or three ounces of oil in the rectum at bedtime is most useful. In some cases it will be necessary to revert to the diets recommended for chronic colitis of which these conditions are often a part. The use of salines is also useful in keeping the caput as free of feces as possible, and a moderate dose of a mild saline cathartic in the early morning is helpful.

INTESTINAL AUTO-INTOXICATION.

The entire subject of auto-intoxication is far from clear, particularly in its clinical bearings, and there may be found great difference of opinion among biological chemists as to the significance of the products of intestinal fermentation and putrefaction in their relation to conditions of actual disease or pathological states. Thus Taylor[1] says that intoxication by resorption of the digestive juices by products of normal digestion and by abnormal products of digestion is not proven experimentally and probably does not exist and in "normal bacterial disintegration of food-stuffs in the alimentary tract no known toxic substance is found," for the products of carbohydrate fermentation, formic, acetic, butyric, valerianic, proprionic, lactic, succinic acids and a trace of oxalic acid are not toxic. So too, according to Taylor, although protein putrefaction yields phenol, skatol, indol and cresol from animo-acids and hexone bases, none of these are toxic. Also there is "no constant relation between the protein ration and the output of aromatic substances, and a high urinary output of aromatic substances indicates active putrefaction in the colon, which may be innocuous or not. On the other hand, a low output need not indicate a low degree of bacterial activity in the intestines and need not speak against a bacterial intestinal intoxication.

Cytolytic degeneration seems allied to the process of fermentation, the functions of the tissues are disturbed by the cytolyses and an auto-intoxication may result, also the products of tissue degeneration may be toxic themselves, so that according to Taylor again it is not possible to separate auto-intoxication from the general pathology of metabolism.

In so-called gastro-intestinal auto-intoxication there is no constant relation, according to the same authority, between constipation, excess of indican and conjugate sulphates in the urine, nor does the degree of these substances bear any relation to the severity of the symptoms.

Combe,[2] on the other hand, is an enthusiastic supporter of the gastro-intestinal origin of certain toxic states of the organism and marshalls his proofs in very clear and logical order. We all know that bacteria play a large part in the digestive processes and the questions are asked:

1. Is the microbic intervention useful to the body?
2. Is it indispensable?
3. Can it become harmful?

1. The answer to the first is positively affirmative, as the bacteria digest foods as do the enzymes and in some instances digest portions of the food (cellulose) which the enzymes cannot.

2. The bacteria are also indispensable as proven by Nuttall, Thierfelder[3] and Schottelins[4] who showed that animals

[1] Osler's Mod. Med., vol. ii, 503.
[2] Auto-intoxication.
[3] Ztschr, f. phys. Chem., vol. xxii, 71.
[4] Arch. fur Hyg., vol. xxiv, 210.

born and raised aseptically did not thrive or, in many instances, live at all.

3. In answer to the third question as to the possible harmful qualities of bacteria in digestion, Combe gives positive assent, although it has been strongly combated by the German school, who admit the symptomatology and the probable focus but find the proofs insufficient. He further fortifies his position by pointing to the autotoxic and detoxifying powers of Nature's three lines of defense against intoxication found in the intestinal epithelium, liver, glands of internal secretion and external secretion as *e. g.*, the kidneys, through which intestinal toxins are constantly eliminated.

Phenol, indol and skatol are all formed in the intestine as a result of putrefaction of nitrogenous food-stuffs, principally meat. Phenol is formed in the large intestine as a result of bacterial activity in the presence of stasis there, but when small in amount is oxidized in the organism or is eliminated by the bowel and only when the formation exceeds the oxidizing powers is it excreted by the urine. Indol is formed in the small intestine as a result of stasis in this part of the bowel and never when the stasis is in the large intestine. It is oxidized into indoxyl, which combines with sulphuric acid in the liver to form indozyl sulphuric acid; this appears in the urine as a salt of potassium, potassium indoxyl sulphate or indican. This substance in turn is oxidized into sulphuric acid and indoxyl, the latter into indigo red or indigo blue if an oxidizer is present.

Both indol and phenol excretions depend on:
1. The composition of the food (which varies).
2. On the degree of peristalsis.
3. On the power of absorption.
4. On putrefaction intensity.[1]

It is strongly disputed whether indicanuria has any effect in producing symptoms of so-called auto-intoxication but there seems little doubt but that it is at least the index for other conditions which result in symptoms, and the association of marked indicanuria and evidence of renal irritation (as a trace of albumin, casts, etc.), is too definite to be dismissed without adequate explanation, particularly as relieving the indicanuria often results in a return to a normal urinary output. The effect of the indican perhaps while not deleterious in itself may be to cause renal irritation and consequent reduction in the kidney's power for excretion of other toxic substances at present unknown but standing in

[1] Combe; Auto-intoxicatiom, p. 61.

a causal relation to the symptoms of intoxication. At the same time there is no end of clinical evidence that when symptoms of a toxemia are present in connection with considerable amounts of indol in the urine, relief is seldom or never obtained until measures are adopted to restrict its formation (diet) and to favor its elimination (catharsis and intestinal irrigation).

On the other hand, there are undoubtedly many cases of indicanuria which are entirely without symptoms, so that while the specific variety of auto-intoxication depends on chemical, physiological and pathological facts too intricate to be as yet made out with clearness and it is not possible to speak of treatment based on specific etiological factors, we know something of the course of development of the intestinal poisons from fermentation and putrefaction[1] and the clinical conditions that lead directly to it, as well as the factors that modify it.

Dyspepsia and stasis either gastric or intestinal; diseased conditions of the intestinal walls with consequent lessening of the defense mechanism; parasites; diminished activity of the antitoxic organs; bad eating habits, hurry, working too soon after a meal, all may be of etiological importance.

Dietetic Indications for Intestinal Auto-intoxication.— When one comes to consider the necessary factors in diminishing nitrogenous intestinal putrefaction one finds that Combe[2] sums up the indications as follows:

1. Modify the intestinal culture medium in which the proteolytic bacteria thrive by.

(*a*) Introducing an antiputrefactive lactofarinaceous diet.

(*b*) Introducing antagonistic bacteria into the intestinal medium.

2. Diminish the vitality of the proteolytic bacteria in the intestine by means of germicidal medicines (there is as yet no known way to accomplish this satisfactorily).

3. Evacuate the proteolytic bacteria and their products by intestinal lavage.

The first indication, namely, that of modifying the culture medium is the one with which we are particularly concerned and leads us to a study of diet for this condition.

General Indications for Diet:
Nitrogenous Foods.

1. Diminish these as much as possible, keeping to the low level of physiological requirement, 40 to 60 gm. (1⅓ to 2 oz.) of protein, per diem.

---

[1] Forchheimer: vol. ii, 664.   [2] Auto-intoxication, p. 234.

2. Absolutely prohibit those forms of nitrogenous foods that favor the development of putrefactive bacteria, particularly animal protein except milk, *e. g.*, meat, fish and eggs.

3. To choose among these milk in one of its many forms, whole, skimmed, zoolak, koumyss, buttermilk, kefir, loppered milk, cream or pot cheese.

Fatty Foods.

1. Avoid meat fat as increasing putrefaction.

2. Give fat best in the form of fresh butter and cream.

Farinaceous Foods.

1. Give as large a proportion of farinaceous foods as possible, saturate the intestines with them, giving five or six meals in the proportion of five times as much farinaceous as protein foods, whenever the latter are given.

2. In auto-intoxication from acute enteritis an exclusive farinaceous diet must be given for several days.

3. In auto-intoxication due to chronic enteritis, the diet should be lactofarinaceous giving later a little meat or eggs.

4. In ordinary auto-intoxication milk mixed with farinaceous food is best, for the lactose of the milk on account of its lactic acid-forming abilities is a strong antiputrefactive element.[1]

Foods to Especially Avoid.—Bouillon, meat soups, meat juices and jellies, meat extracts, white of egg or dishes which are made of it. Milk, unless mixed with farinaceous food. High or tainted meats or those which decompose rapidly, game, rare or raw meats, fish, shell fish.

In severe auto-intoxication absolutely no meat should be taken and when it is begun later, only in small progressive quantities, not forgetting that it should be taken with five times its bulk of farinaceous foods.

Foods to take.

Fruits raw or cooked.

Vegetables, thoroughly cooked and soft, all farinaceous foods, as rice, noodles, macaroni, puddings, purée of vegetables, bread, yolk of eggs. Sauerkraut is a valuable antiputrefactive food.

Modified Sample Menus. Farinaceous without Meat.

7.30 A.M. Cereal prepared with water or milk. Rolls and fresh butter.

10.00 A.M. Some form of gruel made with milk or water.

12.30 P.M. One or two yolks of eggs, raw or boiled, macaroni, rice, farina with salt and fresh butter. Farinaceous pudding. Rolls and butter. Later fruit and soft green vegetables.

[1] Combe: Auto-Intoxication.

3.30 P.M. The same as at 10.00 A.M.

7.00 P.M. Same variety as at 12.30 P.M.

10.00 P.M. Infusion of chamomile, peppermint, fennel, or anise.

After eight to ten days of this, add potatoes, purée or baked. Whortleberry juice or jelly.   No fluids with meals.

Later tea, coffee, cocoa, vegetables, and fruits, may be added in the order named with a little meat, first at one and then at two meals, watching the effect.

In choosing a diet one must also be somewhat guided by the conditions so often associated with intestinal auto-intoxication, e. g., stasis, chronic constipation, torpid liver or actual hepatic disease and circulatory disorders.   Jack[1] recommends loppered milk diet in auto-intoxication associated with emaciation or not, given with well-cooked fruit and cereal, thus one pint of loppered milk with buttered-toast or a cheese or butter sandwich with baked apple or stewed fruit every two hours. After ten or eleven days increase the diet.   When on regular diet again he advises taking as much as five pints of the loppered milk—one pint at each meal and one between meals.   (This is probably too much for the average case.)

A sample diet covering the most usual associated condition, viz., that of chronic constipation or intestinal stasis might be chosen somewhat as follows:

Early morning, one-third or one-half glass of grape juice with equal amount of water.

Breakfast: Glass of milk or buttermilk with cereal and cream (tea or coffee later).   Bread and fresh butter. Fruit.

Midmorning: One-half glass of buttermilk and slice of bread.

Dinner or Supper: Cream vegetable soup made without stock or thickened with flour.   Yolk of two or three eggs poached or scrambled; macaroni, cream cheese, potato, rice, baked farina, green vegetables (that grow above ground).   Glass of milk or buttermilk.   Bread and fresh butter.   Farinaceous pudding with fruit sauce or stewed figs, prunes, apricots, pears, cherries or peaches.

Midafternoon: Cream cheese and crackers.

At Bedtime: One-half to one glass of buttermilk with two or three toasted crackers and several dates or figs.

[1] Buffalo Med. Jour., 1917-18, xcix, 501.

This should be kept up for a long enough time to get rid of the subjective symptoms and any abnormal urinary findings, and then little by little one may add a little meat and other foods, gradually returning to a normal dietary but for a long time keeping the protein at a low level as already indicated before.

The treatment should be begun with a mercurial purge and the use of some laxative or mineral oil continued for some time. When the symptoms are severe great assistance is obtained from high colon irrigations with normal saline or a 1 per cent. solution of ichthyol.

General bodily exercise regularly every day and hygiene are all of great assistance in ridding the gastro-intestinal tract of the toxic materials.

In some instances a complete change of life, a trip to Europe or elsewhere, taking the patient out of his usual routine may be necessary to accomplish the end desired. The usefulness of this has been proven more than once in the writer's experience.

HEMORRHOIDS.

Hemorrhoids are caused by a dilatation of one or more of the veins at the anal ring which at any time may be thrombosed. The dilatation is due either to a temporary and local obstruction to the return venous flow, as in constipation, or fecal impaction, or just mere straining at stool, or to a permanent interference with the return flow, as seen in cirrhosis of the liver or chronic cardiac disease.

The dietary prevention of the temporary venous obstruction is very important and one can do much to obviate the production of hemorrhoids by giving a diet which will be laxative such as is recommended in chronic constipation, including as it does a large amount of cellulose in green vegetables and fruits, fresh and dried; oils, fats and liquids in excess.

When the hemorrhoids develop as a result of straining and tenesmus in prolonged diarrhea, a diet to control the looseness will be of use as in chronic diarrhea, unless one can find the direct cause of the diarrhea and correct it.

In the cases of hemorrhoids dependent on hepatic or cardiac disorders it will be necessary to insure regular bowel movements, using an anticonstipation diet so far as one can in consideration of the underlying causes. Measures directed toward the relief of the hepatic or general intestinal congestion are necessary in addition to the suitable diet.

HIRSCHSPRUNG'S DISEASE.

In this disease, which is a chronic or congenital dilatation of the colon, there are certain dietary indications which are designed to combat rather the symptoms (which are often secondary to the condition, such as chronic constipation and stasis with at times symptoms of toxemia) than the dilatation itself. There is one exception to this, namely, that foods which are particularly prone to be stored up in the colon and increase the dilatation should be avoided, as for example an excess of tough cellulose.

The diet recommended for chronic constipation is best suited to this disease with the precaution that all vegetables and fruits should be soft when fed and not given in indigestible bulk, although the total quantity of such foods should be great.

It would seem as if in this disease the regular use of mineral oil might accomplish much by its lubricating qualities, and certainly deserves a trial, which, with massage of the colon, may help to preserve the muscular tone of the intestine.

A surgical procedure is the only permanent way of relieving Hirschsprung's disease, either as a colectomy or iliosigmoidostomy.

CHAPTER XXIII.

DISEASES OF THE ACCESSORY DIGESTIVE GLANDS

THE action of these glands and their secretions are so indissolubly connected with the processes of digestion that the consideration of one implies consideration of both. We have dealt with dietetics of diseases of the digestive tube separately, but as a matter of fact, unconsciously we are compelled to take account of the state of the accessory glands in doing so, and of making allowances for their integrity or lack of it. On the other hand, there are certain diseases or pathological states of these glands that arise, which demand attention aside from the questions of digestion, as well as the bearing of these conditions on the normal utilization of food-stuffs, and with some of these we are now particularly concerned.

DISEASES OF LIVER AND GALL-BLADDER.

It is much to be regretted that the dietetics of hepatic diseases cannot be more serviceable as curative agents and still more to be regretted that most people are not willing to exercise the common sense and self-restraint in drinking and eating, the failure of which in so large a measure is responsible for the frequency of diseased conditions in these organs.

In other words, dietetics here are much like locking the stable door after the horse has been stolen, for the dietetic prophylaxis is all important. After the damage is done patients are willing to go anywhere and spend any amount to be rid of their troubles or do anything that offers a chance in the prevention of a return or continuance of their symptoms.

In the matter of diets for hepatic disorders and disease we could act a good deal more intelligently if we had a simple and reliable method for testing hepatic functions, for if our choice of a diet could be made to depend on definite knowledge of just what food elements were poorly metabolized by the liver, we could choose a diet especially adapted to the individual case.

The methods in vogue for testing liver functions are too uncertain or too complicated to be of much practical use, although there is no doubt but that there is progress being made in this direction.

414

Strauss used 100 to 150 gm. levulose to test liver functions, a resulting levulosurea indicating a disturbed hepatic function. As a matter of fact, most diseased livers respond to this test, but in many of the cases of cirrhosis the glycogenic function is perfectly well preserved and we get no resulting levulose in the urine.

Opie[1] found that when the liver was poisoned by certain substances as, *e. g.*, chloroform, the susceptibility to intoxication is greatest after a diet of fats, less after meats and least in animals fed on carbohydrates. This by analogy can be used in choosing the diet in threatened cholemic states where the liver cells are failing in their power to functionate, overwhelmed as they are by the poisons in the system, here carbohydrates should be given fully and may even be given subcutaneously, as a 5 per cent. solution of glucose.

Dietetic Prophylaxis.—This question is practically a statement of the etiology of many abnormal liver conditions and while it is to be feared that few will heed advice until experence has taught its bitter lesson, it is certainly a necessary thing to state how most of these diseases may be avoided, excepting of course those due to direct infectious agencies.

It is only necessary to remind the reader of the physiology of the liver to see that almost everything absorbable that is ingested finds its way sooner or later to the liver, which is endowed with extraordinary powers. These powers may be spoken of as the detoxifying, lipogenic, glycogenic and urea-forming functions. In a normal liver these operate to perfection, but in disease are more or less disturbed or permanently disabled. For the exact mechanism by which this is accomplished, one is referred to Physiology, and all that is necessary here is to enumerate the "don'ts" of dietetics to point the way to a preservation of normal functioning.

The excessive ingestion of any one of the food elements, protein, carbohydrates and fat will lead eventually to disturbed liver function, and a continuance of this results in permanent damage to the cells. Among the articles of food especially to be avoided are condiments of all sorts, alcohol, vegetables rich in irritating oils, such as garlic, radish and horse-radish and the continued use of phosphorus or arsenic in course of treatment. This does not mean that one must go through life without the use of any condiments, for a little at times can be successfully detoxified by the liver, but taken in large amounts or continuously they form a very distinct danger to the integrity of the cells by chronic irri-

[1] Jour. Exp. Med., 1914, xxi, 1.

tation and the production of connective tissue. Alcohol is, of course, the chief offender and it hardly seems necessary to mention this point, it is so generally known and recognized even by the laity. Spirits as whiskey, gin, brandy, etc., are especially bad and all other alcoholic drinks directly in proportion to their alcohol content. When taken on a full stomach and largely diluted they are of course. least irritating, but the dilution does not lessen the absorbability of the alcohol but merely spreads it over a longer time, giving the liver a better chance to handle it. Especially bad are undiluted spirits on an empty stomach, as cocktails or neat spirits taken as an appetizer before meals, as here the absorption is quickest and most complete and is apt to be regularly repeated. While the spirits have a tendency to produce cirrhosis, the beers do so also, but to less extent, and their damaging effects are seen as well in the deposition of excessive amounts of fat in and about the liver cells and as a fatty degeneration of the cell itself. With the new prohibition laws it is probable that cirrhosis of the̅ liver will become comparatively a rare condition.

Acute Hepatic Congestion.—This is caused frequently by overeating and drinking and from a dietetic point of view requires starvation or semistarvation until the appetite, which is usually completely lost, returns. During this day or two of starvation water can be given freely, and as soon as the patient is able to take food he may be given small amounts of milk, skimmed or whole, diluted with alkaline waters; also gruels, cream soups, milk toast and soft cereals, custards, soft green vegetables, chicken and so back to full diet, giving the articles in about the order listed.

This condition of acute congestion of the liver is usually designated by the layman as a "bilious" attack, at all events that covers the situation, although nobody knows just what a "bilious" attack is, it seems to be so many things to different people.

Acute Catarrhal Jaundice or Gastroduodenitis with Jaundice.—In this condition we have not only the catarrhal inflammation of the bile ducts but primarily of the stomach and duodenum, so that the catarrh of this part of the digestive tract must be taken into account in the choice of a diet. Fortunately the same diet fits both conditions. As fat is very badly digested in this, it is best to reduce it to a minimum until the jaundice is largely over; to this end skimmed milk is an ideal diet, although here again a day or two of starvation at the outset may be quite the most serviceable procedure, provided water is given in large amounts. After the skimmed milk we can give broth, gruels and soft foods generally in progressive order. An early morning saline laxative is essential, particularly when constipation is marked, but all cases are benefited by it, as it has a favorable influence on the gastric and duodenal catarrh. According to Forchheimer jaundice causes a hyperchlorhydria in direct proportion to its intensity, and the diet must be chosen with this in view, avoiding stimulating acid or irritating foods.

Chronic Hepatic Congestion.—This is usually passive and due to cardiac disease with failure of compensation. The diet should be light, non-stimulating and attention directed to the cause of the congestion.

Portal Cirrhosis.—Although this disease does occur occasionally in children and young adults without known cause, it is for the most part, par excellence, the disease of retribution and can usually be traced to chronic hepatic irritation from overindulgence in irritating foods and drinks, especially alcohol. Where the diagnosis is fairly certain and especially in the earlier stages, it is necessary to institute at once a rigid milk cure (as milk is nourishing and absolutely non-irritating), given continuously and alone for from four to six weeks,[1] 2 or 3 quarts per diem, diluted with soda water, Vichy or Apollinaris or flavored with tea, coffee or cocoa. This diet reduces intestinal putrefaction to a minimum, so causing less hepatic irritation, the fat is in emulsion and absorption can take place in spite of an intestinal catarrh.[2] When nausea or vomiting are sources of trouble, skimmed milk often agrees better than whole milk.[3]

After this period of milk diet one may add eggs, gruel, cereals, fresh green vegetables, stewed fruits. Much sugar is forbidden, as it is apt to cause fermentation, fats too, often give rise by fermentation to the formation of acetic, lactic or butyric acids and should be avoided.

After a month of this diet Osler recommends a return to the milk period again for a time, alternating with the additional diet as indicated. Of course all the foods that belong to the irritating class are to be permanently studiously avoided. Besides those already mentioned one must include meat or strong meat broths, neither of which should be taken for a long time in order to keep the production of urea down to the minimum.

Occasionally the milk may be advantageously given in the form of the Karell cure, particularly if the cirrhosis is compli-

[1] Osler's Modern Med., vol. iii, 444.
[2] Rolleston: Diseases of Liver, p. 297.
[3] Herter Lectures on Chem. Path., 1902, p. 88.

cated by ascites. The low salt content of this diet (1.3 gm. per day) acts as one of the salt-poor diets does in nephritis and often helps in the removal of the fluid, at least in part.

Einhorn recommends duodenal feeding in cirrhosis on account of its sparing the portal congestion; reports on its usefulness are, however, meager.

Biliary Cirrhosis.—Here we have more often an extension, *via* the bile ducts, of a direct infection of the biliary system, the cause often originating in the intestine.

The diet is much the same as that recommended for portal cirrhosis, although the milk diet may not need to be so rigorously or so long continued. Constipation must be especially combated and is best managed by a morning saline laxative. After the milk period of feeding is over we may give sago, zweiback, rice, potato, fish, chicken, etc., avoiding all the irritants as in all other diseased states of the liver.

Fatty Liver.—Since the chief cause of fatty infiltration of the liver is the excessive ingestion of alcohol or fats, the natural recommendation for prophylaxis would be to take less or none of either. The fatty degeneration of the liver will hardly be affected by diet, except as it may modify the acute infection which is the cause of the degeneration.

As a matter of fact fatty infiltration and degeneration usually go hand in hand; one or the other predominating, depending upon the etiological factors.

When one has a well-developed case of fatty liver due primarily to infiltration, it is necessary to oversee the patient's diet with great care. If the individual is obese it will be necessary to institute a reduction diet cure combined with suitable exercises (see Obesity). In this way a certain amount of excess fat can be removed in the general course of reduction and with the improvement in the patient's general condition in consequence of this it is also probable that the fatty infiltration will become less marked unless it has already gone on until the liver tissue has become very fat, as occurs in the more severe cases.

Overeating and alcohol are especially to be forbidden, although this is true, too, of all the conditions already described. Fat food must be interdicted and only a moderate amount of carbohydrate allowed. In hot climates a vegetable diet with milk is particularly recommended. Where there is fever, meat must be restricted, otherwise it may be allowed in moderation,[1] and all the lighter proteins are well borne, as fish, eggs, milk and cheese, if not too rich.

[1] Quincke, Hoppe, Seyler: Die Krankheit d. Leber, p. 122.

As has been already said, when the fatty liver is part of a general adiposis the patients must be treated as for obesity with the hope that much of the excess of fat can be gradually removed as the patients return more nearly to their normal condition and weight.

Acute Yellow Atrophy of the Liver.—Since the admitted cause of this condition is a toxemia, not always due to the same agent, the treatment consists in prophylaxis so far as possible. Any form of jaundice, therefore, particularly that occurring in a pregnant woman, should always be viewed with suspicion.

When the condition has been diagnosed the diet plays a not inconsiderable part in the treatment and since there is apt to be an acid intoxication present the giving of cereal gruels other than oatmeal is important, which with milk should form the basis of the diet. The drinking of a large amount of an alkaline water or even plain water, to which sodium bicarbonate is added or not, is recommended by Kelly.[1]

Amyloid Liver.—The etiological factor in this disease is some focus or foci of chronic suppuration, and the diet should be constructed with an idea of increasing the food consumption to the maximum, compatible with health, in order most successfully to combat the chronic infection, which should, of course, be treated surgically if possible. All fat foods, such as cream, butter, fat meats; concentrated carbohydrate foods, as breads, cereals, macaroni; sugars and honey are especially good. The protein of the diet should be increased to approximately 120 gm. if the patient can take this amount, for combined with exercises this amount of protein will favor the formation of tissue and thus increase the active protoplasm.

Cholelithiasis.—From the dietitian's point of view nothing can be done to aid in the removal of gall-stones when already formed, although much has been written on the possibility of dissolving gall-stones *in situ*. Their partial disintegration and occasional complete disappearance does take place experimentally, when gall-stones are placed in a dog's bladder, either in its normal condition or when an experimental inflammatory condition has been produced in the gall-bladder, but this is very different from the conditions under which the stones form in the human subject and when formed seldom, if ever disappear spontaneously. This does not mean that the gall-stones may not "go to sleep" so to speak, and remain quiescent for years or permanently, as this often

[1] Osler: Modern Medicine, 1st. Ed., vol. iii, 477.

happens in the experience of every physician. While diet
has little or nothing to do with the disappearance of stones
when already formed, it has much to do with their formation
in the first place, and still more to do with their recurrence
after operation, for statistics show that a fair number of
patients in whom the gall-bladder is not removed at time of
operation suffer from recurrence of gall-stones.

Naunyn, Kehr, Aschoff and others regard the formation
of gall-stones as merely an incident in disease in which infection,
bile stasis and inflammatory manifestations are the principal
factors[1] and it is against these factors of disease that dietetic
treatment should be directed, rather than against their
results. Dietetic indiscretions, long continued, that lead to
catarrh of the stomach, duodenum and gall-bladder tend to
produce gall-stones indirectly by affording means for the
access of bacteria[2] to the biliary tract, so that little need be
said to press home the importance of diet as a preventive
measure.

While a large majority of gall-stones are formed of cholesterol, almost every one has at its center a bacterium of one
sort or another, so that infection is perhaps the first and
chief necessity in the production of stones. Lime salts are
frequently superimposed on the cholesterol stones, as well,
and bile pigments, particularly bilirubin, form part of many
stones.

Prophylactic or Postoperative Diet.—There are no new
principles involved in choosing a diet to prevent reformation
of gall-stones, and with certain exceptions it is probably as
much a matter of the quantity of food ingested as the quality. These exceptions will, of course, include all foods or
drinks that tend to produce gastro-intestinal catarrh or those
which have a direct effect on the liver by virtue of their
intrinsic irritating character and the fact of their being
carried directly to the liver by the portal system. Such
foods and drinks have already been spoken of in connection
with portal cirrhosis and include condiments as peppers,
mustard, curry, spices, salty foods, alcohol in all forms and
very hot foods or drinks and ice-water in large amounts.

Meats.—Only easily digestible meats should be taken and
"high" meats, pork, fatty meat and fish, such as goose, duck,
mackerel and blue fish should be avoided.

Fats.—Some dietitians condemn the use of all fats, but
there does not seem to be any reasonable basis for such complete prohibition. Fat is an essential food element and is a

[1] Anderson: Canada Med. Assn. Jour., 1914, iv.
[2] Osler: Modern Medicine, iii, 444.

necessary part of any mixed diet. What should be avoided is fat that is particularly indigestible, such as all those that melt only at a higher temperature than the body, *e. g.*, mutton fat, salt fat, as bacon or pork, or excess of even simple fat is to be avoided. There is no objection to sweet butter, cream in moderation and vegetable oils and meat fat in great moderation that has a low melting-point, as beef fat.

Carbohydrates.—Sugar should be restricted as liable to ferment. and cause indigestion; pies, preserves, candy, rich cakes, syrup, etc., are all to be avoided. Aside from these restrictions one may eat almost anything provided it is not in excessive amounts sufficient to cause overloading of the digestive tract.

All means to stimulate the flow of bile are especially indicated and to this end it is often better to give five small meals a day, than three larger ones, as each time food is taken, bile is expressed from the gall-bladder.

Vegetables and Fruit.—All vegetables that do not ferment are allowable but the cabbage family, radishes, horse-radish are barred, also according to Tibbles' peas, beans, lentils and carrots as containing phytosterol, a vegetable form of cholesterol, the principal constituent of gall-stones. Fruits that are not too sour may be taken, but they are possibly better borne stewed with a little sugar.

Exercises.—Exercises that tend to stir up the liver are all good, such as horseback riding and calisthenic exercises which include bending and compression of the liver area.

Alcohol.—As already stated patients are better off without any alcohol whatever, but when it is insisted upon, they may take light Rhine wines, well diluted with an alkaline water, such as Vichy, and only with meals and in the greatest moderation. Not over 3 or 4 ounces of wine with one meal a day. *Spirits*, all forms are particularly bad as tending to produce a catarrh of the stomach and intestines, besides irritating the liver cells.

Acute Cholecystitis and Colic.—During the attack usually nothing can be taken by mouth often not even water. Later when the stomach is not rebellious, one had best begin with milk diluted with an alkaline water, Vichy, soda or Apollinaris. This should be kept up until all signs of inflammatory reaction have disappeared, although possibly thin cereals may be begun awhile before this, but milk should form the basis of the diet. Later solid food may be taken as outlined in other hepatic conditions. Here again a mild saline cath-

---

[1] Food in Health and Disease, p. 384.

artic should be given in the morning regularly for a time as recommended for catarrhal jaundice and to which a small amount of sodium salicylate may be added to promote the flow of bile; possibly the sulphates are best for this laxative purpose.

In all forms of gall-bladder disease from cholecystitis to stone there is great necessity for drinking water very liberally, and patients should be given a definite amount of water to take in the twenty-four hours.

PANCREATIC DISEASE.

The point at which disease of the pancreas touches dietetics is when the function of the gland is interfered with, so that we find an insufficient, deficient or excessive secretion. Heretofore it has been possible only to arrive at abnormal conditions of the secretion by watching the effects on food digestion, and numerous tests sprang up for determining which element of the secretion was deficient, so we had tests for tryptic digestion, that for pancreatic amylase and pancreatic lipase. Since the introduction by Einhorn of the duodenal tube it is possible in many cases to obtain samples of pancreatic juice, sufficiently large for chemical analysis and to make satisfactory biological tests of its digestive capability. Einhorn and Rosenbloom[1] have done this very satisfactorily from a clinical stand-point and have determined the composition of the normal pancreatic juice. There are variations in the secretion of a purely functional nature, as well as variations due to pathological changes. Deficiency of trypsinogen produces azotorrhea or meat indigestion, lessened lipase a steatorrhea or fat indigestion, and diminished amylopsin results in carbohydrate fermentation. When we have a new growth or interference with the pancreatic internal secretion, pancreatic diabetes is the result with an alimentary glycosuria and hyperglycemia.

Still another result of pancreatic and intestinal disturbance is the production of that curious condition of arrested development known as infantilism, where the subjects develop mentally, but physically they do not increase much in size, although they may take on the adult characteristics. Besides a disturbance in pancreatic secretion in infantilism the intestinal flora is an entirely abnormal one.

Acute Pancreatitis.—In acute pancreatitis there is usually little time to resort to diet for the patients are for the most part in shock. If they survive this initial period, then they

[1] Arch. Int. Med., December, 1910.

may continue to improve, in which case diluted milk, gruels and other liquids (without meat stock) and farinaceous foods generally may be added to the diet, and later chicken and soft vegetables.

Chronic Pancreatitis.—Here the pancreatic secretions may be disturbed in any one of the directions indicated, *i. e.*, there may be a failure or·diminution of the trypsinogen, steapsin or amylopsin with resulting characteristic evidences of this failure in the so-called pancreatic indigestion. It is here that we are apt to encounter the cases of marked steatorrhea characterized by stools with yellow masses of fat, fluid or semisolid, which if not accompanied by jaundice may amount to an average loss of 64 per cent. of the ingested fat. If there is mild jaundice the loss will be greater (72 per cent.) and if the jaundice is marked and bile is completely shut off the loss will amount to 87 per cent.[1] Naturally when this condition obtains the diet must be made up almost exclusively of carbohydrate and easily digestible protein, although by giving artificially prepared pancreatic extract it is usually possible to give a minimum amount of simple fat. In this form of pancreatic deficiency sweetbreads, lean meats, cheese, fowl, breads, macaroni, baked potato, rice and other cereals, sugars, soft vegetables and fruits only if there is no accompanying diarrhea, which is regularly present in the cases of extreme deficiency of steapsin.

When there is a diminution or absence of trypsinogen we find azotorrhea present, in which condition striated muscle fibers can be found in the stools, a condition often associated with marked intestinal putrefaction of protein and with an accompanying indicanuria. Under these circumstances the diet should be largely carbohydrate with some fat in the form of butter, eggs and thin cream. Milk will be fairly well digested if the gastric secretions are approximately normal, or failing this the deficiency in trypsinogen may be supplied again by the pancreatic extract. Cream cheese may also be used to supply protein, besides the vegetable protein. All forms of farinaceous foods may be used in large amounts together with soft green vegetables and stewed fruits. In fact almost any food low in protein will be well digested.

When the amylase is deficient in the pancreatic secretion marked fermentation of the stool will take place in the fermentation tube, so that here it is necessary to reduce the starches to the minimum and give them preferably malted or with a diastatic ferment to compensate for the loss of the natural ferment.

[1] T. Brugsch: Lehrbk, klin. Untersuch. Method., p. 371.

In the condition of achylia of the stomach the starch in moderate amount will be digested by the ptyalin of the saliva, but with normal or increased gastric acidity, this is soon stopped and the starches pass into the intestine imperfectly dextrinized.

In selecting a diet for these cases any of the simple fats and protein foods may be given, but the carbohydrates best tolerated are those partly malted, as malted breakfast food, toast dried to a brown crisp, dry and partially malted cereals in flakes. Next best are fine cereals well-cooked, such as farina, wheatena, cream of wheat and well-boiled rice. Potato and breads are best left alone unless each meal is followed by some artificially prepared diastase and this may be necessary even with the carbohydrates already partially prepared by previous malting.

Where the internal secretion of the pancreas is disturbed and we have a glycosuria the diet must be in accordance with the dietary principles recommended for diabetes mellitus, although here, too, artificial diastase helps in the starch digestion. But these cases are practically diabetics and should be so treated.

In carcinoma, cyst or other pancreatic disease the diet should be chosen with reference to the functional integrity of the gland or the lack of certain of the digestive elements, as we have just seen in chronic pancreatitis.

CHAPTER XXIV.
DIET IN DISEASES OF THE SKIN.

IN order to prescribe a rational diet for any disease it is necessary to understand its etiological factors, at least to some extent. It is therefore unfortunate that thus far there are very few skin diseases in which any definite general metabolic changes are known. With the skin lesions caused by parasites, irritants, etc., we have as dietitians no concern, as food plays no part either in their production, course or cure. It has long been the custom to place the blame for many skin lesions at the door of the digestive canal and in some instances rightly, though often without adequate scientific basis of fact, to be sure, and only on the strength of clinical evidence. There is therefore a vast field as yet inadequately explored, and until painstaking nutritional studies are made on more diseases, we can for the most part only prescribe diets on the basis of bedside experience. The dermatoses due to disturbed metabolism may be divided as Johnson[1] says into:

1. Disorders due to derangement of digestion.
2. Disorders of intermediary nitrogen metabolism.
3. Disorders due to anaphylaxis.

The alimentary eruptions von Noorden[2] divides into:

(a) Acute alimentary eruptions from dietetic causes, such as the urticarial erythemata of the vesicular and bullous types, which may be produced by strawberries or other fruits, asparagus, cabbage, fish, cheese, spices and in some even by fresh eggs.

(b) The chronic alimentary eruptions, for example, pellagra, ergotism and scurvy, although we believe now that both pellagra and scurvy are dependent for their production in some way on lack of vitamines.

Of the disorders of digestion which give rise to eruptions we have changes in gastric secretion, notably hyperacidity, which give rise to vasoconstriction of the skin vessels, as seen in loss of hair.[3]

In disorders of intermediary nitrogen metabolism Johnson found that the N partition gave evidence of disturbance shown by a "decrease of urea and a corresponding increase

[1] Jour. Cut. Dis., 1912, p. 136.
[2] Path. of Metab., vol. iii, 759.
[3] Quart. Jour. Med., 1915, viii, 156.

of rest nitrogen, and when this was marked, symptoms could be looked for.'' A change in the nitrogen partition occurs in eczema, prurigo and dermatitis herpetiformis, particularly in the beginning of the attack. It is not all sure, however, that the lack of nitrogen balance is merely a symptom. In the class of dermatoses due to anaphylaxis we have a definite protein hypersensibility in certain individuals which results in such conditions as urticaria and angioneurotic edema. These diseases are of course of alimentary origin, as already explained, but they may occasionally occur from parenteral protein intoxication.

Tidy, on the other hand, concludes from a study of nitrogen metabolism in dermatoses, that:

1. Changes in the nitrogen excretion in various dermatoses are the result of the condition of the skin and are not connected with the cause of the disease.

2. Retention of nitrogen is apparent, not real, and is accounted for by the abnormal excretion of nitrogen by the skin.

3. Changes in the nitrogen excretion may precede the eruption and it is possible that these may survive it.

In spite of these findings Tidy suggests that a low protein diet is worth a trial in dermatoses which are associated with disturbances of nitrogen excretion.

Although authorities differ in their findings, enough has been said to show that the storm center is about the metabolism of the protein molecule and that carbohydrate and fat enter very little into the discussion of etiology, except in so far as they may give rise to some form of gastro-intestinal disturbance more from quantity than quality. One notable exception to this is, that according to some authorities, fat stands in the first place in the etiology of eczema, particularly in infants. The relation of diet, therefore, to diseases of the skin is undoubtedly, in many instances, a most intimate one, but too little has yet been done, with one or two possible exceptions, to place the question on a basis of established fact.

PSORIASIS.

This is one disease of which considerable study has been made by Shamberg[1] and his collaborators, to determine the metabolic changes. In their investigations the complement-fixation test was not found to be positive, nor was any organism to blame, but a marked nitrogen retention was found throughout the period of the experiment and it was felt that

[1] Jour. Cut. Dis., October, 1913, p. 708.

a definite relationship between the amount of nitrogen in the food and the cause of the disease was established. The corresponding clinical evidence corroborated this, as the patients improved on a low protein diet and became worse on a high protein allowance; this finding was verified in a number of patients. The retention of nitrogen in these cases resembled that seen in convalescence and in one instance amounted to 4.89 gm. nitrogen per day. Curiously enough, however, these patients suffer from what Shamberg calls "nitrogen hunger" and patients with "severe psoriasis present a state of remarkable protein undernutrition." This is because the retained protein goes into making the psoriatic scales which are almost pure protein. The success of the low protein diet in these cases is due to the fact that we can reach the point in diet at which the protein goes only to the vital organs at the expense of the scales, so that the latter do not grow. The amount of protein is therefore only sufficient to cover the wear and tear of the body and leaves nothing to supply the rapidly growing scales. Shamberg ends his conclusions by saying that "the low nitrogen diet has a most favorable influence on the eruption of psoriasis, particularly when it is extensive, almost to the point of the disappearance of the eruption." A high protein diet on the other hand, has an unfavorable influence on the disease and commonly causes its extension. The practical application of these findings in choosing a diet is therefore plain; one should keep the protein down to the low level determined by Chittenden: 45 to 60 gm. (1 ⅓ to 2 oz.) of protein per day or for a short time on even less, of which the following menus are examples.

Low Protein Diets in Psoriasis.

	Grams.	Ounces.
Bread	245.5	8
Sugar	63.0	2
Coffee (breakfast)	210.0	7
Custard	76.0	2 ½
Milk	250.0	8 ⅓
Coffee (lunch)	125.0	4
Potato	150.0	5
Lima beans	80.0	2 ⅔
Coffee (dinner)	210.0	7
Apple dumpling	131.0	4 ⅓
Candy	27.0	

Total nitrogen in food, 8.83 grams = 55 gm. protein.
Fuel value of the food, 1929 calories.

	Grams.	Ounces.
Bread	164.0	5½
Sugar	89.0	2¾
Coffee (breakfast)	210.0	7
Sweet potato	135.0	4½
Quince preserve	73.0	2⅓
Apple turnovers	118.0	4
Coffee (lunch)	310.0	10⅓
Potato	175.0	6
Peas	80.0	2¾
Apple pie	141.5	4¾
Coffee (dinner)	210.0	7

Total nitrogen in food, 7.31 grams = 45 gm. protein.
Fuel value of the food, 2057 calories.

	Grams.	Ounces.
Bread	221.5	7¼
Sugar	77.0	2⅓
Banana	92.5	3
Coffee (breakfast)	210.0	7
Baked potato	165.0	5½
Apple sauce	114.0	4
Coffee (lunch)	210.0	7
Succotash	75.0	2½
Mashed potato	200.0	6½
Chocolate cake	80.0	2¾
Ice-cream	73.0	2½
Coffee (dinner)	210.0	7

Total nitrogen in food, 7.63 ounces = 47 grams protein.
Fuel value of the food, 2065 calories.[1]

Foster's experience, that he could get much more rapid results in psoriasis by making the patiets vegetarians, is easily explained on the basis of facts already submitted.

ECZEMA.

This skin disease is of great importance, as it constitutes, according to Bulkley, one-third of the entire number of skin diseases and its dietetic management is at times exceedingly satisfactory. Eczema is caused by a number of different factors but in many it can be traced to dietetic faults of (1) eating too much; (2) insufficient food; (3) improper food;[2] (4) Hypersusceptibility to certain proteins.

1. In those who eat too much food the cutaneous glands are constantly overstimulated, resulting in a change in the secretions, and as Thompson says, after long irritation the skin finally succumbs to a definite eruption.

2. When one is run down from insufficient food, skin lessions are more apt to develop, particularly since with malnutrition from poverty there are usually added unclean personal habits.

[1] Chittenden: Physiological Economy in Nutrition, p. 62.
[2] Thompson: Practical Dietetics, p. 685.

3. Everyone knows the effect of improper foods, those rich and indigestible, and in persons ingesting such foods eczema is prone to develop.

4. Certain infants are susceptible to particular proteins and give a skin reaction thereto which is really of an anaphylactic nature.[1]

In adults as well as in children, one or more of these causes may be operative, and a careful scrutiny of the patient's actual dietary is necessary before coming to a definite conclusion as to just which causes are at fault in a given case.

Acute Eczema.—The consensus of opinion is that a limited and simple diet is indicated in acute eczema and in fact this rule is applicable to all acute inflammatory skin lesions. Such a restriction is best accomplished by placing the patients either on an exclusive milk diet or with cereals, bread, butter, and fresh green vegetables or on the so-called rice diet which Bulkley recommends from large experience. Bulkley's diet consists exclusively of rice, bread and butter and water for at least five days, after which other foods are gradually added. The rice should be thoroughly cooked for from thirty to sixty minutes in water, not with milk. It can be dried out a little after cooking if it is more palatable in this form. Butter and salt are to be eaten on the rice, which should be taken very slowly, accompanied by thorough mastication. The bread should be stale. According to Bulkley the rationale of this diet lies in the fact that acute eczematous manifestations are due to retained nitrogen waste products, and giving a diet that is of low nitrogen content, allows the kidneys to excrete the retained matter, and when this is accomplished the acute stage of the eruption comes to an end.

At the end of five days it is advised to return gradually to a mixed diet, taking first one regular mixed meal at midday and the rice diet morning and night.

If this is successful a light breakfast is given, such as cereal with butter, eggs and bacon and possibly a little weak tea or coffee,[2] soft green vegetables, farinaceous puddings, whole meal bread, eggs, milk, chicken, fresh fish are then added. Many authorities forbid fruit in any form while others allow it stewed without sugar and still others fresh, if ripened nearby and not picked green.

Chronic Eczema.—In chronic eczema the question as to "too much," "too little" or "improper food," comes up, in a way, for consideration much more than in the acute form.

[1] C. H. Smith.
[2] Bulkley: Diet and Hygiene in Diseases of the Skin, p. 70.

Here much can be done to bring about a favorable progress of the disease by cutting down the food of the glutton, feeding up the poorly nourished and regulating the diet of those who habitually eat indigestible or improper foods.

Among articles of food that should not be touched by these patients are spices, condiments, alcohol, fried foods, rich gravies, pastry, sweets, cake, cheese, salt food, ham, nuts, corned beef, salt pork, much meat and meat soups, salads and twice-cooked meats and curries.

The low (Chittenden) level of protein is advisable for those who habitually overeat. These prohibitions also hold for the "after-diet" in acute cases.

Eczema in Nurslings.—Here the dietetic and hygienic faults are the mother's, and attention to her intake, exercise, and bathing, will often result in the relief of the infant's eczema. There are commonly two varieties seen:

1. In overnourished, fat babies who have shown evidence of eczema since birth.

2. In those babies who have previously thriven, but who develop gastro-intestinal trouble and eczema, seen especially when they are weaned and put on an improper milk mixture.

In the first group the mothers are usually found to overeat or take too much alcohol and too little exercise. In the second group the babies' stools indicate indigestion, which, if rectified results in a cure of the eczema. Finckelstein has obtained good results by feeding nutrose (casein preparation) before each feeding or by giving buttermilk twice a day with some additional carbohydrate.[1] In artificially fed children with eczema Holt advises giving food moderately high in fat and low in protein and if not successful he reduces both fat and protein. In some instances, according to C. M. Williams, it is advisable to withdraw milk entirely from the diet and substitute wheat jelly, thin gruels, beef juice and eggs. Also careful attention must be given to the regulation of the times of feeding. Still other children are benefited as soon as they can be placed on mixed feedings, this is particularly true in the chronic form. It is also true here, as in adults, that those children who are overfed will do better if the food is reduced both in quantity and quality and, *vice versa*, the undernourished fed more liberally.

Meyer found that children with chronic eczema showed salt retention which in turn leads to water retention predisposing to eczema. On this basis Finckelstein fed a salt-free milk diet with high protein and carbohydrate with good results.

[1] Lyman: Arch. Ped., 1915, xxxii, 175.

This salt-free milk is prepared by removing the salts by washing the casein in water then mixing the curd with four-fifths water and one-fifth whey with the addition of 40 to 50 gm. of salt-free carbohydrate. This is known as "eczema soup."

This is not applicable to all cases, but does best in fat babies with a moist, "weeping," impetiginous eczema, when protein digestion is poor, as shown by curds and undigested stools.

Reducing the percentage of the protein in the food will often result in clearing up the eczema.[1] In certain cases cutting out all sugars and carbohydrates and putting the children on a skimmed milk diet, does much to clear up the disease—this of course is almost another way of saying to starve the children moderately. Of course if the eczema is due to protein susceptibility no measure will be definitely efficient until the offending protein is discovered and eliminated from the diet. This diagnosis is made by testing the skin reactions as is done in asthma and urticaria.

Since there is apt to be a very high urinary acidity in all chronic cases of eczema this should be rectified by giving large amounts of water plain or alkaline.

The dietary regulations given are good so far as they go and in some instances are sufficient for a cure, but almost all cases require local treatment as well.

ACNE ROSACEA.

The underlying condition in acne rosacea is a vasomotor instability affecting particularly the blood supply of the skin of the nose and cheeks, resulting in abnormal flushing of these parts of the face.[2] Such a condition can be brought about temporarily, even in normal persons, by hot drinks as soups, tea, etc., particularly in an overheated room. Alcohol is of course the greatest etiological factor in the production of chronic rosacea, although it by no means follows that all chronic cases can be traced to this as a cause. The alcohol acts largely through the gastritis which it causes; gastric hyperacidity from other causes being also frequently responsible for the production of acne rosacea. Chronic indigestion, gastric or intestinal, associated with the putrefaction of animal protein and often accompanied by high percentage of indican in the urine, acts much in the same way and must be kept in mind when prescribing a diet.

[1] Lyman: loc. cit.
[2] G. T. Jackson: Diseases of the Skin.

The proper diet in rosacea is one from which are excluded all the known etiological factors, *e. g.*, alcohol, hot tea, coffee, soup, spices, condiments, fried food, rich sauces, gravies, made-over dishes, pastry, heavy sweets, rich cake, and everything known by the individual to be a possible cause of gastro-intestinal indigestion. Patients should themselves notice the effects on the skin of any particular kind of food and learn to avoid those things which cause flushing. Of the greatest importance is the patient's general hygiene—baths, exercise, fresh air and water drinking—all of which is equally true in both acne rosacea and acne vulgaris.

ACNE VULGARIS.

In acne vulgaris the ducts of the sebaceous glands become closed, the plugs consisting almost entirely of epithelial cells with practically no foreign substances in them. A secondary staphylococcus infection is then engrafted on this, as the opsonic index is low to the staphylococcus, and results in pustulation or at least deep skin infection which may be only inflammatory, short of the production of pus. One factor which probably favors the infectious element is the fact that in acne vulgaris the percentage of blood sugar is higher than normal. This form of acne is most frequently seen in young people at puberty and often disappears after a few years, although in some cases it is of exceedingly prolonged duration and taxes the ingenuity of the dermatologist.

Where the patients are found to be excessive eaters, the quantity of food should be cut down and will often give relief, in some cases Jackson obtained the best results on an exclusive milk diet. On the other hand, when the acne is an accompaniment of malnutrition the patients should be liberally fed and everything done to improve their general health with consequent raising of their opsonic index. Tea, coffee and alcohol and all indigestible foods are forbidden. The amount of fat food should be limited and much the same restrictions insisted upon as indicated for acne rosacea. Williams[1] bars cheese, pickled food, sausage, cabbage, cauliflower, griddle cakes, oatmeal and pastries, fresh bread and salads. Sweets are especially to be forbidden as favoring a still further increase in the percentage of blood sugar, as well a large use of carbohydrates in general.

ERYTHEMA.

Erythema occurs in so many forms; simple erythema, erythema nodosum, multiforme, urticarial and hemorrhagic erythema—all of which are undoubtedly varying skin re-

[1] Food and Diet, p. 337.

actions to a variety of toxic ingesta, and it is difficult to know just where to begin a discussion of the subject from a dietetic point of view. Many persons learn early in life what foods will produce these effects and avoid them; again persons seem susceptible at one time to a certain food and not at another, so that to know just which form of food is responsible for a particular attack, often presents a problem of some difficulty. Where erythema multiforme is seen with urticaria it is probably of gastro-intestinal origin; if with purpura it is more apt to be due to some focus of infection or from a ptomaine toxemia.[1] Of course, it goes without saying that where a certain form of food is at fault that food should be avoided in future and the best method of treatment in addition to this advice is an initial thorough emptying of the digestive canal combined with the simplest sort of diet possible, in order to keep down intestinal putrefaction with its accompanying by-products, which are most often at fault. To this end a lactovegetarian and farinaceous diet is best and is usually promptly efficient in the transient forms, such as in acute urticaria, so often caused by fish or shell fish. In the more prolonged types, such as erythema multiforme, it is often necessary to continue such a diet or at least a very bland and unirritating diet for a considerable length of time or until the eruption is entirely cleared up.

In chronic urticaria we have a difficult problem and from a dietetic point of view an almost hopeless one unless we are fortunate enough by a process of exclusion to find some particular food which is at fault. Testing the skin reactions with the different proteins sometimes shows which protein is at fault. Often, however, this is impossible and the most one can do in diet is to give simple and easily digested foods which, at least, will not increase the trouble by adding intestinal indigestion. Since urticaria is thought by some to be always an anaphylactic phenomenon, the dietetic suggestions detailed under Asthma may prove most helpful in arriving at a proper dietary regimen. (See p. 323.)

Erythema accompanying infection cannot, except secondarily, be influenced by diet, but at least nothing should be given to increase the skin irritation and avoidance of the class of so-called food irritants, such as condiments, spices, garlic, and alcohol, should be insisted upon.

PRURITUS.

Pruritus in any of its forms is an itching condition and may be due to many causes, ranging from an inherited irritable skin to that due to hemorrhoids or fissure, tobacco in excess,

[1] Anthony: Jour. Cut. Diseases, 1912, p. 112.

renal poisoning, diabetes, cold, ascarides, etc.[1] Most of these conditions, it will be readily seen, are not amenable to dietetic relief and yet we can do much to add to the discomfort of an already irritable skin by an improper diet.

When the itching is intense and the skin at all generally hot and inflamed it is a good plan to put the patients on a very bland lactovegetarian diet for a few days, as is true of all acute inflammatory skin lesions. Later avoidance of the stimulating class of foods such as condiments, is indicated; Jackson especially interdicts the use of alcohol, tea, coffee and tobacco; some of the worst cases are seen in heavy smokers, and the condition is distinctly aggravated by even moderate smoking.

"Prurigo and lichen urticatus are closely related to urticaria and are accompanied by a highly susceptible vasomotor or sensory nerve system set in action by a variety of excitants which often elude one's investigation."[2]

In these conditions the diets suggested for rosacea and urticaria are useful.

DERMATITIS.

Dermatitis Herpetiformis.—Hardouin found retention of urea in the system just before the eruption in 8 cases, so that this is undoubtedly the local manifestation of a general metabolic disturbance and as retention of purine bodies probably lies in a causal relation to the disease it would be appropriate to prescribe a diet similar to that advised in gout or at least a very low purine diet, accompanied by effectual elimination through all the exits. Other investigators found normal urinary excretion and cultures and experimental inoculations of the liquid from the bullæ negative and think much points to a deranged nervous system as the cause of dermatitis herpetiformis. During the acute stage the diet should be simply milk; tea, coffee and alcohol are forbidden—when the inflammatory condition has subsided vegetables, farinaceous foods and eggs may be added to the diet, returning gradually to a normal diet, excluding indigestible and purine-rich foods.   (See Diet in Gout.)

Exfoliative Dermatitis.—Probably the best results are obtained with a milk diet and in addition the use of colonic irrigations. Jackson (G. T.) advises flaxseed tea several times a day. After the acute stage is over a diet as in eczema is valuable.[3]

[1] Jackson: Disease of the Skin, p. 450.
[2] Sutherland's Dietetics.
[3] Thompson: Practical Dietetics, p. 685.

Ferunculosis.—Ferunculosis should be treated dietet-ically like acne vulgaris and the same rules hold good. As it is especially prone to develop following severe illness during the period of convalescence, the indications are usually for a full nourishing diet, but simple withal. The feeding of one or two yeast cakes daily is often of great service.

Comedones.—Comedones are due to the blocking of the sebaceous gland ducts by a disordered secretion and are often accompanied by gastro-intestinal disturbances. The diet should conform to the actual digestive disorders present in an individual case and besides careful hygiene of the skin, elimination should be increased by copious water drinking.

Hyperidrosis.—Since the sweating which accompanies hyperidrosis is caused by a vasomotor disturbance, general hygiene plays a part in the cure, with which must be included of course, and although there is no specific diet that is indicated, patients with hyperidrosis should avoid digestive risks and generally keep to a very simple diet. When the hyperidrosis is accompanied by obesity, uricacidemia or some nervous condition, these should receive their appro-priate hygienic and dietetic treatment.

CHAPTER XXV.

DISEASES OF THE GENITO-URINARY SYSTEM.

In attempting to discuss the food factor in nephritis. it must be kept in mind that the relation of diet to nephritis is two-fold—(1) in its causation role, about which we know little; (2) in its relation to rational treatment and dietetics of the disease, about which we know more but still too little. That food does often stand in an important role as the causation of nephritis must be admitted, although as yet we have but a glimmering of its true significance—but when we stop to think of the known drugs and foods which directly irritate the epithelium in greater or less degree, such as cantharides, turpentine, lead, arsenic, salicylic acid, mustard, peppers, the oil from garlic, onion and celery and numerous other substances— it is but a short cry to the possibility of repeated minimal irritation by foods less well recognized as renal irritants. The analogy of liver cirrhosis is sufficient for purposes of comparison, and while the liver is damaged in the attempt it makes to detoxify the irritating alcohol, hot sauces, etc., the kidney must run an equal risk in its excretion of most of the products of protein metabolism. That this is so has been increasingly evident and we have come to recognize still another form of renal irritant in repeated anaphylactic shocks as demonstrated by Longcope by the injection into animals of protein after previous sensitization to these same proteins. After a large secondary dose of protein, acute degeneration of the renal epithelium is seen, or if less acute, one finds collections of round cells about the vessels and in the intermediate zone. If the process is long continued there is found a connective tissue increase and glomerular lesions. These changes are not confined to the kidney but are seen in the parenchyma of other organs. It can therefore be seen that a patient may unconsciously be constantly receiving mild, unfelt anaphylactic shocks from certain food proteins to which he is sensitive, with resulting renal changes. Again, any food that has a tendency to produce acid or to lower the alkaline reserve of the blood, will result in damage to the kidney. Among such foods may be mentioned excessive protein or fats, also inorganic acids.

So presumably anything that reduces the alkaline reserve causes a damage to the cell protoplasm, which if constantly repeated may well result in nephritis. Besides the lessened alkalinity of the blood, Auld suggests demineralization (calcium loss) and impaired metabolism as results of an acid excess. The subject of acidosis in nephritis is one about which much discussion and experimentation has been had. There is no doubt but that in the later stages of chronic nephritis there is a definite lowering of the alkaline reserve due to the accumulation of retained phosphates and there is no doubt but that this condition further cripples the kidney. The index of the acidosis is the concentration of carbon dioxide in the alveolar air as this corresponds with that in the blood. Dietetically, therefore, all foods that tend to reduce the urinary acidity are valuable in nephritis, provided there are no contra-indications from other view points. To this end, potatoes, apples, bananas, raisins, oranges, cantaloupe, sweet potatoes and carrots are especially good, for through them considerable amounts of the desired alkaline bases are gotten into the system. Blatherwick[1] showed that vegetables, fruits (the foregoing particularly) as a class on burning leave base or alkaline elements Na K Mg. Cal. while meat, fish, cereals (especially oatmeal), peanuts, plums, prunes and cranberries are not good as they cause acid production, the last four named, due to their benzoic acid content.

When we are in the presence of complications, such as edema or marked nitrogen retention, it may be necessary to modify the use of the foods especially recommended above but at least these suggestions apply strongly to the period in chronic nephritis before complications supervene and will surely help to put off their evil day.

Gross overeating is undoubtedly a cause of kidney change probably of a fibroid nature, as we know that the same cause acts in producing arteriosclerosis, in which process the kidney shares, as do other organs. Taken then all together, there are definite ways in which food may act in the production of renal changes, although it is often a matter of great difficulty to decide in a given case just which cause is primarily at work, after the exclusion of the more usual causes of renal irritation, such as the infectious diseases, intestinal toxemia, focal infection, etc.

The newer studies in kidney functions have brought to light many facts which have helped us to understand findings which were for so long obscure. Unfortunately they have not yet gone so far that we can classify all cases of nephritis, acute and chronic, to our entire satisfaction, but

[1] Arch. Int. Med. xiv, 409.

enough has been accomplished by experimentation to justify certain therapeutic conclusions that have proven of great value.

The factors which must be taken into especial consideration in dealing with the dietetics of nephritis have to do with the excretion of various substances derived from the digestion of foods, and the different behavior of the diseased kidney from the normal kidney with respect to their elimination. One starts with the premise that the healthy kidney can perfectly eliminate water, nitrogenous products of protein combustion, certain inorganic salts, notably sodium chloride, and organic compounds, which result from bacterial activity. When one then begins to classify the cases of nephritis with respect to the individual's power to excrete these substances, one soon finds that they are almost never found to be of one simple type, since the structures of the kidney are all more or less involved, the excretion of one, two or all classes of constituents of normal urine may be interfered with, so that the kidney's behavior to the excretion of these various substances is not absolutely fixed. In spite of this fact, most of the cases may be grouped separately according as the excretion of one or another urinary constituent is chiefly interfered with. With experimental nephritis it is somewhat different; we can by means of various kidney poisons, artificially introduced into the animal's body, produce what is practically a pure type of tubular, glomerular or interstitial nephritis. It has been by watching the elimination of the normal urinary constituents under one or another form of artificially produced nephritis that we know as much as we do in regard to the behavior of the kidney toward the normal urinary constituents with respect to their elimination. In this connection the effect of certain foods on the behavior of the kidneys in eliminating dyes is the subject of much experimentation by Salant[1] and others with certain conclusions which are of great interest clinically.

1. Small doses of tartrate of soda injected subcutaneously produced an inhibition of elimination of phenolsulphophthalein. When rabbits were fed on oats (acidophylic) it never went back to normal.

2. Evidence of disturbed renal function was seldom obtained with much larger doses if the rabbits were on a diet of young carrots. Large doses of the tartrate gave some decrease in elimination but excretion went back to normal.

3. If the tartrate was injected gradually in increasing doses, no impairment of function was noted even with very

[1] Proc. Soc. Exp. Biol. Med., 1917–18, xv, 8.

large doses (4 to 6 gm. per kilo) if carrots were used alone as diet. This was not so with a diet of oats.

For a full discussion of the various diagnostic methods to determine the renal function founded upon the results of experimental nephritis, such as the sulphophenolpthalein test, salt test, potassium iodide test, lactose test, the determination of the Ambard coefficient, water test and diet test days, the reader must be referred to any one of the newer editions of standard text-books on internal medicine. In order to know just which type of renal hypofunction a given case belongs to, some of these tests must be made and together with the history and clinical findings a fairly accurate idea can be obtained as to which function or functions of the kidney are disturbed and the diet arranged accordingly.

Kidney Dietary Tests.—Water Excretion.—It is a simple matter to determine the water excretion by ordering a definite amount of water for the twenty-four hours and measuring the actual fluid intake and urinary output; thus if 1500 c.c. (50 oz.) are taken and 1200 c.c (40 oz.) or thereabouts represents the output for twenty-four hours, the water excretion is considered normal under ordinary conditions of temperature and humidity, as the 300 c.c (10 oz.) discrepancy between intake and output is lost by bowel, skin and lungs.

Salt Excretion.—This is determined by noting the daily salt output both as to concentration (percentage of NaCL in the urine) and the total twenty-four-hour output on a known salt intake. For this purpose one of the salt-poor diets are used with a known salt content, to which a definite amount of salt is added after weighing. This should be done for several days and accurate daily estimations made. Normally the kidney should be able to concentrate chlorides up to 0.6 to 0.9 per cent. with a total daily excretion of practically the entire intake.[1]

Nitrogen.—The determination of nitrogen excretion is somewhat more difficult, but it can be done if the patient is placed upon a fixed nitrogen diet and the daily nitrogen balance determined. For this a well-equipped laboratory is necessary, while for the determination of water and salt excretion very little is needed in the way of apparatus. Schlayer's nephritic test day, as modified by Mosenthal,

---

[1] *Test for the Amount of Salt in the Urine.*—Dilute 10 c.c. of urine with 900 c.c. of water and add one or two drops of 25 per cent. nitric acid. This mixture should be made alkaline with a 10 per cent. solution of sodium carbonate adding a few drops of a 10 per cent. potassium chromate for an indicator. Titrate with tenth-normal silver chloride solution. Every c.c. of silver solution used equals 0.00583 gm. of sodium chloride.

gives the information desired in the matter of water, sodium chloride and nitrogen excretion in the most convenient way as follows:

DIRECTIONS FOR SCHLAYER'S NEPHRITIC TEST DAY
(Mosenthal).

Needed in the Ward.

7 wide-necked bottles, each labelled.

1 bottle to hold 1000 c.c. for night specimen.

6 bottles to hold 500 c.c. for two-hour specimens during day.

Salt in capsules, each capsule to contain 2.3 grams sodium chloride.

Preceding day's diet should be "soft salt-free" with fluids limited to 1500 c.c.

Test Day.—All food is to be salt-free, from diet kitchen.

Salt for each meal will be furnished in weighed amounts (one capsule containing 2.3 grams, sodium chloride with each meal.)

All food or fluid not taken must be weighed or measured after meals and charted.

Allow no food or fluid of any kind except at meal times as directed.

Note any mishap or irregularities that occur in giving the diet or in collection of specimens.

Meals to be given at the following hours:

Breakfast,   7.45 A.M.
Dinner,   11.45 A.M.
Supper,   4.45 P.M.

No fluids between meals or during the night.

Collection of urine during the day every two hours, and from 7.45 P.M. to 7.45 A.M.

Empty bladder at the following times:

No. of specimen:	7.45 A.M. discard		
1	9.45 A.M. save in separate bottle		
2	11.45 A.M.	"	"
3	1.45 P.M.	"	"
4	3.45 P.M.	"	"
5	5.45 P.M.	"	"
6	7.45 P.M.	"	"
7	7.45 P.M. to 7.45 A.M.	"	"

Label each bottle with period of collection, number of specimen and name of patient and send to laboratory.

Breakfast, 7.45 A.M.—Chart food or fluid not taken.

Boiled oatmeal, 100 grams; sugar, one-half teaspoonful; Milk, 30 c.c.;

Two slices of bread (30 grams each); butter, 20 grams;
Coffee, 160 c.c.; milk, 40 c.c.; sugar, one teaspoonful;
Milk, 200 c.c.;
Water, 200 c.c.

Dinner, 11.45 A.M.—
Meat soup, 180 c.c.;
Beefsteak, 100 grams;
Potatoes (baked, mashed or boiled), 130 grams;
Green vegetables as desired;
Two slices bread (30 grams each); butter, 20 grams;
Tea, 180 c.c; milk, 20 c.c.; sugar, one teaspoonful;
Water, 250 c.c.;
Pudding (tapioca or rice), 110 grams.

Supper, 4.45 P.M.—
Two eggs (cooked in any style);
Two slices of bread (30 grams each); butter, 20 grams;
Tea, 180 c.c.; milk, 20 c.c.; sugar, one teaspoonful;
Fruit, stewed or fresh, one portion.
One capsule of salt with each meal = 3 x 2.3 grams.

FINDINGS IN A CASE OF CHRONIC HYPERTENSIVE NEPHRITIS.

Time.	Amount c.c.	Sp. gr.	Sodium chloride. Per ct.	Total.	Nitrogen. Per ct.	Total.	Approximate intake.
7.45 to 9.45	155	1013	....	....	..	....	Fluids 1760 c.c.
9.45 to 11.45	97	1011	....	....	..	....	Salt 8.5 gms.
11.45 to 1.45	98	1014	....	....	..	....	Nitrogen 13.4 "
1.45 to 3.45	255	1010					
3.45 to 5.45	43	1015					
5.45 to 7.45	325	1011					
Total day	983	....	.16	1.57	.37	3.63	
Night	800	1014	.215	1.72	.48	3.85	
Total 24 hours	1783	....	....	3.29	..	7.49	
Intake	1760	....	....	8.5	..	13.4	
Balance	—23	....	....	+5.21	..	+5.91	

The figures show a negative water balance, but retention of both chlorides and nitrogen.

In discussing the various urinary elements and their excretion, from the clinical point of view, we have a number of questions to be kept in mind.

Water.—It was long thought that the giving of large amounts of water in any form of nephritis was the best thing one could do for the patient, with the idea of washing out the poisonous products of incomplete or even complete metabolism. Von Noorden differed from this view and showed that in certain cases the kidney could not eliminate water as well as it could other substances and the only effect of giving it in large amounts was to increase the edema, or if there was no edema, to overfill the circulatory apparatus, putting an extra strain on the heart and bloodvessels.

In the normal individual there is a loss of water through skin and pulmonary excretion of approximately one-fifth of the intake, so that if a patient is given 2000 c.c. (66 oz.) of fluid, *i. e.*, 1500 c.c. (50 oz.) as fluid direct and about 500 to 750 c.c. (16-25 oz.) in the food taken (which Mohr calculates to be about the amount of fluid contained in the ordinary diet) only 1600 to 1700 c.c. or there about will be excreted by the kidney (53 to 56 oz.) and the rest is lost in the ways already referred to. When in nephritis the amount excreted is still markedly less, then one may be sure that one is dealing with a nephritis which finds difficulty in eliminating water, the unexcreted balance being held in the serous cavities, subcutaneous tissues or circulation. The question may well be asked, What then is the optimum amount of water to give in nephritis? To this no hard-and-fast rule can of course be given, but Mohr[1] found by experimentation that "in any form of nephritis the maximum amount of solids were eliminated if the patient passed from 1250 to 1500 c.c (42 to 50 oz.) of urine." Miller[2] further states that when the kidney is able to excrete the normal amount of fluid and there is no evidence of edema, 1500 to 2000 c.c (50 to 66 oz.) of fluid is quite enough to give in twenty-four hours. When there is difficulty in water excretion then the total amount of water best to give must be determined in accordance with that particular patient's capability as determined by daily measuring the intake and the urine, the doing of which is only a detail of general management.

Salt.—In the consideration of the salt excretion, two classes of salts are to be considered; the chlorides, of which sodium chloride is the most important example, and the sulphates and phosphates, both of which latter behave much as the nitrogenous products do and not as the chlorides. If the patients have no subcutaneous edema the chloride elimination is normal even if the nitrogen elimination is poor. In other words, nephritis with edema invariably shows salt retention.[3]

Strauss puts the principles involved thus: "The human organism holds fast with extreme tenacity to the percentage

[1] Beiträge Zur Diatetik der Nierenkrank. Ztschr. für klin. Med., 1903, p. 1377.

[2] Forchheimer's Therapeutics, vol. iv, 34.

[3] Ibid., vol. iv, 22.

concentration of the fluids in sodium chloride." This is done by a regulating mechanism of which the kidney stands in the first rank. When more than enough salt is taken by a healthy person it is promptly eliminated and when the organism is starved, as in extreme vomiting, the output of salt in the urine is at once diminished in order to keep the blood concentration at about 0.6 to 0.9 per cent.[1] Strauss also reached the conclusion that the chloride retention in nephritis with edema was of renal origin and that withdrawal of salt from the diet (all but the necessary 1.5 or 2 gm. per day) was necessary for treatment. The three factors on which he based his views were: (1) that in unilateral nephritis lower chloride values are found in the urine from the diseased kidney; (2) in an exacerbation of the disease the value of sodium chloride excreted often falls off; (3) that only dropsies were helped by remedies which caused not only an increased water output but at the same time a polychloruria. Dechlorination according to the same authority consists of two elements: (1) a salt-poor diet; (2) salt elimination from medicaments.

The minimum of salt which is necessary to maintain the normal molecular salt concentration, as already stated, is about 1.5 gm. per day, but as it is almost impossible to construct a salt-poor diet with much less than this amount, there is no practical danger of actual salt starvation, provided there are enough calories in it to meet nutritional demands.

Nitrogen.—When we turn to nitrogen elimination we find that in the mild types of nephritis the nitrogen elimination is delayed as compared with the normal person. This delay being caused (judging by experimental nephritis) by injury to the glomeruli.[2] When one has to do with a more severe nephritis it is found that the nitrogen compounds are retained in the blood and tissues. These facts are of paramount importance in prescribing definite amounts of protein food, for with the more severe cases accompanied by nitrogen retention we must reduce the protein intake not only to the nutritional minimum but below this for a short time.

Goodall[3] discovered that by placing chronic nephritics on a low protein diet the blood-pressure fell and on examining the blood of these cases that had been so dieted he found the non-protein nitrogen lowest and he therefore concludes that the general condition and bood-pressure were improved

[1] Strauss: Post Graduate, 1913, xxviii, 532.
[2] Manakow: Duetsch. klin. Med., April, 1911.
[3] Boston Med. and Surg. Jour., 1913, clxviii, 761.

when the end-products of protein metabolism in the blood were lowest. Frothingham and Smillie[1] tried diets in chronic nephritis of low, medium and high protein content and concluded "that in certain types of chronic nephritis the nitrogenous content of the diet should be carefully watched in order to prevent an increase in non-protein nitrogen in the blood. The exact effect of an increase in blood nitrogen produced by a high nitrogenous diet is not known at present, but presumably it is unfavorable to the best interests of the patient, since in some it increases their discomfort. A diet low in nitrogen content will frequently keep down to normal the non-protein nitrogen of the blood in chronic nephritis. In uremia the non-protein nitrogen is always high." To this last statement there are known exceptions.

While the foregoing facts represent the general opinion in regard to kidney function and the influence of the various food-stuffs in the matter of excretion, another school of clinicians, of whom Martin Fischer is perhaps the best known, take exception to almost all of these ideas and contradict flatly many of the foregoing statements in fact, most of them; thus for example Fischer recommends in all cases of nephritis that large amounts of water should be given even if apparently the patient is not excreting the normal proportion of the fluid intake. This is done to dilute the body acids so that they can be excreted, for "a kidney that is killing itself clearly needs water to rid itself of the poisons that are killing it."[2] Too much water he admits sometimes increases the swelling of the kidney and washes out valuable salts, but these objections are overcome by giving certain salts with the water, notably sodium chloride and sodium carbonate.[3]

If ordinary dried sodium carbonate is obtainable only one-third as much as the crystallized should be used.

In regard to the use of the salt-poor diets Fischer and his school, as championed by Lowenburg[4] feel that the salt-poor diet may lead to albuminuria and nephritis which Fischer explains as being "due to the low salt content of the body occurring as a result of food without salt," which as already stated he believes washes out the salts naturally present. This salt starvation leads to renal acidosis and this to neph-

[1] Arch. Int. Med., 1914, xv, No. 2, 225.
[2] Martin Fischer: Nephritis, Cartwright Prize Essay, 1911.
[3] The solution Fischer uses is:

Sodium carbonate (crystallized)	20 gm.	⅔ oz.	
Sodium chloride	14 gm.	½ oz.	given by rectum.
Water q. s. ad	1000 c.c.	quart	

[4] Jour. Am. Med. Assn., November 28, 1914, p. 1906.

ritis as represented by albuminuria, cloudy swelling, casts and edema.[1] Lowenburg's conclusions in regard to NaCl based on Fischer's teachings are:

1. Sodium chloride neither produces nor increases water retention in nephritics and non-nephritics.

2. It is curative in cases of edema from any cause provided the kidneys are not too much damaged.

3. When combined with alkalies and plenty of water it exerts a beneficial effect on the symptoms of nephritis.

4. The best method of giving the salt is in an alkaline solution by rectum or intravenously (not hypodermically).

The answer to Fischer's objection, that a salt-poor diet causes sodium chloride starvation and low salt content in the body, is, that first, in severe nephritis the salt concentration in the blood is above normal and second that it is practically impossible as already explained, to give a salt-poor diet which contains less than 1 or 1.5 gm. sodium chloride, sufficient for the body needs for a considerable time, and at best a salt-poor diet of the lowest salt content is only a temporary expedient and a matter usually of not over ten to fourteen days.

In dealing with the actual diets recommended for the various types of nephritis and their complications, the classification of renal diseases must necessarily be a simple one and a division into acute and chronic nephritis with or without nitrogen, salt, or water retention, one or more in combination, is about as far as we can go at present. The older method of ordering diet merely upon the basis of the supposed pathological changes in the kidney is no longer useful in the light of our present knowledge of renal function.

Albuminuria.—Albuminuria being a symptom of renal irritation may be produced in a great variety of ways. It may be toxic in origin from chemical irritants that may have been ingested, *e. g.*, turpentine, cantharides, mercury, etc., or from the toxemia arising from bacterial infection in the course of any of the acute or chronic infections, or as an early manifestation of primary renal disease or finally as a part of a general asthenia characterized by visceroptosis, small heart and ordinarily designated as an orthostatic albuminuria.

When the albumin in the urine is a symptom of actual renal irritation, chemical or bacterial, it is necessary to treat the causal conditions by removal of poisonous materials from the food and to furnish such a dietary that no unnecessary strain shall be put upon the renal epithelium. For this

[1] Loc. cit.

purpose a milk or lactofarinaceous diet is best, milk alone being used for the more serious cases and farinaceous additions being made in the milder grades. When the albuminuria is a part of a general acute or chronic infection, the diet must conform largely to the requirements of the particular infection at fault, but in general the milk or lactofarinaceous diet fills the requirements perfectly and must be kept up as long as the signs of renal irritation persist.

Where there are difficulties in the excretion of water, salts or nitrogen, as shown by edema or any evidences of acute uremia, it is often best to use either the Karell diet or one of the soft salt-poor diets, or with impending uremia a day or two of starvation, giving only water combined with hot packs, and colon irrigations, to relieve the internal congestion.

In the ordinary milk diet, when that is applicable to these cases, we may order from 1500 to 2500 c.c. (3 to 5 pints) of milk per day given in 180 to 240 c.c. (6 to 8 ounces) dosage, every two hours.

As the albuminuria and other evidences of any inflammatory reaction subside and remain in abeyance, other articles of diet may be added—all farinaceous foods, vegetables, except those which contain irritating oils such as onion, garlic and celery; and lastly when things have settled back to what is practically a normal condition, a small amount of meat may be allowed.

In the case of orthostatic albuminuria it is not necessary to diet strictly, for it has practically no effect on the quantity of albumin in the urine, all that can be done is to avoid an excess of any food or drink, particularly meat products and alcoholic beverages.

Acute Nephritis.—In cases of acute nephritis from whatever cause (except mercury poisoning, *q. v.*) the diet must be exceedingly sparing, and it is often best in acute uremia, provided there is no water retention, to give nothing but water for twenty-four hours in rather considerable amounts, relieving the kidney from the necessity of excreting nitrogen except that of endogenous origin. In these cases water excretion is often low, not so much as a result of any impermeability of the kidney to water as from conditions arising in any disease accompanied by fever, which is usually present in acute cases. The various methods to get water into and out of the system are advisable in certain cases, such as water by mouth, hot colon irrigations, hypodermoclysis, saline infusion (in very severe cases), hot packs and catharsis. All these methods both spare the kidneys and at the same time act favorably by flushing them out; just which methods shall be used must depend on the severity of the case. If the less serious cases and on the second day in serious cases feedings may be begun; Tyson[1] recommends 2 ounces of milk every two hours for a few days. This is of course a modified form of the Karell diet which will be described under chronic nephritis. The quantity of milk can be increased as the urine secretion rises and to it may be added within several days farinaceous articles of diet, especially bread, cereals and barley gruel, all served with a moderate amount of sugar. Nothnagel recommends adding fats, as butter and cream, then light green vegetables; these latter according to most American usage are chosen chiefly from those varieties which grow above ground.

Practically all authorities agree that a prolonged and exclusive milk diet is distinctly a bad thing, as it results in anorexia, coated tongue and often in intestinal indigestion with diarrhea. There is no doubt, however, that milk should form the bulk of the diet in the acute cases, although it is well not to give a daily total of protein over 30 to 40 gm. at first, gradually increasing this perhaps to 70 to 80 gm., depending on excretion and the size of the patient. This lactofarinaceous vegetarian diet fills the requirements of food value, variety and bulk, with the minimum of renal irritation. The appetite can usually be trusted to take approximately sufficient food with the restrictions exercised particularly in the protein foods as indicated, and although the total caloric value of the food will necessarily be low at first, it is better so, and as the appetite returns the quantity may be increased at will. Fischer's explanation of the benefit from a lactovegetarian diet is that it contains much fluid and that the salts in the vegetable fruits produce carbonates in the blood which in turn counteract renal acidosis. He also explains in the same manner the usefulness of the old empirical alkaline mixtures given for nephritis, such as the potash salts.

If these cases are prolonged and become subacute, developing edema and difficulty with salt and water excretion, they had best be put on one of the salt-poor diets, although according to Fischer even these cases need to have water in large amounts which if given by rectum and combined with sodium chloride and sodium carbonate, as already stated, reduce the general body acidity and results in the disappearance of the edema. As yet this plan has not met with general acceptance, although there are some favorable reports.

[1] New York Med. Jour. January 31, 1914, p. 223.

Most of the acute cases complicating or following infectious diseases fortunately clear up with care and gradually they may be returned to a normal diet, taking care for months that all irritants are excluded from the diet, such as much meat or meat soup, celery, garlic and onion, which on account of irritating oils are injurious. Alcohol is best left absolutely alone and is not to be recommended for any purpose. If patients refuse to do entirely without alcohol, some of the light white or red wines when diluted with carbonated waters are preferable, but strong liquors, beers and ales should not be taken under any circumstances.

Certain cases of acute nephritis, particularly those of idiopathic or unknown origin tend to continue indefinitely and trail off into a subacute condition or one that becomes chronic. These, in their early stages are treated as are the other acute cases and when they may be said to have become chronic they follow the dietary rules of that class.

Diet and Treatment for Acute Toxic Nephritis From Mercury Poisoning.—Mercury is not infrequently taken with suicidal intent or by mistake for headache tablets; unless the poison is at once removed a severe form of toxic nephritis is set up if the dose is large, resulting eventually in complete anuria, coma and death unless relieved. The following treatment for these cases has been devised by Lambert and Patterson[1] on the basis of laboratory experimentation of K. C. Vogel.

The first indication is to give the patient the whites of several eggs as soon as it is known that mercury has been taken unless it is possible to perform lavage at once which should of course be done, leaving in a pint of milk after the lavage. Lavage should usually be performed as soon as the patient is seen.

The following routine is instituted as soon as the patient ceases to vomit, the termination of which may be hastened by regular lavage.

1. "Every other hour the patient is given 250 c.c (8 ounces of this mixture: Potassium bitartrate, 4 gm. (1 dram); sugar, 4 gm. (1 dram); lactose, 15 gm. (½ oz.); lemon juice, 30 c.c (1 oz.); boiled water, 500 c.c. (16 oz.). Eight ounces of milk are given every alternate hour."

2. The drop method of rectal irrigation with a solution of potassium acetate, 4 gm. (1 dram) to the pint (500 c.c.) is given continuously. The amounts of urine secreted under this treatment are often very large.

3. The stomach is washed out twice daily.

4. The colon is irrigated twice daily in order to wash out whatever poison has been eliminated that way.

5. The patient is given a daily sweat in a hot pack.

[1] Arch. Int. Med., November, 1915, p. 870.

The colonic drip enteroclysis is kept up day and night without interruption. When one dose of mercury has been taken, the treatment may be stopped after two negative examinations of the urine for mercury. For the less severe cases treatment had best be kept up for one week. When large or repeated doses have been taken or where an old kidney disease is present the treatment should be kept up for three weeks, as the mercury is very slowly eliminated by the kidneys, stomach and bowel.

Chronic Nephritis.—The diet in chronic nephritis in its various forms is a trying matter, for the cases are apt to run for years with occasional acute exacerbations, and great care is constantly required in order to prevent the recurrence of symptoms from injudicious diet and hygiene. In the acute cases of nephritis dieting is more stringent but of comparatively short duration and the need for long-continued watchfulness is less imperative. The dietary treatment of the acute exacerbations, occurring in the course of chronic nephritis, is the same as in the acute cases and afterward the cases must be fed and managed with the idea in mind that they may live a fairly long life.

Before turning directly to the subject of specific diets it seems worth while to give some attention in a short paragraph to the general management of chronic nephritis from a dietetic point of view.

Dietetic Management of Chronic Nephritis.—1. As most cases of chronic nephritis have distinct limitations in regard to their excretory power of nitrogen, salts and water, it is absolutely necessary for their most intelligent dietary treatment that these limitations be determined, at least approximately.

2. Since in these cases diet is a matter of months or years, it is necessary to make sure that any diet chosen is palatable, supplies the full requirements in protein, fat, carbohydrate salts, and calories adjusted to the requirements of the particular case and avoiding undue increase in weight.

3. In the long-standing cases it is not necessary to exclude meat absolutely except possibly in the cases with high arterial tension. Most authorities agree with Hare[1] in thinking that the removal of red meat from the diet for a long period is harmful. Since it is the extractives which seem to contain the pressor substances, meat soups are much better excluded from the diet and boiled meat is more to be desired than meat broiled or roasted, as the boiling removes a large

[1] Therapeutic Gazette, 1914, p. 615.

29

proportion of the extractives. Boiling in two waters is better still.

4. The diet, so far as possible, must be kept laxative, as many cases of chronic nephritis are made distinctly worse when there is constipation.

5. Von Noorden recommends once a week the giving of an extra one or two liters of water for the sake of its flushing effect. On these days the food is best limited to not over half the usual allowance. Of course when the patient is not excreting the ordinary daily allowance of water, it would be of doubtful utility to give this extra amount, although again Fischer insists that a kidney that is not secreting water in normal amount needs more water, provided it contains the necessary salts and alkali.

6. The use of vegetables, fruits in large amount as already explained is of the greatest value in furnishing alkaline basic salts.

Diets in Chronic Nephritis.—When in chronic nephritis there are no particular evidences of renal insufficiency, the diet should be distinctly of a prophylactic nature and should contain only the mild foods and unirritating substances. Such a diet may contain:

Oysters, fresh fish, cream soups, vegetable purées made without meat stock. Eggs in limited number, not over one or two a day. Green vegetables, exclusive of those already mentioned as irritating to the kidneys. Fruits of all sorts. Meat, a little once a day (if there exists no contra-indication in hypertension) simply prepared. There is little difference between light meat or dark meat, mammalian meat, or that of fowl, except the latter probably contains a lower percentage of extractives. Fats, butter and oil, mild cheese, farinaceous products such as cereals, breads, preferably stale, simple puddings and desserts. Milk, cream. Vichy, cider if sweet, grape juice or other unfermented fruit juices. Tea and coffee in moderation, avoiding other articles likely to disturb digestion. Alcohol has been disposed of under acute nephritis and what was said there applies equally to chronic nephritis and needs no discussion—it should not be used.

Diet for Cases with Nitrogen Retention (Chronic Uremia.) —In these individuals there is the very distinct indication to feed small quantities of concentrated food with low total nitrogen content Miller[1] recommends for this purpose cream in a total daily amount of one pint, or one-quart half milk, half cream. This pint of cream furnishes 12.5 gm. protein, 92.5 gm. fat, 22.5 gm. carbohydrate and about

[1] Forchheimer's Therapeutics, vol. iv.

1000 calories, or for the quart of half milk—half cream, protein 29 gm., fat 112 gm., carbohydrate 47 gm., 1350 calories; to be sure an amount entirely inadequate to the general nutritional needs but sufficient for temporary use. These cases of chronic or acute uremia often do surprisingly well on this diet for a few days, extra water being allowed and given by mouth, hypodermoclysis, rectum or intravenously, with or without venesection.

Nothnagel praises a milk diet in these uremic or "near uremic" conditions and recommends a liter of milk in twenty-four hours, then when better, increasing it to one and a half to two and a half liters per day. This is carried out for two weeks when the conditions are acute. At all other times an exclusive milk diet is unsuitable, but should constitute a considerable proportion of the daily ration plus vegetables, fruits and farinaceous foods.

This condition of uremia with failure of nitrogen excretion Fischer ascribes to extreme renal acidosis and this condition of acidosis unquestionably exists as proven by estimations of CO_2 in the expired air. Acting on this theory cases are given alkalies by mouth, rectum or intravenously, often with marked benefit (?) in the diminution of the uremic symptoms.

When the immediate danger of uremic coma or convulsions is past one may increase the quantity of milk allowed, adding cereals at first, then vegetables, etc., gradually build-up the diet unless there are contra-indications on account of an existing edema with salt retention or water retention or both, when the limitations of diet for these conditions must be observed.

In nephritis with nitrogen retention, but without difficulty in water elimination, Foster has shown it is often advantageous to push the water ingestion up to 3000 to 4000 c.c. (3 or 4 quarts), as in this way more nitrogen is swept out, for such patients cannot concentrate their urine and the only way of accomplishing elimination is by this method. One prerequisite, however, is a fairly competent circulatory apparatus.

Diet in Water Retention. Edema.—This seldom occurs alone but is usually a part of a total picture of sodium chloride and water retention together. It was formerly thought that the water retention was primary, but later the chloride retention assumed the leading role and the water retention went with it hand in hand in order to keep the chlorides at their normal concentration of a 0.6 to 0.9 per cent. solution. In these cases the salt-poor diets are often useful, or the Karell diet may be used to advantage.

The details of this latter are as follows:

For first five to seven days: 200 c.c. (6½ oz.) milk every four hours, at 8, 12, 4, and 8. No other fluids allowed.

Eighth day: Milk as above and in addition,

10 A.M. One soft-boiled egg.

6 P.M. Two pieces of dry toast.

Ninth day: Milk as above and in addition.

10 A.M. One soft-boiled egg and two pieces dry toast.

6 P.M. One soft-boiled egg and two pieces dry toast.

Tenth day: Milk as above and in addition,

12 NOON Chopped meat (?), rice boiled in milk, vegetables.

6 P.M. One soft-boiled egg.

Eleventh and *Twelfth* days, same as tenth day.

No salt is used at all throughout the diet. Salt-free toast and butter used. Small amounts of cracked ice are allowed with the diet.

This method gives the kidney little water to excrete and later it may resume secretion probably as a result of its rest. On the other hand, cases are sometimes seen in which the fluids have been limited to 800 to 1000 c.c. (27 to 33 oz.) but without therapeutic success, improve as soon as water is pushed, giving an extra 2000 c.c. or even more.

Diet in Salt Retention.—Although this has been discussed slightly in connection with acute nephritis, it is in the chronic forms that we are apt to meet the long-standing and persistent cases with edema, due to chloride retention, accompanied of course by water retention and where some form of diet poor in salt is indicated. Having determined the daily output of salt on a fixed salt diet, as well as the elimination time for some definite extra amount of salt, say 10 gm., we are in a position to know what form of salt-poor diet is indicated. Where no means exist for determining the chloride excretion it may be concluded with considerable confidence that when one finds edema complicating nephritis, in the presence of a fairly competent heart, it is due to primary chloride retention.

If one finds sufficient indication for the use of milk from the character of the urine, *e. g.*, much albumin, blood cells and casts, we can remember that the chloride content of one liter of milk is 1.6 gm., and if one uses the Karell diet of course in the 800 c.c. there would be only 1.2 gm., of salt for the first few days of milk. When it is not necessary to use solely a milk diet even for a few days one can make use to advantage of one of the salt-poor diets, beginning with No. 1, then No. 2 or No. 3, gradually working toward a modified normal dietary exclusive of the renal irritants.

In using the salt-poor diets it is necessary to keep in mind the fact that many cases in whom the edema is due unquestionably to chloride retention do not begin to clear up on the salt-poor diet as rapidly as one could wish or might expect, but that in many instances the diet has to be continued for a week or longer before the rapid emptying of the tissues of salt and water takes place. Still other cases are even more resistant.

The explanation of this fact is not always clear but it seems likely that sparing the kidney for some time finally results in a restoration of its power to excrete salt.

While these salt-poor diets are primarily designed for use in the diet of nephritis, other conditions accompanied by edema, such as chronic cardiac diseases, are often greatly benefited, and in fact collections of fluid in the serous cavities are frequently favorably influenced by one or another of these forms of salt-poor diet.

In this diet, the cereals—butter, bread, etc.—used are all prepared withoLt salt.

Salt-poor Diet No. 1.

Breakfast.	Gm.	Oz.
Farina	60	2
Bread	30	1
Butter (unsalted)	30	1
Sugar	10	⅓
Egg (1)	40	1⅓
Coffee	175	5⅔
Prunes, stewed	60	2
	405	13⅓

Dinner.	Gm.	Oz.
Rice	60	2
Farina	100	3⅓
Bread	30	1
Butter (unsalted)	20	⅔
Sugar	10	⅓
Tea	175	5⅔
	395	13

Supper.	Gm.	Oz.
Toast	15	½
Egg (1)	40	1⅓
Bread	30	1
Butter (unsalted)	15	½
Sugar	10	⅓
Custard	100	3⅓
Baked apple	60	2
Tea	175	5⅔
	445	14⅔

Approximate Values.

Protein 36 gm. (1⅕ oz.); fat 65 gm. (2⅙ oz.); carbohydrate 160 gm. (5⅓ oz.); calories 1350; chlorids 1. gm.

Salt-poor Diet No. 2.

Breakfast.	Gm.	Oz.	*Dinner.*	Gm.	Oz.
Egg (1)	40	1⅓	Egg (1)	40	1⅓
Farina	60	2	Bread	60	2
Bread	65	2⅙	Butter (unsalted)	35	1⅙
Butter (unsalted)	30	1	Farina	100	3⅓
Coffee	175	5⅔	Sugar	10	⅓
Prunes or baked apple	60	2	Rice	60	2
			Tea	175	5⅔
	430	14		480	15½

Supper.	Gm.	Oz.
Toast	15	½
Egg (1)	40	1⅓
Butter (unsalted)	30	1
Bread	60	2
Custard	100	3⅓
Baked apple	60	2
Prunes	60	2
Tea	175	5⅔
	540	17½

Approximate Values.

Protein 51 gm. (1⅔ oz.); fat 100 gm. (3⅓ oz.); carbohydrate 250 gm. (8⅓ oz.); calories 2150; chlorids 1.4 gm.

Salt-poor Diet No. 3.

Breakfast.	Gm.	Oz.	*Luncheon.*	Gm.	Oz.
Bread	30	1	Potato or young carrots	50	1⅔
Egg (1)	40	1⅓	Bread	30	1
Wheat or corn cereal	60	2	Rice	80	2⅔
Orange juice	200 c.c.	6⅔	Tomato	100	3⅓
Sugar	25	⅚	Butter	20	⅔
Butter	20	⅔	Raisins	15	½
Cream	50	1⅔	Sugar	10	⅓
			Ice cream	100	3⅓

Supper.	Gm.	Oz.
Bread	40	1⅓
Butter	30	1
Wheat or corn cereal	60	2
Cream	50	1⅔
Raisins	10	⅓
Sugar	35	1
Potato or young carrots	50	1⅔
Egg (1)		

Approximate Values.

Protein 37 gm. (1⅙ oz.) (5.9 gm. nitrogen); calories 2000; chlorides about 1 gm. (15 grains).

Salt-poor Diet No. 4.

Breakfast.	Gm.	Oz.	*Luncheon.*	Gm.	Oz
Bread	60	2	Bread	40	1⅓
Orange juice	200 c.c.	6⅔	Butter	20	⅔
Butter	40	1⅓	Egg (1)	40	1⅓
Cream	30	1	Potato or carrots	125	4
Farina	50	1⅔	Cream cheese	20	⅔
Sugar	30	1	Sugar	30	1
Coffee or tea	180 c.c.	6	Rice	50	1⅔
			Cream	30	1

Supper.	Gm.	Oz.
Bread	50	1⅔
Butter	35	1
Farina	50	1⅔
Cream	40	1⅓
Cream cheese	30	1
Olive oil	15	½
Lactose	8	¼
Sugar	30	1
Potato or carrots	75	2½

May have in addition moderate amount of tomatoes, lettuce, cabbage, cauliflower, spinach (fresh), beets, carrots, squash, oranges, grape-fruit, peaches, grapes, apricots, pears, melons, jams.

Approximate Values.

Protein 35 gm. (1⅛ oz.) (5.6 gm. nitrogen); calories 2600; chlorides about 1 gm. (15 grains).

Salt-poor Diet No. 5.

(Higher protein.)

Breakfast.	Gm.	Oz.
Bread	60	2
Orange juice	200	6⅔
Butter	30	1
Eggs (2)	80	2⅔
Wheat or corn cereal	90	3
Fresh fruit	50	1⅔
Cream	40	1⅓
Sugar	50	1⅔
Tea or coffee	150 c.c.	5

Luncheon.	Gm.	Oz.
Bread	40	1⅓
Butter	10	⅓
Potato or carrots	80	2⅓
Meat—choice of:		
Lamb chop or	100	3⅓
Steak or	100	3⅓
Chicken	125	4
Fish	70	2⅓
Rice	80	2⅔
Cream	20	⅔

Vegetables from list.

Supper.	Gm.	Oz.
Bread	50	1⅔
Butter	30	1
Cream	40	1⅓
Lactose	8	⅓
Cereal	30	1
Stewed fruit	100	3⅓
Olive oil	20	⅔
Eggs (2)	80	2⅔
Sugar	30	1
Tea	150	5

The same list of accessory fruits and vegetables that was given with Diet No. 4 is available here.

Approximate Values.

Protein 69 gm. (2⅓ oz.); nitrogen 11 gm. (⅓ oz.); chlorides 1-1.5 (15-23 grains); calories 3000.

Table of Salt Content of Common Foods.

	Per cent.
Milk	0.18
Beef broth	0.735
1 egg	0.086
Chicken broth	0.35
Pea soup	0.499
Ordinary white bread (not salt-free)	0.701
Rice	0.748
Boiled potato	0.058

```
Chicken .    .    .    .    .    .    .    .    .    .    .    .    0.01
Beef .    .    .    ..    .    .    .    .    .    .    .    .    0.04
Lamb chops    .    .    .    .    .    .    .    .    .    .    0.97    (Coleman)
Pickerel .    .    .    .    .    .    .    .    .    .    .    0.10
Cod .    .    .    .    .    .    .    .    .    .    .    .    0.59
Salmon .    .    .    .    .    .    .    .    .    .    .    0.46    Schall-Heisler
Haddock    .    .    .    .    .    .    .    .    .    .    .    0.59
Oatmeal gruel    .    .    .    .    .    .    .    .    .    .    0.075
Macaroni    .    .    .    .    .    .    .    .    .    .    .    0.07
Beans    .    .    .    .    .    .    .    .    .    .    .    .    0.0058
Carrots .    .    .    .    .    .    .    .    .    .    .    .    0.029
Apple sauce    .    .    .    .    .    .    .    .    .    .    0.0025
```

Conclusion.—Thus it will be seen that if care is taken in determining the type of nephritis, whether acute or chronic, and as well, which of the functions are principally disturbed, much can be done by dietary regulation to spare a diseased kidney unnecessary labor, and at the same time furnish the organism with the food distinctly appropriate to the needs of each individual case.

PYELITIS.

Whatever the cause of the irritation in the pelvis of the kidney may be, whether from calculus or infection, the dietetic indications are plain enough. As soon as the trouble is recognized the patient should be put on a milk diet with a certain allowance of farinaceous gruel and large amounts of water urged, either as plain water or mild, alkaline drinks, such as Vichy or Vichy and water, equal parts, or water with 1 gm. (15 grains) of bicarbonate of soda added to each glassful. (If urotropin is used to combat the infection, nothing should be used to reduce the natural acidity of the urine, as this drug is only decomposed in an acid medium.) As soon as the fever is over one may give a lactofarinaceous diet with green vegetables and later return to a mixed diet, but with the meat strictly limited to a very small portion, not more than once a day. No condiments of any kind should be allowed and alcohol in every form is contra-indicated.

If nephritis occurs as a complication of the infection the diet should be regulated in much the same way except that the return to mixed feeding should be delayed until all signs of the acute process in the kidney substance have subsided. Attention must be given to preventing constipation, and for this purpose some of the mild saline laxative waters may be used or aloes and podophylin, cascara, etc. If edema develops as a consequence of nephritis it will be necessary to make use of one or other of the salt-poor diets, as detailed under nephritis.

One important fact to remember is, that a continued flushing of the kidney pelvis by large quantities of ingested fluid removes the products of irritation and helps greatly in the healing process.

CYSTITIS.

Practically the same dietetic rules given for pyelitis hold good in cystitis for the difference in the location of the infection does not cause any change in the dietetic requirements. A bland diet at first, largely fluid, and always containing considerable amounts of liquid, is the factor of chief importance; the same abstinence in the use of alcohol and condiments or irritants is observed as in pyelitis.

GONORRHEA.

Even with a specific infection of the anterior and posterior urethra and possibly the complicating cystitis and prostatitis the diet conforms very largely to that already recommended for pyelitis and cystitis. In the early stages a milk diet for a few days, to reduce the irritation, combined with alkaline drinks, to change the reaction of the urine to alkaline, will make the patients much more comfortable. The diet may then be enlarged by the use of all farinaceous and vegetable foods, eggs, milk products, cheese, etc., and, when the inflammatory process reaches the subacute stage, the addition of meat once a day is entirely allowable.

Foods to be particularly avoided are: all forms of spiced and highly seasoned food and condiments, alcohol in any form whatever, strong tea and coffee, acid fruits, tomatoes and asparagus.

It should be remembered that a discharge that is almost cured may be readily started again by an indulgence in irritating foods or drink. This is especially true of the use of alcohol. If it should seem necessary for any reason to take some form of alcoholic drink, a diluted light claret or white wine is best, using an alkaline water, such as Vichy or Apollinaris as a diluent. However, too much stress cannot be laid upon the avoidance of any alcohol.

NEPHROLITHIASIS.

The majority of calculi belong to one of three classes, uric acid, phosphates or oxalates. Uric acid and oxalate calculi are found in acid urine, phosphatic calculi in alkaline urine and these latter are more apt to come secondary to infection and fermentation.

The diet must be simple, avoiding all rich foods and sauces or a great variety at one meal and should be sufficient for the needs of the body but with no surplus.

If the stone is of uric acid, a purine-free or low purine diet should be insisted upon, omitting meats, particularly glandular organs, soups and all highly seasoned foods. Sugar and fat may be taken moderately. Hindhede has shown that vegetable eaters urine has an increased ability to dissolve uric acid so that presumably a low purine and high vegetable diet does most in preventing uric acid stone formation.

When the stone is of the oxalate variety all the foods that contain oxalic acid in excess should be left out of the diet, notably strawberries, rhubarb, figs, apples, peas and spinach. Most of the other vegetables except beans and peas are also theoretically best left alone, as they all contain an excess of lime, rendering the oxalate more insoluble. As a matter of fact however, the fruits and vegetables containing an excess of oxalic acid are the ones to be curtailed.

Meat, in all except glandular form, is allowed freely. This same general dietary rule holds for phosphatic calculi.

In all but phosphatic stones the use of alkaline mineral waters is allowed and does good not by virtue of dissolving the stone, but by flushing the kidneys, rendering the urine less acid with the consequent lessened chance of further calcareous deposit.

It is best to keep the urine faintly acid or neutral but not alkaline, in the latter instance it favors the deposit of phosphates either a calculi or as a coating to a uric acid calculus.

Water in large amounts is recommended to dilute the urine and flush the kidneys, so preventing much of the further deposition of salts.

AMYLOID KIDNEY.

There are no special indications for diet in this condition so far as the amyloid disease itself is concerned, but since in this condition the excretory power of the tubules is diminished the nitrogenous foods should be kept at rather a low point, 40 to 60 gm. (1 ⅓ to 2 oz.), per day while the total food value of the diet should be high to help combat the chronic infection almost always present somewhere in the body, which is the active cause of the amyloid degeneration.

CHAPTER XXVI.

DISEASES OR PATHOLOGICAL STATES DUE TO DISTURBANCES OF NORMAL METABOLISM.

OF course in all diseases there are disturbances of metabolism, so in setting apart a classification such as this we mean merely that in the following diseases the abnormal anabolism or catabolism assumes the chief role, notwithstanding everything else. On this account it is not always easy to say just which diseases shall be included in this class, and as in the other classifications it is more than probable that a certain amount of rearrangement will be necessary as time passes.

In all these states the resultant conditions are more comparable to the results of hyperfunction or hypofunction of certain sets of glands which control growth and body exchange, rather than to actual disease, although the line is often not sharply drawn between the two, for that which starts merely as a functional disturbance may progress to the proportions of a fatal disease, e. g., alimentary glycosuria and severe diabetes.

DIABETES INSIPIDUS.

This disease, characterized by the passage of large amounts of urine of low specific gravity, is probably due to a functional or organic disease of the brain and there is also a possibility that the center in the medulla which controls the renal blood supply as well as excretion, is affected.[1]

Disease in or about the hypophysis is often associated with diabetes insipidus and Frank[2] has suggested the theory that excessive function of this gland is the cause of the disease. The injection of pituitrin often helps these cases, which would rather make it seem as if a hypofunction of the gland were more probable than excessive secretion.

"Minkowski[3] advises that the amount of chlorides and specific gravity of the urine be determined after the ingestion of considerable salt. If both increase relatively more than the urine does, he believes that the power of excreting a concentrated urine is still possessed by the kidneys. · Therefore diminishing the amount of water drunk by the patients

[1] Ref. Handbook Med. Sc., 3d ed., p. 516.
[2] Berl. klin. Wchnschr., xlix, 9.
[3] Therapeutic die Gag., 1910, p. 1.

will help them. If the amount of urine increases relatively the more, a salt-free diet and one poor in protein will be a help."

In choosing a diet it is necessary to avoid foods that cause indigestion or flatulence, particular restriction being placed on sugar, for when an excess of this is taken it tends to raise the percentage of sugar in the blood, which aggravates the polyuria. Cold drinks which are diuretic must be given up, as cold milk, beer, cider, also watery fruits. A salt-poor and low protein diet tend to diminish the quantity of urine when the kidneys do not concentrate the urine normally.

DIABETES MELLITUS.

In perhaps no other disease is diet such a matter of vital importance as in diabetes mellitus, for as time has gone on and one after another procedure or drug has been vaunted as a cure only to be cast aside as entirely wanting, diet has remained as the one factor which is capable, if properly employed, of resting the glycogenic function of the liver, and in all but the most severe and necessarily fatal cases is also capable of bringing about a condition more or less approaching the normal. By its proper employment the mild cases are clinically cured, the moderately severe are rendered mild and the most of the very severe are changed to cases of moderate severity.

An extended discussion of the pathological physiology and disturbed metabolism of diabetes is not necessarily a part of a book on dietetics but it is necessary to discuss the important changes of metabolism if one is to appreciate, to even a small degree, the importance and significance of diet in the varying phases of this disease.

Interest naturally centers about carbohydrate metabolism which formerly was thought to be the only matter of importance and that the metabolism of protein and fat in no way entered into the question for the diabetic. Following this, the importance of fats in the production of acidosis was discovered, and last of all the fact that the body could synthesize sugar out of protein. With this last the whole question of diet in diabetes was revolutionized at a stroke and an explanation was at hand as to why certain cases failed to become sugar-free on a meat-fat diet. Another significant change of thought has been that formerly attention was focussed on the glycosuria as the most important index of a disturbed sugar metabolism, whereas now the hyperglycemia, which always accompanies glycosuria, except in the few cases of so-called renal diabetes, occupies chief attention, since it is found that many cases of diabetes get rid of their glycosuria and would formerly have been pronounced cured but are found to retain their hyperglycemia, thus still showing evidence of a disturbed sugar metabolism.

When we come to study the various aspects of the sugar question we do not find unanimity of opinion. Claude Bernard, Lowe and von Noorden believing that diabetes is due to disturbance of sugar production, while Naunyn and Minkowski believe it due to a disturbance of sugar burning.[1] Hepatic disorders or pathological states were blamed in time past while now the liver is believed by most to be little more than the organ which stores sugar or glycogen and is "played upon" so to speak, by other organs by which the process of sugar excretion by the liver is stimulated or depressed. If we will refresh our memories by reference to normal physiology and then its application to diseased states, we will get a better idea of the question which is so well put by von Noorden.[2]

The liver is the organ which renders sugar available for an immediate source of energy and maintains the sugar content of the blood at 0.075 to 0.1 per cent. If the liver produces more sugar than is required by the tissues, there is an increased amount of it in the blood (hyperglycemia) under which condition some escapes in the urine. If, on the other hand, the liver does not supply enough sugar to the blood, the muscles are the first to suffer and the individual feels fatigue, as occurs after severe labor.

In a condition of alimentary glycosuria the amount of sugar ingested is excessive and cannot be used up, so is excreted in the urine. In order to prevent this, however, the liver stores the sugar as insoluble glycogen which forms a reserve supply. By the action of glycogenase, also found in large amounts in the liver and more or less universally in the body, the glycogen is reconverted into soluble sugar again and so goes into the blood. If for any reason the ordinary supply of carbohydrate is withheld the liver can form sugar out of the protein and fat.

In health the supply and demand for sugar in the blood are exactly balanced and regulated, *i. e.*, the liver does not split up more glycogen for the use of the body than necessary. There are at least two factors which according to von Noorden influence the function of sugar making, viz., the pancreas and the suprarenals, the former a depressant, the latter excitants to sugar formation. According to this

[1] Berl. klin Wchnschr., 1913, p. 2161.
[2] Am. Jour. Med. Sc., 1913, cxlv, 1.

theory, from the pancreas there goes to the liver a specific secretion (an internal secretion, presumably from the islands of Langerhans) which acts as a depressant to sugar formation in the liver. If the pancreas is removed, so is this break in sugar production, and the diastase acting unhindered causes an excessive sugar output from the liver, which is excreted in the urine. This, von Noorden says, is really a severe diabetes.

Adrenalin excites the production of sugar by the liver and a small amount of it is constantly being excreted by the suprarenals and absorbed by the blood. Therefore the suprarenals antagonize the action of the pancreas in its relation to sugar production and these two glandular systems really control the sugar production by the diastase in the liver. The suprarenals do not act alone, for "they are especially under the control of the nervous system." The Claude Bernard center in the medulla is the point from which go out impulses that stimulate the suprarenals to hyperfunction through the sympathetic nerves and thereby cause glycosuria. The pancreas is not independent either, for it is under the control of the thyroid and when the thyroid overfunctionates the pancreatic function is paralyzed and the glycogenase in the liver again acts unhindered, resulting in the overproduction of sugar and glycosuria. So in Grave's disease we see glycosuria and in myxedema increased sugar tolerance. The pancreas is also probably affected by other factors as yet unknown.

This theory is visualized by the diagram on page 463. The arrows represent the direction of the stimuli and the plus or minus signs whether the stimulus is an excitant or depressant on the next organ.

Besides the disturbance in carbohydrate metabolism we have to consider carefully that of protein and fat.

The Relation of Protein Metabolism to Glycosuria.— Protein metabolism in the mild forms of diabetes probably proceeds normally and requires no further discussion, but in the more severe varieties we have other factors that must be taken into consideration. In 1913, Cammidge[1] called attention to the fact that in estimating the degree of toxicosis in diabetes, one should take into consideration the complete picture and that three stages should be distinguished. In two of the three "the defect in metabolism is confined to a more or less complete inability to make use of the sugar derived from the carbohydrate foods, but amino-acids are still available as a source of energy and the body makes use

[1] Lancet, 1913, ii, 1319.

of these supplemented in the milder forms by a certain amount of sugar derived from starchy foods and fats, for its needs. In the third form, to which the name 'diabetes' is confined by some writers, the power to metabolize amino-acids is diminished, with the result that these bodies appear in the urine and gradually increase in amount as the metabolic defect becomes more pronounced. Even in the most serious cases, however, some of the amino-acids are diaminized and converted into dextrose, thus contributing to the sugar excreted in the urine, while the fatty acids of others are imperfectly oxidized and give rise to the 'acetone bodies' (acetone, aceto-acetic acid and β-hydroxybutyric acid) that are passed at the same tmie. Estimations of the amino-acids, 'acetone bodies' and sugar give therefore a much more complete picture of the state of the metabolism than any one of these taken alone, and by considering them in conjunction with the effects produced by a diet of which the qualitative and quantitative composition is known, we can determine the stage that has been reached and the probable expectation of life."

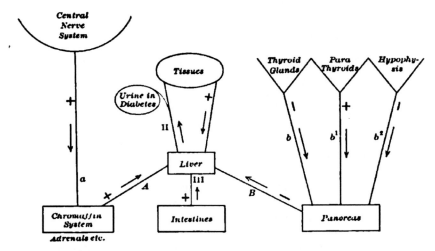

These findings go with the clinical observation that when the diabetes is severe, the protein should be curtailed and intervals of a meat-free diet given.

Animal food is rich in those forms of protein which the disturbed organism finds it difficult to break down and utilize, while vegetable proteins are poor in these constituents and a larger proportion of amino-acids which can be made use of to supply the energy needed by the tissues. Egg protein is more like vegetable protein in this respect and can be used safely where other animal protein is forbidden. Milk however, is like the meat protein.

When we find a patient with amino-acids in the urine we must determine whether they are from the food or from breaking down of their own tissues. and if from the food whether they can still take care of the protein from egg and vegetable. If omitting animal proteins results in freeing the urine of amino-acids, as is the case in gout, the prognosis is better and the outlook with proper diet of getting rid of glycosuria is good, but if we are not able, by regulating the diet, to get rid of the amino-acids the outlook is poor. This constitutes the third or true diabetic stage.

The Nitrogen Balance in Diabetes.—Cammidge[1] in calculating the intake and output of nitrogen in a severe case of diabetes found that with an intake of 12 gm. nitrogen and 52 gm. carbohydrate, the urine showed 31.8 gm. nitrogen with high acetone bodies, ammonia nitrogen, calcium and magnesium and 229 gm. sugar. This demonstrated that the patient was forming sugar from his own tissues. This together with the abnormal excretion of amino-acids, uric acid and creatinin showed that there was a high degree of tissue waste accompanied by defective protein metabolism. When in this case the nitrogen intake was reduced to 3 gm. still keeping the sugar value of the diet at nearly the same level, resulted in the fall of sugar excretion to less than one-half its former amount, the blood sugar fell from 0.3 to 0.2 per cent. and the alveolar carbon dioxide rose to 4.6 per cent. from 0.75 per cent. before; the β-oxybutyric acid also fell from 19.7 to 3.6 gm. accompanied by a clinical improvement. Sufficient has been said to leave no doubt in the mind that the sugar excretion is markedly influenced by protein metabolism and that it is not possible in severe diabetes to make up a deficiency of carbohydrate in the diet by feeding large amounts of protein. Until this fact was learned it was not understood why a diabetic continued to excrete sugar on a carbohydrate-free diet and that it was not until the protein was reduced or changed from a meat to an egg protein that the patient began to be sugar-free.

In this connection reference should be made to coma occurring in some cases of severe diabetes due to a perverted protein metabolism not associated with a ketonuria. Kraus,[1] Rumpf[2] and Lepine[4] and others showed that cases of diabetic coma occurred without any increase of organic acids in

[1] Lancet, 1915, ii, 1187.
[2] Zeit. f. Heilk,. 1906, x, 1899.
[3] Berl. klin. Wchnschr., 1895, xxxii, 185, 669, 700.
[4] Rev. d. med., 1887, xii, 224; 1888, xiii, 1004.

the urine and Rosenbloom[1] reports 3 cases of typical coma occurring in severe diabetes with no carbohydrate tolerance, and even with a restricted protein intake the glycosuria was not diminished. They were observed weeks or months during all of which time the urine contained an average normal amount of ammonia nitrogen, no ketone bodies nor was there any evidence of kidney disease. All 3 cases died in typical diabetic coma. Here we have an effect from abnormal protein metabolism which must be taken into account when dealing with severe diabetes, and its clinical application to dietetics is plain.

Relation of Fat Metabolism to Glycosuria.—As is well known the normal end-products of fat metabolism are water and CO_2; the body fats are chiefly palmitic, stearic, and oleic acids, all of which contain an even number of carbons in their respective molecules. Although protein can add to the formation of acetone bodies, they arise mainly from fat. The complete breaking down of the fatty acids is not altogether an independent process, as it is largely dependent on the presence of carbohydrate in the diet as well as upon the ability of the organism, to metabolize carbohydrates. [2]

Fat does not act as a stimulant to sugar production as does protein but is a source of sugar, although it is only used by the liver in making glycogen when other supplies fail. In severe diabetes, however, the body fat is used in large amount so resulting in emaciation. [3]

In severe diabetics with no carbohydrate tolerance the butyric acid molecule formed in intermediary metabolism of the fatty acids becomes incompletely oxidized only to β-oxybutyric, aceto-acetic acids, and acetone which last is derived from the two former acids. Ringer believes that "one of the functions of the glucose molecule in normal metabolism is to make β-oxybutyric acid, which arises constantly in the catabolism of the higher fatty acids, combustible," and he concludes that if we could find fats with an uneven number of carbon atoms they would be oxidized into glucose instead of acetone bodies. In these conditions of perverted fat metabolism and ketonuria, although we speak of acidosis, by this is meant the accumulation of acid bodies in the blood and tissues sufficient to neutralize enough of the sodium bicarbonate there present to reduce the alkaline reserve to a level below normal; it does not mean that blood and tissues become actually acid in reaction. [4]

[1] New York Med. Jour., August 7, 1915.
[2] Ringer: Tr. Assn. Am. Phys., 1913, xxviii, 469.
[3] Von Noorden: Am. Jour. Med. Sc., 1913, cxlv, 1.
[4] Stillman: Med. Rec., 1916, lxxxix, 390.

Although ketonuria is more apt to be extreme when there is no carbohydrate tolerance, it is a fact that considerable amounts of acid bodies may be excreted when the carbohydrate tolerance is 20 to 30 gm. In long fasting, man shows a fall in his respiratory quotient while the diabetic shows some tendency to a rise. Such observation leads to the belief that the diabetic even in the severest cases burns some sugar or some other body substance to compensate for it. Joslin[1] says there is much experimental evidence that the other body substances are the acids. β-oxybutryric acid has a high caloric value and yields a high respiratory quotient.

Hyperglycemia.—Before proceeding to the discussion of diets in diabetes a word about hyperglycemia is in place, the various causes of which as given by Dock[2] are as follows:
1. Excessive ingestion of sugar.
2. Reduction of liver function.
3. Exaggeration of the glycolytic function of the liver.
4. Reduction of the glycolytic function of the muscles.
5. Exaggeration of the glycolytic function of the muscles.
6. Reduction of formation of fat from glucose.
7. Reduction of combustion of glucose in the muscles.

Since in diabetes mellitus one or more of these functions may be disturbed we see what a various etiology of hyperglycemia there may be, and it is a much more accurate index of perverted metabolism in diabetes than is glycosuria.

While an increase of blood sugar over the normal (0.07 to 0.14) per cent. is usually unfavorable in diabetes, Mosenthal[3] says that diabetic patients by raising the fasting or basal blood sugar percentage, tend to adjust their carbohydrate metabolism in such a manner that they are able to utilize the food offered them to better advantage. While a low blood sugar is usually considered best it may not be desirable in all cases of diabetes mellitus to reduce this.

According to Williams and Humphrey[4] the renal threshold for blood sugar tends to rise with the age of the patient,—younger diabetics have a low or normal threshold and when the diabetes is mild or quiescent the point at which the kidneys eliminate sugar is stationary, but when the disease becomes progressive the threshold tends to rise. Before death the blood sugar renal threshold may reach great heights with little or no sugar in the urine.

[1] New York Med. Jour., 1915, ci, 628.
[2] Int. Cong. Med., 6 Med., p. 234.
[3] Johns Hopkins Hosp. Med. Bull., 1918, xxix, 94.
[4] Arch. Int. Med., xxiii, 537.

Dietetic Treatment of Diabetes.—The dietetic treatment of diabetes mellitus resolves itself into the questions as to how much carbohydrate the individual can utilize and how a tolerance for carbohydrate can be obtained or increased.

If, as Allen says, we compare the glycosuria to a gastro-intestinal indigestion, due to either a functional or organic disturbance, we see at once that what is needed is rest for the deranged function, followed by a gradual system of dietetic reëducation, principally so far as the carbohydrates are concerned, until step by step the body can take care of slowly increased amounts of this food element.

The avoidance of overstrain of the glycogenic function must be kept ever in mind, for if during the process of reëducation sufficient food is given to again precipitate the glycosuria this puts off the further advance disproportionately and if it is continued, quickly results in the loss of the bettered function obtained by previous careful dieting. In other words "over-strain weakens while rest strengthens any damaged function.[1]

Mosenthal[1] studying the maintenance diet in diabetes found the standard in one of two criteria.

1. The caloric requirement as determined by the height-weight formula of DuBois & DuBois[2].

2. The nitrogenous equilibrium as the lowest possible food standard of maintaining physical and mental well-being.

On this basis the loss of weight found favorable nowadays in diabetes comes from fat and not from vital protein. He further investigated the food value of protein, fat and alcohol in nitrogenous equilibrium of diabetes and concluded that "the addition of an equal number of calories of protein, fat or alcohol to a low caloric carbohydrate-free diet in cases of diabetes results in the assimilation of considerable amounts of nitrogen when protein is used, a favorable N balance in only occasional instances with fat and no change in N equilibrium when alcohol is given. This would point to a high protein diet as the most desirable low caloric carbohydrate-free diet by which to conserve the body tissues and furnish a maintenance diet for the diabetic."

On the basis of what is known in regard to the relation of amino-acids to sugar production the high protein diet advised by Mosenthal would better be of the protein with little or no purine (see Purine Content of Various Foods).

[1] Foster: Diabetes Mellitus, p. 183.
[2] Arch. Int. Med., 1918, xxi, 269.
[3] Ibid., 1916, xvii, 863.

In considering the details of dietetic management we have two principal methods of treatment, one the European, best exemplified perhaps by the von Noorden routine, and the other an American method, known as Allen's fasting cure for diabetes. While there are of course numerous modifications of these methods and to a certain extent they are modifications of each other, the von Noorden cure puts the emphasis on first finding the carbohydrate tolerance, if any, by beginning with increasing or diminishing amounts of carbohydrate with a certain amount of modified starvation in severe cases, for a day or two. Allen's method lays stress on the fasting phase of the treatment, the reduction of weight of the patient and keeping the total caloric value of the food low when feedings are begun. The fats are kept particularly low, for if given in any considerable quantities the carbohydrate tolerance is reduced. The fast is persisted in until the urine becomes sugar-free and the ketone bodies usually drop, but do not as a rule disappear until the patients are fed after their fast. When the patient is sugar-free, carbohydrate is allowed in small amount and gradually increased to tolerance, quite as much emphasis being also put on the protein and fat tolerance in their relation to hyperglycemia.

Von Noorden Method.—For a differentiation of the treatment we may arbitrarily divide diabetics into three classes of cases.

1. Those in whom the sugar excretion is less than 50 gm. without ketonuria.

2. Those in whom the sugar excretion is more than 50 gm. also without ketonuria.

3. Those in whom the sugar excretion is more than 50 gm. with ketonuria.[1]

The first step is the determination of the individual's carbohydrate tolerance if such be present. In the very mild cases associated with overeating of sweets and starches it is usually only necessary to order a rational diet curtailing these food elements to promptly and permanently render these people sugar-free. On the other hand any glycosuria even a so-called alimentary form due to excessive ingestion of sugar-forming foods must be viewed as a real diabetes, although mild, and with potency for developing into a severe grade if neglected. (Even these mild cases should be taught to examine their own urine with Benedict's solution once in so often in order to be sure that the sugar does not recur.)

[1] Foster: Diabetes Mellitus, p. 188.

In all but these very mildest cases it is necessary as the first step, to determine the individual's carbohydrate tolerance. This is done by gradually reducing the patient's carbohydrate allowance until after about five days they are put on a standard strict diet containing only 15 gm. of carbohydrate in the green vegetables allowed. To this is added a definite carbohydrate allowance in the form of white bread (55 per cent. carbohydrate), Huntly and Palmer biscuits, 5 gm. Uneeda biscuit, 4.6 gm. carbohydrate each.

A convenient method is to allow with the Standard Strict Diet 25 gm. carbohydrate in any one of these three forms, at each meal, testing the urine of the second twenty-four hours. If it still contains sugar, reduce the carbohydrate allowance one-half and so by a process of reduction or addition, in case the tolerance is over the 75 gm. carbohydrate, the point at which sugar just fails to show in the urine is reached. The amount of carbohydrate that will accomplish this constitutes the carbohydrate tolerance. When this is determined the patient is put on a diet which contains not over one-half the tolerance. The reason for this being that while the urine may become sugar-free on the full tolerance, the hyperglycemia does not disappear so easily and ordinarily needs a greater reduction in the carbohydrate to reduce this to normal. After the patient has been on this tolerance for some weeks it is safe to gradually increase the amount of carbohydrate and determine its utilization by frequent urinary tests. In this way over a period of months by resting the disturbed function it is usually possible to materially increase the amount of carbohydrate beyond the original tolerance and gradually bring the patient up to an improvement which allows of a fair diet. In order to vary the diet as much as possible it is necessary to know the actual carbohydrate content of the different foodstuffs and to construct a diet that shall not be monotonous. The use of the table of carbohydrate equivalents will materially aid in doing this. One prerequisite of success is the actual weighing of the foods, in the mild cases only of the carbohydrate foods, in the more severe the protein and fats must also be weighed.

Standard Strict Diet:

Breakfast: Eggs, two; ham, 90 gm. (3 oz.); coffee (without sugar); butter, 15 gm. (½ oz.), this used on bread or biscuit; if no carbohydrate is allowed, cooked in with the eggs; cream, 45 c.c. (1½ oz.).

Luncheon: Meat (chops or steak), 120 gm. (4 oz.); green vegetables allowed from list, 2 tablespoonfuls; wine, white or red (2 claret glasses), 6 ounces, or brandy or whiskey (2 tablespoonfuls) 1 ounce; butter 15 gm. (½ oz.), cooked with the vegetables or on bread if allowed.

Afternoon tea with 15 gm. (½ oz.) cream (no sugar).

Dinner: Clear soup; fish, 90 gm. (3 oz.); meat (fowl, beef or mutton), 120 gm. (4 oz.); green vegetables, 2 tablespoonfuls (see list); salad, with 15 gm. (½ oz.) of oil with dressing; cream cheese, 30 gm. (1 oz.); red or white wine or whiskey as at luncheon; coffee, small cup; butter, 30 gm. (1 oz.) on the fish, meat or green vegetables in case no bread is allowed.

Bedtime: A cup of bouillon with a raw egg.

This represents: Protein, 112 gm. (3⅔ oz.); nitrogen, 18 gm. (270 grains); fat, 160 gm. (5½ oz.); calories, 2200.

Standard Diet with Restricted Protein.

Breakfast: Eggs, two; bacon, 15 gm. (½ oz.); coffee, with cream, 45 gm. (1½ oz.); butter, 20 gm. (⅔ oz.).

Luncheon: Egg, one; bacon, 15 gm. (½ oz.); meat (ham steak or chops), 60 gm. (2 oz.); salad, with 15 gm. (½ oz.), oil for dressing; wine, white or red, 2 claret glasses, 180 c.c (6 oz.), or whiskey or brandy, 2 tablespoonfuls, 30 c.c (1 oz.); butter, 40 gm. (1⅛ oz.).

Afternoon tea with 15 gm. (½ oz.) cream.

Dinner: Clear soup; meat (mutton, beef, turkey or chops), 90 gm. (3 oz.); vegetables from list, 2 tablespoonfuls; salad with 15 gm. (½ oz.) oil; cream cheese 30 gm. (1 oz.); wine, red or white, 2 claret glasses, 180 c.c. (6 oz.) or whiskey or brandy as at luncheon; coffee; butter, 30 gm. (1 oz.).

Bedtime: Bouillon with one egg.

This represents: Protein, 70 gm. (2⅓ oz.); nitrogen, 10 gm. (150 grains); fat, 180 gm. (6 oz.); calories, 2500.

Green Days:

Breakfast: Egg, one; cup of coffee, without cream or sugar.

Dinner: Spinach with one egg, hard-boiled; bacon, 15 gm. (½ oz.); salad, with 15 gm. (½ oz.) oil; wine, red or white, 250 c.c. (8 oz.) or whiskey or brandy, 30 c.c. (1 oz.).

4.30 P.M. Cup of broth or beef tea.

Supper: Egg, one, best scrambled with a little tomato or butter; bacon, 15 gm. (½ oz.); cabbage, sauerkraut, string beans, cauliflower or asparagus; wine, red or white, whiskey or brandy as at dinner.

Give 15 to 30 gm. (½ to 1 oz.) of bicarbonate of soda in the twenty-four hours. This diet represents the following values: Protein, 32 gm. (1 oz.); nitrogen, 5 gm. (75 grains); carbohydrate, 5 gm. (⅙ oz.); fat, 65 gm. (2 oz.); calories, 575.

In any of these diets if there are reasons for not using bacon, beef 30 gm. (1 oz.) may be substituted for it.

Oatmeal Days:

Porridge made from oatmeal, 250 gm. (8 oz.); butter, 250 gm. (8 oz.), salt and pepper. The oatmeal should be boiled all night in a double boiler with the butter and whites of six eggs added next morning.

"This constitutes the food for one day and may be eaten as gruel, mush or fried mush, divided into seven equal parts, one part to be taken every two hours." Two cups of black coffee and 180 c.c. (6 oz.) of red or sour white wine or 30 c.c. (1 oz.) of whiskey or brandy may be taken during the day.

This represents: Protein, 63 gm. (2 oz.); nitrogen, 16.8 gm. (½ oz.); carbohydrate, 170 gm. (5⅔ oz.); fat, 212 gm. (7 oz.); calories, 3300.

General Diabetic Diet List.

May take—Soups: Meat soups and broths. Egg, cheese or allowed vegetables may be added.

Meats: All kinds of fresh, smoked and cured meats (except liver), poultry. Pate de fois gras, no sauces that contain flour.

Fish: Every kind (except shell fish), dried, fresh, smoked or pickled.

Egg: Cooked in any style but without flour.

Fats: Lard, butter, oils, suet.

Cheese: Swiss, English, cream, pineapple cheese.

Vegetables: Cabbage, cauliflower, celery, chicory, cress, asparagus, beet tops, sprouts, cucumber, eggplant, endive, lettuce, Kohlrabi, okra, pumpkin, radish, rhubarb, sauerkraut, spinach, tomatoes, string beans, vegetable marrow.

Salads and Pickles: Made of above vegetables, unsweetened.

Mushrooms and truffles.

Cream: If allowed in tolerance, 90 c.c. (3 oz.) per day.

Condiments: Pepper, salt, curry, cinnamon, mustard, nutmeg, caraway, capers, vinegar.

Desserts: Custards, ice-cream, ade mwith eggs and cream. Lemon water-ice, jellies made with gelatin. No sugar to be used but saccharine only for sweetening and flavored with brandy, coffee, vanilla or lemon.

Beverages: Tea, coffee sweetened with saccharine. Whiskey or distilled liquor, 150 c.c. (5 oz.). Red or white wine (sour) up to 500 c.c. (1 pint) per day.

Foods Prohibited Except as Allowed in Accessory Diet:

Sugars or sweetening other than saccharine, saxin, garantose, dulcin.

Puddings, preserves, cake, pastry or ice-cream.

Bread, biscuit, crackers, toast, etc.

Cereals of all kinds, macaroni, potatoes, or other underground vegetables, as carrots, parsnips, beets, turnips, also beans, peas and corn.

Fruit, fresh or dried.

No flour allowed in soups or gravies.

Ale, beer, porter, sweet wines, sparkling wines, cider, milk, chocolate, cocoa, sweet drinks, liquor.[1]

TABLE OF CARBOHYDRATE EQUIVALENTS.
Carbohydrate equivalents.

White bread:

Grams	4	8	16	25	32	40
Drams	1	2	4	6	8	10
Equals						
Potato . . . . . . Gms.	22	44	88	132	176	220
Hominy (cooked) . . . "	25	50	100	150	200	250
Oatmeal (cooked) . . . "	40	80	160	240	320	400
Rice (cooked) . . . . "	15	30	60	90	120	150
Farina (cooked) . . . "	25	50	100	150	200	250
Shredded wheat . . . "	5	10	20	30	40	50
Indian-meal mush . . . "	27	54	108	162	216	270
Macaroni . . . . . "	30	60	120	180	240	300
Corn bread . . . . "	10	20	40	60	80	100
Barker's gluten food, A . "	102	204	408	612	816	1020
Barker's gluten food, B . "	74	148	296	444	592	740
Barker's gluten food, C . "	54	108	216	224	432	540
Almond meal . . . . "	65	130	260	390	520	650
Gum gluten (ground) . . "	12	24	48	72	96	120
Soja-bean meal . . . "	50	100	200	300	400	500
Casoid flour . . . . "	55	110	220	330	440	550
Pure gluten biscuit . . "	50	100	200	300	400	500
Protopuff No. 1 . . . "	45	90	180	270	360	450
Protopuff No. 2 . . . "	12	24	48	72	96	120
Salvia sticks . . . . "	25	50	100	150	200	250
Milk (whole) . . . . "	112	224	448	672	896	1120
Cream . . . . . "	112	224	448	672	896	1120
Grapefruit weighed with skin "	187	375	750	1125	1150	1875
Rice pudding . . . . "	14	28	56	84	112	140
Tapioca pudding . . . "	15	30	60	90	120	150
Beets (cooked) . . . "	65	130	260	390	520	650
Custard (baked) . . . "	30	60	120	180	240	300
Carrots . . . . . "	65	130	260	390	520	650
Corn (canned or green) . "	22	44	88	132	176	220
Egg plant . . . . "	90	180	360	540	720	900
Parsnips . . . . . "	35	70	140	210	280	350
Green peas . . . . "	30	60	120	180	240	300
Turnips . . . . . "	56	112	224	336	448	560
Baked beans . . . . "	22	44	88	132	176	220
Apples . . . . . "	45	90	180	270	360	450

Thus 4 gms. of white bread (by which the tolerance was determined) contains the same amount of carbohydrate as do 22 gms. of Potato, 40 gms. of Oatmeal, 30 gms. of Macaroni, etc.

[1] These diets are adapted from Janeway, in Musser and Kelly's Therapeutics.

	Equals						
Bananas . . . . . Gms.	20	40	80	120	160	200
Oranges . . . . . "	40	80	160	240	320	400
Peaches . . . . . "	50	100	200	300	400	500
Pears . . . . . . "	50	100	200	300	400	500
Prunes . . . . . "	24	48	96	144	192	240
Watermelon . . . . "	225	450	900			

Method of using the table of carbohydrate equivalents; Take for example a case with a carbohydrate allowance of 32 gm. (1 oz.).

Proto puff No. 1	45 gm.	= 4 gm.	carbohydrate
Potato	22 "	= 4 "	"
Oatmeal	40 "	= 4 "	"
Beets	33 "	= 2 "	"
Orange	40 "	= 2 "	"
Rice pudding	56 "	= 16 "	"
	236 "	= 32 "	"

Foster's System of Carbohydrate Units.—For the milder grades of the disease Foster has devised a system of carbohydrate units, each unit representing 10 gm. of carbohydrate. Of course these quantities are not absolutely accurate but are approximately so and when the tolerance has been determined the allowance of carbohydrate can be conveniently taken from this table without weighing, the patients learning soon to remember the units.[1]

Soups:

Bean	Average portion equals	1 unit
Clam chowder	" " "	1 "
Cream of corn	" " "	1 "
Pea puree	" " "	1 "
Potato	" " "	1 "

Vegetables:

Beans, baked	2 tablespoonfuls "	2 units
Beans, butter	2 " "	1 unit
Beans, lima	2 " "	2 units
Beans, kidney	2 " "	2 "
Beets	2 " "	1 unit
Corn, canned	2 " "	2 units
Corn, green	1 ear "	2 "
Onions	2 onions "	1 unit
Green peas	2 tablespoonfuls "	1 "
Potato, baked	1 medium-sized "	2 units
Potato, boiled	1 " "	3 "
Potato, mashed	2 tablespoonfuls "	2 "

Fruits:

Apple	1 medium-sized "	2 "
Blackberries	2 tablespoonfuls "	1 unit
Cantaloupe	One-half "	2 units
Currants	3 tablespoonfuls "	1 unit
Huckleberries	2 " "	1 "
Orange	1 medium-sized "	2 units
Peach	1 " "	1 unit
Pear	1 " "	2 units
Plum "	2 " "	1 unit
Raspberries	3 tablespoonfuls "	1 "
Strawberries	4 " "	1 "

[1] Foster: Diabetes Mellitus, p. 201.

Cereals:

Bread	Slice 3 x 4 x ½ in.	Equals	2 units
Hominy, boiled	1 tablespoonful	"	1 unit
H. O. (oatmeal), boiled . . .	2 tablespoonfuls	"	1 "
Macaroni, boiled	2 "	"	2 units
Macaroni, baked with cheese . . .	2 "	"	2 "
Oatmeal, boiled	2 "	"	1 unit
Rice, boiled	1 "	"	2 units
Shredded wheat biscuit	1 biscuit	"	2 "
Spaghetti, baked with tomato . . .	2 tablespoonfuls	"	2 "

Sample Diet.

Sample Diet (six units allowed, *i. e.*, 60 gm. carbohydrate):

Breakfast: Bacon and eggs; cereal (equal to 1 unit), with tablespoonful of cream.

Lunch: Clear soup; meat and green vegetable; bread, ½ slice (1 unit); mashed potato (2 units).

Dinner: Soup; meat and green vegetable; baked beans (2 units); salad and cheese.

Foster suggests that this table of units should not be used when the glycosuria is over 70 gm.

Procedure in the Medium Severe Cases (over 50 gm. glucose in urine).—If the case has no carbohydrate tolerance and does not become sugar-free on the Standard Strict Diet without added carbohydrate, the next step is to put the case on the Standard Strict Diet with restricted protein. If after two or three days the glycosuria does not clear up, put on two green days, then back on Standard Strict Diet with restricted protein for a few days. If this results in freeing the urine of glucose then the regular Standard Strict Diet may be used and if the urine still remains sugar-free it may be possible to add carbohydrate, preferably in the form of green vegetables as recommended by Joslin, using weighed amounts of vegetables containing 5, 10, 15 or 20 per cent. of carbohydrate (p. 481). These are ordinarily better borne than any form of bread or biscuit, although bread may be tried tentatively in definite, small amounts. Often this routine will result in freeing the urine of sugar and with care a certain amount of carbohydrate tolerance may be developed, but in any case the total amount of carbohydrate allowed should be kept distinctly below the point of tolerance for the reasons already explained.

In these cases the use of the table of carbohydrate equivalents or Foster's carbohydrate units will be found useful.

Severe Cases with Marked Ketonuria.—The best plan is to put the patients at once on the oatmeal diet for several days, two to ten, without regard to the sugar in the urine, at the same time giving considerable amounts of bicarbonate of soda, enough to render the urine alkaline, which should be attained if possible. If the acidosis diminishes but the sugar content of the urine remains high, patients are often benefited by two green days and from this to the Standard Strict Diet with restricted protein, then the full Standard Strict Diet, if the acidosis remains in control.

Von Noorden recommends what he calls a "set of days" consisting of two days restricted protein diet, two days of green diet and three days of oatmeal diet. We then return to the restricted protein diet or even full protein, but if sugar again appears the "set" is repeated. Often the patients become sugar-free and acid-free on this plan when a little carbohydrate can again be tried, preferably in vegetable form.

When the acetonuria is extreme or coma threatens, von Noorden found "alcohol days" of great benefit and recommends giving 90 to 150 c.c. (3 to 5 oz.) of whiskey daily well diluted and no food. This often diminishes the ketonuria and the general condition is much improved. The alcohol diet is limited to one or two days and then the oatmeal days, etc., are again tried as before. This is practically a fasting cure and in some form has been found by many observers to be of great service under these conditions.

Instead of using oatmeal some clinicians prefer to use potato days or bread-and-butter days, or as Falta recommends, a rotation of the different starchy foods taking one at a time.

Potato Diet:[1]

Breakfast: One baked potato with butter; one cup of coffee, cream, 25 c.c. (1 oz.).

Luncheon and Dinner: Potato boiled, butter; green vegetable; whiskey or wine.

Bread-and-Butter Diet:[2]

Breakfast: Two pieces of bread or toast, buttered; yolks of two eggs, cooked.

Luncheon and Dinner: Two slices of bread and butter; green vegetable, with oil or egg sauce; a rasher of bacon; wine, whiskey or coffee.

Allen's Treatment of Diabetes Mellitus.—This treatment, based on results of extensive animal experimentation, has only been used for human diabetes during the past three or four years and although apparently very successful it has not as yet stood the test of time nor has it been used long enough to judge of the late results years after treatment was begun. As already stated in this form of treatment emphasis

[1] Foster: Diabetes Mellitus, p. 186.
[2] Loc. cit.

is placed upon an initial fast period sufficient to clear up the glycosuria and acidosis, if that is present, and it has been found practically without exception that fasting from two to ten or twelve days at the outside will accomplish these ends.

As Allen says in speaking of this treatment in dogs: "It was found that the grave condition of diabetes yielded to an initial fast of days or weeks with a subsequent diet which kept the animals at a low level of weight and metabolic activity. Anything that tended to increase the weight or metabolism brought back the glycosuria and acidosis. If the animal was allowed to go down by glycosuria with emaciation, weakness and death, it was found that degenerative changes took place in the islands of Langerhans and if this decline was prevented the islands remained intact."

The two cardinal points in Allen's treatment are:

1. An initial fast to the point of clearing up the glycosuria accompanied by a reduction in weight which should be permanent.

2. The subsequent diet which does not allow of a return of the glycosuria but if by chance there is a return an immediate fast day or two is given to clear it up again.

Before speaking in detail of the method, it is necessary to emphasize one point upon which Allen lays great stress and which is entirely contrary to the older teachings, namely, that a loss of weight is of distinct advantage, as it tends to increase carbohydrate tolerance and makes the patients feel much better, which suggests the possibility that the weakness and many of the other symptoms are due to an intoxication and more than likely from the unexcreted end-products of protein metabolism. If these patients are made to gain by adding fats to the diet or trying to give larger amounts of food, as is the custom with the older forms of treatment, at once glycosuria and the acidosis returns. This loss of weight is of course of greatest benefit in those cases who are rather overweight to begin with, but even the moderately well-nourished or spare individuals bear the fast advantageously with the consequent loss of weight, although surprisingly enough the diabetic does not seem to lose weight as rapidly as in starvation of the normal man, due to the fact that a certain amount of energy is derived from the burning of the ketone bodies. As in severe diabetes there is more or less of a breakdown all along the line, Allen urges limiting the total caloric intake and the body mass to correspond to the assimilative function. He therefore warns against efforts to maintain patients on a high level of diet or weight.

In a few cases the starvation causes alarming symptoms of nausea and vomiting which disappear on feeding and when a second fast is instituted, after a few days or a week or two, these patients stand it perfectly well and become sugar-free. The old theory that a dangerous acidosis is engendered by a prolonged fast has absolutely to be given up as untrue.

During the fasting period, the patients being kept in bed, are allowed the following diet:

Whiskey, black coffee, bouillon, water, tea. Thrice-cooked green vegetables (whereby all starch is removed) may be given, but are not a necessary part of the diet in the period of starvation. They merely give a sense of fulness to the patient.

The whiskey given in amounts of 50 to 120 c.c. per day (1 ⅔ to 4 oz.) is not an essential part of this period but may be used and if so furnishes 7 calories per c.c. It has no influence on sugar formation and aside from this the other articles allowed have practically no food value. (Whiskey is said not to have any influence on acetone formation in normal individuals.)[1]

Twenty-four to forty-eight hours after the urine becomes free of glucose, cautious feeding is begun, individualizing the diet as much as possible, but it is absolutely essential that the patient remain sugar- and acid-free. In the feeding, one usually begins by using carbohydrates most easily by prescribing 100 to 200 gm. (3⅓ to 6⅔ oz.) of green vegetables (cooked once) of the 5 and 10 per cent. classes according to Joslin's classification. (See page 481).

This is increased in amount daily until possibly a trace of glucose appears which is at once cleared up by a fast day. This marks the patient's carbohydrate tolerance. Next the protein tolerance is determined in the same way by giving the whites of one or two eggs, then meat is added until either glycosuria appears or the patients reach a fair, physiological protein allowance, or one tests the protein tolerance first, then the carbohydrate; in either case in finding the tolerance only one food element is used at a time, protein or carbohydrate. If for example in a given case we were to have a protein tolerance of 60 gm. (2 oz.) protein and 20 gm. (⅔ oz.) carbohydrate, such a patient would be put on a diet with probably 50 gm. protein and 10 gm. carbohydrate which is gradually increased. In other words, just as we saw in the von Noorden regimen, the patients do best when they are allowed only about one-half their carbohydrate tolerance at first, which can be gradually increased.

[1] Jour. Am. Med. Assn., September 9, 1916, p. 84.

Geyelin's method of using the Allen treatment in the Presbyterian Hospital, New York is somewhat as follows:

The patient is arbitrarily placed on a low caloric diet consisting of 15 gm. (½ oz.) carbohydrate; 30 gm. (1 oz.) fats; 30 gm. (1 oz.) protein (diet No. 1). This is continued for a few days to determine the effect of this low food intake in overcoming the glyosuria. This is a more agreeable diet than a virtual fast, but if after from one to four days of this diet the glycosuria is not decreasing or is perhaps increasing a definite fast is instituted (diet No. 2). As soon as the patient is free from sugar, a diet of from 10 to 20 gm. (⅓ to ⅔ oz.) carbohydrate is given with 30 gm. (1 oz.) protein and 30 gm. (1 oz.) fat. Keeping the carbohydrate at a constant level (10 to 20 gm.) the protein and fat are increased 10 gm. (⅓ oz.) daily, until sugar appears, or until the protein intake has reached a level of 1½ gm. (22 gr.) per kilo of body weight and the fat 100 to 150 gm. (3⅓ to 5 oz.). If on this diet the patient is still sugar-free the carbohydrate is increased 10 gm. (⅓ oz.) daily until sugar appears in the urine, a fast day is then given. After the urine is again clear of sugar, the diet is arranged with the same protein and fat content, but with only one-half to two-thirds the carbohydrate tolerance as determined by the point at which we found the patient "spilled" sugar in the urine.

If glycosuria appears while the patient is on a fixed low carbohydrate diet and while the protein and fat are being increased, a fast day is given; following the fast the protein and fat intake is lowered from 10 to 20 gm. (⅓ to ⅔ oz.) and kept constant while the carbohydrate is gradually increased 5 gm. (75 gr.) daily until glycosuria again appears. Another fast day is then given after which the increase in protein and fat is again begun as before. Later the carbohydrate is also gradually increased 10 gm. (⅓ oz. a day).

For the most part the increase in carbohydrate is best made with once boiled vegetables, at first of the 5 per cent. class and later of those with higher percentage of carbohydrate. It is not until the carbohydrate tolerance is considerable that we allow any actual starch in the form of bread or bread substitutes.

The increases in diet can be worked out most conveniently from the food tables (pp. 671 and 677)

In the more severe cases with only moderate acidosis at most, the patient's diet is gradually decreased in carbohydrates until after a few days they are fasted and put on diet No. 2 or No. 1. This results as a rule, in converting a severe into a moderately severe case.

If coma is impending, the best plan is to give the patient a plain saline infusion into the vein and urge them to take from 5 to 10 gm. (⅙ to ⅓ oz.) of salt by mouth with the idea of inducing a subcutaneous edema and so storing the ketone bodies in the tissues. In addition glucose is given by mouth, particularly if the patients have been starved of carbohydrates.

After the danger of coma is passed the cases are treated as are those of medium severity.

STANDARD STRICT DIET (GEYELIN).

DIET No. 1:

15 gm. carbohydrate, 30 gm. fat, 30 gm. protein.

Breakfast:
2 eggs.
1 cup coffee, 200 c.c. (6½ oz.) and saccharin, no cream.

Luncheon:
Tomatoes (fresh) 200 gm. (6½ oz.) (7.8 gm. (117 gr.) carbohydrate).
Broth, 200 c.c. (6½ oz.).

3 P. M.:
White of one egg.
Broth, 200 c.c. (6½ oz.).

Supper:
String beans (canned), 200 c.c. (6½ oz.); 7.2 gm. (108 gr.) carbohydrate.
Butter, 7 gm. (¼ oz.).
Two eggs.
One cup of tea, no cream.
Next day 25 gm. (⅚ oz.) carbohydrate.

To increase diet No. 1, 10 gm. carbohydrate add 250 gm. (8 oz.) cooked beans at luncheon (once boiled).

For the following day 35 gm. (1⅙ oz.) carbohydrate. To increase 10 gm. (150 gr.) more carbohydrate add 180 gm. (6 oz.) of once boiled cabbage at 3 P.M. Feeding.

For 45 gms. (1½ oz.) carbohydrate add 250 gm. (8 oz.), raw or canned tomatoes for breakfast. For 55 gm. (1¾ oz.) carbohydrate add 180 gm. (6 oz.) cabbage.

All vegetables are to be served salt-free.

DIET FOR FAST DAY.

DIET No. 2:

Breakfast:
Cup of coffee, 200 c.c. (6½ oz.), saccharin.
No milk or sugar.
Thrice cooked 5 per cent. vegetables.
200 gm. (6½ oz.), *e. g.*, string beans, spinach, cauliflower, etc., with vinegar Q. S.

Mid. A. M.:
Salt-poor broth, 200 c.c. (6½ oz.).

Luncheon:
Salt-poor broth, 200 c.c. (6½ oz.).
Cup of tea or coffee, 200 c.c. (6½ oz.) or more if desired.
5 per cent. vegetables, 200 c.c. (6½ oz.).
Whiskey or brandy, 30 c.c. (1 oz.) if desired.

Supper:
Same as luncheon. Using other of the 5 per cent. vegetables.

Bed-time:
Salt-poor broth.
Water.

In those cases accompanied by old age, obesity or nephritis, it is better to omit the initial fast at first and put them directly on a 15 : 30 : 30 food formula (diet No. 1.), as food fasting sometimes causes these patients to pass rapidly into coma. If this brings about a sugar-free urine, that is favorable, if not, then it may be advisable to try a fast, watching the ketonuria carefully.

Allen says that "fat is less urgently needed except in very weak and emaciated patients and can be added gradually."[1] In the severe cases it is necessary to test in this way the tolerance for all classes of foods, carbohydrate, protein and fats one at a time. Carbohydrate is given if possible, but is kept safely below the limit of tolerance. Protein must be kept fairly low, sometimes very low. With a dangerously low protein tolerance the working rule has been to exclude all carbohydrate, then feed as much protein as possible without glycosuria. Experience seems to indicate that every patient can tolerate his necessary minimum of protein and that glycosuria appears only when this is exceeded. The severe diabetic is often thin and weak because he cannot metabolize enough food to be strong and well, but as long as his weakened function is not overtaxed he seems to be able to retain such weight and strength as he has, at least for a considerable period. Any attempt to build him up with any kind or quantity of food beyond that which he is able to metabolize perfectly, apparently hastens a fatal result.[2]

The mild or moderately severe cases are usually c'eared of their glucose and acetone with a fast of one or two days, the subsequent period of observation being devoted to an education of the patient in food values (after determining the carbohydrate tolerance), for these cases can usually take a full allowance of protein and fat. With the really severe cases, of course, the intitial fast is usually necessarily of longer duration and with no carbohydrate tolerance the feeding of the proper amount of protein becomes a nice problem. With perseverance, almost all the cases can be taken along to a point where they can take their minimum of protein, some fat and later probably a little carbohydrate which if the progress be fortunate, may be gingerly increased.

There is still a small class of cases that resist every effort at reaching a maintenance diet and who must inevitably perish of their disease, fortunately these are few and the favorable reports of Allen's treatment makes it seem probable that they may be still further reduced in numbers.

[1] The Treatment of Diabetes, Boston Med. and Surg. Jour., February 18, 1915.
[2] Loc. cit.

The best results in this treatment are naturally obtained in hospitals or sanatoria where everything is readily controlled; but Geyelin has had marked success with this treatment in ambulatory cases at the Vanderbilt Clinic, New York City. The patients are taught when leaving the hospital how regularly to examine their own urine with Benedict's solution and to take one fast day every seven, ten or fourteen days, according to the severity of the case when under treatment.

Allen recommends exercise in the cases which reach a fair tolerance, not only light but very active and vigorous exercises, as tending to keep the patients in better physical condition and actually increasing carbohydrate tolerance. One fact needs repetition, when after a fast of eight to ten days the urine does not become sugar and acid-free it is well to give a food protein in small amount, 30 to 50 gm. (1 to 1⅔ oz.). This usually increases the sugar, but if after a day or two of this diet a fast is again instituted the urine usually becomes promptly sugar- and acid-free. This is shown by the illustrative case on January 20th to 23d, although of course this is not a severe type of case, as it serves well for the illustration of the method and of charting. A separate sheet is kept on which the actual foods and their amounts are recorded.

The following short resume of Allen's treatment given by Joslin[1] is of value for its clearness and forms a good working basis for those wishing to use this treatment.

Strict Diet. Meats, Fish, Broths, Gelatin, Eggs, Butter, Olive Oil Coffee, Tea and Cracked Cocoa.

(Foods Arranged Approximately According to Per Cent. of Carbohydrates.)

Vegetables, 5 per cent.		10 per cent.	15 per cent.	20 per cent.
Lettuce	Cauliflower	Onions	Green peas	Potatoes
Spinach	Tomatoes	Squash	Artichokes	Shell beans
Sauerkraut	Rhubarb	Turnip	Parsnips	Baked beans
String beans	Egg plant	Carrots	Canned lima	Green corn
Celery	Leeks	Okra	beans	Boiled rice
Asparagus	Beet greens	Mushrooms		Boiled
Cucumbers	Water cress	Beets		macaroni
Brussels	Cabbage			
sprouts	Radishes			
Sorrel	Pumpkin			
Endive	Kohl-rabi			
Dandelions	Broccoli			
Swiss chard	Vegetable			
Sea kale	marrow			

[1] Am. Jour. Med. Sc., 1915, cl, 492.

31

Date	24 hr. volume c.c.	Sp. gr.	Ace-tone	Dia-cetic	β-oxy-butyric	Output glucose %	Output glucose Total gm.	Total calories. Diet	Na Cl bal. gm.	Total N urine	D M N.	Am-monia N.	Weight	Reac-tion	Blood CO2	Miscellaneous
Jan. 14-15	1480	19	++ Ft. tr.	+	..	+1.20	17.82	0	xx	7.03	2.5	3.41	46.9 103.2	ac.	—	—
15-16	2395	21	tr.	o	..	+	21.39	0	xv	9.02	2.37	4.63	46.9 103.2	ac.	34.3	..
16-17	2975	19	+	+	..	+	11.9	350 alc. cal.	xx	9.81	1.52	4.54	Not weighed	ac.	..	Whiskey, 120 cc.
17-18	3715	14	+	+	11.6	+	11.14	350 alc. cal.	xx	7.645	1.46	3.99	Not weighed Unable to stand	ac.	..	Whiskey, 120 cc.
18-19	4050	14	++	+	..	+	10.0	350 alc. cal.	xx	10.178	1.03	4.20	Not weighed	ac.	38.675	Whiskey, 120 cc.
19-20	3830	10	Ft. tr.	Tr.	7.12	+ Very Ft. tr.	Trace only	350 alc. cal.	xx	6.97	..	2.57	Not weighed	Ft. acid	..	Whiskey, 120 cc.
20-21	2290	13	Tr.	Tr.	5.77	Ft. tr.	W	262 alc. cal.	xx	7.37	..	2.29	Not weighed	ac.	..	Whiskey, 90 cc. Pro., 20; whiskey,
21-22	3125	14	Tr.	Ft. tr.	5.7	Ft. tr.	W	262 alc. cal.	xx	5.108	..	1.9	Not weighed	Ft.	39.90	90 cc.
22-23	4120	13	Tr. Ft. tr.	Tr.	..	o	o	82 pro. 262 alc. cal.	xx	8.10	..	2.19	Not weighed	ac.	..	Whiskey, 90 cc.
23-24	2700	15	Ft. tr.	Tr.	2.4	o	o	82 pro. 0 alc. 123 pro. cal.	xx	7.41	..	2.59	Not weighed	Ft.	..	Pro., 20; 0 whiskey.
24-25	1640	10	Ft. tr.	Tr.	..	o	o	205 pro.	xx	6.53	..	2.05	Not weighed	ac.	42.35	Pro., 30.
25-26	2820	15	+ Ft. tr.	Tr.	..	o	o	205 pro.	xv?	10.94	..	1.38	Not weighed	ac.	..	Pro., 50.
26-27	2330	15 15	Tr. Tr. ? Ft. tr.	Tr. o ?	..	o o ?	o o	287 369 pro.	xv	..	..	..	Not weighed	ac. Ft.	..	Pro., 70.
27-28	+	18 ?	Ft. tr. Ft. tr.	o	..	Tr. Ft. tr.	..	451	xv	..	..	..	Not weighed	ac. Ft.	39.20	Pro., 90.
28-29	2420	13	o Ft. tr.	o	..	o	..	0	xv	..	..	..	Not weighed	ac.	..	Pro., 110.
29-30	3335	14	o Ft. tr.	o	..	o	o	41.0	xv	..	..	..	Not weighed	..	..	First day a thrice cooked veg.
30-31 Feb. 31-1	2660 1729	15	o	o	..	o	..	413	xv	..	..	..	Not weighed	ac. Ft.	..	Pro., 10 gms. given. Partial taste 3b veg. Fat Pro.,

Fruits

Ripe olives (20 per cent. fat)	Lemons	Apples	Plums
Grapefruit	Oranges	Pears	Bananas
	Cranberries	Apricots	
	Strawberries	Blueberries	
	Blackberries	Cherries	
	Gooseberries	Currants	
	Peaches	Raspberries	
	Pineapple	Huckleberries	
	Watermelon		

Nuts

Butternuts	Brazil nuts	Almonds	Peanuts
Pignolias	Black walnuts	Walnuts (English)	
	Hickory nuts	Beechnuts	
	Pecans	Pistachios	
	Filberts	Pine nuts	40 per cent.
			Chestnuts

Miscellaneous: Unsweetened and unspiced pickles, clams, oysters, scallops, liver, fish roe.

Reckon actually available carbohydrates in vegetables of 5 per cent. group as 3 per cent., of 10 per cent. group as 6 per cent.

Joslin's Resume of Allen's Treatment—*Fasting.*—Fast until sugar-free. Drink water freely and one cup of tea and one cup of coffee if desired. If sugar persists after two days of fasting, add in divided portions 300 c.c. clear meat broth.

Alcohol.—If acidosis (diacetic acid) is present, give 0.5 c.c. of alcohol per kilogram body weight daily until acidosis disappears. Alcohol is best given in small doses every three hours.

Carbohydrate Tolerance.—When the twenty-four-hour urine is sugar-free, add 150 grams of 5 per cent. vegetables, and continue to add 5 grams carbohydrate daily up to 20 grams, and then 5 grams every other day, passing successively upward through the 5, 10 and 15 per cent. vegetables, 5 and 10 per cent. fruits, potato and oatmeal to bread, unless sugar appears or the tolerance reaches 3 grams carbohydrate per kilogram body weight.

Protein Tolerance.—When the urine has been sugar-free for two days, add 20 grams protein (three eggs) and thereafter 15 grams protein daily in the form of meat until the patient is receiving 1 gram protein per kilogram body weight or if the carbohydrate tolerance is zero, only ¾ gram per kilogram body weight. Later, if desired, the protein may be raise to 1.5 gram per kilogram body weight.

Fat Tolerance.—While testing the protein tolerance, a small quantity of fat is included in the eggs and meat given. Add no more fat until the protein reaches 1 gram per kilogram body weight (unless the protein tolerance is below this figure), but then add 25 grams fat daily until the patient ceases to lose weight or receives not over 40 calories per kilogram body weight.

Reappearance of Sugar.—The return of sugar demands fasting for twenty-four hours or until sugar-free. The diet preceding the reappearance of sugar is then resumed except that the carbohydrate should not exceed half the former tolerance until the urine has been sugar-free for two weeks, and it should not then be increased more than 5 grams per week.

Weekly Fast Days.—Whenever the tolerance is less than 20 grams carbohydrate, fasting should be practised one day in seven; when the tolerance is between 20 and 50 grams carbohydrate, 5 per cent. vegetables and one-half the usual quantity of protein and fat are allowed upon the fast day; when the tolerance is between 50 and 100 grams carbohydrate the 10 per cent. and 15 per cent. vegetables are added as well. If the tolerance is more than 100 grams carbohydrate, upon the weekly fast day the carbohydrate should be halved.

Bread is seldom prescribed, because it is so easy for a patient to overstep the limits. Many patients use bread substitutes, such as Huntley and Palmer's Akoll Biscuits, Barker's Gluten Flour[1] (Brand A), Hepco Flour,[2] Lyster Bros. Diabetic Flour, Whitefield, New Hampshire. The quantity of fat which it is necessary to give a severe case is considerable. A diabetic weighing 60 kilograms requires at least 30 calories per kilogram body weight to be up and about the hospital, with an occasional walk. Since in the severe cases not more than 10 grams carbohydrate, representing 40 calories, can be given in this form, and seldom more than 75 grams protein (1.25 grams per kilogram body weight) which would amount to 300 calories more, the balance of the diet must be made up of 150 grams fat, amounting to 1350 calories, and even more unless 15 grams alcohol are given, which would amount to 105 calories.

QUANTITY OF FOOD REQUIRED BY A SEVERE DIABETIC PATIENT WEIGHING 60 KILOGRAMS.

Food	Quantity, grams.	Calories, per gram.	Total Calories
Carbohydrate	10	4	40
Protein	75	4	300
Fat	150	9	1350
Alcohol	15	7	105
Total			1795

[1] Herman Barker, 433 Broadway, Somerville, Mass.
[2] Waukesha Health Products Co., Waukesha, Wisconsin.

Should the patient remain sugar-free and the weight be maintained upon this diet, gradually the quantity of fat could be lowered and the carbohydrate increased. A very few of the patients have a tolerance for between 200 and 300 grams of carbohydrate. With most the tolerance is below 100 grams, and with the majority it is under 50 grams.

The patient should have one day of restricted diet each week, no matter how mild the case. This is done partly to spare the function which controls the carbohydrate metabolism, but also to remind the patient of what a strict diet really is. The patient is told to gain little or no weight, and as Allen advises, not to come up to his former weight. The severer cases examine the urine daily, and the milder ones once a week. The patients are instructed to lead less strenuous lives. Unfortunately, they feel so well that often this advice is disregarded, and he believes that all of us err in allowing our patients to do too much. They should have nine hours in bed at night and should have a quiet hour of rest each day, no matter how well they feel.

Diabetic Special Receipts.—The curtailment of the carbohydrates in diabetes is the most difficult problem to deal with and it is usually upon this rock that patients wreck their treatment unless they are exceptionally determined. With the newer method of giving the carbohydrate largely in the form of the 5, 10, 15 and 20 per cent. vegetables there is introduced a considerable food bulk which is satisfying and makes the loss of concentrated carbohydrate foods such as bread, cereal, etc., less disturbing. But there is in addition the necessity of supplying a variety in the diet and the cry for bread substitutes is more or less universal.

The following bread substitutes and "near" carbohydrate recipes are given to assist those who must make up the diabetic's menus.

Akoll Biscuit (Huntly and Palmer).—Carbohydrate, 2.7 per cent.; nitrogen, 7 per cent. Each biscuit weighs 5.1 gm. and contains 0.14 gm. carbohydrate and 0.41 gm. nitrogen.

Soja-bean Meal Biscuit, made from soja-bean meal, to be procured from Thos. Metcalf Co., Boston, Mass. Sugar, 9.34 per cent.; starch, none; protein, 44 to 64 per cent.; fat, 19.43 per cent.

Gluten-meal Biscuit, made of Barker's Gluten Food A, procured from H. B. Barker, Somerville, Mass. Carbohydrate about 4 per cent.; nitrogen, 13 per cent.

Gluten Biscuit and potato-gluten biscuit procured from Battle Creek Sanitarium Food Co. Carbohydrate, 10 per cent.; nitrogen, 12 per cent.

Casoid Biscuit, procured from Thos. Leeming and Co., New York City. Carbohydrate, 0 to 2 per cent.; nitrogen, 10 per cent.

Proto Puff No. 1, procured from Health Food Co., Lexington Avenue, New York City. Carbohydrate, 10 per cent.; nitrogen, 12 per cent.

Diabetic Milk (Wright).—Take a definite quantity of milk and dilute with three or four volumes of distilled water to which glacial acetic acid has been added, *e. g.*, 6 to 12 c.c. (1½ to 3 drams) to 500 c.c (1 pint) of water. This precipitates the casein and fats.

Allow it to settle and strain through cheesecloth, wash repeatedly. Redissolve the curd in a 1 per cent. solution of the following mixture, sufficient to make the original amount of milk used.

Potassium chloride	9.9
Sodium chloride	11.5
Monopotassium phosphate	13.8
Dipotassium phosphate	10.0
Citrate of potassium	5.9
Dimagnesium phosphate	4.0
Magnesium citrate	4.4
Dicalcium phosphate	8.0
Tricalcium phosphate	9.6
Calcium citrate	25.5
Calcium oxide	5.5
Sodium carbonate	40.0

Analysis of Wright's Diabetic Milk (Granat)

Specific gravity	.1011	
Carbohydrate	0.015	per cent.
Protein	1.907	"
Fat	3.600	"
Ash	0.200	"
Total solids	5.722	"
Sodium chloride	0.110	"

Special Recipes for the Use of Oatmeal.—(On oatmeal days the oatmeal porridge may be varied with these.)

Oatmeal Griddle Cakes.—Into the beaten white of one egg stir 100 gm. (3⅓ oz.) of cooked oatmeal and 5 gm. (⅙ oz.) (full teaspoonful) of melted butter. Cook on hot griddle. Eat with butter and cinnamon.

Oatmeal Popovers.—Into the white of one egg, beaten up, stir 100 gm. (3⅓ oz.) of cooked oatmeal. Mix well. Bake for twenty minutes in hot popover pan. Serve with butter.

Oatmeal Muffins.—Finely ground oatmeal 130 gm. (2 half-pint cups). Add one heaping teaspoonful of baking powder and one-half teaspoonful of salt. Mix well, and add 1⅓ cups of cold water and add melted butter or lard 30 gm. (1 oz.). Beat well and bake in a very hot oven in buttered muffin pans.

Soja-bean Meal Biscuits.—1 cup cream, 2 eggs, 1 teaspoonful baking powder, salt q. s. Use enough soja-bean meal to make a batter, not very thick. Make into eight cakes and bake.

Soja-bean Pancake.—Sift one tablespoonful of soja-bean flour with a little salt, add water until a thin batter is made, then beat in thoroughly the yolk of an egg, then mix in the beaten white of an egg. Cook brown on a hot griddle.

Baked Custard.—3 tablespoonfuls of cream; 1 egg; 5 tablespoonfuls of water; 2 or 3 saccharin tablets (or less) to taste; 10 drops of vanilla essence. Beat well; bake in buttered dish for twenty minutes; grate a little nutmeg on top.

Ice-cream.—3 tablespoonfuls of water; 3 tablespoonfuls of cream; 2 tablespoonfuls of coffee with 2 or 3 saccharin tablets dissolved in it; 1 egg. Mix in sauce pan and beat until thick. Cool and freeze.

Cranberries, stewed and sweetened with saccharin to taste.

These special recipes are largely adapted from Janeway's Treatment of Diabetes, in Musser and Kelly's *Therapeutics*.

Bran Biscuits (Rockefeller Institute Recipe .—Bran, 60 gm.; salt, one-fourth teaspoonful; agar-agar (powdered), 6 gm.; cold water, 100 c.c. (½ glass).

Tie the bran in cheesecloth and wash under cold water tap until water is clear. Mix agar in the water cold 100 c.c. (½ glass) and bring to the point of boiling. Add to washed bran the salt and agar-agar solution. Bake in a moderate oven from forty-five to fifty minutes.

Lyster Brothers[1] put up a Prepared Casein Diabetic Flour for gems, muffins, etc., which is said to be practically starch-free.

CARBOHYDRATE CONTENT OF FOODS COMMONLY USED IN DIABETIC DIETS. UNDER 5 PER CENT. CARBOHYDRATES.[2]

	Per cent.		Per cent.
Casoid Baking Powder . . .	0	Soson	1.1
Dr. Bouma Sugar-free Fat-milk	0	Rose's Diabetesmilch . . .	1.2
Van Abbott's Diabetic Table		Casoid Sugarless Marmalade .	1.2
Jelly, Orange . . .	0	Energin	1.3
Whiting's Sugar-free Milk . .	0	Casoid Sugarless Jam . . .	1.5
Rademann's Johannisbeer Saft		Kalari Biscuit	1.7
ohne Zucker	0.9	Casoid Dinner Rolls . . .	2.1
Kalari Batons ('09)	0.9	Casoid Flour	2.2
Glidine	1.0	Tropon	2.7
Roborat	2.9	Barker's Gluten Food "A" .	4.1
Gericke's Aleuronat	3.1	Bauer's Sanatogen	4.2

[1] Lyster Brothers, 105 Barnard Street, Andover, Mass.

[2] J. P. Street: Eighteenth Report of Food Products, 1913, Conn. Agri. Experiment Station.

	Per Cent.		Per Cent.
Jireh Diatetic Pine Nuts	3.4	Kellogg's Pine Nuts	4.2
Rademann's Preserved Fruits, "entzuckert"	3.5	Kellogg's 80 per cent. Gluten Biscuits	4.4
Kellogg's Protose	3.6	Amthor's Weizen-Protein	4.8
Hundhausen's Aleuronat (pure)	4.0	Bischof's Gluten Flour	5.0

5 TO 10 PER CENT. CARBOHYDRATES.

	Per cent.		Per cent.
Casoid Biscuits No. 2	5.6	Barker's Gluten Food "C"	7.7
Rademann's Preserved Fruits "in eigenem Saft"	5.7	Casoid Biscuits No. 3	7.8
Casoid Biscuits No. 1 ('13)	5.8	Gumpert's Ultrabrot	7.8
Barker's Gluten Food "B"	5.9	Kellogg's 80 per cent. Gluten ('12)	7.9
Kellogg's Nuttolene	6.3	Van Abbott's Almond Flour	7.9
Nashville Nutcysa	6.3	Casoid Biscuits No. 1 ('06, '09)	8.0
Huntley and Palmer's Akoll Biscuits	6.5	Kellogg's Almond Butter	8.2
Nashville Nutfoda	6.8	Fromm's Uni Bread	9.0
Rademann's Preserved Fruits "ohne Zucker"	7.0	Plasmon	9.3
Muller's Tomatoes fur Diabetiker	7.3	Gumpert's Ultramehl	9.4
Kalari Batons ('13)	7.4	Metcalf's Vegetable Gluten ('13)	9.8
		Groetzsh's Pfeffernusse	9.8

10 TO 15 PER CENT. CARBOHYDRATES.

	Per cent.		Per cent.
Kellogg's Pure Gluten Biscuit ('06)	10.2	Kellogg's 80 per cent. Gluten ('09)	12.6
Hundhausen's Aleuronat (less pure)	10.6	Van Abbott's Gluten Flour	12.5
Gumpert's Diabetiker-Stangen	11.0	Van Abbott's Gluten Butter Biscuits	12.7
Health Food; Pure Washed Gluten Flour ('13)	11.1	Nashville Nut Butter	13.0
Health Food; Alpha Diabetic Wafers	11.3	Van Abbott's Euthenia Biscuits	13.2
Loeb's Imported Gluten Flour	11.8	Kellogg's Nut Butter	13.9
Health Food No. 1; Proto Puffs	11.9	Bischof's Diabetic Gluten Bread	14.3
Kellogg's Potato Gluten Biscuit ('06, '09)	11.9	Fromm's Litonbrot	14.3
Kellogg's Nut Meal	12.1	Gericke's Sifarbrot	15.0
Van Abbott's Walnut Biscuits	12.3	Jireh Diabetic Baking Powder	15.0
		Peanut Butter (range 12-20)	15.0

15 TO 20 PER CENT. CARBOHYDRATES.

	Per cent.		Per cent.
Fritz's Litonbrot	15.4	Groetzsch's Esschokolade	17.2
Van Abbott's Caraway Biscuits	15.9	Hundhausen's Aleuronatzwieback	17.7
Van Abbott's Diabetic Rusks	16.0	Callard's Ginger Biscuit	18.1
Casoid Chocolate Almonds	16.1	Callard's Prolactic Biscuit	19.3
California Paper Shell Almonds	16.3	Rademann's Erdnuss-Brot	19.7
Callard's Cocoanut Biscuit	16.4	Fritz's Braunes Luftbrot "B"	19.8
Van Abbott's Ginger Biscuits	16.7	Groetzsch's Diabetiker-Salzbrezeln	20.0
Rademann's Diabetiker-Chokolade	16.9		
Health Food Almond Meal	16.9		

20 TO 25 PER CENT. CARBOHYDRATES.

	Per cent.		Per cent.
Goldscheider's Sinamylbrot	20.2	Rademann's Litonbrot	21.6
Callard's Almond Shortbreads	20.7	Rademann's Diabetiker-Chokolade-Biskuit	21.9
Callard's Casoid Rusks	20.8		

	Per Cent.		Per Cent.
Rademann's Diabetiker-Makronen	20.8	Fritz's Mandelbrot	23.1
Plasmon Cocoa	20.9	Cereo Soy Bean Gruel Flour	23.7
Health Food Protosoy Diabetic Wafers	21.2	Health Food Salvia Sticks	24.0
Jireh Patent Cotton Seed Flour	21.3	Health Food Protosoy Soy Flour	24.5
Casoid Lunch Biscuit	21.6	Metcalf's Soja Bean Meal	25.0

25 TO 35 PER CENT. CARBOHYDRATES.

	Per cent.		Per cent.
Jireh Soja Bean Meal	25.8	Fromm's Luft Bread	30.7
Gericke's Dreifach-Porterbrot	26.0	Van Abbott's Gluten Bread	30.9
Groetzsch's Kochschokolade	26.1	Spencer's Almond Paste	31.6
Brusson Chocolate with Added Gluten	26.4	Van Abbott's Midolia Biscuits	31.6
Rademann's Diabetiker-Stangen	27.0	Van Abbott's Gluten Semola	32.4
Rademann's Diabetiker-Dessert-Geback	27.5	Fromm's Conglutin-Diabetiker-Schokolade	32.7
Nashville Malted Nut Food	27.5	Frank's Protein-Roggenbrot	33.0
Gumpert's Doppel-Diabetiker-Zwieback	27.6	Van Abbott's Gluten Biscottes	33.0
Metcalf's Vegetable Gluten ('06)	28.1	Health Food No. 2; Proto Puffs	33.3
Health Food Pure Washed Gluten Flour ('06)	29.5	Frank's Protein-Weizenbrot	33.5
		Ferguson Gluten Bread	33.6
		Gum Gluten Breakfast Food	34.2
		Gericke's Sifarbiskuits	35.3

Diet for Diabetics with Gout.—When gout accompanies or complicates diabetes the necessity for regulating the diet in conformity with the necessities of both diseases is evident. When a case of diabetes with very low carbohydrate tolerance has a fairly good protein tolerance, and one naturally comes to rely on the latter for furnishing a fair number of calories, in the presence of gout, care must be exercised with regard to the sort of protein that is ordered. If the case shows very mild evidences of gout it may only be necessary to curtail an excess of purine bodies by entirely eliminating stock soups and giving only meats with the lowest purine content, such as fish and chicken, either but once a day or once every other day. When the case is more pronounced it is necessary to eliminate the purines from the diet as much as possible, using the animal albumins which are purine-free, such as egg albumen and cheese principally and the vegetable proteins contained in beans, peas and lentils. In this way we can secure the required amount of albumin which is purine-free or nearly so, in conformation with the requirements of gout.

Exerting care in the selection of foods it is thus possible to construct a diet which is suitable for both diabetes and gout.

Diabetes in Elderly People or in the Young.—In many text-books these extremes of life are treated dietetically somewhat differently from the ordinary average adult. In elderly people it is often felt that a small amount of sugar (below 2 per cent.) is no particular menace and therefore need not be treated very rigorously particularly if the subjects are obese. As a matter of fact every case of glycosuria has potentialities of disaster and if untreated tends to grow progressively, although often very slowly, worse; on this account they should all be made and kept sugar- and acid-free (ketonuria). In the mild cases this is usually a simple matter, in the more severe they should be treated more vigorously and not treated lightly as of little importance as is so often done. One great reason for this care being the fact that such elderly people with even a mild diabetes are prone to intercurrent infections, gangrene, etc., all of which are rendered much less probable if the hyperglycemia can be reduced to normal.

In diabetes in the very young there is the necessity for the most painstaking care, as these cases tend to grow progressively worse, most of them ending fatally.

Allen's treatment offers the best plan of attack and some really remarkable cases are on record in which this treatment has at least put off indefinitely the fatal acidosis. While it is not such a difficult matter to render them sugar- and acid-free, it is usually extremely difficult to get them up to a fair maintenance diet and almost impossible to keep them nourished in accordance with the demands of the growing organism. It should be nevertheless tried and every effort made to prolong life with the hope that the disturbed function may again be reestablished.

Diet for Obesity with Diabetes.—As in the case with gout associated with diabetes we must find certain means by diet for controlling the obesity factor in this case.

In mild cases regulating the diet on the caloric basis by giving a diet one-fourth to one-third lower in calories than would be ordinarily required by a person of the same height we can without difficulty reduce the patient; all foods that are allowable so far as the diabetes is concerned may be used but in reduced amount. In the more severe cases of diabetes there is usually no difficulty in reducing patients, for with Allen's method of treatment fasting is the means by which the glycosuria and ketonuria are cleared up, and the patients readily lose about one pound a day or thereabout. When feedings are again begun the patients continue to lose weight, since for a considerable time, while testing out the protein, fat and carbohydrate tolerance, they are on an insufficient diet. The dietary regulation of this complication of diabetes must receive especial attention in that it is recognized that a too rapid withdrawal of carbohydrates often hastens an impending acidosis. These patients should never be jumped from ordinary diet to fasting diet but the reduction must be made gradually extending over several days watching the ketonurea as a guide to the rapidity of carbohydrate reduction.

As has already been pointed out this loss of weight is a distinct advantage and care must be exercised not to allow it to increase to the former proportions.

Diet in Diabetes Complicated by Nephritis.—It is unfortunately true that many cases of diabetes are complicated by nephritis, particularly among older people. This always adds a difficult factor to the situation and in choosing a suitable diet for such cases it must be first determined which disease is of chief importance. If for example the nephritis presents the picture of an acute disease, the diet must conform to that useful in such a condition (more or less regardless of the diabetes, although of course, one would naturally omit from the diet all food which is primarily carbohydrate). In this condition one should rely upon an exclusively milk diet for a time, later adding egg albumen and fats in the form of cream and butter and as the patient showed an improvement in the renal condition, an attempt may be made to increase the diet along the lines best suited to diabetics. Of course a day or two of starvation at the outset would be good for the diabetics and would rest the kidneys, as well, water alone being given or the so-called "fasting" diet, (p. 477), but a return to milk diet would probably cause a reappearance of the glycosuria unless the case were very mild.

If the nephritis is a chronic affair of some time standing, one must treat primarily the diabetes, taking care in planning the diet that the protein ration shall be kept as low as possible to maintain nitrogenous equilibrium and that no purine containing protein shall be used or at most only those animal proteins that contain the lowest percentage of purine bodies (see Purine Bodies). In such cases it is well to place as much reliance on the fats as the metabolism will stand with the hope that the carbohydrate tolerance may be increased rapidly. At best it is often a nice point to select a diet which is suitable to both conditions, but with care it can usually be done unless the diabetes is of the most severe variety.

OBESITY.

In America there are fewer cures for obesity undertaken than abroad, for, probably partly on account of national characteristics, partly on account of the climate and partly because our leisure class is not so large as one formerly found abroad, there are fewer obese people here. Whatever the causes fewer people take up seriously the matter of reduction of weight than one finds on the other side of the water.

The Causes of Obesity.—The causes of obesity may be divided into: first, lack of exercise. Second, overfeeding. Third, hereditary constitutional causes.

For certain reasons, not thoroughly understood, the tendency to obesity may not, and in fact usually does not, show itself until toward middle life, at which time all three factors seem to be the most active in its production. There are, of course, numerous cases of obese youngsters of both sexes, usually from constitutional causes, such as hypopituitarism in which there is an increased tolerance for carbohydrates, but these are the exception and do not fall into the class of cases that apply for relief of their obesity *per se.*

Most persons in adult life attain to the use of what von Noorden calls their "maintenance diet," *i. e.*, their regular dietary which suffices, without effort on their part, to keep them at an average, even weight If these people reduce their activities without reducing the total quantity of food, the result will be an increase in weight, which if maintained long enough will result in obesity. Or these same people on their maintenance diet may entirely change their mode of life and under ore mattractive surroundings unconsciously eat more with the same result, so far as increase in weight goes.

There are always exceptions to these conditions and one often sees a spare individual who eats much more than would suffice to fatten him, but who does not get fat. So, too, some obese persons are comparatively small eaters and in old age with metabolism at "slow speed" weight is maintained often on very little food.

So far as the constitutional causes go, hypopituitarism has already been spoken of. Hypothyroidism is a fairly frequent cause for increase of weight and may develop at any time, but usually at middle life or in women at the climacteric, for in men diminished thyroid secretion is an extremely rare cause for obesity.

What it is that makes an obese parent pass his or her fat characteristics to the children is still a mystery.

Given a case of increased fat deposition, what must be our criteria for saying whether such an individual should undertake a reduction cure or not, as many may think that they are overweight and yet when judged by the average, are found to be within normal limits? The method most in vogue is to judge the normal by the relation of height to weight, for which numerous tables have been prepared. In America the tables prepared by one of the life insurance companies are much in use; or abroad, Tibble's table answers the same purpose.

AVERAGE WEIGHTS FOR MEN AND WOMEN, AS COMPILED BY THE METRO-POLITAN LIFE INSURANCE COMPANY.

Men.			Women.		
Height, Ft.	In.	Weight, Lbs.	Height Ft.	In.	Weight, Lbs.
5	1	120	4	10	108
5	2	125	4	11	112
5	3	130	5	..	114
5	4	135	5	1	118
5	5	141	5	2	123
5	6	145	5	3	126
5	7	150	5	4	129
5	8	154	5	5	133
5	9	159	5	6	137
5	10	164	5	7	142
5	11	169	5	8	146
6	..	175	5	9	150
6	1	181	5	10	154
6	2	188	5	11	158

NORMAL WEIGHT OF MALES AT VARIOUS AGES.[1]

Height.		Ages.							
Ft.	In.	15 to 24 years. Lbs.	25 to 29 years. Lbs.	30 to 34 years. Lbs.	35 to 39 years. Lbs.	40 to 44 years. Lbs.	45 to 49 years. Lbs.	50 to 54 years. Lbs.	55 to 59 years. Lbs.
5	0	120	125	128	131	133	134	134	134
5	1	122	126	129	131	134	136	136	136
5	2	124	128	131	133	136	138	138	138
5	3	127	131	134	136	138	141	141	141
5	4	131	135	138	140	143	144	145	145
5	5	134	138	141	143	146	147	149	149
5	6	138	142	145	147	150	151	153	153
5	7	142	147	150	152	155	156	158	158
5	8	146	151	154	157	160	161	163	163
5	9	150	155	159	162	165	166	167	168
5	10	154	159	164	167	170	171	172	173
5	11	159	164	169	173	175	177	177	178
6	..	165	170	175	179	180	183	182	183
6	1	170	177	181	185	186	189	188	189
6	2	176	184	188	192	194	196	194	194
6	3	181	190	195	200	203	204	201	198

Having this standard before us we can decide quickly whether a given individual is overweight or not, so far as can be said for a healthy man or woman, although conditions of disease may indicate the necessity for a reduction of weight below that which is normal in health.

The Conditions for which an Obesity Cure is Indicated are:
1. Those people whose weight is excessive for their height.

[1] Tibbles: Food in Health and Disease, p. 465.

2. Those who although within the normal limits but who on account of some disability or occupation would be better off with less weight.

3. Those who have serious circulatory diseases are almost invariably improved if relieved of excessive weight. This refers especially to cardiovascular renal diseases.

4. Those who have a fairly high grade of chronic emphysema or bronchitis.

Of those who fall in the first class, there is little more to be said, if the excess of weight is considerably above the average, they would be better for having less.

Those in the second class may be those with some disability of their locomotive apparatus or who, on account of their occupation, must remain a little underweight, *e, g.,* dancers, acrobats, etc.

Of those in class three, more needs to be said. There is every reason to feel, and from clinical experience to know, that cases of chronic renal or cardiovascular disease, whether valvular or muscular, are much better off if their excessive weight is removed and are brought even below their normal weight for their height. The results in this direction are often brilliant and it should be insisted upon in all such cases that an earnest attempt be made to reduce the weight. The results are seen in a lessened tendency to dyspnea, edema and palpitation, all present in cases of circulatory disease complicated by obesity and to a less extent even in cases with normal circulatory apparatus, but accompanied by obesity.

In cases of hypertension the results are often even more brilliant and if we can reduce these patients we almost always reduce the blood-pressure to a greater or less extent and often very markedly. The most convincing statistics on this are published by Gaertner, showing the relation of the decline in blood-pressure to the decrease in weight (p. 495).

There is one class of cases in whom the question comes up as to whether or not they should be subjected to a reduction cure, namely old people who are more or less obese. The general concensus of opinion for these people is that they should not undergo a marked reduction unless they have serious cardiac, circulatory, renal or pulmonary complications, for if otherwise healthy they will naturally tend to grow thinner as they approach extreme old age, at least this seems to be the rule and they bear reduction cures rather badly.

The Objects of a Reduction Cure are:

1. To effect a slow consumption of the previous fat deposits.

No.	Sex.	Age.	Weight, Kg.	Height, Cm.	Blood-pressure, mm. Hg.
1	F.	32	114	161	165–115
2	F.	31	82	164	115– 90
3	M	49	103	170	200–155
4	F.	16	77	167	165–130
5	M.	67	90	168	165–120
6	F.	37	82	157	105– 95
7	M.	34	105	174	100– 90
8	F.	51	91	153	120–100
9	M.	40	88	177	110– 95
10	M.	31	102	169	120–100
11	F.	33	117	162	130–100
12	F.	52	79	163	140–100
13	F.	28	90	164	110– 90
14	F.	26	106	176	116–100
15	M.	44	96	176	150–108
16	F.	40	84	166	130–100
17	M.	53	87	175	140–118
18	F.	42	103	155	145–100
20	F.	55	74	157	140– 95
21	F.	52	80	161	135–115
22	M.	66	114	170	145–118
23	M.	44	81	174	150–120
24	F.	22	115	170	130–115
25	F.	38	72	159	180–110
26	F.	42	93	167	140–128
27	M.	39	105	181	115–110
28	F.	23	92	157	110– 95

2. The maintenance of the normal metabolic processes.[1] There are two types of obese persons:

1. Plethoric type, occurring in healthy, often athletic persons, with an exaggerated normal appetite. After forty they are apt to develop serious organic trouble. They often show increased blood-pressure.

2. Anemic type, occurring for the most part in women who are flabby and anemic and who suffer from all sorts of disorders but who are less to develop serious troubles than the plethoric individuals.[2]

Having decided upon a reduction cure in any patient, what are the steps and methods by which this may be best accomplished? It is here that we meet with a bewildering array of methods for the reduction of obesity, probably any one of which will result in the object sought, some methods being more applicable to one temperament or set of conditions, another to a different kind, and the cases must be individualized to some extent, even in the use of any one method.

In the lesser degrees of obesity where only slight, or at most, very moderate reduction is sought, it is usually enough to regulate the patient's diet by cutting out certain classes of foods, e. g., sugars, much starchy or fat foods, and increasing

[1] Anders: New York Med. Jour., 1914, c. 1.
[2] Saundley: Med. Press and Circul., 1914, N.S., xcviii, 112.

the bodily exercise; but where anything like a severe reduction cure is indicated, it is often necessary to weigh all the food as otherwise the error is too great and our efforts are not successful, the method and the physician both coming in for the blame.

In the treatment of the plethoric type of obesity we can use more stringent methods as to diet and more vigorous exercises. In the anemic type the reduction must be made possibly more slowly and carefully with attention fixed on the upbuilding of the patient's blood and general condition, as well as on the details of the reduction.

Reduction Cures.—Von Noorden Cure.—Among all the methods to be found none appeals more strongly to the intelligence than the reduction cure recommended by von Noorden, as it places the emphasis on the regulation of food intake as affecting: first, slight obesity; second, moderate obesity and third, marked obesity.

The assumption is made that a patient weighing 70 kilos (154 pounds) requires for ordinary activities 37 calories per kilo or 2590 calories in all as his "maintenance" diet; if this patient weighs 100 kg. (220 lbs.) this is 30 kg. over what he should weigh for his height, and while the 2590 calories are enough to maintain him at 70 kg. (154 lbs.) it would require 1110 extra calories to feed these 30 kg. extra. The ideal weight for his height being 70 kg., his maintenance diet is therefore 2590 calories, so that in calculating the calories necessary for any individual, account must be taken of the maintenance diet for that particular person from which must be taken one-fifth, two-fifths, or three-fifths of the maintenance allowance, *e. g.*,

1st. Degree of reduction diet four-fifths of the demand, 2000 calories.

2d. Degree of reduction diet, three-fifths of the demand, 1500 calories.

3d. Degree of reduction diet, three-fifths to two-fifths of the demand, 1500 calories down to 1000.[1]

It is easy to arrange Diets I and II, for all that is needed in Diet I is to omit all visible fat, such as oil, butter, fat meat, etc., to have vegetable and farinaceous dishes made with little fat and to prohibit the use of alcohol.

In Diet II dishes made from flour, stewed fruits, milk and soups containing flour must be forbidden as well. The results of these diets are slow, but if lived up to, the reduction will come gradually.

In Diet III, the foods should be chosen from this list:

[1] Disorders of Metabolism and Nutrition, von Noorden, Obesity, p. 31.

"Coffee, tea without milk or sugar; meat broth (fat skimmed off) with vegetables; lean meat or fish (total weight 250 to 350 gm. (8 to 12 oz.) weighed cooked); lean cheese; abundant green vegetables and salads, prepared with as little fat or oil as possible; vinegar, lemon, pickles, tomatoes, celery, radishes (abundant raw fruit with small percentage of sugar, as apples, peaches, strawberries, raspberries, currants, blueberries, sour cherries, grapefruit, early oranges, etc.); coarse bread (bran or graham bread) in quantities of from 40 to 70 gm. (1⅓ to 2⅖ oz.) per day only; potatoes prepared without fat, in quantities of from 80 to 150 gm. (2⅖ to 5 oz.), mineral waters *ad libitum;* wine in weak persons up to 200 c.c., but preferably omitted altogether; eggs, one or two; skimmed milk; buttermilk."[1]

The diet must be calculated in calories necessary for the individual, and von Noorden advises against this third degree of reduction except under direct supervision of the physician, best in a sanatorium.

Fat and Carbohydrate Restriction.—The fats must be restricted to 30 gm. (1 oz.) per day, but considerable carbohydrate in fruit, potatoes, bread and buttermilk are allowed. Von Noorden says that it is not necessary to go below 100 gm. (3⅓ oz.) of carbohydrate in a day's ration and he usually permits 120 gm. (4 oz.). This fairly generous supply of carbohydrate contributes to sparing of the body albumin better than 53 gm. of fat, although the latter has the same caloric value.

Hunger should not be allowed, for it will result in the failure of the cure or else a rapid return to overeating as soon as the cure is over. This may be accomplished by feeding foods of considerable bulk but of low food value.

Protein Allowance.—The diet allows a fair amount of protein, 120 to 180 gm. (4 to 6 oz.) which is necessary to spare the body albumin. On the basis of what has been said von Noorden builds his minimal and maximal diets as follows:

	Minimal.	Maximal.
Protein	120 gm. (4 oz.) 492 cal.	180 gm. (6 oz.) 738 cal.
Fat	30 gm. (1 oz.) 280 cal.	30 gm. (1 oz.) 280 cal.
Carbohydrate	100 gm. (3⅓ oz.) 410 cal.	120 gm. (4 oz.) 492 cal.
	1182 cal.	1510 cal.

A sample of the von Noorden Diet:[2]

Breakfast: Lean meat, 80 gm. (2⅖ oz.); bread, 25 gm. (1 oz.); tea, one cup with milk, no sugar.

[1] Von Noorden, ibid.
[2] Osler's Practice.

32

Midforenoon: One egg.

Luncheon: Soup, 1 small portion; lean meat, 160 gms. (5⅓ oz.); potatoes, 100 gms. (3⅓ oz.); fruit, 100 gms. (3⅓ oz.).

Afternoon:

3 P.M.   Cup of black coffee.

4 P.M.   Fruit, 200 gm. (6⅔ oz.).

6 P.M.   Milk, 250 c.c. (8 oz.).

Dinner: Meat, 125 gm. (3⅙ oz.); bread (graham), 30 gm. (1 oz.); fruit, small portion as sauce *without* sugar; salad, vegetable or fruit, radishes, pickles.

Banting's Cure (very severe):

Breakfast, 8 A.M.; 150 to 180 gm. (5 to 6 oz.) meat or broiled fish (not a fat variety of either); a small *bis-cuit* or 30 gm. (1 oz.) dry toast; a large cup of tea or coffee without cream, milk or sugar.

Dinner, 1 P.M.: Meat or fish as at breakfast, or any kind of game or poultry, same amount; any vegetables except those that grow under ground, such as potatoes, parsnips, carrots or beets; dry toast, 30 gm. (1 oz.); cooked fruit without sugar; good claret, 300 c.c. (10 oz.). Madeira or sherry.

Tea, 5 P.M.: Cooked fruit, 60 to 90 gm. (2 to 3 oz.); one or two pieces of zweiback; tea, 270 c.c (9 oz.) without milk, cream or sugar.

Supper, 8 P.M.: Meat or fish, as at dinner, 90 to 120 c.c. (3 to 4 oz.); claret or sherry, water, 210 c.c. (7 oz.).

Fluids restricted to 1050 c.c (35 oz.) per day.

Oertel's Cure.—In Oertel's obesity cure great stress is laid upon the condition of the heart and any circulatory changes, large meals being distinctly apt to embarrass either.

The object of the diet is to furnish food and exercise so that the patient may burn his own body fat, but not allow any destruction of protein which is not fully supplied by the diet.

Each case must be studied with a view to seeing what function must be safe-guarded while the process of reduction is in progress.

Oertel's calculations for the needs of the body are:

	Protein, grams.	Fat, grams.	Carbohydrates, grams.	Calories.
Minimum . . .	156 (5⅛ oz.)	25 (⅚ oz.)	75 (2½ oz.)	1180
Maximum . . .	170 (5⅔ oz.)	45 (1½ oz.)	120 (4 oz.)	1608

Restriction of fluid is an essential part of the treatment and while he allows 1500 c.c (1½ quarts) in average cases, it may be best to reduce it to 1250 or 750 c.c (41 to 25 oz.).

Solid foods must be taken alone and fluids between meals, five or six meals are given in the day.

Exercise is regarded as of equal importance with diet, and ordinarily out-of-door exercise of five hours per day is insisted upon, beginning with what the patient is up to and gradually increasing. In European health resorts hill-climbing is much in vogue, there being four different grades, as follows:

First.   incline from   o to 5 degrees.
Second.   "   "   5 to 10   "
Third.   "   "   10 to 15   "
Fourth.   "   "   15 to 20   "

At first the patient takes only the first or second climb, avoiding overexertion and walking about from one to two hours, not taking into account the down-hill return.

If necessary, from the patients condition, the first walking must be on level ground, and where even this causes cardiac or respiratory distress it is especially useful to have them given resisting exercises to all muscles, beginning with 5 to 10 movements to each set, increasing the amount of resistance and the number of movements up to 20 to 25 for each set of muscles. If there is angina, great caution must be used in all exercises, not to allow anything that will materially raise the blood-pressure.

After sufficient reduction in weight has been accomplished Oertel puts patients on an "after-diet" as follows:

Breakfast: Coffee or tea with milk, 150 to 200 c.c. (5 to 6½ oz.); bread, 75 gm. (2½ oz.).

Midmorning: Soft eggs, one or two, or 30 to 40 gm. (1 to 1½ oz.); meat, 100 gm. (3⅓ oz.); wine or port, 50 c.c. (1⅔ oz.); a little bread.

Dinner: Soup, 100 c.c. (3½ oz.); meat or fowl (not fat), 150 to 200 gm. (5 or 6 oz.); fish, cooked without fat, 100 gm. (3 oz.); dessert, fruit, 100 to 200 gm. (3 to 6½ oz.); light wine or beer, 160 to 250 c.c (5 to 8 oz.); water.

Midafternoon: Coffee or tea, 150 to 200 c.c. (5 or 6 oz.); water, 250 c.c. (8 oz.); bread, 30 to 60 gm. (1 or 2 oz.).

Supper: Meat as at dinner, or eggs; bread, 30 gm. (1 oz.); small amount of cheese, salad or fruit; wine or beer, 300 to 500 c.c. (10 to 16 oz.), with water or not.

Ebstein's Dietary.—Ebstein modified existing obesity cures by allowing a considerable amount of fat but notably restricting the carbohydrates, forbidding all sugar, sweets and potatoes, but allowing 180 to 210 gms. (6 or 7 oz.) of bread. Vegetables that grow above ground are allowed and all sorts of meat, especially is fat meat permitted. Fats are allowed, 120 to 180 gms. (4 to 6 oz.) per day. Three meals with the heartiest at midday.

> *Breakfast:* One large cup of black tea, without cream or milk, or sugar; white or brown bread, 60 gms. (2 oz.) with plenty of butter.
>
> *Dinner:* 2 P.M. Clear soup, meat 120 to 180 (4 to 6 oz.) with gravy and fat meat is especially recommended; vegetables in abundance (as noted above); small amount of fresh or stewed fruit (without sugar) or salad; two or three glasses of light white wine. Shortly after dinner a cup of tea is allowed with sugar or milk.
>
> *Supper:* 7.30 P.M. Large cup of tea, without sugar or milk; one egg with or without a small portion of meat, preferably fat. Occasionally a little cheese or fresh fruit

Total values: Protein, 100 gm. (3⅓ oz.); fat, 85 gm. (3 oz.); carbohydrate, 50 gm. (2⅜ oz.).

Schweninger's Dietary.—Absolutely no fluids are allowed with meals but must be taken at least two hours afterwards.

> *Breakfast,* 8.00 A.M. Meat, eggs or milk.
>
> *Lunch,* 10.30 A.M. Fish or meat with 90 c.c. (3 oz.) light wine.
>
> *Dinner,* 1.00 P.M. Meat, vegetables and fruit.
>
> *Supper,* 7.00 P.M. Meat, stewed fruit or salad and 90 c.c. (3 oz.) white wine.

As little bread as possible to be taken. Exercise is to be taken frequently during the day, in fact some time after each meal.

Germain-See Diet.—The chief recommendation in this diet is that fluids are forced and no wine allowed.

Tibble's Milk Cure:[1]

> *Breakfast:* Milk, 500 c.c. (1 pint).
>
> *Lunch:* Meat, 180 gm. (6 oz.); plate of boiled vegetables (bread and potatoes are not allowed); junket, 250 gm. (½ pint).
>
> 5 P.M.: Junket, 250 gm. (½ pint); two cups of tea, very little sugar.
>
> *Dinner:* Milk, 500 c.c. (1 pint); two apples, 1800 calories.

Tibbles has used this with great success.

Total values:

Protein.	Fat.	Carbohydrate.	Calories.
100 gm. (3⅓ oz.)	60 gm. (2 oz.)	50 gm. (1⅜ oz.)	1800

[1] Tibble: Diet in Health and Disease, p. 462.

Salisbury Method.—In cases of obesity with carbohydrate dyspepsia accompanied as it is by a great amount of flatulence, it is always advantageous to reduce the carbohydrate intake to a minimum. At times it may be necessary to go still further and put such a patient on a diet that offers no substance for fermentation. Such a diet is Salisbury's. In this only finely chopped beef and hot water or weak tea are allowed.

One hour before breakfast a pint of water is to be drunk hot, also one and a half hours before dinner and supper.

Breakfast: 180 to 250 gm. (6 to 8 oz.) finely chopped meat, made into cakes or broiled. A pint of water, plain or flavored with a little tea, coffee or orange juice, without sugar.

Dinner and *Supper* the same as breakfast.

If patients are faint between meals, broth or a little chopped meat is allowed. The amount of meat is increased up to one pound (500 gm.) at each meal, but no more. This can be kept up for a considerable length of time, but ordinarily a few days or a week is sufficient, after which other meats may be allowed, also eggs, rice, baked potato and a little stale or toasted bread.

Later green vegetables are added and gradually the patient returns to a full mixed diet, keeping down the carbohydrate intake to the minimum and permanently excluding all sugars and sweets.

Tower-Smith's Modification of Salisbury Diet.—*First stage* fourteen days. The diet is restricted to three pounds of lean beef, one pound of codfish and six pints of water, preferably hot. This is divided into four meals. The water should be taken as follows:

1. One pint early morning.
2. One pint half an hour before breakfast.
3. One pint an hour before midday meal.
4. One pint before the afternoon meal.
5. One pint before the evening meal.
6. One pint at bedtime.

Condiments are allowed. The meat contains 286 gm. (9½ oz.) protein, 43 gm. (1½ oz.), nitrogen.

Second stage. Twenty-one days.

The water is now but four pints, the beef and fish together but three pounds. Any meat-free fat or fish of the non-fatty variety may be used. Bread, as before 60 to 90 gm. (2 or 3 oz.). Dry white wine or tea is also allowed.

No person with organic disease should take this cure, and if not carefully carried out it may result in the production of mental disturbance amounting at times to mania.

Galisch's Cure.[1]—The principle of this diet is to give very little food at night so that during sleep the body has less food to store up.

Diet.—Early A.M. Tea with white bread and butter.

10 A.M. One egg with a little bread and butter.

1 P.M. Meat and vegetable, a little sauce, potato, salad and stewed fruit.

Afternoon: Coffee with zweiback or white bread and a little butter.

Evening: A small piece of bread and butter. A little beer or wine.

At breakfast and dinner enough is allowed to satisfy the appetite, but during the afternoon for a few days the patients are very hungry, this disappears, however, when more breakfast is taken.

When the patient is down to normal weight, more food is cautiously allowed at night. Brauer recommends at the outset a Karell cure for ten days, then an after-cure given in bed.[2]

Folin-Denis Method of Reduction.[3]—Since the essence of the successful reduction method in obesity lies in keeping the intake of energy below that of the output, complete fasting would theoretically, at least, accomplish this purpose most promptly. Unfortunately this is not possible without the production of symptoms such as headache, nausea and dizziness which indicate abnormal metabolic conditions. It was found that these symptoms could be easily made to disappear if even a little food was given. On account of these symptoms it has been the habit to underfeed the obese in reduction cures rather than starve them in order to cause a loss of weight due to the actual oxidization of the body fat.

In the course of observations on the voluntary fasting of two exceptionally obese patients of the Massachusetts General Hospital in Boston, Folin, and Denis noted "the usual development of the indications of 'acidosis,' that is, an increased elimination of acetone, aceto-acid and particularly of β-oxybutyric acid and ammonia in the urine. In one of the subjects the figures were exceptionally high, amounting to over 18 grams of β-oxybutyric acid and no less than 2.5 grams of ammonia-nitrogen during the fourth day of starvation. The appearance of such products in these amounts is in accord with the widespread scientific belief that the

---

[1] Med. Klin., 1912, viii, 1909.
[2] Deut. med. Wchnschr., 1913, xxxix, 1336.
[3] Jour. Biol. Chem., 1915, xxi, 183.

'acetone bodies' are derived chiefly from incompletely oxidized fat. When the obese are compelled to depend on their store of fat for maintenance, one might reasonably expect these intermediary products to 'crop out.'"

In order to relieve the subjective symptoms associated with this fasting acidosis, Folin and Denis interrupted the period of complete starvation by a period of very moderate diet, just sufficient to cause the disappearance of the "acetone bodies" from the urine.

Thereupon a second fast was begun. Here the striking observation was made that the acidosis did not manifest itself anew until the third day of this fast, and the patient felt well until the fourth day. After an interspersed repetition of "low" diet a third fast was begun five days later. Here again the onset of acidosis was even slower than during the second period. These facts, supported by confirmatory evidence in a similar case, have suggested to the observers that with regard to the complete oxidation of body fat in starvation, the human organism is capable of at least a certain amount of adaptation, and that it is this individual factor rather than the tendency to obesity or the extent of the fat deposits in the body which chiefly determine the onset and the degree of acidosis. Folin and Denis conclude that one of the effects of repeated fastings is habituation to the complete oxidation of mobilized body fat, and a consequent retardation of the development of acidosis.

These results suggest, in the words of their discoverers, that one perfectly safe, rapid and effective method of reducing the weight of very obese persons is by a series of repeated fasts of increasing duration, the ammonia or β-oxybutyric acid determination being used as a guide to the length of each fast.[1]

This might be said to be the last word in obesity cures.

Exercise and Massage.—Exercise and massage form part of the treatment in every case. Massage does not remove fat but only helps to keep the muscles in good condition. Exercise often with extra clothing helps to burn up the excess of fat, but patients must be careful that the increased appetite which follows exercise does not cause them to regain at the next meal all they have lost.

Water in Obesity.—Just a word in closing on this mooted subject. Water *per se* does not increase weight unless there is chloride retention, but it acts indirectly to increase weight by making the swallowing of food more easily accomplished so that one is apt to eat more; water also increases the appe-

[1] Jour. Am. Med. Assn., October 23, 1915, p. 1462.

tite. Denning,[1] who investigated this question, found that the amount of water taken exerts very little effect upon either the production or loss of fat. Von Noorden probably voices the rational view of the question in saying that the restriction of water is not important except in four conditions: (1) In cases with weak circulation; (2) at the commencement of an obesity cure to make a mental impression on the patient, for by restriction of fluids loss of weight is greater; (3) when reduction of water causes less appetite for fat-producing foods (*e. g.*, water after sweets); (4) when the sweat excretion is excessive, the water intake should be reduced to 1100 c.c. (2¼ pints) per day.

GOUT.

Although a detailed discussion of the etiology of gout is not a part of a book on dietetics, a certain understanding of the causes producing this disease are essential to an intelligent application of dietary principles, so that even at the risk of repeating what many of the readers already know, enough must here be incorporated to accomplish this end.

The final word has not been said in the biochemistry of gout and we are a long way still from understanding much about it, yet it can be definitely stated that whatever else may be at fault, the inability of the organism to properly metabolize the food purines is primarily disturbed, according to most authorities. In some, instances, possibly in most, there is also an accompanying failure in excretion due to deficient renal function; indeed many authorities assert that this renal complication is the chief factor in the precipitation of gouty symptoms. So long as elimination is good great increase of uric acid productions can occur without there being any resulting gouty symptoms. This actually is shown to be the case in lobar pneumonia and acute leukemia, where the percentage of uric acid in the blood is often very high, yet no symptoms referable to it are found, as the excess is prevented from backing up, through sufficient elimination. That the amount of uric acid in the blood is the index of a disturbed purine metabolism is course of generally believed but that uric acid is the only substance at fault seems improbable. Of course the cogeners of uric acid, xanthin, hypoxanthin, guanin, theobromine, etc., are all included in the generic term "uric acid." Hence we see that it probably takes at least two factors to account for gouty manifestations. First, increased uric acid production through

[1] Zeit. f. Diet und Physik, Therap., ii, 292.

perverted metabolism of purine bases and second, a deficient excretion. In certain cases of clinical gout the excretion of exogenous uric acid is not always delayed as shown by Magnus-Levy, Wintraud, Rommel, Pratt and Rosenbloom.[1]

McClure[2] after a study of uric acid in gout comes to the following conclusions:

(1) More than 3 mg. of uric acid per 100 c.c. of blood with the patient on a purine-free diet is a symptom of gout but is not diagnostic of the disease.

(2) No relation exists between the amount of uric acid and total non-protein nitrogen found in the blood of gouty persons.

(3) A marked retention of non-protein nitrogen is not frequent in gout.

(4) The excretion of exogenous uric acid by normal, by arthritic and by gouty persons varies greatly both in amount and duration.

(5) The retention of exogenous uric acid is a symptom of questionable importance in the diagnosis of gout.

The source of blood uric acid is twofold:

1. That derived from catabolism of the body tissue nucleins (the nuclei of cells) called endogenous uric acid.

2. That derived from the foods, called exogenous uric acid.

Naturally there is always a certain amount of uric acid in the blood even on a uric acid-free diet due to the breaking down of cell nuclei. This, however, should not exceed 0.5 to 1 mg. per 100 c.c. of blood and is of no pathological importance, provided elimination is sufficient. In severe nephritis, even though the uric acid production is not increased, the difficulty in excretion results in a uricacidemia. This, however, does not by any means invariably produce gouty manifestations and in fact few cases of chronic Bright's show them. This fact seems to prove that there is still another element in the production of gout that has thus far eluded us. Duckworth[3] says that gout is caused by an excess of uric acid in the blood but further states that it is the result of a special disturbance of the nervous system, there being a trophic center for joints in the medulla and the sudden precipitation of an attack is due to nervous causes, given the underlying uricacidemia and poor elimination.

Ebstein showed that in the deposition of the sodium biurate in the joints a destructive process always precedes the

[1] Jour. Am. Med. Assn., 1918, lxx, 285.
[2] Tr. Am. Assn. Phy., 1917, xxxii, 186.
[3] Jour. Advance Therap., New York 1913.

deposition of the salts due to the local effect of the circulating uric acid. Today it is easier to believe that this preliminary destructive process may be rather due to some process of chronic infection and the association of this with what are apparently gouty lesions must not be forgotten. Infection may play a much more important role than we have been wont to imagine and may supply the missing link in the chain of evidence that might connect the uricacidemia with the arthritic changes. This is admittedly an elusive factor in the production of gout for which the nervous system is blamed by some. In other words uricacidemia plus chronic infection may result in the deposition of biurate of soda in the connective tissues, so-called "gout"— whereas chronic infection plus certain other unknown conditions may result in arthritis of other kinds—the so-called chronic rheumatoid arthritis, etc.

Garrod[1] says that there are only three established *facts* in gout.

1. The deposits in the tissues are sodium biurate.

2. The blood contains an excess of uric acid.

3. Except during attacks there is no excess output of uric acid in the urine (although there is an increased percentage of it in the blood almost constantly).

In patients past forty-five or fifty, it is frequently the custom to ascribe almost all irregular and unexplained aches and pains to gout, but undoubtedly innumerable cases of non-gouty arthritis, luetic lesions and occasionally tuberculous joints are treated as gout, so that a careful diagnosis is of special importance if one wishes to be successful in the dietetic handling of this disease. There is also another reason for an accurate diagnosis, in that to put a patient on a purine-poor diet for a prolonged period, without adequate cause, is not without its dangers, for nowadays we have come to know that some disease conditions are brought about by a lack of certain food elements in the diet and one has only to mention scurvy and beriberi, both due to the absence of accessory food substances sometimes called "vitamines" to realize that a continuous diet which almost entirely leaves out these useful food factors may result in damage to the organism and "until these factors are known and reckoned with, rules of diet on scientific lines are not possible."[2]

So much then for a brief theoretical discussion of the underlying facts which must govern us in the construction of a gouty diet, the object of which is to prevent the development

[1] Lancet, 1913, i, 1790.
[2] Garrod: Lancet, 1913, p. 1790.

of a gouty condition and to control the active symptoms of an acute attack. We see that the best we can do is to give a diet which will not increase the uric acid in the blood, on account of there being a disjointed eliminative system, but at the same time keeping in mind that a gouty person cannot stand protein starvation any better than anyone else, although such an one is probably improved by keeping the protein of the diet somewhere near the low level suggested by Chittenden, not over 50 to 70 gm. protein per day. This latter provision is also important, as with a complicating contracted kidney there is apt to be more or less nitrogen retention. Another further consideration in the regulation of the diet is the fact that we must keep in mind the general nutrition of the patient, who, if already poorly nourished will hardly improve if his nutrition is still further disturbed by an insufficient diet. One must also diet with reference to complicating obesity or glycosuria both not infrequently accompanying conditions of gout.

Before proceeding to a discussion of the foods and actual dietaries in gout, it would be quite worth while quoting von Noorden's[1] and Schleip's[2] methods of making a diagnosis of actual gout by the dietary regulation. Their practice is to put a patient on a purine-free diet for five days and estimate the urinary uric acid. The normal person on such a diet should daily excrete an average of 0.45 gm. uric acid (endogenous). If during this period less uric acid is excreted each day than is normal, gout may be suspected. A definite amount of purine-containing food is then added for two days, 400 gm. of beef, weighed raw (or 50 gm. thymus gland). The 800 gm. of beef (or 100 gm. thymus) (the supply for two days) are equivalent approximately to 1.4 gm. uric acid, of this 0.7 gm. may be expected to show in the urine in twenty-four hours after the last day on which the meat was taken. If this extra uric acid elimination is below 0.7 gm. or is delayed in elimination over several days, the uric acid from this amount of beef or thymus is too much and is beyond the individual's tolerance. If this is so, repeat the test, using one-half the amount of meat; when the tolerance is found it shows how much purine food can be given daily with the expectation of complete elimination and without causing a uricacidemia. As compared with the normal individual, Pratt has shown that a dose of 100 gm. of meat for a gouty person causes the blood uric acid curve to rise and remain up much longer.

[1] Gout, p. 73. [2] Berl. klin. Wchnschr., 1905, 42, 1297.

Umber's[1] elimination curve is deterimned in much the same way, as the initial steps are the same but only 200 gm. of meat are given, or one can use 25 gm. thymus. The length of time for complete elimination is noted. Normally this excess uric acid should be eliminated in twenty-four hours. In mild cases of gout it may be delayed over three or four days, in more severe cases five or six days may be required before the normal limit is reached. The number of days it takes to eliminate the extra with a return to the normal level will indicate the period there should be between purine days. This will often show that a mild case of gout should take meat or purine food only twice a week and more severe cases only once a week or at even longer intervals. Clinically this plan of giving meat or purine food only once every few days has long been in use and has been found a satisfactory way to allow purine food. The use of thymus instead of beef is advised by Fine, for in such large amounts as 400 to 800 gm. of beef, the excess of meat alone is apt to delay the elimination of the uric acid. As already indicated 50 gm. of thymus yields the same amount of uric acid as 400 gm. of meat.

The diagnosis of uricacidemia is made now so easily by means of the direct examination of the blood for uric acid by Folin's method, that it can readily be determined whether an excess of uric acid is circulating in the blood or not. The longer method described is therefore less useful for diagnostic purposes than it is for the determination of the length of time required for uric acid elimination and its degree after a definite dose of purine.

Foods in Gout.—The actual dietary management of acute or chronic forms of gout will be given under a separate heading, but it is necessary to indicate here not only the best forms of protein, fat and carbohydrate, but what is quite as important, those forms which must be especially avoided. Protein food derived from glandular organs is especially to be avoided as containing the higher percentages of nucleic acid, derived from cell nuclei in which such organs abound. Soups made with meat stock may all be labeled "poison" for gouty people, containing as they do such a high percentage of extractives, almost a solution of purines. In fact these patients might much better eat the meat from which the soup is ade mthan the soup itself and a safe rule for them is to forget that such a thing as a clear or meat soup exists. Rich gravies and sauces should also be omitted from the diet as should condiments of all sorts. Only the simple hydrocarbons should be taken, such as butter, cream and vegetable oils.

[1] Lehrbuch d. Ernahrung u. d. Stoffewec. Krankht., Berlin, 1909.

Carbohydrates.—Rich or concentrated sweets should be avoided as tending to disturb digestion and cause flatulence, but a moderate amount of simple sweetened food is allowable as palatable, of high caloric value and purine-free. All foods that have a well-earned reputation for indigestibility, quite independent of their constituents, must be avoided.

Salt.—While it is not necessary to resort to extreme limitation of common salt, it should be kept at the lowest possible level compatible with palatability, for Lindsay[1] says that sodium has the effect of throwing sodium biurate out of solution from the blood, and it is known that the deposit of sodium biurate occurs in a distinct ration to the amounts of sodium salts in the various tissues in the body. The joints and tendons which are most highly sodium-containing are the most frequent sites of the uratic deposits, Hence keeping down the soda intake to the lowest level reduces, theoretically at least, the chance for a deposit of sodium biurate in the joints.

Alcohol.—Undoubtedly the gouty patient is better without any alcohol whatever, unless he has been a steady user of it, in which case a little whiskey, well diluted, preferably with an alkaline table water, is allowable. The writer has seen cases in which the entire withdrawal of alcohol, in patients accustomed to taking considerable quantities caused a decided increase in the symptoms, which were made distinctly less when a small amount of alcohol was again allowed. Any use of alcohol should be discontinued as soon as possible, and sweet wines, beers or champagne are especially bad, and should never be allowed. German clinicians, however, allow light Rhein wines in moderation, but the gouty subject is better without any form of alcohol.

Coffee, Tea and Cocoa contain considerable purine. This is changed in the digestive processes into bodies which have very little do do with uric acid and while small amounts of these beverages are allowable, any excess of them tends to disturb digestion and should be interdicted. Tea and coffee should not be boiled but made as a fresh infusion if used at all. Many recommend the use of one of the "caffeine-free" coffees (see p. 249). Having discussed the "dont's" of gout, we may now consider what foods and in what proportion they are allowable in the construction of a gouty diet. From what has already been said it is clear that the object sought in prescribing a gouty diet is to either omit all purine foods or to keep them down to a low level, preferably a known low level. Many so-called purine-free

[1] Gout, Oxford Press. 1913.

foods in reality contain a very faint trace of purine which, however, may be disregarded from a practical stand-point.

Diet in Acute Gout or Podagra.—During the first twenty-four to forty-eight hours of an acute attack in sthenic individuals, it is a wise plan (after a thorough emptying of the intestinal canal) to starve the patients completely, giving them only large amounts of water (preferably salines) provided they have not a coexisting high blood-pressure when less water should be allowed, but in any instance enough should be taken to act as a tissue diluent and for its flushing effect. If patients absolutely insist on food, a glass of milk may be given four times a day but nothing else. During this period, if accompanied by proper medication large amounts of uric acid may be eliminated. The patients may then be put on a purine-free diet, preferably a liquid or semisolid diet, consisting of milk, eggs, either plain or as junket and custard, limiting the milk to 1000 c.c. and the eggs to three and giving a little every three hours. This limitation of the protein is advisable because there is usually or often an accompanying contracted kidney which alone is capable of causing a nitrogen retention. After the acute symptoms have passed one may give a soft purine-free diet and later modify this according to the plan for chronic gout.

Purine-free Foods.—Eggs (including caviare), milk, bread (only white, not graham or entire wheat bread), butter, biscuits, cereals (hominy, rice, farina), cream, sugar, syrup, jam and marmalade, cake, cream soups, potatoes (have slight amount of purine), cauliflower, cabbage, lettuce, egg plant.

Desserts.—Nuts, cheese, ice-cream, water ices, cake, rice, bread, farina, cornstarch or tapioca puddings, custards.

Drinks.—Sweet cider, grape juice, unfermented fruit juices generally.

Soft Purine-free Diet. Use for Main Diet. (Vanderbilt Clinic.)

6.00 A.M. Milk, 180 c.c. (6 oz.).

8.00 A.M. *Breakfast*—Milk, 180 c.c. (6 oz.); one and a half slices of bread and one pat of butter; two tablespoonfuls of cream of wheat or wheatena with 60 c.c (2 oz.) cream and 2 tablespoonfuls of sugar; one soft-boiled egg.

12.30 P.M. *Dinner*—Milk, 180 c.c. (6 oz.); one soft-boiled egg; potato with cream, 30 c.c. (1 oz.) and pat of butter; lettuce or young cabbage with dressing; 1½ slices of bread, with one pat of butter.

3.30 P.M. Milk, 180 c.c. (6 oz.).

6.00 P.M. *Supper*—One soft-boiled egg; milk, 180 c.c. (6 oz.); 2½ tablespoonfuls of rice with cream, 30 c.c. (1 oz.) and one tablespoonful of sugar; crackers with one pat of butter; one cube of cheese (2 inches); one cup of weak tea with cream, 30 c.c. (1 oz.), and one teaspoonful of sugar.

9.00 P.M. Milk, 180 c.c. (6 oz.).

This gives: Protein, 80 gm. (2⅖ oz.); fat, 112 gm. (3½ oz.); carbohydrate, 207 gm. (7 oz.); calories, 2300.

In chronic gout we are not compelled to combat the severe pain and discomfort seen in the acute form which necessitates a drastic dietary regimen to help in cutting it short, so that we may proceed more leisurely to an accurate determination of just which foods an individual case will do best upon. It is here that we cannot do better for our guidance than refer freely to von Noorden's clear statements. Just as in diabetes we put the patient on a strict carbohydrate free food until the urine is sugar-free and then by adding small amounts of carbohydrate, determine the carbohydrate tolerance, so in gout we must put a patient on a purine-free diet and then by additions of purine-containing foods, determine his tolerance for purine.

1. The purine-free diet is also called the main diet.

2. The accessory diet consists of foods containing purines.

For the main diet it is convenient to use the soft-purine-free diet already given and this should be used for several days or until the low level of uric acid output is reached either presumably or as determined by analysis of the urine. When this point is reached then we may make use of the accessory diet to some extent.

In the accessory diet von Noorden takes 100 gm. (3⅓ oz.) of roast beef as the unit and reckons other meats, fish, fowl, etc., on this basis as follows:

100 gm. (3⅓ oz.) of roast beef, veal, mutton, lean pork, ham, tongue, venizon, rabbit contain the same amount of purine as 200 gm. (6½ oz.) fish, except the salmon family, or 200 gm. (6½ oz.) lobster or crab, or 24 oysters, or 2 pigeons, or 1 spring chicken, or ½ capon, or 1 guinea hen, or ½ duck, or ¼ goose.

So in ordering the accessory diet, we can advantageously use one or more portions of these various purine-containing foods.

When we have found by trial how much of the accessory diet the patient can eat without getting gouty symptoms, (which can also be checked up by urinary estimations of uric acid), it is always a good plan to put in one or two purine-free diet days a week, depending on the patient's tolerance, comparable to the diabetic fast or green days. Just as there are some cases of diabetes who cannot take any carbohydrate food or only minimal amounts without showing sugar in the urine, so some cases of gout can stand little or no purine food without presently showing symptoms. These cases must walk a narrow dietetic path, so far as the use of purine foods is concerned, and many do well only so long as they are kept on a purine-free diet. Complicating obesity or diabetes must be treated according to the principles laid down for these conditions in addition to their gouty diets and often it is no easy matter to take proper account of all these complications without fairly starving the patient. Often the most prominent condition must be dieted first without much reference to the other conditions present.

It must also be remembered that in a small percentage of cases no form of dieting seems to do good and the patients go on from bad to worse, as they are unable to dispose of even the purine products of their own metabolism.

There are certain individuals in whom it seems fairly certain that gout is present in some degree and in whom it is wise to institute a diet suitable for such mild cases which will not impose too great a dietary hardship, while at the same time keeping the purines down to a very low level. This would be distinctly useful in conditions which seem almost certainly due to a uricacidemia (although there are no definite joint symptoms), such as gouty skin lesions, long-standing catarrhs of the respiratory tract, etc., mostly in middle-aged or really old people. Of such a diet the following is an example, made up of the purine-free articles of diet or those with a small amount of purine prepared in the least objectionable way.

Diet in Gouty Diathesis.

Breakfast: Fruit, cooked or raw; cereal, any one, but preferably wheat preparations; white bread, toast, rolls or muffins and butter; eggs, cooked as desired except fried; cup of weak tea, cocoa or coffee, largely milk, with sugar; a little marmalade if there is no indigestion.

Luncheon or Dinner: Soup, cream or purée of vegetables (no meat); egg, entrée; meat or fish, never more than once a day, in small amounts, the meat best boiled in two waters—beef, mutton, chicken, ham; vegetables potatoes (white or sweet), cabbage, spinach, egg plant, corn, sprouts, beet tops, lettuce, rice, macaroni, noodles, cauliflower, string beans, celery, (peas, lima beans or white beans, if there are no active symptoms), no stock to be used in sauces: desserts, fruit cooked or raw; all simply prepared desserts, not too sweet, ice-cream, simple cake, American, cream, Swiss or Pot cheese; beverages, milk, unfermented fruit juices, *e. g.*, grape juice, apple juice, cider, alkaline mineral waters in small amount; plain water.

Mineral Waters.—Much has been written on the subject of the efficiency of cures at the various mineral spas or the taking of either the natural or artificial mineral waters at home and at one time or other many of the mineral springs, alkaline or saline, have enjoyed considerable vogue and still do. The first indication is for the use of considerable amounts of water for the mechanical effect of "flushing the system" and also for the beneficial effect on coexisting gastro-intestinal catarrh or hepatic congestion, but there is little evidence that these waters otherwise effect the elimination of uric acid, and on the contrary, prolonged use of them often acts in the reverse way and therefore should be discouraged. Short courses of water cures may be taken at Vichy, Marienbad, or Carlsbad, but should not be long-continued. In the United States, Saratoga, Hot Springs, Va., and White Sulphur Springs furnish treatments very similar.

THE PURINE BODIES IN VARIOUS FOODS.[1]

Fish:		Vegetables (Continued)	
Cod	0.5	Beans (Haricot)	0.63
Salmon	1.1	Asparagus	0.21
Halibut	1.0	Cabbage	0.0
Meat:		Lettuce	0.0
Beef	1.3 to 2.0	Cauliflower	0.0
Fat	1.1	Onions	0.09
Mutton	0.96	Tapioca	0.0
Fat	0.0	*Special foods:*	
Veal	1.1	Milk	0.0
Fat	0.0	Butter	0.0
Pork	1.2	Eggs	0.0
Fat	0.5	Cheese (fat)	0.0
Ham	1.1	*Drinks:*	
Meat soups, varying large amounts:		Beer	0.12
Chicken	1.2	Ale	0.14
Vegetables:		Porter	0.15
Potatoes	0.02	Per pint (500 c.c.)	
Rice	0.0	Tea	1.2
Flour (white)	0.0	Cocoa	1.0
Bread (white)	0.0	Chocolate	0.7
Oatmeal	0.53	Coffee	1.7
Peas	0.39	Claret	0.0
Lentils	0.38	Sherry	0.0
		Port	0.0

[1] J. Walker Hall: The Purin Bodies in Food-stuffs, etc., London, 1903. 2d edition, revised.

33

Radio-active waters have come into great popularity and in some quarters hopes have run high in consequence, some authors praising it extravagantly as of distinct value in doses of 1000 Mache units a day, increasing to 5000 to 10,000 m. u. The theories that account for its usefulness as summarized by Burnham[1] are:

1. Activation of ferments causing the oxidation of the uric acid and its further disintegration into CO_2 and ammonia.

2. Direct action on the uric acid, the emanations causing its solution and disintegration.

3. Increased activity of the kidneys by means of which excess uric acid is excreted by the blood.

On the other hand, Chace and Fine[2] conclude that radium emanation in concentration of at first 0.5 and later 100 m. u. per liter of air, radium drinking water and injection of soluble radium bromide in none of their cases showed any influence whatever upon the uric acid concentration of the blood, nor was the output of uric acid in the urine definitely increased.

DIET FOR LEANNESS OR FATTENING CURES.[3]

In discussing this subject von Noorden says that the average layman at a glance will undertake to say whether a certain individual is normally well developed, too thin or too fat; but as a matter of fact there are other factors which must be considered in arriving at this apparently simple diagnosis. Thus a person with tuberculosis who is somewhat overweight is better so, a person with chronic nephritis or cardiac disease who is somewhat underweight is better off so and under no circumstances should be the subject of further increase in weight. It is also important in arriving at the necessity of a fattening cure to know whether the muscle substance or the adipose, or both, are too little.

The first thing of importance in any given individual is to know their maintenance diet, *i. e.*, a measure of which may be taken as the diet which will keep him in nitrogenous equilibrium and at an even weight. Of course this means that a certain number of calories will constitute a fattening cure for one man, whereas for another who is naturally larger or whose work is more arduous it would not even be a maintenance diet. Given the maintenance diet it is important in planning a fattening cure to know about what increase in

[1] Med. Rec., New York, 1913, lxxxi, 117.
[2] Washington Med. Jour., 1912, 3, xi, 23; Jour. Pharm. and Exp. Therap., 1914, vi, 219.
[3] Adapted largely from von Noorden, "Fattening Cures."

weight may be counted upon by giving extra calories. Von Noorden on the basis of much material has come to the following conclusion:

Daily surplus of food or fattening additions.	Results in a possible average weekly increase in weight of:
500 to 800 calories	600 to 1000 gm.
800 to 1200 "	800 to 1200 "
1200 to 1800 "	1200 to 2000 "

This surplus of food or fattening addition von Noorden calls the "sum of the nutritive units (calories) administered in excess of the calculated nutritive demands (maintenance diet) of the individual."

The two essentials in a satisfactory fattening cure are to increase, first, the nitrogen surplus, and second, the adipose tissue. One without the other does not make a satisfactory result.

In a usual fattening cure with a fair protein ration (100 to 120 gm. daily) and a fair caloric surplus (30 to 40 per cent. above the calculated amount of the maintenance diet), one may expect a daily retention of nitrogen of from 1 to 3 gm., or if the caloric surplus is 40 to 60 per cent. above the maintenance diet one may expect a retention of from 2 to 6 gm. nitrogen per day. Nevertheless this added nitrogen does not tend to "stick" but is rather soon gotten rid of when the excess diet is reduced, and it must be concluded that we are "not justified in concluding that by overfeeding alone, without the coöperation of other factors, a material increase of 'flesh' (genuine breathing protoplasm) can be forced." "The real accumulation of flesh seems to be dependent on altogether different factors and seems to presuppose a specific predisposition on the part of the organism to accumulate flesh, we find a ready tendency to the increase of flesh in:

"1. The growing organism.

"2. During convalescence, following the sacrifice of protein.

"3. In muscles (and glands) that are stimulated by exercise (labor hypertrophy)."

The increase of adipose tissue is the other factor to be considered in fattening cures and is a much more simple matter, as it can be calculated quite accurately on the basis of the intake of the surplus over and above the maintenance diet, except in certain individuals.

Foods to be Used in Fattening.—Any of the food elements, protein, carbohydrate or fat are capable of increasing the weight.

Protein.—We cannot get patients to take continuously excessive amounts of protein, as it is apt to disturb digestion when given in amounts of 150 gm. (5 oz.) **per day; the** optimum in fattening cures probably lies between 100 to 120 gm. (3⅓ or 4 oz.) of protein.

If, as following severe illness or to accomplish **severe mus-** cular work, it is advisable to increase the protein **allowance** above 100 gm. (3⅓ oz.) it can best be done by adding some of the more concentrated protein foods, as their **bulk is** smaller and there is usually less strain put upon all **the excre-** tory organs. Von Noorden's list of foods and amounts containing 100 gm. (3⅓ oz.) protein is helpful in choosing an additional protein allowance.

100 gm. (3⅓ oz.) of albumin is contained in the *following* foods:

Eggs (without the shell), 900 gm. (30 oz.).

Veal, chicken (weighed raw,) 500 to 550 gm. (16⅔ to 18 oz.).

Fish (weighed raw), 500 to 600 gm. (16⅔ to 20 oz.).

Beef (weighed raw), 480 to 550 gm. (16 to 18 oz.).

Cow's milk, 3000 to 3500 (3 or 3½ qts.).

Cream cheese, 400 to 450 gm. (13 to 15 oz.).

Sanatogen, 105 gm. (3⅓ oz.).

Tropon, 110 gm. (3⅔ oz.).

Somatose, 120 gm. (4 oz.).

Carbohydrate.—Carbohydrates being palatable and of great variety, are extensively used in all fattening cures *except* where there is diabetes present or some form of carbohydrate indigestion. People differ both as individuals and as races in their ability to take carbohydrates. The average diet in health contains somewhere about 180 gm. (6 oz.) carbohy- drate per diem and if a little care is taken in selecting the more concentrated forms as much as 320 gm. (10⅔ oz.) can easily be given patients. This additional 140 gm. (4⅔ oz.) represents 570 calories. It is possible in selected cases and with care to increase this allowance up to 400 to 500 gm. The result of this one-sided carbohydrate diet is much the same as the excessive protein diet, *i. e.*, the excess fat or excess protein stored up does not last but when the large amount of carbohydrate is stopped the weight rapidly de- clines, hence von Noorden advises against giving more than 300 to 320 gm. (10 or 11 oz.) carbohydrate per diem with the one exception that patients who can take grape-juice can secure an additional 550 calories in a bottle containing 750 c.c. (25 oz.).

Cereal with cream, represents a good way to get in extra calories, and grapenuts are especially recommended by von Noorden, who estimates that 40 gm. (1⅓ oz.) of grapenuts moistened with hot water and 40 gm. (1⅓ oz.) of butter added, served with 60 c.c. (2 oz.) of 40 per cent. cream represents about 660 calories.

If we wish especially to increase the protein of the body the giving of large amounts of carbohydrate is essential, as it spares the protein combustion. The following list of foods contain 100 gm. (3⅓ oz.) of carbohydrate, besides other food elements and forms a convenient method of making additions to the diet. Each 100 gm. of carbohydrate represents 410 calories.

Oatmeal, 150 gm. (5 oz.).
Cornmeal, 140 gm. (4⅔ oz.).
Rice, 130 gm. (4⅓ oz.).
Macaroni, 135 gm. (4⅓ oz.).
Bread, 180 to 200 gm. (6 or 6⅔ oz.).
Zweiback biscuits, 120 to 135 gm. (4 to 4⅓ oz.).
Potatoes, 600 gm. (20 oz.).
Sugar, 100 gm. (3⅓ oz.).
Honey, 140 gm. (4⅔ oz.).
Peas (dry, 200 gm. (6⅔ oz.).
Fresh fruit, 1000 gm. (30⅓ oz.).
Chesnuts (without shell), 130 to 140 gm. (4½ or 4⅔ oz.).
Grape juice, 500 to 600 gm. (16⅔ to 20 oz.).
Beer, 1800 to 2000 gm. (60 oz.).

Fat.—This is the most readily available source of energy and represents the highest caloric value in the smallest bulk. People who need a fattening cure are usually poor fat eaters, else they would probably not be in need of fattening, for as a rule they do not spontaneously take over 100 gm. (3⅓ oz.) of fat per diem. With care this can usually be raised to a total of 250 gm. (8 oz.) of fat which alone represents 2350 calories. It is possible at times to give even more than this, but as a rule this is sufficient. As a matter of fact the fattening cure is really a process of education in the eating of fat for these people, as otherwise they are quite likely to relapse and the success of the "cure" both immediate and remote largely depends on the physician's ability to accomplish this. When gastro-intestinal disturbances are at the bottom of the nutritional disturbance it is more difficult to use fats in such quantities.

Bacon, cream, butter and milk are all fat-containing foods of great availability and should form a large part of a fattening cure diet. Olive oil or peanut oil are also valuable fatteners.

Alcohol.—The use of alcohol as a routine in fattening cures is not to be recommended, as many people are better without any on one ground or another, and everyone is **injured by** larger doses.   Alcohol never becomes a part of the **organism** but has a fuel value of 7 calories per gm.   "When 9.3 gm. alcohol are given 7 gm. less of fat are oxidized **than would** have been the case if no alcohol had been administered." Its toxic properties, as already indicated, preclude its extensive use, although theoretically it should be a **good fat**-tening substance.   Probably the best wines to use **are those** containing 15 to 20 per cent. of alcohol)—Madeira, **sherry** and port which may be allowed in amounts of 50 c.c. (1⅔ oz.) at one or two meals or heavy beer or ale may be substituted occasionally, if it can be obtained.

The inclusion of prolonged rest in bed as a routine in **fatten**-ing cures, is not necessary but in certain cases of nervous exhaustion, and digestive disorders accompanied by **leanness** it is certainly indicated.   In other cases it may be **valuable** as a preliminary measure but only for a short time, as active bodily exercise is essential if one wishes to build up not only fat but also muscle and leave the patient at the end of the cure an efficient machine and not a Strassburg goose.

To recapitulate the suggestions for diet in leanness, it is recommended to construct a dietary containing—protein, 100 to 120 gm. (3⅓ or 4 oz.); carbohydrate, 300 to 350 gm. (10 to 11⅔ oz.); fat, up to 250 gm. (8⅓ oz.).

Alcohol if used at all 50 to 100 gm. as a 15 per cent. wine.

The procedure is to add a certain excess of food to the maintenance diet and gradually to increase it as the patient is educated up to taking larger amounts of food, as for the most part patients in need of fattening are those who are either naturally very small eaters or who have become so from one or another reason.

When the rest cure plus the fattening process is to be combined, Weir Mitchell's plan is of the greatest use in properly selected cases where leanness is complicated by neurasthenia or severe gastro-intestinal disturbances (*q. v.*).

PHOSPHATURIA.

The occurrence of a cloudy urine due to the precipitation of phosphates is of common occurrence and has received probably more attention than its significance warrants, due no doubt to the fact that when noted by introspective or neurasthenic persons it has caused great mental disturbance regardless of a symptomatology; other people letting its presence pass either unnoticed or at least without anxiety.

Phosphaturia is due to a spontaneous separation of the earthy phosphates, *i. e.*, calcium and magnesium phosphates of the urine and is liable to occur in any urine which is concentrated and neutral or particularly alkaline in reaction. This does not mean that the separation of the phosphates denotes a pathological increase in their excretion, for as Herter[1] says "it is difficult to say what constitutes an excessive excretion of earthy phosphates but at all events in most cases of phosphaturia there is no evidence of such excess," and the chief pathological significance of its separation is the neutral state of the urine that permits it. In other words, the turbidity of the urine when due to phosphates is often wrongly thought to be caused by an increased elimination (phosphaturia), while it is more likely caused by a decreased acidity of the urine and should be called an alkalinurea.

"The average excretion of P_1 is 1 to 5 gm. per diem and comes in small part from the oxidation of the phosphorus of protein material, *i. e.*, endogenous, and to a greater extent from the phosphates of the food, *i. e.*, exogenous. The extent to which this latter controls the phosphate excretion in the urine depends upon the relative abundance of alkali and alkaline earthy phosphates."[2] The phosphates of the alkali earths are absorbed with difficulty and are therefore for the most part eliminated directly through the feces.

Newberg[3] classifies phosphaturia as follows:

Physiological Phosphaturia.—A diet rich in alkaline carbonates or one which has an excess of salts of vegetable acids or alkaline albuminates leads to diminished urinary acidity. This often is found in healthy people taking large amounts of vegetables or alkalies (often seen during alkaline treatment for gout or gastric hyperacidity), or a diet rich in lime and magnesia may act in the same way as one containing alkali, all producing a phosphaturia. It may also occur physiologically in an increased urinary alkalinity due to decreased excretion of acids in the urine. This is seen when on a diet that is largely protein where acid is withdrawn from the system to form the hydrochloric acid of the gastric juice so it will often be found in cases of hyperchlorhydria and gastric hypersecretion for the same reason.

Nervous and Sexual Phosphaturia.—This is ascribed variously as the cause or effect of nervous states, nervous causes effecting the secretory functions of the kidney and its selective action resulting in a phosphaturia. Phosphatic diabetes is also of nervous origin which together with essential phosphaturia is included under the neurasthenic variety.

---

[1] Chem. Pathology, p. 127.
[2] Myers and Fine: Essence of Path. Chem., p. 32.
[3] Von Noorden: Metabolism and Practical Medicine.

Juvenile Type.—This is at times a nervous affair and at others a real anomaly of phosphaturia as proven by metabolism experiments by Soetbeer, depending presumably on a disturbance of secretion of the mucous membrane of the large intestine and is often associated with calcium carbonate in the urine, called calcuria. Other cases are found without the associated calcuria.

Finally disturbances of phosphorus and calcium metabolism as in rickets, osteomalacia and functional disturbances of the sexual organs and of the thyroid also act to bring about a phosphaturia.

From what has been said it can be seen that so far as we know phosphaturia is of comparatively slight clinical importance and should concern us as dietitians but mildly, *i. e.*, in its being responsible for any general symptomatology. We do know that it is increased by a diet of potatoes, fruit and all fresh green vegetables, as already indicated, and decreased by abstaining from these articles of food, giving largely milk, eggs, cheese, cereals and legumes.[1]

When there have been symptoms caused by the calcuria, as in Soetbeer's type, limiting the articles rich in lime, brings the calcuria promptly down to normal. Directly trying to increase the urinary acidity by food or giving inorganic or organic acids has proven practically valueless,[2] although benzoic acid enjoys some reputation for this, it cannot be kept up indefinitely on account of consequent digestive disturbances.

The presence of phosphorus in the body tissues led to giving foods rich in phosphorus in conditions of phosphaturia thinking that this represented an excessive loss of phosphate from the system particularly in nervous disease, but it was found that the insoluble phosphates of the food were excreted by the feces and the soluble phosphates by the urine and anyhow as a regular thing in a mixed diet we take in more phosphates than we need to replenish those lost in the body's metabolism.

Phosphates and Calculi.—One additional factor relative to phosphates in the urine must be considered and this is in connection with the formation of calculi. This occurs in the presence of ammoniacal fermentation of the urine in the bladder, during which process phosphates may be precipitated on uratic stones or the phosphates and carbonates of lime may be found together.

[1] Friedenwald and Ruhräh: Dietetics, p. 454.
[2] Minkouski, Von Leyden: Handb. d. ernahrungs Therap. 2d auf, 1904, p. 319.

In a combination of a series of cases of 223·calculi, 36 or 16 per cent. were phosphatic. 72, or 37 per cent. were oxalate of lime often mixed with urates.

Phosphaturia, however, is not to be confused with the deposition of triple phosphates from an alkaline fermentation of the urine.[1]

Diet Recommended for Calculi.—The object is to render the urine as acid as possible in the hope that phosphatic calculi will be dissolved, and to this end Tibbles recommends tartaric and citric acids and fruits containing these and benzoic acid, such as is contained in lemons, limes, grapefruit, oranges, gooseberries, strawberries, currants, cherries, grapes, plums, green gages, etc.[2]

The dietetic treatment of stone, however, is more of a theoretical possibility than a clinical probability and the most that can be done after the removal of the calculi from the bladder is to combat the vesical catarrh and make the attempt to keep the urine acid by the means suggested but without very definite hope of success.

OXALURIA.

Calcium oxalate is the form in which oxalic acid appears in the urine, the oxalic acid coming from the decomposition of oxaluric acid, combines with calcium to form the oxalate of lime crystals. When there is gastric indigestion, particularly of the subacid type with the overproduction of mucus, oxalates are apt to be found. Also, the ingestion of certain vegetables, such as rhubarb, tomatoes, sorrel, cabbage, celery, grapes, currants, strawberries, gooseberries, plums, raspberries, cranberries, apples, pears, figs, pepper, cocoa, tea, coffee, if in large amounts, will result in oxaluria. Again, when too much wine or champagne, moselle, beer or ale are taken, the same result is often seen. Consumption of citrous fruits is also a source of oxaluria, and if much more food is eaten than is required by the organism.

The real significance of the oxalates is in their relation to "stone" either in the kidney or bladder, which is apt to occur when there is an overproduction of mucus in the bladder in the presence of calcium oxalate crystals.

Diet in Oxaluria.—When uch moxalate of lime is found in the urine it is necessary to put the patient on a thorough, sensible hygienic regimen, ordering only the simplest food, free of the substances known to contain an excess of oxalates, as already detailed; to avoid overfeeding and overdrinking

[1] Osler's Mod. Med.   [2] Tibbles: Food in Health and Disease, p. 404.

and in fact doing anything to disturb digestion, which should be the chief care. A vegetarian diet if in muse ust be changed to a mixed diet and the protein ration kept at a medium high amount, *i. e.*, about 100 to 120 gm. (3⅓ or 4 oz.). Where the patient is also gouty, the purine bodies should be kept at the lowest possible level and the total protein is better for being mininimal amount. In fact it is necessary to keep in mind all concomitant digestive or metabolic disturbances and construct as nearly a perfect diet as possible. According to Klemperer it is wise to keep foods rich in calcium at a low level—among these milk holds chief place, but according to Johnston-Lavis[1] there is sufficient lime even in a restricted calcium diet to furnish calcium for the oxalic acid in necessary amount for combination, so that it is not imperative that we should be so careful of the calcium intake, as an excess above the small amount required to form calcium oxalate does no particular harm.

Mineral Springs.—The Spa treatment for oxaluria at one of the European resorts offers certain advantages, as here the patients are on a guarded dietary, live according to rule, exercise regularly and drink the waters probably with much the same effect as they would if they lived the same hygienic life and drank rain water. Vittel water enjoys the highest reputation for this particular metabolic disturbance; Contrexeville coming next. In America, Saratoga and Hot Springs, Va., draw a fair number of persons needing Spa treatment.

DIET IN OLD AGE.

Much has been written on the dietetics of old age and it seems a pity that so many people as they grow older do not take the trouble to consult their physicians about a diet, for it is certainly a rare occurrence to have an elderly patient come for advice in this, unless there are some symptoms pointing to disease for which the patient thinks he should have a diet. It is unquestionably true that more damage is done by these people by overeating than by any other form of excess, for illnesses which might run a favorable course are prone to terminate fatally in the habitually overfed individual of advanced years. Among the conditions especially unfavorably influenced by either obesity or excessive eating in the aged are chronic cardiovascular disease, chronic emphysema and bronchitis, chronic nephritis and hypertension, and he that would live to an advanced age must be free of all unnecessary handicaps.

[1] Brit. Med. Jour., 1911, p. 966.

The natural tendency of elderly people is gradually to curtail the quantity of their food and to simplify its quality, for a person reaching old age has gotten there, to some extent at least, by a life of more or less abstemious living, so that the rational sequence of events is, for such an one to live more and more simply. The exceptions to this while numerous, of course, only tend to emphasize the rule already stated. In nothing is this curtailment better seen than in the modern tendency to reduce the intake of animal protein, especially meat. This is no doubt the result of constant reiteration on the part of many physicians, the newspapers, magazine articles, etc., and while it has its good side, it is not at all certain that the entire withdrawal of meat is advantageous in an elderly person otherwise healthy. Many of the most famous nonagenarians and a few centenarians have taken meat daily during the entire time and we have seen that the consensus of opinion is that a vegetarian diet does not tend to good resistance to disease, but rather the opposite. Conari who lived to be a hundred and wrote a treatise on longevity, was a mixed feeder, taking a considerable proportion of his daily ration in meat of various sorts, eating about 12 ounces of food daily made up chiefly of bread, wine, broth, eggs, veal, mutton, partridge, chicken, pigeon and fish. When disease of the kidneys and bloodvessels is prominent it is a different matter and meat must here be reduced below that allowable for the ordinarily healthy old person.

The reduction usually seen in the diet of old people is secondary, of course, to a general diminution in their digestive powers, both secretory and motor, for in many old people the free HCl and pepsin are either absent or much diminished and probably to some extent accounts for the lessened appetite for meat. The stomach and intestine tend to greater dilatation and lessened peristalsis, in many cases there is constipation and in some undue absorption of digestive by-products, so that they soon learn that too much food favors the accumulation of waste. Metchnikoff sums up the pathology of old age as a "sclerosis affecting all the organs but especially the bloodvessels."

Food Requirements of the Aged.—When we come to study the actual food requirements of the aged we find practical unanimity in the lessened amount of food needed to furnish energy for these people, the actual amount in a given case depending on the person's activities.

Murel[1] emstiates the maintenance diet of old people as follows:

[1] Rev. Soc. Science Hyg. Aliment, 1906, p. 763.

Age.	Protein per kilo.	Energy per kilo.
Adult	1.50 gm.	35 to 38 calories
50 to 70 years	1.25 "	30 to 35 "
70 years and over	1.00 "	25 to 30 "
Extreme old age	0.75 "	20 to 25 "

These estimations are for people at rest, not at work. When one studies the relative values of food requirements for persons of different age and occupation, as compared with that required by a man in full vigor at moderate work, the same diminution is seen in the requirements for old age.[1]

Man, period of full vigor at moderate work	= 100 gm. protein	
" " " hard work	= 120 "	
" " " sedentary occupation . .	= 80 "	
Woman, period of full vigor at moderate work . . .	= 80 "	
" " " sedentary occupation .	= 70 "	
Man or woman at hard work	= 100 "	
" old age	= 90 "	
" extreme old age . . . . . . = 70 to 80 "		
Boy, fifteen or sixteen years old	= 90 "	
" thirteen or fourteen years old	= 80 "	
" twelve years old	= 70 "	
" ten to twelve years old	= 60 "	
Girl, fifteen or sixteen years old	= 80 "	
" thirteen or fourteen years old	= 70 "	
" ten to twelve years old	= 60 "	
Child, six to nine years old	= 50 "	
" two to five years old	= 40 "	
" under two years old	= 30 "	

So, too, when one investigates the actual dietaries used by old people, they will be seen to conform very largely to these figures. Thus, for example, Forster found that among a number of elderly people the following figures applied:[2]

	Protein.	Fat.	Carohbydrates.	Calories.
Men	92	45	332	2149
Women	80	49	260	1875

There is no doubt but that metabolism proceeds at a much slower pace in old age than earlier, and the food requirements are less, both in so far as nitrogenous food is concerned as well as in the total energy requirement, and in practice one constantly sees old people living on a diet which would be hopelessly inadequate in both, particularly for a younger person of the same weight and height, nevertheless maintaining weight and vigor in a normal degree.

Just what part the internal glandular secretions have to do with this is not clear but presumably the lessened thyroid secretion in old age accounts to some extent for the lessening of metabolism.

[1] Langworthy: Year Book of Department of Agriculture (U. S. A.), 1907.
[2] Hutchinson: Food and Dietetics, p. 46.

Gurier[1] following the metabolism of five old people concluded :.

1. That the amount of protein consumed by old men may be diminished if considerable fat and carbohydrate is given to replace it.

2. The assimilation of nitrogen by old men is less than normal, in these instances varying between 86.17 and 91.15 per cent; that of young men on similar diet being 94 per cent. and it made little difference whether the nitrogen was furnished in meat and milk or beef tea and vegetables.

Sonden and Tigerstedt[2] found by metabolism experiments that, as measured by the respiration apparatus, old men and women excreted a less amount of CO_2 per square meter of surface area than young or middle-aged people. There was practically no difference in the CO_2 excretion of the two sexes, which is contrary to that which is found in those of younger years, where in men the CO_2 excretion is greater than in women of the same surface area.

Since the lessened food requirements are thoroughly demonstrated the only question that arises is where the greatest reduction should be made.

The fact that the natural tendency for old people is to eat less of meat, the frequent absence or diminution of HCl and pepsin in the gastric secretion already alluded to, makes it quite evident that the curtailment should be largely in this direction. Some authorities going so far as to say that no large meat eaters live to a great age. The low physiological requirements of nitrogen as determined by Chittenden[3] are certainly applicable here and should be adhered to or at least not greatly exceeded (roughly 45 to 65 gm. protein per day), as giving the kidneys less excretory work, while the larger bulk of the diet can be made up of carbohydrates and fats.

Foods Especially Desirable for the Aged.—Sir Henry Thompson wrote that "indigestion was not a disease but an admonition," so that when one suffers from indigestion it proves that one has not yet found one's ideal diet and at no age is this more true than in old age, where great care is necessary to avoid the disastrous results of gross dietary indiscretions, which with a weakened heart or bloodvessels might very well be serious.

According to the same eminent authority, half the chronic diseases seen in advancing years are due to dietetic errors, a large portion of which might by care be easily avoided.

[1] Tibbles: Food in Health and Disease, p. 175.
[2] Skand: Arch. Physiol., 1895, p. 1.
[3] Physiol. Economy in Nutrition.

Animal Food for the Aged.[1]

Tender chicken, game or meats.

Potted chicken and sweetbreads.

White-meated fish, flounders, sole, smelts, halibut, cod.

Bacon, grilled; eggs, lightly cooked or beaten up with milk.

Nutritious soups, chicken purée, fish purée, beef tea, mutton, or chicken broth.

Milk in all forms when well digested.

Milk and Vichy.

Vegetable Foods for the Aged:

Smooth bread and milk.

Cereals.

Puddings of ground rice, tapioca, arrowroot, sago, macaroni with milk and eggs served with a little jelly. Stale bread and butter, rusks.

Artificial foods, predigested starches.

Farinaceous foods should be subjected to high temperature for a long period to break the starch granules.

Vegetable purées of all kinds.

Stewed or baked fruits, fruit jellies, pulp of ripe fruits.

If fruits are too acid, neutralize with a little soda, as less sugar will be demanded with consequently less fermentation and acidity.

Lactose is better than cane-sugar for sweetening.

Butter, cream and oil are allowed for fats.

Bread, whether white or brown, should be toasted quite brittle, the amount for a meal, 3 to 5 ounces when fresh, then toasted. Fresh butter, 3 or 4 ounces.

Weak tea is best for breakfast with considerable milk, sugar if it agrees, taken five minutes after the meal, not with it, and he is very insistant that no liquid should be taken with meals, but directly afterward and between.

He recommends two hours of quiet sedentary occupation after breakfast, then an hour or more of exercise with a little rest. Rest twenty to thirty minutes before luncheon, recumbent. One and a half hours' rest after luncheon, then a drive, visit, whist, billiards or light exercise.

A cup of tea at five, without food. A light evening meal at 7 P.M. without meat or rich foods of any kind.

This list agrees well with the general consensus of opinion and it will be seen from it that meat is by no means forbidden. It should preferably be used but once a day, best at the midday meal, but unless there is some contra-indication as gout or hypertensive nephritis, it need not be excluded.

[1] Yeo: Food in Health and Disease, p. 287.

It must be borne in mind that elderly people cannot be starved to any greater advantage than other people and on the other hand at no time in life should greater care be taken to prevent overfeeding. For the most part the appetite must be trusted, as few old people will voluntarily agree to diet according to a specific weighed quantity of food, but where this is seen to be excessive and particularly in the direction of protein food a definite menu should be written out giving particular amounts of each article to be taken at a meal.

Preparation of Food for the Aged.—Since with advancing years the teeth are apt to be gradually eliminated, the proper preparation of food becomes of increasing importance, certain authorities point to this loss of teeth as a physiological process and say that it is a mistake to replace them by artificial teeth, as their wearers are apt to overeat and that their loss is Nature's way of curtailing the intake or at least of necessitating its soft consistency.

On the other hand, it is a fact that most teeth in advancing years are lost through infection and decay which would not occur if we lived on a rational dietary requiring much more chewing and that in the aged among savages the teeth may be worn down to stumps, but are seldom missing. Nevertheless, we are confronted by the undoubted fact that in the majority of cases the teeth of old people are either wanting or are at least in poor condition for fulfilling their normal function, so that we have the alternative of either supplying artificial teeth or giving food that does not need any chewing. There can be little doubt but that making good the deficiency by artificial teeth is the correct procedure with due care in the preparation of food, and improvement in digestion is often dated from the time that people secure adequate means of chewing their food.

Food should be prepared without too much of a rough element in the form of connective tissue and cellulose, so that meats should be tender and well cut up before eating and vegetables thoroughly cooked or divided.

The starch foods should be thoroughly cooked in order to break the cellulose envelope of the starch grain. This also applies to vegetables, although with good teeth there is no objection to soft raw fruits, and salads, if not rich. It is also necessary to guard against taking large quantities of animal fat with a high melting-point, such as mutton fat, which often causes digestive disturbance by its overslow disintegration. With these few precautions it is not necessary to soften the food for elderly people except in extreme old age; however, where the muscular power to chew satisfactorily is lacking the food should all be thoroughly softened and the individual urged to slow insalivation.

Diet Routine in Old Age.—Sir Henry Thompson[1] in his classical monograph recommends four meals a day for the aged. Breakfast at 8.30 A.M., luncheon 1.15 P.M., dinner at 7 to 7.30 P.M., and a light supper at 11.00 P.M. in the following manner.

"The animal foods supplied for breakfast and at lunch may include eggs or fish cooked in various ways. At luncheon a little tender meat or fowl may be taken, unless it is preferred to reserve them for dinner, in which case fish and farinaceous pudding may be substituted. This last-named meal should generally commence with a little good consommé; often substituting a vegetable purée, varying with the season and made with light meat stock or broth; or a good fish soup as a change. Then a little fowl or game and a dish of vegetables, according to the time of year. Finally, perhaps, some light farinaceous pudding with or without fruit, should close the meal, which is to be a light one in regard to quantity.

"Lastly, supper; a very light refreshment may be advantageously taken the very last thing before entering bed, at about eleven o'clock or so, as it favors sleep. Elderly men require some easily digested food to support them during the long fast of night. It is well-known that the forces of the body are at their minimum at 4 or 5 A.M. and this may be well provided for by taking about 5 or 6 ounces of consomme with one ounce of thin toasted bread, served in the bedroom."

The question of the use of alcoholic beverages often comes up for consideration in connection with the diet of the aged and needs a word of explanation. Probably no good is done by their use that might not be better done by other means, e. g., food, hot milk, hot tea, etc., so that it is never necessary to recommend alcohol for the aged, although when chilled on coming into the house and when it is not possible for one to go to bed with hot-water bottles, etc., a drink of diluted spirits taken hot induces capillary dilatation, diaphoresis and often relieves an internal congestion better than by other means. Aside from this, the aged are better without alcohol. If, on the other hand, they insist upon it, the best form is a claret or white wine diluted with alkaline water or a very little whiskey or brandy taken in the same way.

It is not necessary or worth while to set down sample dietaries for old people, as no two people would probably want

[1] Diet in Relation to Age Activity.

the same assortment of foods, old age being famous for insisting on individual likings, but with the foregoing explanation and suggestions in mind anyone can construct a diet suitable for an elderly person. Fletcher's Dietary Routine is certainly valuable for many elderly persons. (see p. 649).

OSTEOMALACIA.

Since in this disease the bones undergo softening due to a disturbed calcium and phosphorus metabolism it would seem as if feeding foods rich in these substances or even giving them in medicinal does would be a rational procedure. As a matter of fact while this may be tried and is usually done, the fault lies in an excessive excretion of these substances rather than to the fact that the diet does not contain sufficient for metabolic needs, so that it is much like trying to fill with water a barrel that has several holes in the bottom. At the same time since the output of these elements is excessive unless we add a certain surplus in the diet, the system becomes more or less completely drained of calcium and phosphorus; in other words, we can keep the barrel partly full of water by pouring in at the top in spite of a leaky bottom.

To this end we can give the calcium-containing foods, such as milk, oatmeal, green vegetables and fruits, while to help in replacing the phosphorus loss, fish and cod-liver oil are very good.

Adrenalin by injections or fed by mouth seems to do good in certain cases, probably by means of its effect on metabolism. If all other means fail and as a procedure of last resort castration may be done, which results in a retention of calcium and phosphorus in the system from a changed body metabolism.

34

CHAPTER XXVII.

DIET IN THE BLOOD DISEASES.

THE ANEMIAS.

THE relation of diet to diseases of the hemapoietic system must, of course, in the very nature of things, be an intimate one. Nevertheless, although this is so, comparatively little is known about the etiology of the diseases characterized by marked blood changes nor how diet might modify them, except to a minor degree. That malnutrition, from whatever cause, is accompanied by a greater or less degree of anemia is common knowledge and these changes may be qualitative as well as quantitative.

Toxemia is a convenient phrase to cover our ignorance and while doing so, it is more than likely at the bottom of much of the so-called primary anemia, and secondary as well; in fact all anemias must be secondary, but when the probable cause is too elusive, it is easier perhaps in the present state of our lack of knowledge to distinguish between primary of unknown origin and secondary of known origin, or better, whose chief accompanying condition of disease is recognized. Of the simple primary anemias, chlorosis is the chief example; those primary cases which are severe and often fatal with still greater differences between their blood picture and that of normal blood are called pernicious anemia. In both forms of primary anemia there are marked changes in blood production as well as destruction. In the secondary anemia, while we are able to tell the accompanying condition which is doubtless responsible for the anemia, we do not know how it acts to bring about blood destruction, for in secondary anemia there is apparently little interference or change in the blood-forming functions, but the agencies that destroy the blood are all important and keep the patients anemic until conditions are changed or causes removed. Chlorosis or "green sickness" occurs for the most part in young girls, often without apparent cause, but is very apt to show itself at puberty or when a complete change is made in residence or work, as in the case of young immigrants. Of the dietary cases we find that many chlorotics eat a very small amount of protein and fat and too much carbohydrate, or the total amount of food is too small. In other cases the diet contains too large a proportion of foods that are actually injurious, such as vinegar, coffee, tea, highly spiced or seasoned food.[1]

The habit of taking large amounts of tea, while not a proven etiological factor, is so frequently an associated condition that the suspicion seems justified that there is definite connection between the two. In these cases there is very apt to be found more or less tissue hydremia, as shown by subcutaneous edema, and when present in marked degree, even in the absence of any direct renal complication, special salt-poor dietetic rules apply. There is little difficulty in making the diagnosis of chlorosis in a typical case or even when complicated by edema, but when as often happens, there are marked gastric symptoms, one is often at a loss to know whether the case is one of simple anemia or of peptic ulcer with a complicating anemia, for ulcer symptoms may be more or less exactly simulated. The author has in mind one case which was treated for ulcer by two dietary cures without relief to the pain, which promptly disappeared, followed by complete recovery when iron was given. Just what the association is between the anemia and symptoms of ulcer it is not possible to say, but it is quite usual to find a hyperchlorhydria in chlorotics which by causing pylorospasm may give rise to the pain. Whatever the cause the facts are important enough to be kept in mind.

Treatment of Chlorosis.—In considering the treatment of chlorosis one must take into consideration the following recommendations, all of which are important.

1. Rest, and rest in bed for severe cases.
2. Treatment for gastro-enteric associated conditions, notably constipation.
3. The giving of iron in some form.
4. Diet.

While this volume has little to do with general treatment of disease there are certain conditions in which diet plays in some respects a minor role, except it be a part of a general plan of attack, and chlorosis belongs to this class.

Rest.—There are many cases of obstinate chlorosis and secondary anemia, which in spite of every other means do not progress satisfactorily unless complete rest is added to the regimen. This means rest in bed and in the fresh air and sunshine as much as possible. This procedure alone is capable of changing the result to a successful issue.

The treatment of gastro-intestinal conditions is exceedingly important and in certain cases accompanied by marked constipation, the relief of this complication by appropriate

[1] Sutherland: System of Diet. p. 627.

diet see section on Constipation, p. 397) often results in a disappearance of the anemia. Where there are symptoms of so-called toxic absorption, such as headache, asthenia with or without marked urinary evidences of intestinal putrefaction (*e. g.*, increased ethereal sulphates and indicanuria), high colon irrigations plus a laxative diet are exceedingly valuable measures and may alone solve the problem.

Iron.—In practically every case of simple or secondary anemia the giving of iron in some form is to be considered and leads naturally to the question of iron metabolism. Much time and investigation has been expended on this question and even yet there is no unanimity of opinion as to just how it acts in restoring the blood elements to their normal condition. From the theoretical stand-point a full mixed diet contains sufficient iron, in organic combination, to satisfy the demands of the system, but whatever the perversion of metabolism, the time comes when the destruction of blood proceeds more rapidly than its regeneration and the organism is no longer able to make use of the natural food iron in sufficient quantity or sufficiently rapidly to preserve the normal balance, and anemia results.

Theories of the Action of Iron.—There are at least three chief theories of the action of iron:

1. That the system can make direct use of inorganic iron as such but in exceedingly small quantities, which is either directly absorbed or acts as a stimulant to the hemapoietic organs.

2. That the body can only make use of organic iron in one or the other of these ways.

3. That either organic or inorganic iron furnishes an element to the intestinal contents which prevents the destruction of the normal food iron albuminate and releases it, so to speak, for its proper use in blood building.

Austin[1] says "from the work of Abderhalden, Müller and Tartakousky it seems probable that iron in the organic form as an albuminate of iron may be absorbed and utilized for hemoglobin formation, but that in this form it is no more effective, but probably less effective than is the iron which is a natural constituent of such foods as lima beans, peas, spinach, red meat, yolk of eggs, etc." He also doubts that inorganic iron stimulates the blood-forming organs, although a true stimulation of these organs may in certain instances be possible.

The iron in the blood is found as hemoglobin and the total amount of iron in the blood of an adult is 3 gm.[2]

[1] Therap. Gaz., 1914, 3 S., xxx, 846.
[2] Tibbles: Diet in Health and Diseases, p. 81.

There is also much iron in the liver and spleen which exists in the liver as compounds of iron with nuclein and protein. After the exhibition of inorganic iron all but a very small part appears in the feces.

For the percentages of iron in different foods see p. 96.

Diet in Chlorosis.—In choosing foods especially good for chlorosis one should, theoretically at least, take those forms which are highest in natural iron compounds, although of course it is not practicable to confine the diet exclusively to these articles. All foods should be fresh, not cooked over, salted, tinned or dried.

When there are gastro-intestinal symptoms it is best to put these patients on a fluid or semifluid diet until the symptoms subside and then to increase to a light diet and finally to a full diet somewhat as follows, as outlined by Sutherland[1] choosing largely from the iron-rich foods.

Diets in Anemia (Chlorosis):

4.00 A.M.	Milk, 300 c.c. (10 oz.). (Hot or cold.)
8.00 A.M.	Bread and milk, 450 c.c. (15 oz.).
11.00 A.M.	Egg flip, 300 c.c. (10 oz.).
1.00 P.M.	Milk pudding with milk, 450 c.c. (15 oz.); (corn flour, ground rice, seminola, sago, tapioca, arrowroot custard).
3.00 P.M.	Benger's food, 300 c.c. (10 oz.) or malted milk.
5.30 P.M.	Milk pudding or bread and milk, 300 c.c. (10 oz.).
8.00 P.M.	Milk, 300 c.c. (10 oz.).

Light Diet.

4.00 A.M.	Milk, 300 c.c. (10 oz.).
8.00 A.M.	Milk or weak tea with milk, 300 c.c. (10 oz.); bread and butter, 60 gm. (2 oz.); white fish, boiled, with white sauce, 120 gm. (4 oz.) or an egg.
11.00 A.M.	Milk, Benger's food or malted milk, 300 c.c. (10 oz.).
1.00 P.M.	Chicken or white soup, 300 c.c. (10 oz.); bread, 30 gm. (1 oz.); potatoes, 60 gm. (2 oz.); vegetables, 30 gm. (1 oz.); milk pudding, 300 c.c. (10 oz.).
5.30 P.M.	Milk or weak tea with milk, 300 c.c. (10 oz.); bread and butter, 60 gm. (2 oz.); an egg or white fish, 120 gm. (4 oz.).
8.00 P.M.	Milk, 300 c.c. (10 oz.); cream, 300 c.c. (10 oz. daily.

[1] System of Diet and Dietetics, p. 617.

Full Diet.

4.00 A.M.	Milk, 300 c.c. (10 oz.).
8.00 A.M.	Milk or weak tea with milk, 300 c.c. (10 oz.); bread and butter, 120 gm. (4 oz.); white fish, 120 gm. (4 oz.), or an egg.
11.00 A.M.	Milk, Benger's food or malted milk, 300 c.c. (10 oz.).
1.00 P.M.	Soup, 300 c.c. (10 oz.); meat, boiled or roasted 180 gm. (6 oz.); bread, 60 gm. (2 oz.); potato, 60 gm. (2 oz.); milk pudding, 300 c.c. (10 oz.).
5.00 F.M.	Milk or weak tea with milk, 300 c.c. (10 oz.); bread and butter, 120 gm. (4 oz.); an egg or white fish, 120 gm. (4 oz.).
8.00 I.M.	Milk, 300 c.c.; (10 oz.) cream, 300 c.c. (10 oz.) per day.

There seems to be a general consensus of opinion that blood pigment is increased by a diet with a large amount of protein; scraped beef sandwiches, meat broths thickened with scraped meat, giving as high as 150 to 180 gm. (5 or 6 ounces) of albumin in a day. Seé gives 14 ounces of raw meat daily. Green vegetables also being rich in iron are to be used in large amount and many think that claret, Burgundy, Madeira, porter and stout[1] help to increase the formation of hemoglobin. Whether this is so or not is not possible to say, but often such addition to the diet increases the appetite and aids digestion if taken in very moderate amounts.

Von Noorden advises protein-rich food because the readily available carbohydrates go to the liver first and recommends five meals per day as follows:

Breakfast: Two or 3 ounces (60 to 90 gm.) meat; one or two slices toast or unsweetened rusks; small cup of tea with very little cream or sugar.

Mid-A.M.; Two eggs, toast, butter, glass of milk and a little sherry.

Luncheon: Preceded by one-half hour rest, then a full meal, without soup, if the appetite is poor. No fluid with this meal. Rest afterward.

Mid-P.M.: Cooked or raw fruit with zweiback or bread. If there is already too much acidity he gives tea, cocoa, toast followed by a glass of milk and cream.

Supper: Any simple food.

Bedtime: Beer or milk.

[1] Thompson: Practical Dietetics, p. 537.

When there is edema present it is necessary at times to limit the fluid and salt intake to the point of a salt-poor diet, such as is used in nephritis. The anemia in these cases is due to a certain extent at least to too much blood plasma and chloride retention.

Secondary Anemia.—The treatment of secondary anemia consists in doing all one possibly can to remove the underlying cause or mitigating it as much as possible if it is not possible to remove it, *e. g.*, in the case of a chronic nephritis. The other essentials of treatment are the same as those already outlined for chlorosis.

Pernicious Anemia.—Since the causes of pernicious anemia are not definitely known it would seem out of place in a work on Dietetics to spend too much time on the discussion of the various theories advanced. The blood picture which is found in cases of bothriocephalus latus is so precisely that of pernicious anemia that the finding of a hemolytic element in the parasite seemed to establish this form of anemia as due to hemolysis, and by analogy it was sought to trace cases other than of bothriocephalic origin to intestinal hemolysins. In pursuance of this theory Hopkins[1] extracted the stools in various diseases and tested for hemolysins with the following conclusions:

1. The extract from stools of primary anemia did not show the presence of hemolysins with any degree of consistency.

2. The extract from stools of renal and gastro-intestinal cases did show hemolysins in approximately 50 per cent. of the cases.

3. Normal stools gave negative results.

These conclusions do not bolster up the hemolysis theory to any satisfactory degree, at least as far as pernicious anemia goes. Finding the associated achylia gastrica as such a frequent accompaniment of pernicious anemia at first led to the conclusion that the gastric atrophy stood in a causal relation. But as the achylia and atrophy are frequently found without pernicious anemia this had to be given up. Friedenwald[2] after analyzing a series of cases concluded that "it is quite probable that the poison which produces the hemolysis is the same which is also responsible for the alteration in the gastric secretion."

Again the spleen was thought to be concerned with the production of the disease or on account of its being the "graveyard" of the red cell the removal of the spleen was

[1] Proc. Path. Soc., Philadelphia, 1913, xv, 46.
[2] Alumni Assn. Coll. Phys. and Surg., Baltimore, 1912, 3, xv, 97.

practised. Some cases seemed to improve but eventually
the disease progressed. Whatever the actual causes of
pernicious anemia are, there is no doubt but that blood
destruction by some means is excessive and fatal and the
stimulation of the blood-forming organs is also great, as
shown by the putting into the circulation great numbers of
immature blood cells apparently in an attempt to compensate, as Nature so often does.

In the absence of positive knowledge as to the etiology of
pernicious anemia any attempt to prescribe a diet based on
physiological needs is out of the question and all that one can
do is to take cognizance of associated conditions of the alimentary canal from the teeth and gums, clear through to
the rectum and eliminate every possible pathological condition that is found, such as removal of bad teeth, treatment of
pyorrhea, the use of artificial gastric juice (dilute hydrochloric acid and pepsin), regular intestinal emptying with
cathartics and high colon irrigation and in addition the use
of duodenal lavage by allowing one or two quarts of saline to
flow into the duodenum through a duodenal tube on a fasting stomach. This latter procedure seems to do good, but
not unquestionably so.

The actual diet best for pernicious anemia is more or less
problematical and no case has been cured by it. At the same
time it is of distinct value in keeping the patient's condition
up to the highest point of efficiency for the particular individual. The food should all be nourishing and patients forbidden to fill up on non-essentials; the iron-containing foods
as in chlorosis are good but in view of the usually deficient or
absent gastric secretion meat once a day is all that is indicated, finely cut and without connective tissue. Thompson
recommends fresh fruit, green vegetables, oranges, lemons,
grapefruit, apples, beans, lettuce, celery, potatoes and meat
once daily, all with a large amount of water between meals.
Carbohydrates are rather better borne than proteins and
should form the bulk of the meal. On the other hand Barker[1] recommends a meat diet at first, followed by a diet rich
in protein urging the patients to eat regardless of appetite
or the effect on digestion. He also recommends dilute
hydrochloric acid shortly after meals, and pancreatin and
calcium carbonate each 45 gr. (3 gm.) three hours later.

Many authorities recommend very highly the feeding of
bone marrow from the long bones of ox or sheep given in
doses of half an ounce to an ounce and a half, spread on bread
well-seasoned with pepper, Worcestershire or tomato sauce

[1] Johns Hopkins Bull., 1918, xxviii, 355.

or added to bouillon. When not possible to obtain the marrow fresh, one of the preserved preparations may be used. Whether the use of marrow is actually favorable it is not possible to say but it at least cannot do harm and is worth a trial.

Posthemorrhagic Anemia.—This is most often a sequence of some acute surgical condition which demands interference. When established in an acute form the indications are, of course, to make up the deficiency of the liquid portion of the blood by means of saline enemata, hypodermoclysis, intravenous saline infusion or blood transfusion. These procedures are all best when the likelihood of further hemorrhage has been prevented by appropriate medical or surgical treatment. During convalescence the diets as suggested for chlorosis are recommended, giving a large amount of protein in the form of meat and eggs, milk and beef juice, together with green vegetables and fresh fruits.

LEUKEMIA.

From a dietetic point of view this disease is of scant importance so far as the particular foods go that might be of benefit in combating the condition, because we know nothing of its etiology. Presumably a mixed diet with considerable protein and moderate amount of carbohydrate with green food is best, but the time comes in many of these cases when the mouth and gums are in such a pitiable condition, bleeding, ulcerated and painful that the taking of any kind of food becomes a hardship and even drinking water is almost impossible. Under such circumstances one may feed by gavage concentrated liquid foods. (see Suralimentation, p. 550). These may be given by putting the tube to a point below the larynx or by merely slipping a catheter into the back of the mouth and letting the food pass in slowly through a funnel, provided the act of deglutition is not in itself painful. When even this is too painful the tube may be passed to the stomach or nearly so, or a small catheter passed through the nose, to a point below the larynx and liquid food poured in.

HEMOPHILIA.

For a long time it was thought that a deficiency of calcium in the blood was at the bottom of the etiology of hemophilia, but the conclusion has been reached that in this disease the lack of calcium has nothing to do with its causation and the addition of calcium to the blood does not hasten clotting.[1]

[1] Addis: Jour. Path. Bact., 1911, xv, 427.

Hess concludes that typical hereditary hemophilia is not associated with a deficiency of calcium.[1]   One typical hemophyliac did show a definite calcium deficiency from a functional point of view and quantitative estimations of calcium in the blood showed a deficiency below the normal.

Since some apparent benefit has followed the giving of calcium lactate to cases of hemophilia it would seem indicated to include in the dietary as much calcium-containing food as possible, such as milk, zoolak, buttermilk, cheese; in fact, milk in any form; oatmeal, bread and fresh herbaceous vegetables.   Aside from this possible indication the diet for the hemophiliac should be in accordance with any concomitant symptom, such as anemia, gastro-intestinal disturbances, nephritis, etc.

PURPURA HEMORRHAGICA.

This condition is really only a symptom and is characterized by subcutaneous or submucous hemorrhages without known cause, although it occurs as an associated condition with such diseases as severe and terminal nephritis, arthritis, sepsis and profound anemia and is here presumably of toxic origin.

The dietetic necessities of this disease, if there are such. are entirely unknown and one can do little more than regulate the diet in accordance with diseases with which purpura is associated.

[1] Johns Hopkins Hosp. Bull., 1915, xxvi, 372.

CHAPTER XXVIII.

DEFICIENCY DISEASES.

DEFICIENCY diseases are those pathological states of the body due to a lack of certain accessory substances in the food called vitamines. Vitamines are of recent discovery and are still few in number so far as is yet known. So far as actually demonstrated this class includes scurvy, beriberi and xeropthalmia certainly, probably rickets and osteomalacia and possibly pellagra and sprue. Where the regular food supply contains these vitamines, no disturbances of this nature arise but if foods lacking in vitamines are fed, the subject rapidly develops one or another form of disease, depending on the vitamine that is lacking. Whether the vitamines are interchangeable is not yet known, e. g., whether a certain deficiency disease can be cured by the vitamines concerned with another disease entity. They probably are not interchangeable. There is still comparatively little known of the entire subject.[1]

SCURVY.

Scurvy is distinctly and exclusively a dietetic disease and is probably due very largely to the lack of vitamines in the food, but there is also undoubtedly an element of individual predisposition, for with a number of individuals under exactly the same conditions of diet in which the fresh food principles are lacking, only a certain number will contract scurvy. This is particularly well seen in children under a year old. Before antiscorbutic substances were known it was a very common thing to find scurvy wherever persons lived on a monotonous diet lacking in freshness, e. g., on long cruises, jails, almshouses, etc., but since the prevention of the disease has become so generally known the cases arise only sporadically in people who are on such a diet. The pasteurization or sterilization of milk has long been thought to account for many cases and there is no question but that they predispose to scurvy. Hess was able to produce scurvy in infants almost at will by putting them on a diet of pasteurized milk and to cure them promptly by antiscorbutics added to the diet. On the other hand, the New York Board of Health have about 55,000 babies to whom they yearly supply

[1] For a fuller discussion of these deficiency diseases see p. 102, Part I.

pasteurized milk through the milk stations, and of this number only 5 developed any signs of scurvy in 1915 (Sobel). This is largely due to the fact, no doubt that few of the mothers limit the babies' diet to milk, but after six months are apt to give vegetables, beef juice, soup, etc., all good antiscorbutics. Even breast-fed children develop scurvy at times.

In metabolism experiments on a case of scurvy, Bauman[1] found the total sulphur metabolism normal. Chlorine and sodium were retained during the period when fruit juice was added to the scorbutic diet, but excreted in excess of the intake during the preliminary period. More potassium, calcium and magnesium were retained during the fruit-juice period.

Diet in Scurvy.—The prophylaxis of scurvy consists of breast feeding when possible, and when this is impossible, in feeding raw milk and in the early addition of fruit juice (usually sweet orange juice) to the infant's diet. If the milk supply is such that it must be heated to make it safe, pasteurization is preferable to boiling, as pasteurization probably injures the antiscorbutic properties of milk less than boiling. Infants fed on the various proprietary infant foods, especially those that are made up without milk, are liable to develop scurvy. If one of these foods has to be used for any length of time orange juice should be added to the diet as soon as possible. Potato juice, made by mashing raw potato into a pulp with cold water and straining through cheesecloth, may be used to dilute the milk, and acts as does orange juice.

When scurvy is present the infant's diet should be changed so as to furnish those articles of food which we know will effect a cure. All heating of the milk should be stopped and a good raw milk used in making up the food. If the milk is diluted with a cereal water, the latter should be cooled before mixing with the milk. Some fruit juice should be begun at once. Sweet orange juice is the best and it may be diluted with water and sweetened if necessary. Better results will be obtained if as much as two ounces is given each day. A good method is to give one ounce an hour before the forenoon feeding and the other before the late afternoon feeding. It should not be withheld because of loose undigested stools. Other fruit and vegetable juices have antiscorbutic properties, but they have no advantages. Mashed potato (one tablespoonful each day) may be added to the diet of older infants, and the use of potato water instead of

[1] Tr. Assn. Am. Phys., 1912, xxvii, 514.

cereal water as a diluent has been suggested by Hess and Fish.[1] In general the antiscorbutics are most abundant in citrous fruits and cabbage leaves, less in tubers. There is enough vitamine in one pound of potato, less of cabbage, or one orange to protect from scurvy.[2]

The effect of heat on the antiscorbutic properties of various foods is different. Lemon, orange and raspberry juices are little if any affected by a temperature of 100° C. for considerable periods of time. Vegetable juices are more easily affected by heat. The experimental evidence regarding the effect of heat on the antiscorbutic properties of milk is conflicting, but clinical evidence seems to show that heat does damage these properties and furthermore that the damage varies directly with the degree and duration of the heating.

After six months one may readily add the orange juice, lemonade, soup made with carrots, potato, beef juice, broths and potato water.

In older children and adults who are so situated dietetically that they are apt to develop scurvy, prevention by taking any one of the antiscorbutic articles of diet is, of course, the only sensible procedure. When scurvy has actually developed, fresh vegetables, fruits, especially oranges, lemons, limes and apples (underdone) and raw meats will all effect a cure. Certain dried fruits and vegetables are also good antiscorbutics—*e. g.*, dried apples, dried tomatoes, strawberries, etc. Lime juice has an especially high reputation as an antiscorbutic and can easily be taken on trips where there is any danger of the development of scurvy. The main thing about a diet to prevent any danger from scurvy is that all the food shall be fresh, or if a part of it is necessarily dried, salted, or smoked, to always provide a certain amount of fresh food element.

BERIBERI.

The discovery of the cause of beriberi and its practical application to the diet of Eastern peoples has been one of the romances of medicine and deserves reading for its historical interest alone.

Beriberi, which is a toxic polyneuritis, has been abundantly proven to be a "deficiency" disease, due to a lack of some element in the food which, although known to exist, has never been actually demonstrated—the name vitamine given to this substance is not equally agreeable to all scientists, but is more or less in general use. In each deficiency disease

[1] Am. Jour. Dis. of Child., 1914, viii, 385.
[2] Brit. Med. Jour., 1918, i, 183.

the absence of the specific vitamine is responsible for the disease.

While beriberi occurs for the most part among people who make their diet largely of polished rice, it is not found exclusively among rice eaters, but may also develop on a diet of white bread, sago, or in fact any food naturally poor in vitamines, or made so by prolonged cooking, or cooking under pressure (Funk). It has also occurred among companies of men living on a mixed diet composed largely of tinned food, in which these vitamines were necessarily lacking.

Cases have occurred following relapsing fever and has followed prolonged feeding on condensed milk. Osler says it sometimes follows any prolonged wasting disease, such as chronic dysentery and tuberculosis.

A polyneuritis in birds[1] can be produced by a diet of polished rice; or a synthetic vitamine-free diet, such as casein, lard, sugar and salts, will cause beriberi as rapidly as a polished rice diet.

Caspari and Moszkouski consider beriberi purely a toxic disease, but their results can be turned to account in proving the vitamine theory. This avian polyneuritis is readily cured or prevented by giving rice polishings or a watery extract of rice polishings, for the preventive vitamine is found in the pericarp of the rice grain. If the rice is prepared in such a way as to leave this on, beriberi does not occur, provided a liberal general diet is also allowed. Other substances besides the rice pericarp were found to be capable of preventing beriberi and among these are ox cerebrum, cerebellum or liver, cow's milk, husked filberts and cheese—oddly enough human milk was less protective than cow's milk. Yeast vitamines have also proven most efficient in curing polyneuritis. "Beriberi occurs thus on a stagnant diet with a negative or insufficient supply of beriberi vitamines." (Funk.)

The dietary treatment is a simple matter from a prophylactic point of view and avoidance of a polished rice diet combined with a liberal supply of nitrogen and "fresh" foods is entirely capable of preventing its occurrence. This was well illustrated in the Japanese Navy, where formerly beriberi was very prevalent, and simply by giving unpolished rice and a larger proportion of nitrogenous foods, the disease has entirely disappeared from the service.

When once the disease is established it is a matter of great difficulty to influence its course, as anatomical changes occur and are not to be easily overcome. Hence, though we may

[1] Eijkman: Virchows Archiv., 1897, cxlviii, 523.

give foods high in beriberi vitamines, the progress toward health is slow and sometimes no result at all is accomplished toward a cure by dietary regulation. On the other hand, mild cases are not infrequently relieved and undergo spontaneous restitution.

The diet should contain a fairly high percentage of protein, 120 to 150 gm. (3 to 4½ oz.), largely made up of fresh milk, eggs and meat that is lightly cooked; green vegetables, fruits, farinaceous food of all sorts and rice polishings mixed with the cereals, one or two tablespoonfuls at least twice a day. On such a diet as this, even without the rice polishings, beriberi will not occur, and if once established such a diet combined with rest in bed and general hygiene will do all that is possible to favor a cure.

Xeropthalmia.—Xeropthalmia is the most recent condition definitely to be classed among the deficiency diseases and is a rare disease due apparently solely to the lack of fat soluble A in the diet. It is observed in adults principally who have been on a monotonous diet with practically no animal fat such as egg, milk or butter fat, and consists of a yellowish discoloration about the eyes which later becomes inflammatory and eventually destroys the sight unless checked by proper diet. The remedy is found simply in giving these forms of animal fat with a generally nourishing diet. Vegetable fats such as olive oil, cottonseed oil, etc., do not contain fat soluble A and therefore exert no curative influence.

PELLAGRA.

The etiology of pellagra has been a source of continued thought and experimentation for many years and first one and then another theory has been advanced in explanation. The spoiled maize theory, the bad hygiene and poor sewerage disposal theory, the infectious theory, the theory that it is an acidosis the result of a carbohydrate or alcohol diet with practically no protein[1] and finally the theory that traces its origin to a dietetic fault whereby pellagra is brought about by lack of vitamines in the diet are a few of the more recent contributions. Jobling[2] studied the alkaline reserve of the blood in pellagra but found it did not vary from normal in either the acute or chronic cases, therefore it is not an acidosis or alkalosis in this. In practically all forms of treatment that have given any degree of success, Goldberger finds that there was a simultaneous change in the diet of

[1] Yarbrough. Med. Rec., 1917, xcii, 892.
[2] Jour. Am. Med. Assn., 1917, lxix, 2026.

the patients toward a better balanced ration. From work which he has done among pellagrins a change in the diet from a one-sided, principally carbohydrate diet, to a better balanced selection of foods, seems to show that this one factor is capable of preventing pellagra, On the other hand, by taking people off a mixed diet and placing them on a one-sided, largely carbohydrate diet, he was able to produce the disease in over 50 per cent. of the squad of prisoners who were the subjects of the experiment. His conclusions are certainly more in line with the modern conception of the deficiency diseases, such as beriberi and scurvy, and deserve to be quoted and are as follows:[1]

Goldberger's Conclusions.—1. "Diet is the common factor in the various methods of treatment recently advocated. The marked success claimed for each of these methods must logically be attributed to the factor (diet) which they have in common.

"2. The value of diet in the prevention of pellagra has been tested at two orphanages and at an asylum for the insane, endemic foci of the disease, marked increases in the fresh animal and leguminous protein elements of the institution were made. Of the group of pellagrins on the modified diet at the insane asylum, 72 remained continuously under the observation up to October 1, 1915, or at least until after the anniversary date of their attack of 1914, not one of this group has presented recognizable evidence of a recurrence, although of a group of 32 controls 15 have had recurrences. Pellagra may therefore be prevented by an appropriate diet without any alteration in the environment, hygienic or sanitary, including the water supply.

"3. The reverse was demonstrated on voluntary convicts, who were promised their freedom, by feeding a one-sided diet, chiefly carbohydrate (wheat, corn and rice), a diet from which fresh animal proteins and legumes were excluded. Six out of 11 developed pellagra, none of the controls did.

"4. For practical purposes of preventive medicine it would seem to be of fundamental importance to recognize that the pellagra-producing dietary fault, whatever its intimate nature or however brought about, is capable of correction or prevention by including in the diet suitable proportions of fresh animal and leguminous protein food."

A house to house study of pellagrins and non-pellagrins showed the following factors:

1. A physiological defective protein supply.

2. A low inadequate supply of fat soluble and water soluble vitamines.

[1] Jour. Am. Med. Assn., February 12, 1916, p. 471.

3. A defective mineral supply in the diet.[1]

Goldberger concludes his observations by saying that "a definite conclusion as to the intimate mechanism involved in bringing about or preventing the disease by diet cannot be drawn from the available data." On the other hand the report of a commission on pellagra comes to this conclusion:

1. That it is the result of a distinct poison dependent indirectly at least on poor sanitation.

2. That while devitalizing influences such as poor food, over-work, disease, etc., may render individuals susceptible, they do not produce the disease singly or combined.[2]

The Thompson-McFadden Commission places the blame entirely on poor sanitation.

Although his conclusions have been strenuously combated it would seem as if so far they offer the best method at one's command for combating this strange disease, time and further experience being necessary to establish the apparent facts on a firm basis.

Funk's[3] belief is that "beyond doubt pellagra has a close connection with maize." According to his theory it is due to a lack of vitamines in maize as it is milled, whereby the pericarp is removed—comparable to beriberi in its relation to polished rice. It is certainly a fact that pellagra occurs principally in sections of the country where maize forms from 74 to 84 per cent. of the daily ration. Nevertheless many people who have eaten corn products so extensively do not contract the disease and pellagra develops at times in people who have never eaten corn. There was no marked dietary fault among 500 cases of pellagra which occurred in Illinois, an observation, which if correct, is the strongest proof presented against Goldberger's theory.

Diet in Pellagra.—Since at present it is not possible to state the absolute undisputed cause of pellagra it would seem the wisest plan in choosing a diet for these people to place the patients in the best possible hygienic surroundings, avoid maize in every form and furnish a general mixed diet with 100 to 125 gm. (3⅓ to 4¼ oz.) of protein, largely made up of animal and leguminous protein with a total caloric value of 30 to 35 calories per kilo. Fresh vegetables and fruits are also essential unless there is diarrhea, in which case no vegetables rich in cellulose should be used, but only purée vegetables, principally purée of beans and peas or lentils.

[1] Goldberger. New York Med. Jour., 1918, cvii, 1146.
[2] Jour. New Med. Assn., 1918, x, No. 4, 165.
[3] Practitioner, 1913, i, 940; and Biochem. Bull., 1916, v.

35

Milk is perhaps the most important single food in balancing a diet in preventing or curing pellagra according to Goldberger, and where a deficient supply of lean meat and green vegetables only is available one and one-half pints of milk (sweet or buttermilk) should be given two or three times a day. This in addition to the customary diet will practically in all instances protect from an attack of pellagra.[1] Tisdale[2] eliminates all carbohydrate from the diet giving a large amount of protein food. If there is nausea or vomiting only milk, meat broths and fresh fruit juice are given, salt solution by enema and hypodermoclysis is also good. In severe diarrhea an examination of gastric chemistry should be made, and if deficient, dilute hydrochloric acid and pepsin are given. In some cases there may be a deficiency of pancreatic enzymes and it is often a good plan to give these in enteric coated pills or capsules.

Goldberger recommends the following minimum diet as preventive of pellagra:

Breakfast: Sweet milk, daily, oatmeal boiled, with butter or milk, q. 2. d. Boiled hominy or mush with meat gravy or milk every other day. Light bread or biscuit(¼ soy bean meal) with butter, daily.

Dinner: Meat, fish, fowl, maccaroni and cheese once a week.

Dried beans or cow peas two or three times a week.

Potatoes (Irish or sweet) four or five times a week.

Rice two or three times a week with stew or beans.

Green vegetables (cabbage, Gallards turnips, greens, spinach, snap beans, okra, all especially good), three or four times a week.

Corn bread (¼ Soy meal) daily. Butter-milk.

Supper: Light bread or biscuit (¼ Soy meal) daily. Butter-milk, daily. Stewed fruit (apples, peaches, prunes, apricots), three or four times a week on days when no green vegetable is given for dinner. Peanut butter twice a week. Syrup once or twice a week.

[1] Pub. Health Rep., 1918, xxxiii, 487 (Washington).
[2] Jour. Florida Med. Assn., 1916, xiv, 137.

CHAPTER XXIX

DIET IN DISEASES OF THE NERVOUS SYSTEM.

THE dietetics of organic nervous diseases are with a very few exceptions exceedingly unsatisfactory, while in some of the so-called functional cases more may be expected.

The etiology of so many diseases of the nervous system is either obscure or so impossible of influence by diet (*e. g.*, lues), that it leaves but a small field in which to diet these cases successfully in the light of their causation. Among the organic conditions that may be helped or influenced by diet are neuritis, epilepsy, insanity and apoplexy. Among the functional cases are neuralgia, periodic headaches, migraine, neurasthenia, chorea and digestive neuroses.

ORGANIC NERVOUS DISEASES.

Neuritis.—In order to treat any form of neuritis successfully, it is absolutely necessary to make an etiological diagnosis. Is it due to a toxicosis of some sort as lead, alcohol, gout, arsenic, following infectious disease, or is it due to an infection or pressure? When the exciting cause is found and removed the battle is already more than half won. Little need be said regarding the role alcohol plays in the production of neuritis and that its use should be interdicted at once. Patients with alcoholic neuritis are usually undernourished and need special attention on this account or they are the subject of a chronic alcoholic gastritis and have to be dieted with this in view (see p. 347).

As the course of alcoholic neuritis is often of months' duration and usually much sleep is lost on account of the pain, ample opportunity is given for these people to get in a bad state of subnutrition.

In a gouty neuritis, diet also plays a distinct therapeutic role and should be treated as any case of gout, giving a purine-free diet at first and later one with a low purine content (see Gout, p. 504).

Where the neuritis is of obscure origin but the patient is either in a condition of over- or undernutrition too much importance cannot be placed on the necessity for regulation of the diet to meet either of these conditions, as without this, other therapeutic measures will doubtless fail. In these cases as well, constant attention to the intestinal functions is necessary and elimination promoted there by rectal salines or colon irrigations or both, as undoubtedly a certain number of cases of obscure neuritis have their origin in a faulty bowel elimination.

The dietetics of lead or arsenical neuritis have only to do with preventing the ingestion of these poisons and so not interest us otherwise except when as a result of a chronic toxicosis the general nutrition suffers. Neuritis due to lack of accessory substances in the food or vitamines, *e. g.*, beriberi has been dealt with separately in the Chapter on Deficiency Diseases.

What has been said of neuritis applies equally to the neuralgic states, and these are especially seen in individuals who are overfed and underexercised.

Epilepsy.—Epilepsy has been rather a dietetic storm center, much having been written pro and contra on the influence of diet as modifying either the frequency or severity of the attacks. Those who insist upon the influence of diet point to the fact that epilepsy is frequent among carnivorous animals but rare in herbivora, Turner and Stewart[1] saying that "a vegetable diet, salt starvation and above all a purine-free diet permit the bromide salts being reduced to a minimum." On the whole Schloss[2] concluded that the nature of the diet had little or nothing to do with the frequency or severity of the attacks, but he did find in fact that reducing the sodium chloride intake in addition to giving bromides exerted a marked and favorable effect on the attacks. This point seems fairly well established and should always be considered in prescribing a suitable diet for epilepsy. Despite Schloss's contention that diet has no material effect on the epileptic seizures the large majority of clinicians distinctly favor a low protein diet and one particularly low in purine bodies, as Turner[3] has emphasized. The deleterious effect of the high protein is no doubt due to the frequency with which the ingestion of considerable amounts of meat products is accompanied by intestinal putrefaction and absorption of intestinal by-products. An indication of this is indol in the urine, and while this has in itself often no ill-effect, it is frequently the index of other intestinal poisons which may still further lower the threshold of nervous stability, so leading to the easier production of an epileptic seizure.

The prevention, therefore of intestinal decomposition is absolutely indicated[4] and every means should be taken to

[1] Text-book of Nervous Diseases, p. 582.
[2] Wien. klin. Wchnschr., 1901, xiv, No. 46.
[3] Practitioner, 1906, lxxvi, 476.
[4] Dana: Text-book of Nervous Diseases, p. 534.

obviate its production and to assist in its limitation and elimination when present. Among the best means to prevent or relieve this condition is the maintenance of a low protein diet with the emphasis put on the reduction of animal protein, particularly meat, placing the patients for a few days on a strict vegetarian diet and later on a lacto-ovo-vegetarian regimen as already explained under vegetarianism. When the indican, as the index of intestinal poison, is reduced to a minimum, one may again add small amounts of meat, particularly if the patients are able to take a good deal of out-of-door exercise or work, but making meat the least constituent of the protein ration. In addition to proper diet in intestinal decomposition consideration must be given to promoting intestinal peristalsis and the mechanical removal of by-products by colon lavage.

When these dietary regulations are carried out it will be found possible to control the seizures with the minimum amount of bromide salts, particularly if the sodium chloride intake be kept at a low level, even at times to the point of a so-called salt-free diet, particularly in adults.

Aside from these restrictions an epileptic may eat almost anything that is in itself digestible, remembering always that acute or chronic indigestion favors the production of the attacks and included under this must also be mentioned chronic constipation.

A new method of treating epilepsy has been devised by Concklin, of Battle Creek, Michigan. In this the patients are put to bed and starved for from ten to fourteen days, allowing of course all the water desired. After this initial period of starvation they are again gradually fed, beginning with light foods—egg albumin in orange juice, cereals, and so gradually back to a fairly generous diet. In severe cases a second fast is sometimes given for a shorter period. Many cases cease to have attacks after the first forty-eight hours of the fast. The treatment is still in its experimental stage.

Insanity.—Practically the only dietetic problems of importance that arise in connection with the various forms of insanity are the questions of forcible feeding and the prevention of indigestion or actual blocking of the esophagus by bolting large masses of food. The latter is easily guarded against by serving only food that is well-cooked and finely comminuted. As to the question of forced feeding by gavage, there is no question at times as to its necessity since it must be done in cases of mania or extreme melancholia where the patients refuse food. It must not be forgotten however, that even these patients may refuse food on account of lack of appetite or from some actual disability, such as painful deglutition, but when it is decided that forced feeding (or suralimentation as it is called) is needed, the method to be followed is as follows: If the patient is apathetic and will allow the passage of the stomach-tube with little or no restraint it may be passed and fluid food according to the appended formulæ may be used three or four times a day. If, on the other hand, there is active resistance to the process the patients must be forcibly restrained either by strapping to a high-back chair or probably better by restraining them flat on the bed and inserting the mouth gag gently. A very good form of gag is a wooden cork with a hole in it large enough to allow the passage of the stomach-tube through it and insert this cork between the teeth; it should be made with a flange on either end to prevent it from slipping out from between the teeth and of course a string attached to the outer flange to prevent it from slipping down the throat.

The best foods to use for this forced feeding are milk, cream, beef powders, beef meal, pureé of beans and peas, cereals, eggs, cane-sugar and lactose. A convenient basis, for at least some of the feedings, may be found in the milk, cream and lactose formulæ under Diet in Typhoid Fever (p. 575), to which can be added the other foods suggested.

In order to maintain nutrition and body weight it is of course necessary to calculate the food requirements for the patient's normal weight and height and feed accordingly. Debove uses 1000 c.c. (1 qt.) of milk, 100 gm. (3⅓ oz.) of meat powder and one egg, three or four times daily.[1] For a sample formula this is very well but whether or not it is sufficient for a given individual will depend on the actual food requirements, calculated on the ordinary basis, 30 to 40 calories per kilo of body weight. which must always be reckoned out, remembering that the restless insane burn up more food than the melancholic.

Apoplexy.—The dietetics of apoplexy might well be divided into prophylactic diet and that actually to be employed in the presence of a cerebral hemorrhage. In the preventive diet it is necessary to warn patients with high blood-pressure or marked arteriosclerosis or both that they should eat sparingly of all foods but especially of the purines of animal food-stuffs, as tending to raise blood-pressure; they should never take a very hearty meal, particularly at night and should abstain from alcoholic drinks at all times. A diet largely vegetarian or ovo-lacto-vegetarian is best

[1] Thompson: Dietetics, p. 514.

suited to these people, taking the best meal at midday and a light supper.

Continuous and persistent overeating is probably a frequent acquired cause of hypertension and arteriosclerosis and should be discouraged at any time of life, but particularly so late in life where an overindulgence is apt to prove disastrous.

When once an apoplexy has occurred the dietetic indications are to reduce the volume of blood as much as may be and lower blood-pressure. If the patient is plethoric or obese the best way to bring this about is to give no food or even water for several hours after the hemorrhage, but to promote free intestinal evacuation in every way by quick cathartics such as elaterin, croton oil, castor oil or repeated doses of concentrated solution of magnesium sulphate, 1 or 2 drams every half-hour, in 2 ounces of water, until thoroughly effectual. After six to eight hours one may begin with small quantities of milk. Probably one of the best methods is to place these patients on a Karell diet (see p. 310), beginning with 200 c.c. (6½ oz.) milk four times a day for four or five days then gradually increasing to soft foods as indicated in that dietary regimen. This has two advantages in that it gives little bulk and aids in reducing weight with consequent lowering of blood-pressure. This is about all one can do dietetically for these cases, but it is often surprising how effectual the method is in reducing the full bounding pulse so often seen, to one of lower tension and less volume. After the patients are again restored to their new normal, *i. e.*, when either the results of the hemorrhage have disappeared or their permanence demonstrated, then what has already been said in regard to prophylaxis for these cases is indicated.

FUNCTIONAL NERVOUS DISEASES.

Migraine or Periodic Headaches.—Among the most trying conditions a physician is ever called upon to treat, migraine and periodic headache have few peers. At one time or another almost every variety of food has been blamed for these headaches and one can find diets based on the elimination of one or another kind, some authorities vaunting a meat-free diet, others a diet low in hydrocarbons, still another curtailing the carbohydrates. As the etiology is probably various so one dietetic treatment or another fits and relieves the symptoms or not as the case may be, so accounting for similar results by dissimilar diets, *e. g.*, cases with gouty migraine may be helped by a purine-free diet; another case with marked digestive acidity and fermentation will be helped most by a diet without sweets and low in starches; so that so far as is possible a correct determination of the etiological factors should be made if dietetic treatment is to be at all helpful in its results.   Many cases with a markedly neurotic habit respond to no particular diet but must be treated generally if any favorable results are to be obtained, *e. g.*, rest, hydrotherapy, exercise, suggestion, etc., diet playing only the usual nutritive role in maintaining a good physical condition.

In short, no specific directions can be given to cover all these cases, as they all respond differently, each must be studied separately and often when one fails to identify the underlying cause, recourse must be had to experimentation, trying first one, then another diet until one becomes convinced that certain omissions are helpful.   In this the patient's feelings are often valuable, for many of them soon learn to know whether one or another class of foods cause them to feel worse or better.   The presence of decayed teeth is often associated with periodic headache and must be borne in mind as an etiological factor.   Heredity, too, is frequently seen to be a factor, as a parent with these headaches is very apt to beget a child who later develops the same trouble. Again, some children who have epilepsy as children, outgrow this and develop periodic headaches which apparently represent another expression of the nervous explosion which in their early youth resulted in a convulsion.

In some cases we find a vegetarian diet with milk gives excellent results, particularly if the cause can be traced to a lithemic condition or a purine-free diet as already outlined, and most of them, unless they have their headaches in spite of hard labor, do best on a low (Chittenden) protein diet. As a matter of interest this condition is seldom seen in the laboring man, but more often in a highly organized and educated man or woman, who lives more or less without regular exercise and with a tendency to overeating.

In some way the impression cannot help but be a strong one that people who work hard. exercise freely, sweat more or less profusely at work are not often subjects of periodic headaches, facts which point the way to a rational work and dietetic cure.

Hare[1] has thought that the best results have been obtained in his experience by reducing the "carbonaceous" material in the diet.   This is accomplished by ordering a diet "mainly protein, 8 to 12 ounces cooked meat or fish with $1\frac{1}{2}$ ounces

[1] Medical Magazine, 1907, xvi, 722.

bread or toast and a little butter. Green non-starchy vegetables are allowed. Tea and coffee with a little milk but no sugar." On this the patients slowly lose weight, which is regularly taken and recorded. The carbohydrates and fats are cautiously increased in the form of bread, butter and milk until the weight remains stationary, "carbon equilibrium being maintained on a minimum intake."

In order to do this satisfactorily it is necessary to weigh the food and it is best to begin two weeks before an attack is expected.

Chorea.—The etiology of chorea is somewhat obscure but occurring as it does, for the most part, after rheumatic infection makes it pretty surely a result of this infection or intoxication. Just how the nervous system comes to be involved is far from clear, but the fact remains that the individuals who are thus affected are usually found to be anemic, poorly nourished, and in need of physical up-building. The diet, therefore, which will accomplish most for these patients is a very nourishing one with emphasis placed upon the feeding of fattening foods in order that their nervous system may take part in the general up-building of the organism. So far as possible then these patients should be placed upon a fattening cure with the addition of considerable quantities of cream, butter and cereals, and other carbohydrate foods without too great an allowance of protein, particularly the meat proteins; eggs cooked in any form, in custards, ice-cream, etc., should be freely used and with the fattening process there should go careful attention to the elimination, rest, light exercise later on, and freedom from all external and internal nerve irritants. In conformity with the latter suggestion the exclusion of tea or coffee from the diet is imperative. Where the digestion is good, it is often advisable to allow a glass of milk with cream or an egg-nog between meals and at bedtime, if this interferes with the consumption of three good meals a day the between-meal feeding should be omitted.

Neurasthenia.—The causes of this protean disease are so numerous and far-reaching that for a complete discussion of the subject one must refer to the standard text-books on neurology. Predisposing causes are largely hereditary and as such outside the consideration of dietetics. There are certain physical conditions which predispose to its development and which are to some extent preventable by proper attention to diet. Thus, any condition of lowered vitality as that following influenza, typhoid fever and other prolonged illnesses or severe operations, all act as causes, and can be, to a certain extent, guarded against, if the lowered vitality can be combated from the start or altogether prevented by proper attention to diet and by guarding against the semi-starvation diets so often resorted to in the conditions named. When one considers the usual immediate causes such as worry, overwork, shocks, accidents, fright, all the forms of chronic unhappiness, and "ingrowing" thoughts, it is plain that diet is not specially concerned, except insofar as a properly fed body is less liable to worry, than one that is poorly nourished. The newer conception of the causation of many of the cases of neurasthenia include attention to various possible chronic intoxications, some of which are doubtless of digestive origin, such as chronic intestinal stasis, chronic constipation, various chronic forms of gastro-intestinal digestive defect, besides the intoxications that arise from localized points of chronic infection often hidden or unsuspected, *e. g.*, chronic tonsillar infection, tooth infections, low grade pelvic infections. In fact *localized* infection anywhere with resulting chronic absorption of the products of bacterial change with the well-*known* effects upon the blood causing an anemia, and the more remote effects upon the nervous system. All these *possible* factors must also be taken into account and weighed when trying to find the cause in a particular case of neurasthenia.

Given a case, therefore, of neurasthenia what can we, as dieticians, do for the patient?

In this decision we must have a clear idea of just how severe a case we have to deal with, for the lighter cases are less drastically treated than those which are severe or advanced, so that we may divide them into mild, medium severe, and severe in order to reduce the question to orderly discussion.

The three great essentials of the treatment in these cases are: rest, diversion, diet, and regulated exercise.

In the mild cases it is often only necessary to keep the patients in bed for half the day, let them rest and read and above all in a room to which air is freely admitted by open windows, or even better, out of-doors on a protected porch. The remainder of the day they may go about their affairs with caution, resting before dinner and getting to bed early. The diet in these cases (particularly if undernourished) should be pushed, giving food frequently and in concentrated form. This may be done by following Keating's[1] diet as follows:

6 A.M. 240 c.c. (8 oz.) strong beef tea, hot.
8 A.M. Half a glass of iron water. Breakfast of fruit, steak and coffee, 240 c.c. (8 oz.). Milk with extract of malt and citrate of iron, quinine 6 grains.

[1] Thompson's Dietetics.

10 A.M. Electricity.

12 NOON Milk, 240 c.c. (8 oz.) with malt.

2 P.M. Dinner with half a glass of iron water, followed by a glass of milk with the malt.

6 P.M. Third dose of iron water with light supper of fruits, bread and butter and cream. Glass of milk and malt.

10 I.M. Beef soup, 120 c.c. (4 oz.) preceded by massage with cocoa oil for one hour.

In the more severe cases it is necessary, in order to get good results, that the patients should be kept in bed and put upon some modification of the Weir Mitchell treatment, its rigor depending upon the severity of the case and the length of time that the routine should be kept up.

Weir Mitchell Diet and Treatment.[1]—The Weir Mitchell treatment for various conditions of malnutrition and neurosis consists essentially in absolute seclusion of the patient, preferably away from home with a nurse who is entirely unknown to the patient, but chosen by the physician for her qualities with special reference to the individual case. The nurse should be changed if she is a misfit with the patient. The patient is kept in bed during the treatment which is from four to eight or more weeks. Massage and electricity (faradic) is given daily in hour or hour and a half periods and feedings which are based on the following routine.

Milk is the food of first importance with Mitchell, for he found that on an exclusive milk diet for a few days patients promptly lost their various digestive symptoms. When neurasthenia is combined with obesity the Karell cure for a fortnight or less is the best method of procedure particularly in the cases of extreme fatness with anemia. Skimmed milk is especially recommended as most favorable to the dyspeptics given two-hourly with or without lime water. The milk should be slowly sipped and when it is disgreeable or nauseating can be flavored with tea, coffee, caramel or salt. If the milk causes "acidity" the use of alkalies is indicated. At first 4 ounces are given every two hours, and as the amount is enlarged the periods may be lengthened to three hours with a total of 2 quarts of milk daily.

For the first few days the patients lose weight but then remain stationary or even gain. Patients on this diet are usually sleepy after a few days. Constipation and coated tongue are usual and have to be attended to, and Mitchell says on a skimmed-milk diet uric acid disappears almost entirely from the urine but reappears as soon as a mixed

[1] "Fat and Blood."

diet is begun. The addition of various farinaceous and milk preparations to the milk diet such as malted milk and Nestle's food, etc., is often useful. Ordinarily after four to seven days a light breakfast is allowed, in another couple of days a chop is given as a mid-day dinner and again in a day or two bread and butter are allowed three times a day. After ten days it is usually possible to allow three full meals, together with 3 or 4 pints of milk given at or after meals instead of water. After ten days Mitchell also orders 2 to 4 ounces of a good fluidextract of malt before each meal. The foods actually used are largely according to the patient's wishes but butter in considerable amounts is urged and a cup of coffee or cocoa is allowed the first thing in the morning.

At the end of the first week a raw meat soup is added, made as follows: One pound of rare beef chopped up and put in a bottle with 1 pint of water and 5 drops of strong hydrochloric aid. This is allowed to stand all night on ice and in the morning the bottle is placed in water at 110° F. and kept for two hours at this temperature. It is then strained through a cloth under pressure and the resulting fluid given in divided doses three times during the day. A little more pleasant taste is obtained by first roasting the meat slightly on one side. When the patients are on full feedings, iron is given, also cod-liver oil, either by mouth or rectum, when there has been much loss of flesh.

Under this regimen the increase of weight and well-being is often extraordinary but there is much dependent upon the physician's attention to details and his ability to carry the patient along psychologically; in other words, the same treatment and regimen will succeed in the hands of one man, and not with another. One criticism that has been offered is that while the patients do gain they lose the additional fat very shortly after they are allowed up.

This is not a fact if the massage has been kept up vigorously and steadily, for this in conjunction with the electricity, prevents the patient's from getting "soft," the added weight being firm and sound.

A convenient routine founded upon the Weir Mitchell diet by J. K. Mitchell is as follows:

7.00 A.M. Cocoa. Cold sponge with rough rub.
8.00 A.M. Breakfast with milk. Rest an hour afterward.
10.00 A.M. Milk, 240 c.c. (8 oz.), peptonized. Massage.
12.00 M. Milk as soup. Reading aloud by nurse.
1.30 P.M. Dinner. Rest one hour afterward.
3.30 P.M. Peptonized milk, 240 c.c. (8 oz.).
4.00 P.M. Electricity.

6.00 P.M.   Supper with milk.
8.00 P.M.   Reading aloud by nurse, half an hour.
9.00 P.M.   Light rub by nurse with drip sheet.
10.00 P.M.   Peptonized milk, 240 c.c. (8 oz.) with biscuits.
During the night a glass of milk is needed.
With dinner and supper give malt extract 240 c.c. (8 oz.)
After each meal some tonic mixture with iron if anemia is present.

Digestive Neuroses.—These are of many sorts and kinds, some referred to the stomach and accompanied either by an excess or diminution of acid values in the gastric secretion or they may be referred to the intestinal tract with constipation or diarrhea or even the passage of mucus as the cardinal symptoms, with or without abdominal pain.

Then there is the well-known type of vomiting occurring in nervous individuals often most trying to deal with. Where these digestive neuroses are severe a Weir Mitchell regimen has a very salutary effect even though it is not necessary perhaps to carry it out to the last letter of detail, but the effect of absolute rest combined with the skimmed-milk diet in increasing amounts is most useful. In fact there are many cases of gastro-intestinal disturbance in which no definite lesion or cause can be determined but in which a graduated milk diet combined with rest seems to produce the desired result, doing away with the symptoms.[1]

Insomnia.—Insomnia has so many causes that it is quite impossible to give off-hand, dietary advice to meet all the general factors. One must make a correct etiological diagnosis before it will be possible to prescribe a diet rationally; for depending upon whether the cause is digestive, nervous or from organic disease such as chronic nephritis, arteriosclerosis, or old age the diet will all have to be reckoned on the basis of the underlying trouble. If we can exclude definite organic disease and digestive errors we have left an idiopathic form of insomnia which is for the most part a functional neurosis. Patients get the habit of not sleeping until a certain hour or not until after a certain hour or of waking up at a particular hour, with great regularity.

There are many methods of general hygiene which must be brought into play in order to bring about the best result, *e. g.*, prevention of exhaustion, bathing, suitable exercise, clothing, air and food, all of which are factors in producing insomnia or of perpetuating it. People drop into the habit of taking drugs with great ease and one constantly finds

[1] For further discussion of digestive neurosis see Chapter on Gastro-intestinal Diseases.

patients taking trional, sulphonal, medinal, veronal, etc., more or less frequently, often with disastrous results so far as the general health is concerned; but with measures for insomnia other than diet we have nothing directly to do and one must be referred to neurological text-books for all such assistance. Diet does play a very distinct role in the treatment of the idiopathic form of insomnia, and it is of course of chief importance in those cases due to a disturbed digestion.

The entire day's dietary for the insomniac should be of the simplest sort, avoidance of all indigestible substances at every meal, making the heartiest meal in the middle of the day. The supper should be light, free of stimulants, tea, coffee, alcohol and tobacco or much meat, as meat products are all distinctly stimulating to most persons. At bedtime it is often a good plan to take a glass of milk, hot or cold, as preferred, sipped slowly. Malted milk or any other flavor may be added to the milk to taste. If milk in any form is distasteful a small cream-cheese sandwich, piece of bread and butter or fruit, in fact any simple article of food may often be taken on retiring with advantage. In certain cases a split of ale in small amount, not over one glass, may produce the same effect.

If the patient falls asleep easily but awakens in the night, particularly toward morning, sleep may often be obtained if a glass of milk or sandwich or hot cocoa (in a thermos bottle), if taken immediately on waking, not waiting to see if sleep will come itself. If one waits, then the chances are that even though the food is taken later, it does not have the same effect and wakefulness continues.

Delirium Tremens.—While it may seem at first that the question of diet does not enter very vividly into the question of delirium tremens, or hyperalcoholization, as a matter of fact it is of the utmost importance, and if properly carried out may readily turn the scale in favor of recovery rather than death. Almost invariably it will be found out on inquiry—or failing this, may be safely assumed—that during the period of excessive alcoholic use the patient has taken little or no food. Excessive drinking and food taking do not go together, so that these patients while they have been supplied with a considerable number of heat units in taking the alcohol (7.2 calories per c.c.) which has somewhat spared the fat combustion, are virtually in a state of nitrogen starvation, besides being poisoned by the products of their own perverted metabolism. What they need, after a thorough purgation, is a large amount of nourishment with a high protein content easily taken and digested. Milk fills these indications particularly well and should be given every hour, preferably hot, and 8 to 10 ounces at a time, depending on the size of the patient. After the first twenty-four hours the amount may be increased or the milk may be modified upward, so to speak, by the addition of cream and lactose, as used in typhoid fever (see p. 575). After forty-eight hours the interval may be lengthened to two hourly feedings and usually, if the case is progressing well, soft solids may then be allowed. This plan of feeding combined with the preliminary catharsis (although we should not wait for the cathartics to act before giving the milk) and proper use of sedatives has in the writer's experience proved its worth many times.

Nervous Anorexia.—Nervous anorexia is a well-known neurosis occurring in people who have undergone some severe mental shock or strain or it may develop as a sequel of any prolonged illness during which the nervous reserve has been unduly depleted. Whatever the cause, the condition is one of absolute anorexia; nothing whatever makes an appeal to the palate and the patient often refuses every kind of food unless actually forced to take it. · Under these circumstances the treatment is divided into general hygiene and diet. Under hygiene comes the general care of the patient; hydrotherapy, suggestion—massage, exercises, etc.— all of which play a most important part in overcoming the underlying causes of the anorexia in a nervous system that is away below par. So far as the dietary management goes, one can try all sorts of ways to tempt the appetite with special foods, attractive preparation and insistence on the part of the nurse. At times the Weir Mitchell routine is of the greatest value, for this attacks the trouble at its source and the simplicity of the dietary regimen lends itself to success with these patients. In those patients who absolutely refuse nourishment one of two methods may be adopted; feeding concentrated foods by gastric gavage three or four times a day as recommended in suralimentation, or by duodenal feeding as recommended by Einhorn. By either method a large amount of food can be furnished independent of appetite which will gradually favorably affect the entire organism, building it up in spite of a complete disinclination to food, with the certainty that if sufficient progress can be made the appetite will presently return of itself and the difficulty in feeding will be at an end.

CHAPTER XXX.

ACUTE AND CHRONIC INFECTIONS.

IN the dietetics of the infections great advance has been made, taking the subject out of the realm of hypotheses and placing it on the solid rock of accurate experimentation, checked by calorimetry and the tracing of the protein metabolism. Great credit is due to Coleman, Shaffer and Du Bois for their painstaking work in typhoid, the results of which have formed the basis of much of our present ability to keep fever patients in a state of good nutrition, while formerly patients with acute infections were kept in a state of semistarvation, with resulting subnutrition amounting in many instances to emaciation. These same patients today, instead of losing 30, 40 or 50 pounds during a six weeks' typhoid, emerge from their illness with minor losses or none and in some instances showing actual gain in weight. The resulting shortening of convalescence and comparative freedom from many of the complications of these infections have been some of the results obtained, and it is not to be doubted that the modern method of feeding in infections has had its decided influence on the prolongation of life.

FEVER.[1]

The body temperature is regulated through two processes, chemical production of heat by an increased or decreased rate of oxidation; and physical loss of heat through conduction, radiation, evaporation, or excretion. There is a critical air temperature, approximately 15° C. (59° F.) at which there is a balance between production and loss which does not affect the body temperature. The metabolism of fasting at the critical temperature represents the heat needed for the performance of the various functions of the body. Below this temperature the heat production, controlled by chemical regulation, rises or falls with variations in the external temperature, while above it heat production is slightly increased, and the regulation depends upon physical means. Between 20° and 30° C.(68° and 86° F.) the heat production

[1] Shaffer and Coleman: Arch. Inter. Med., 1909, iv, 538. Coleman: Tr. XVth International Cong. Hyg. and Demog., 1912, ii, 602. Carpenter: Am. Jour. Physiol., 1909, xxiv, 203. Coleman and Du Bois: and numerous other papers by other investigators.

is practically stationary; regulation is then dependent upon physical regulation, particularly upon increased evaporation.

Factors which will tend to increase heat production and temperature are work, ingestion of food, particularly protein, exposure to various stimuli, such as cold, or the production of toxic substance in the body, as in fevers. Heat loss is increased by dilatation of the surface bloodvessels and excretion of water with subsequent evaporation; these processes are under the control of the nervous system. The rapid movement of the air surrounding the body assists in the removal of heat directly and indirectly through increased evaporation, provided the humidity be low. Conversely the stagnation of air and prevention of loss by radiation and clothing tends to conserve the heat within the body.

The cause of increased heat production in fever is not known; it is closely associated with infection with bacteria and other organisms or the products of their activity, toxins. It may be that the organisms themselves stimulate directly the production of heat. The substances produced as a result of their metabolic activities, particularly on protein, have been held to be the more specific stimulants to metabolism.

The rise of the body temperature above the normal may be taken as an index of the intensity of intoxication, but in children a mild infection may be accompanied by a very high temperature, while in the aged a severe infection may cause only a comparatively slight rise, one or two degrees.

An increase in temperature itself, provided it does not exceed a certain limit, 40 to 42° C. (104° to 107° F.) or, as has been suggested below, the temperature at which certain proteins begin to coagulate is not of itself harmful. This fact has been demonstrated with animals which were kept at a temperature of 40° C. (104° F.), for weeks without showing signs of disintegration; they were even more resistant to staphylococci, pneumococci, or B. coli inoculation than control animals, for they lived longer or even survived the infection.

In fever an increase or decrease in the total metabolism is accompanied by a rise or fall in the body temperature; a subnormal temperature is associated with a rate of metabolism which is below normal. Metabolism in fever has been studied particularly in connection with typhoid fever.

The idea has been prevalent that it was impossible or unwise to feed fever patients sufficient food to prevent loss of protein and that food was poorly utilized in fever. It has

36

been found, however, that when furnished with sufficient energy-yielding food and moderate amounts of protein, fever patients may be able to maintain their body weight and in some cases nitrogen equilibrium. Sufficient food must be given to enable the patient to meet the increased heat production, 40 to 50 per cent. above the normal, without using his own reserves for that purpose.

While a normal man can maintain himself on a diet containing sufficient protein and yielding energy equivalent to but little more than his basal heat production, a fever patient requires a diet containing a quantity of energy-yielding foods far in excess of the expected metabolism, on the basis of his height and weight. Thus, a man producing 40 calories per kilogram per day cannot be brought into equilibrium unless he receive from 57 to 87 calories per kilogram; or a man of 65 kilograms body weight, producing 2400 calories per day, would require from 3600 to 5000 calories to keep him in equilibrium.

In convalescence the energy requirement more nearly approaches the calculated normal. A man who required 77 calories per kilogram to cover his energy requirement during a relapse, needed only 37 calories per kilogram a few days later during convalescence. The table on p. 63 gives the percentage rise in the basal metabolism above the average normal.

Since the protein metabolism is increased during fever even with a diet high in calories a larger proportion of protein is required than for the normal individual. That this is not due to the effect of a temperature rise to 40° C. or increased heat production has been demonstrated on men for short periods of time. Evidence points to some specific action, perhaps a toxic destruction of protein.

Studies of the utilization of food by typhoid fever patients indicate that it is almost as complete as in health. Protein is as fully utilized as in normal individuals. Carbohydrate, when fed in amounts under 300 grams per day, appears in the stools only in traces; above this value 2 or 3 grams of reducing substances may appear. Fat is absorbed in large amounts but the percentage of absorption is slightly lower than the normal, particularly in the early stages of the disease.

Objection has been raised to the ingestion of large quantities of food in fever on the ground that food itself is stimulating and therefore causes an increase in heat production when there is already an excessive liberation of heat. The work of the Russell Sage Institute of Pathology has demonstrated that the rise in heat production usually observed upon the ingestion of food, particularly of protein, occurs only to a limited extent, 2 to 5 per cent., in typhoid fever, due, perhaps, to the increased rate at which the body is already metabolizing. This does not hold for all fevers, however, such as that in exophthalmic goiter. Because protein metabolism in fever cannot be reduced to the level of that of a normal person, protein ingestion in fever often merely serves to replace protein already disintegrating in increased quantity and such protein would not serve to increase the heat production (Lusk). From this work it is evident that there is no objection on a scientific basis to feeding most fever patients, on the contrary, experience seems to point to the desirability of adequate feeding.

Diet in Fever.—In view of the experimental data, especially that presented by Coleman and Shaffer and Du Bois in their studies of metabolism in typhoid fever, we see that in order to maintain a patient's nitrogenous equilibrium it is necessary to give fairly large amounts of protein in the food; an allowance of 80 to 120 gm. is usually sufficient, provided large amounts of carbohydrate and fat are included in the dietary, for both these foods spare the protein combustion. The importance of this fact is realized when consideration is given to the condition of cloudy swelling of the kidneys, associated with any high temperature which renders them less capable of eliminating large amounts of nitrogenous products. Of the end-products of carbohydrate and fat combustion, CO_2 and water, CO_2 is given off by the lungs, and only water has to pass the kidney, a much simpler process than the excretion of nitrogen.

As will be brought out later, the necessity for liberal feeding in fever depends largely on the disease present. If the infection is slight, mild or apt to be short-lived as in influenza, measles, etc., it is not necessary to plan the feeding campaign with such care as when we have a long-continued infection to deal with, as in typhoid, typhus, tuberculosis or other long-standing pus infections, such as empyema. In the latter cases *the necessity for preventing undue tissue loss is of the greatest importance*, for any infection is better fought by a body that is well nourished than by one that is half starved. Besides the protein-sparing qualities of carbohydrates they have another important function in fever, namely, that of favoring the production of the less harmful intestinal bacteria, so overcoming the effects of an excessive protein putrefaction, which is apt to take place when the diet contains a disproportionate amount of protein.

Carbohydrate also has still another important function in fever in that it reduces the tendency to acidosis; always an additional burden in fever when it develops secondary to a low carbohydrate ration.

When we come to discuss the actual constituents of fever diet, we have to take into consideration the usability of the various food elements.

Carbohydrates.—These may be given in considerable amount up to 300 gm. (10 oz.) or more per day, depending on the patient's ability to take them without causing indigestion, beginning with less amounts and gradually increasing up to the limit.

The forms of carbohydrate that appeal to the patient may be used, provided there is no special contra-indication present from the special fever to be fed; cereal gruels, toast and crackers, sago, tapioca, arrowroot and cornstarch. If amylaceous dyspepsia is present the cooked forms may be dextrinized by the use of commercial preparations of diastase, such as takadiastase (10 to 15 drops added to a portion of cooked cereal kept at blood heat for fifteen minutes is usually sufficient) or some of the malted foods may be used, such as malted milk, Mellin's food and malted breakfast food. Besides these we may use the various sugars in addition to the maltose preparations already alluded to, principally lactose and cane-sugar which may be added to cereal or milk feedings to advantage (see Typhoid Diets), and can also be administered with fruit juices, as in lemonade or orangeade.

Protein.—The most easily available form of protein for ill people is some milk preparation given either as raw milk, skimmed milk, buttermilk, ripened milk, whey, Martin's milk, yoghurt, junket, boiled milk, soured milk, koumyss, matzoon, zoolak, cream, Delafield's mixture, peptonized milk, or citrated milk (made by adding 1 or 2 grains of sodium citrate to each ounce of milk). It may also be modified by the addition of water, Vichy, lime water, thin gruels, milk soups, cream, (lactose or cane-sugar). In some invalids the mild cheeses are entirely allowable and constitute a palatable change from the usual routine; for this purpose pot cheese, cream cheese and cottage cheese are principally useful. At most, probably not more than 3 or 4 pints of milk preparation should be given daily. This amount of milk represents approximately 60 to 80 gm. protein, fat and carbohydrate with a total caloric value of 960 to 1280 calories, not, of course, sufficient for complete nutrition. It is posssible in many cases to give even 5 or 6 pints of milk in the day, but such a large bulk of food is apt to disturb digestion and result in an undue amount of feces with the added danger of gastro-intestinal disturbance. If greater caloric value is needed than that furnished by the 3 or 4 pints of milk daily, it is better to bring up the total fuel requirements by the addition of carbohydrates and fats.

Next in value to milk come eggs as a protein supply for the sick. These are capable of preparation in so many forms that although patients tire of an excess of eggs, still a good amount of protein may be given by varied combinations; furthermore the fat of the yolk is one of the most readily assimilable fats that we have. Many patients have an idea that eggs do not agree with them and make them bilious (whatever that may be), but as a matter of fact there are exceedingly few persons who cannot take eggs in some form, the fallacy of their contention, is shown by the fondness of these same people for custards, either baked or frozen. There are, of course, a very few people who cannot take eggs on account of an anaphylactic reaction caused by protein poisoning, but fortunately this is an infrequent occurrence. Among the many preparations of eggs suitable for sick people may be mentioned boiled, poached, scrambled, coddled, raw, beaten up with milk and flavored with sherry, brandy or fruit juice; as custard—baked or frozen—egg whip, egg-nog, egg a la Swisse (baked with a little cheese over it).

Meat protein, except in the form of broth is ordinarily omitted from the fever patient's diet, but if the appetite is good and the temperature low, a little beef may be given in the form of scraped-beef sandwiches. Broths of all kinds or meat jellies are freely allowed and although of little food value are distinctly useful for their appetizing qualities, the patients often relishing other foods better if they are allowed broths.

For the same reason beef juice is often used, besides which it also has a slight stimulating effect upon the circulation. This is particularly seen in children who after beginning beef juice may pass a more or less excited, sleepless night. For the most part glandular meat preparations are by common consent left out of the fever patient's diet, although sweetbreads are allowed early in convalescence. The high percentage of purine bodies in these foods form an objection in that their excretion is an unnecessary and additional burden to the kidneys. Oysters, if small, are often well borne and patients may be given certain kinds of fresh fish; cod, halibut and bass, boiled or shredded, if they wish. As a matter of fact few ill fever cases like the "fishy" taste of this form of protein.

Fats.—The simplest and most easily digested fats are those in natural emulsion, *e. g.*, egg yolk and cream. Next in order is fresh butter. Fat from meat or fish is much less easily digested, although there seems in certain cases to be an exception in favor of crisp bacon fat. From these forms of fat one can easily supply the dietary requirements.

Beverages.—Beverages form a most important part of a fever patient's daily allowances and should receive careful attention. Most fever subjects crave water and take it liberally, but occasionally, a very ill patient or one in delirium cannot ask for water, so that the nurse must be on the lookout to supply a minimum of from 1500 to 2100 c.c. (50 to 70 oz.), fluid in twenty-four hours or in certain cases even more. This allowance may be made up of plain water, Vichy, tea, coffee, milk, cocoa or water flavored with fruit juices, lemons, oranges or grape juice. If milk, in an allowance of 3 pints per diem, representing 1500 c.c., forms the principal food, additional water should be given; at least up to 500 to 800 c.c. or more.

Intervals of Feeding.—Ordinarily a two-hourly period is most convenient for feeding and agrees with the majority of patients, giving water in some form between feedings. There are cases in whom a three-hour period is better borne or even hourly feedings may at times be necessary.

In prescribing an actual diet for fever patients the exact character of the food to be given will depend upon the type of fever, whether part of a short or prolonged illness and upon whether the fever is high or low. In general the short infections may be fed more or less according to the patient's appetite, while those with long-continued and high temperatures must be amply fed, the food for the most part being of a liquid or semisolid character.

The routine for this is perhaps best exemplified by the typhoid diets (*q. v.*) the caloric value of which may be increased at will to meet nutritional demands by addition of either more or other food-stuffs, a good working rule being to furnish 1.5 to 2 gm. protein and 30 to 45 calories per kilo of body weight, the latter being increased still further if necessary, the patient's weight in health being taken as the basis of reckoning. Where no contra-indications exist it is possible in most cases of fever to give some soft solid foods chosen largely from the carbohydrates.

Alcohol.—The use or necessity for alcoholic beverages in fever is a much-discussed question and must be answered from the stand-point of, first, necessity and second, expediency. On the first score, viz., that of necessity, the pendulum has swung far away from giving alcohol as a routine in fever and as an essential part of the diet, so much is this the case that one has only to consult the commissary department of any large hospital to note the comparatively small amount of alcohol now in use. While alcohol is ozidized in the body and to some degree can take the place of fat in sparing protein, it causes surface dilatation of the vessels and some loss of heat possibly from a half to one degree in moderate dosage, so that its food value is thus promptly nullified. Secondly, expediency. The use of alcohol depends somewhat on the patient's former habits, if a regular alcohol user, a moderate amount may be given at first, gradually diminishing it, as many patients who have used alcohol freely develop delirium tremens if it is withdrawn quickly, particularly in fever. On the other hand, ordinarily it is not necessary but may do good in the typhoid state with a brown dry tongue, dry skin and subsultus; under these conditions 3 to 6 ounces per day of good whiskey or brandy may prove very beneficial, otherwise it need not be used except possibly as a mild stimulant to the appetite or occasionally to flavor foods. When real stimulation of the heart is needed it is much better accomplished by other drugs. Abroad we still find wines ordered much more freely than on this side of the water, but even there the routine use of alcoholic beverages in fever is not practised as it formerly was.

During convalescence the diet may be increased as rapidly as the appetite and digestion warrants, using soft solids such as farinaceous dishes of all sorts, scraped beef, fish, soft green vegetable purées, wine jelly, ice-cream, custards and gradually back to a normal dietary with due regard to any possible complications, such as nephritis or any sequelæ of the fever.

TYPHUS FEVER.

In the United States this disease is seldom met with except in the milder form, as in Brill's disease, which is really a mild typhus. Abroad, however, and especially during wars, typhus is often met with in its severe forms, and while diet does not play the nice part that it does in typhoid it is equally necessary to keep these patients nourished to the limit of their capacity, digestively speaking. They can take all the foods recommended for typhoid in the high calorie regimen, and using good quantities of food prevents undue loss of weight which if well digested certainly helps the patient to fight the disease and renders convalescence shorter. In addition to the usual typhoid regimen one may use soft solids more freely, depending upon the patient's appetite. Chopped meat, purée vegetables, eggs in any simple form, cereals, ice-cream, blanc mange, and jellies, may be used to advantage.

During convalescence the foods should be increased in variety and quantity just as rapidly as the patients will take them. Alcohol may be used at any stage but it is not especially useful unless there is a failure of appetite, dry tongue or a typhoid state when a moderate amount of good whiskey or brandy, well diluted, is advisable.

TYPHOID FEVER.

With the advent of antityphoid innoculation this disease bids fair to be largely overcome, but until this is more universally adopted typhoid will be endemic in this country and we shall have need for a proper treatment of the disease. In this treatment diet holds the first place in importance and while America has been blameworthy in its former carelessness of typhoid it has happily been the pioneer in feeding these patients on scientific and rational lines, thus in some way making atonement. Indeed it is interesting to look through the Index Medicus on this topic and find that practically all the literature on advanced feeding during the past few years has been contributed by American physicians.

Older Diets.—There is little use in taking up the reader's time with a discussion of the older methods of feeding where only milk, or milk, eggs and broth have been used, for these methods have been entirely discredited and although these articles still form a part of most typhoid dietaries, their inadequacy, when given alone, has been proven beyond a doubt. It would hardly seem necessary to urge practioners to feed their fever patients more liberally in the light of the generally diffused knowledge on the subject were it not for the fact that some of the older medical authorities, who are hardly to be equalled or excelled in the matter of clinical observation and diagnosis, are so hopelessly incomplete when they discuss the diet of this disease, as *e. g.*, one standard text-book recommends a diet which allows 39 to 54 gm. protein and furnishes 675 to 1000 calories, certainly insufficient if one wishes to maintain even approximately a nitrogenous equilibrium and body weight.

Modern chemistry has taught us that the efficiency of human digestion during fever is reduced not more than 5 to 10 per cent., and that the flow of the digestive enzymes is little, if any, interfered with, provided the organism as a whole, is properly nourished. Carlson, however, of late says that in forms of sufficiently high temperature all types of gastric secretion, continous, psychic and hormone are depressed or at times completely abolished. If the pancreas and intestinal enzymes are not interfered with too much, digestion of properly prepared food will proceed practically normally as is seen in gastric achylia from other causes. Here then is the key-note of feeding these cases; that they shall be sufficiently fed in order to prevent malnutrition. It is to be hoped that we shall see no more sunken and hollow-cheeked typhoid cases reminding one of the Cuban reconcentrados or subjects of the Indian famines.

The object sought in these cases is to prevent loss of body protein and weight as nearly as possible on the principle that a starving organism, of whatever degree, is not the best possible fighting machine. It is not always possible or even best to attempt to attain these objects in certain cases, as there are unquestionably individuals who cannot take the large amounts of food necessary to accomplish this end and we must be content on account of an irritable stomach, complications, etc., to come as near this as possible. Each case, however, should be nourished to the limit of his or her capacity.

Bacteriological and Physiological Basis for More Liberal Diets.—The older clinicians were temperamentally just as generous as those of the present day and only fed sparingly because they concluded that food was incompletely absorbed under such conditions as exist in the intestines of typhoid cases. Du Bois[1] has made a study of food absorption in typhoid on patients who were receiving large amounts of food and has found that absorption in these cases is little altered from the normal and draws the following conclusions, based on careful analyses to wit: That typhoid fever patients can absorb carbohydrates and proteins in large amounts and as well as normal individuals. Early in the disease the absorption of large amounts of fat does not seem quite as complete as in normal individuals. Late in the disease enormous amounts of fat can be absorbed (up to 327 gm. per day in Du Bois's cases.)

Here then we have a catagorical reply to the question of absorption of food in typhoid, so that from this point of view one would no longer be justified in withholding a liberal diet. Having established this fact, it would be fair to ask in what proportion should the food elements be given, *i. e.*, the protein, carbohydrates, fats; to this question the bacteriologist and physiologist have also brought a definite reply.

[1] Med. Surg. Report Presby. Hosp., New York, 1912, p. 175.

Carbohydrates.—Physiology has shown that carbohydrates spare both protein and fat, so that the diet rich in carbohydrates is capable of preventing loss of body protein, if given in sufficient amounts, without crowding the consumption of protein above the average amount. This is in the face of a pretty active catabolism and Folin[1] showed that in starvation nitrogen metabolism can be reduced one-third by the use of carbohydrates.

Then, too, carbohydrates are completely oxidized into water and CO_2 neither of which products cause, in elimination, any strain or irritation to organs whose functions are already somewhat impaired by a parenchymatous degeneration accompanying any high temperature.

They also found that "the greatest amount of heat produced by any patient was 48 calories per kilo a day, the majority giving off about 35 calories. On this basis the high calorie diet gives 1000 to 2000 more calories than are expended in twenty-four hours and if the patients do not receive this, they lose both nitrogen and weight; later in the disease the excess is used in storing fat." It can therefore be seen that carbohydrates should form a considerable proportion of the typhoid's dietary.

From the bacteriological point of view Kendall[2] tried two diets on cats, one protein and one carbohydrate, alternating biweekly. It was found that "the intestinal flora can respond in two ways: First, the flora may become dominantly proteolytic, then fermentative as the diet is changed, and second, in addition to alternations in bacterial types certain organisms can actually change their metabolic activities to accommodate themselves now to a protein now to a carbohydrate regimen. These changes consist essentially of alternations between proteolytic and gas-forming bacteria on a protein diet and acid-forming bacteria on a carbohydrate regimen. The absence of carbohydrate prevents the development of the acid-forming bacteria on a protein diet and the excessive amounts of acid produced by the fermentation of sugar inhibits the growth of the proteolytic and aërogenic forms in the carbohydrate regimen."

The character of the food taken in alters the bacterial flora of the alimentary canal and the toxins as well.[3] If an excess of carbohydrates is given the bacteria grow tremendously, but after a time they manufacture that which inhibits their own further growth and the specific bacterial

---

[1] Am. Jour. Physiol., 1905, p. 66.
[2] Jour. Am. Med. Assn., lvi, 1084.
[3] Interstate Med. Jour., 1913, xx, 413.

toxins are less potent than when the bacteria are grown on protein alone. "The splitting products which the bacteria elaborate from carbohydrate are comparatively non-toxic to the human economy." "On the other hand, when the protein predominates in the food and there is a small amount of sugar present the bacteria grow luxuriantly, manufacturing an extremely potent, specific toxin and produce from the proteins splitting products which are toxic when absorbed from the alimentary canal. Hence in conditions of intestinal infection, especially typhoid, carbohydrates, should constitute a preponderating percentage of the food."

In the high caloric feeding cases tympanites was found to be due to an excess of lactose, diarrhea from an excess of cream in the diet. Torrey found that patients who were able to take large amounts of food without digestive disturbances possessed an intestinal flora largely dominated by the bacillus acidophilus and that patients with an initial putrefactive flora were capable of developing a favorable fermentative flora with a disappearance of tympanities and diarrhea under the influence of diet.[1] The exceptions were among those who could not be liberally fed. Giving a culture of bacillus acidophilus was very satisfactory in tympanities and diarrhea.

These quotations are given in full in order to bring home more sharply the necessity for placing a large reliance on carbohydrates in this condition, for most of the older dietaries were principally protein and a very small percentage of fats or carbohydrates, scarcely more than that contained in milk.

Metchnikoff has recognized these facts in his treatment of auto-intoxication. He reduces the amount of protein in the diet and increases the carbohydrates and feeds lactic acid bacilli to split up the sugar to form acid which will inhibit the growth of the ordinary proteolytic bacteria.

Fats.—There is at least a theoretical objection to the large use of fats in the typhoid's diet in that they do not oxidize as readily as the carbohydrates and the intermediate products of the fatty acids may some time cause serious trouble and produce an acidosis. In clinical support of this theory there is the well-known fact that obese persons stand typhoid very badly. Coleman, however, did not find this a practical objection for after the early part of the disease the fats were as completely utilized as in the normal and in his series the fats furnish one-half the food energy.

Proteins.—So far as the daily protein requirement is concerned, Shaffer and Coleman found that the best results in

[1] Jour. Am. Med. Assn., 1917, lxix, 329.

sparing body protein were obtained on diets containing from 62 to 94 gm. per day. This comparatively low quantity is, of course, only enough if sufficient carbohydrate is allowed to prevent unnecessary protein loss.

Energy Requirement.—Coleman and Shaffer[1] calculated that the theoretical requirement of a typhoid case to be 40 calories per kilo, *i. e.*, approximately 3000 calories for a man of 150 pounds. "but they found that a diet furnishing this amount of energy was not sufficient to establish nitrogenous equilibrium." The best results in the maintenance of nitrogenous equilibrium were on 60 to 80 calories per kilo, *i. e.*, 4000 to 5000 calories per day. Patients of smaller stature requiring more energy per kilo than the average adult on account of the disproportion of surface area to weight.

Having satisfied ourselves on the foregoing grounds that it is not only possible but distinctly advantageous to feed our typhoid cases liberally in the ways indicated, one naturally turns to the practical application of these principles as exemplified in definite dietaries. One can and often must build up a suitable and particular diet for individual cases to meet the special conditions, but in general the following dietaries will be found helpful, as they fulfil the theoretical requirements which have also been proven practical as well. The moderate use of protein in them and the large use of carbohydrates carries the patients through the period of greatest danger without undue loss of body protein or weight.

Results Obtained by Liberal Diet.—An answer to this question scarcely seems necessary to one who has read the fore-going pages but for those who want a definite statement to this end one can perhaps not do better than to quote Coleman's[2] analysis of 444 cases of feeding in typhoid cases. One-half on high caloric diet the other half on a diet of milk with few additional foods with a total caloric value of from 1000 to 1500 calories as follows:

1. Duration. No difference, but long recrudesences, perhaps less common in high caloric (H. C.) patients than in low caloric diets (L. C.).

2. Condition of mouth was better in (H. C.) because patients mental condition was better.

3. Nausea and vomiting in H. C. 19.3 per cent. L. C. 22.6 per cent.

4. Tympanites in H. C. 67.5 per cent. L. C. 31.7 per cent.

5. Diarrhoea in H. C. 16.2 per cent. L. C. 48.6 per cent.

[1] Am. Jour. Med. Sc., 1912, p. 77.
[2] Jour. Am. Med. Assn., 1917, lxix. 329.

6. Nervous symptoms in H. C. 3.6 per cent. L. C. 10.81 per cent.

Long delirium in H. C. 7.65 per cent. L. C. 38.3 per cent.

7. Perforation in H. C. .9 per cent. L. C. 3.15 per cent.

8. Recrudescences in H. C. 6.7 per cent. L. C. 11.3 per cent.

9. Relapses in H. C. 18. per cent. L. C. 14.9 per cent.

10. Mortality in H. C. 8.1 per cent. L. C. 17.6 per cent.

11. Complications. There were 110 complications in 81 cases on H. C. 144 in 19 L. C.

12. Range of temperature not affected.

Before actual dietaries are discussed it must not be forgotten that the early beginnings of the better feeding of typhoid cases dates back a number of years, and much more liberality was allowed by a few men of great clinical experience like Kinnicutt and others, than by the majority of physicians. It has remained, however, for Coleman, Shaffer and Du Bois to demonstrate conclusively the various theories in regard to this question and putting the whole subject upon the plane of scientific accuracy.

Typhoid Diets.—*Proteins.*—Meats are better left out on account of the ease of putrefaction and renal irritation caused by the elimination of meat products. This is also true of all acute febrile diseases.

Eggs.—Egg albumen has been much used but the whole egg is best, the preferable form being slightly boiled.

Fats.—Are best given as cream, butter and yolk of egg.

Carbohydrates.—Starch without cellulose, crackers, toast, cereal, potato, rice, lactose. Fruit juices of all kinds. Apple sauce.

Milk.—In typhoid, milk has been the subject of much discussion, but most patients can take it in some form and can digest it in quantities of from 1½ to 2 quarts a day.

General Directions for Feeding.—The patient's appetite must, of course, be consulted and his taste for particular foods; above all great care must be taken to eliminate promptly any article that disagrees or causes persistent diarrhea, tympanites or vomiting. Feeding hours should be regular and the interval two or three hours. After a patient is first seen and his intestinal canal cleared it is well to begin on a very light diet for a day or two then gradually increase the amount of the daily ration until a full quantity of nourishment is taken.

During the severest part of the illness feedings should be continued night and day, as a very ill patient usually is only momentarily disturbed by taking nourishment.

Among the diets suitable for the first days of the illness and in some cases continued much longer the liquid diets as given are most valuable and supply sufficient protein and are of fair caloric value

TYPHOID FLUID DIET (No. 1).

8 A.M.	Milk and coffee, each 120 c.c. (4 oz.); 240 c.c. (8 oz.).
10 A.M.	Milk, hot or cold, 240 c.c. (8 oz.).
12 M.	Barley gruel, 120 c.c. (5 oz.) with milk, 60 c.c. (2 oz.).
2 P.M.	Milk, 240 c.c. (8 oz.).
4 P.M.	Oatmeal gruel, 120 c.c. (4 oz.) with milk, 60 c.c. (2 oz.).
6 P.M.	Custard with lactose (full cup) or ice-cream.
8 P.M.	Hot milk, 240 c.c. (8 oz.).
10 P.M.	Whey, 180 c.c. (6 oz.), with one whole egg and sherry.
12 M.	Oatmeal gruel, 120 c.c. (4 oz.); milk, 60 c.c. (2 oz.).
2 A.M.	Milk, 240 c.c. (8 oz.).
4 A.M.	Broth, 240 c.c. (8 oz.), with one egg.
6 A.M.	Milk, 240 c.c. (8 oz.).

Values: Protein, 98 gm. (3⅓ oz.); fats, 52 gm. (1⅔ oz.); carbohydrates, 150 gm. (5 oz.); calories, 1900.

TYPHOID FLUID DIET (No. 2).

8 A.M.	Milk and coffee, each 120 c.c. (4 oz.).
10 A.M.	Milk, hot or cold, 240 c.c. (8 oz.).
12 M.	Barley gruel, 120 c.c. (4 oz.), with milk, 60 c.c. (2 oz.).
2 P.M.	Junket with cane- and milk-sugar.
4 P.M.	Oatmeal gruel 120 c.c. (4 oz.), with milk, 60 c.c. (2 oz.).
6 P.M.	Junket with cane- and milk-sugar or ice-cream.
8 P.M.	Hot milk, 240 c.c. (8 oz.).
10 P.M.	Whey, 180 c.c. with one whole egg and sherry.
12 M.	Oatmeal gruel, 120 c.c. (4 oz.) with milk, 60 c.c. (2 oz.).
2 A.M.	Junket with cane- and milk-sugar.
4 A.M.	Milk, 240 c.c. (8 oz.).
6 A.M.	Milk, 240 c.c. (8 oz.); 15 gm. (½ oz.) of lactose added to the four milk feedings.

Values: Protein, 71 gm. (2⅓ oz.); fats, 81 gm. (2⅔ oz.); carbohydrates, 160 gm. (5⅓ oz.); calories, 2300.

In certain cases we cannot increase the value of the diet beyond these limits and although a certain amount of weight is lost the condition of patients remains surprisingly satisfactory. After a few days, however, it is possible for the most part to steadily increase the quantity of food and this may be done by adding any one of the following articles either in addition to the diet already given or by replacing some of the feedings by these articles.

Apple sauce, 1 ounce, 30 calories.
Bread (slice) 1 ounce, 80 calories.
Butter (1 pat), ⅛ ounce, 80 calories.
Cereal (cooked), 1 heaping tablespoonful, 1½ ounces, 50 calories.
Egg (one), 2 ounces, 80 calories.
Egg white (one), 30 calories.
Egg yolk (one), 50 calories.
Lactose (1 tablespoonful), 1 ounce, 36 calories.
Milk (whole), 1 ounce, 20 calories.
Potato (whole), 1 medium, 90 calories.
Potato (mashed), 1 tablespoonful, 70 calories.
Rice (boiled to pulp), 60 calories.
Cream, 20 per cent., 1 ounce, 115 calories.

MODIFIED MILK FLUID DIETS AND FOOD COMBINATIONS AND MENUS.

For 1000 calories a day.   Calories

Milk, 1 quart (1000 c.c.)	700
Cream, 1⅔ oz. (50 c.c.)	100
Lactose, 1⅔ oz. (50 grams)	200

This furnishes eight feedings each containing:

Milk, 4 ounces (120 c. c.)	80
Cream, 2 drams (8 gm.)	15
Lactose, 1½ drams (6 gm.)	24

or

Eggs, 2	150
Lactose, 30 grams (1 ounce)	120
Sugar, 25 (⅚ ounces)	100
Milk, 800 c.c. (26⅔ ounces)	560
Cream, 30 c.c. (1 ounce)	60
Lemon-juice, 30 c.c. (1 ounce)	12
Coffee, 150 c.c. (5 ounces)	00
Tea, 150 c.c. (5 ounces)	00

This furnishes seven feedings, one containing;

Coffee, 150 c.c. (5 ounces)	00
Egg, 1	75
Lactose, 30 grams (1 ounce)	120
Sugar, 5 grams	20

One feeding containing:
Tea, 150 c.c. (5 ounces)............................
Cream, 30 c.c. (1 ounce).........................
Sugar, 5 grams...................................
Four feedings each containing;
Milk, 200 c.c. (6⅔ ounces)......................
One feeding containing;
Egg, 1...
Sugar, 15 grams (½ ounce).......................
Lemon juice, 30 c.c. (1 ounce)...................
Water, 4 or 5 ounces.............................
For 1500 Calories a day;
Milk, 1½ quarts (1500 c.c.).....................
Cream, 1⅔ ounces................................
Lactose, 3⅓ ounces (100 grams).................
This furnishes six feedings each containing;
Milk, 8 ounces (240 c. c.)......................
Cream, 2 drams (8 gm.)..........................
Lactose ½ ounce (16 gm.).......................
or
Eggs, 2...
Lactose, 110 grams (3⅓ ounces).................
Sugar, 25 grams (⅚ ounces).....................
Milk, 800 c.c. (26⅔ ounces)....................
Cream, 120 c.c. (4 ounces)......................
Lemon-juice, 30 c.c. (1 ounce)..................
Coffee, 150 c.c. (5 ounces).....................
Tea, 150 c.c. (5 ounces)........................
This furnishes one feeding containing;
Coffee, 150 c.c. (5 ounces).....................
Egg, 1..
Lactose, 40 grams (1⅔ ounces)..................
Sugar, 5 grams (⅙ ounce).......................
One feeding containing:
Tea, 150 c.c. (5 ounces)........................
Cream, 50 c.c. (1⅔ ounces).....................
Lactose, 30 grams (1 ounce).....................
Sugar, 5 grams (⅙ ounce).......................
Four feedings each containing:
Milk, 200 c.c. (6⅔ ounces).....................
Cream, 17 c.c. large tablespoonful..............
One feeding containing:
Egg, 1..
Lactose, 40 grams (1⅓ ounces)..................
Sugar, 15 grams (½ ounce)......................
Lemon-juice, 30 c.c. (1 ounce)..................
Water, 4 or 5 ounces.

		Calories
For 2000 calories a day.		
Milk, 1¼ quarts (1250 c. c.)	....	1000
Cream, 8 ounces (240 c.c.)	....	500
Lactose, 4 ounces (120 grams)	....	500
This furnishes seven feedings each containing:		
Milk, 7 ounces (210 c. c.)	....	140
Cream, 1 ounce (30 c. c.)	....	60
Lactose, (½ ounce) (18 grams)	....	72
or		
Eggs, 2	....	150
Lactose, 125 grams (4 ounces)	....	500
Sugar, 15 grams (½ ounce)	....	60
Milk, 1000 c.c. (32 ounces)	....	700
Cream, 240 c.c. (8 ounces)	....	480
Cocoa, 5 grams	....	25
Orange juice, 60 c.c. (2 ounces)	....	30
Lemon juice	..................negligible	00
Coffee, 150 c.c. (5 ounces)	....	00
This furnishes one feeding containing:		
Coffee, 150 c.c. (5 ounces)	....	00
Egg, 1	....	75
Lactose, 50 grams (1⅔ ounces)	....	200
Sugar, 5 grams (⅙ ounce)	....	20
One feeding containing;		
Cocoa, 5 grams (⅙ ounce)	....	25
Milk, 120 c.c. (4 ounces)	....	80
Cream, 60 c.c. (2 ounces)	....	120
Lactose, 50 grams (1⅚ ounces)	....	200
One feeding containing:		
Egg, 1	....	75
Lactose 40 grams (1⅓ ounce)	....	160
Sugar, 10 grams (⅓ ounce)	....	40
Orange juice 120 c.c. (4 ounces)	....	60
Lemon juice 1 to 2 teaspoonfuls		
Four feedings containing:		
Milk, 210 c.c. (7 ounces)	....	140
Cream, 45 c.c. (1¼ ounces)	....	90
For 2500 calories a day:		
Milk, 1½ quarts (2500 c. c.)	....	1000
Cream, 8 ounces (240 c. c.)	....	500
Lactose, 8 ounces (240 gm.)	....	1000
This furnishes seven feedings each containing:		
Milk, 7 ounces (210 c. c.)	....	140
Cream, 1 ounce (30 c. c.)	....	60
Lactose, 1 ounce (30 grams)	....	144
or		

37

Calories

Milk, 1000 c.c (32 ounces) 700
Cream, 240 c.c. (8 ounces)........................ 480
Eggs, 3.. 225
Lactose, 165 grams (5½ ounces).................. 660
Sugar, 40 grams (1⅓ ounces) 160
Bread, 1 slice, 30 grams (1 ounce) 80
Uneeda Biscuit, 1................................ 25
Butter, 10 grams (⅓ ounce)...................... 80
Orange juice, 120 c.c. (4 ounces)................. 60
Lemon juice (1¼ ounce).......................... 20

This furnishes one feeding containing:

Coffee, 150 c.c. (5 ounces)....................... 00
Egg, 1.. 75
Lactose, 40 grams (1⅓ ounces)................... 160
Sugar, 5 grams (⅙ ounce) 20
Toast, 1 slice................................... 80
Butter, 10 grams (⅓ ounce) 80

One feeding containing:

Egg, 1.. 75
Lactose, 50 grams 1⅔ ounces).................... 200
Orange juice, 120 c.c. (4 ounces)................. 60
Sugar, 10 grams ⅓ ounce)....................... 40
Lemon juice to taste.
Water.

One feeding containing:

Egg, 1.. 75
Milk, 200 c.c. (6⅔ ounces)...................... 140
Cream, 40 c.c. (1⅓ ounces)..................... 80
Lactose, 25 grams (⅚ ounces).................. 100
Sugar, 5 grams (⅙ ounce) 20
Flavor with vanilla or nutmeg.

One feeding containing

Lactose, 60 grams (2 ounces).................... 240
Sugar, 20 grams (⅔ ounce)...................... 60
Lemon juice 30 or 40 c.c. (1 or 1½ ounces)........ 15

Four feedings each containing:

Milk, 200 c.c. (6⅔ ounces)...................... 140
Cream, 50 c.c. (1⅔ ounces)..................... 100

For 3000 calories a day.

Milk, 1¼ quarts (1250 c. c.) 1000
Cream, 1 pint (480 c.c.)......................... 1000
Lactose, 1 ounce (30 gms.)...................... 1000

This furnishes eight feedings each containing:

Milk, 6 ounces (180 c. c.)....................... 120
Cream, 2 ounces (60 c. c.) 120
Lactose, 1 ounce (30 gm.)....................... 120

or

Breakfast: **Calories**

	Calories
Farina	100
Toast, 1 slice (30 grams before toasting)	80
Cream, 100 c.c. (3⅓ ounces)	200
Butter, 8 grams (⅓ ounce)	60
Lactose, 40 grams (1⅓ ounces)	160
Sugar, 20 grams (⅔ ounce)	80
Coffee, 1 large cup or 2 small cups (300 c.c.)	00

10–10.30 A.M.;

	Calories
Milk, 200 c.c. (6⅔ ounces)	140
Cream, 50 c.c. (1⅔ ounces)	100

Dinner:

	Calories
Egg, 2	150
Potato, medium, about	100
Bread, 1 slice, or roll, 1, about	80
Butter, 30 grams (1 ounce)	234
Apple, 1 medium (pared and cored)	75
Sugar, 15 grams (½ ounce	60

3 to 4 P.M.;

	Calories
Tea, 150–200 c.c. (5–6 ½ ounces)	
Lactose, 50 grams (1⅔ ounces)	200
Sugar, 5 grams (⅙ ounce)	20
Cream, 50 c.c. (1⅔ ounces)	100
Crackers, 3 uneeda, or 2 soda, toasted	75
Butter, 8 grams (½ ounce)	62

Supper:

	Calories
Rice, 25 grams (1 ounce) or farina, cooked with	100
Milk, 100 c.c. (3⅓ ounces)	720
Toast, 30 grams (1 slice)	80
Butter, 8 grams (½ ounce)	62
Sugar, 5 grams (for cereal) (⅙ ounce)	20
Cream, 60 c.c. (2 ounces)	120
Orange, 1 slice	100
Sugar, 5 grams (with orange)	20

Potato baked, served with butter, apple baked with 15 grams sugar and about 8 grams butter. Some patients will eat more butter if unsalted butter is used in the diet.

8 to 9 P.M.

	Calories
Cocoa, 5 grams (⅛ ounce)	25
Sugar, 10 grams (⅓ ounce)	140
Milk, 150 c.c. (5 ounces)	105
Cream, 30 c.c. (1 ounce)	60
Lactose, 25 grams (⅚ ounce)	100

For 3900 calories a day

	Calories
Milk, 1½ quarts (1500 c. c.)	1000
Cream, 1 pint (500 c. c.)	1000
Lactose, 16 ounces (480 grams)	900

Calories

This furnishes eight feedings each containing:

Milk, 6 ounces (180 c. c.)........................ 120
Cream, 2 ounces (60 gm.)........................ 120
Lactose, 2 ounces (60 gm.) 240

Great care must be taken that the physician's enthusiasm for preventing loss of weight should not lead him to allow too great a jump in food quantities.

The steps of increasing the amounts allowed must be gradual or almost certainly the digestive organs will be overtaxed and one must not forget that a patient's appetite is a fair indicator of the amount of food to allow. A high calorie diet forced down a patient with anorexia would most certainly lead to a gastronomic fall.

TYPHOID DIET No. 3.[1] (CALORIES 3910)

This diet is best in later stages or in convalescence.
(9.00 A.M., 1.00, 3.00, 7.00 10.00 P.M. and 1.00 and 4.00 A.M.)

Milk, 6 oz., total, 1260 c.c.; calories, 860.
Cream, 2 oz., total, 420 c.c.; calories, 840.
Lactose, 10 gm., total, 70 gm.; calories, 280. Total calories, 1980.

At 11.00 A.M.:
Egg (one), calories, 80.
Mashed potato (20 gm.), calories, 20.
Custard (4 oz.), calories, 250.
Toast or bread (1 slice), calories, 80.
Butter (20 gm.), calories, 150.
Coffee.
Cream (2 oz.), calories, 120.
Lactose (20 gm.), calories, 80. Total calories, 780.

At 5.00 P.M.:
Egg (one), calories, 80.
Cereal (3 tablespoonfuls), calories, 150.
Cream (2 oz.), calories, 120.
Apple sauce (1 oz.), calories, 30.
Tea.
Cream (3 oz.), calories, 180.
Lactose (20 gm.), calories, 80. Total calories, 640.

At 7.00 A.M.:
Egg (one), calories, 80.
Toast (one slice), calories, 80.

[1] Diets 3, 4 and 5 are taken from Coleman and Shaffer: Am. Jour. Med. Sc. 1912, p. 77.

Butter (20 gm.), calories, 150.
Coffee.
Cream (2 oz.), calories, 120.
Lactose (20 gm.), calories, 80.   Total calories, 510.
Milk-sugar lemonade may be substituted for the milk mixture at 3.00 o'clock.
Approximate values: Protein, 90; fat, 250; carbohydrate, 318; calories, 3910.

TYPHOID DIET No 4.   (CALORIES 5580.)

Milk, 5 oz., 9.00, 11.00 A.M., 1.00 P.M.; 1200 c.c.; calories, 820.
Cream, 2 oz., 3.00, 7.00, 10.00 P.M.; 480 c.c.; calories, 1440.
Lactose, 15 gm., 1.00 and 4.00 A.M., 120 c.c.; calories, 480. Total calories, 2740.
At 11.00 A.M.:
Eggs (two), calories, 160.
Toast (2 slices), calories, 160.
Butter (20 gm.),, calories, 150.
Mashed potato (70 gm.), calories, 70.
Custard (8 oz.), calories, 500.   Total calories, 1040.
At 5.00 P.M.:
Egg (one), calories, 80.
Toast (2 slices), calories, 160.
Butter (20 gm.), calories, 150.
Cereal (6 tablespoonfuls), calories, 290.
Cream (4 oz.), calories, 240.
Apple sauce (1 oz.), calories, 30.
Cream (2 oz.), calories, 120.
Lactose (20 gm.), calories, 80.   Total calories, 1150.
At 7.00 A.M.;
Egg (one), calories, 80.
Toast (2 slices), calories, 160.
Butter (20 gm.), calories, 150.
Coffee.
Cream (3 oz.), calories, 180.
Lactose (20 gm.), calories, 80.   Total calories, 650.
Approximate values: Protein, 122; fat, 293; carbohydrates, 515; calories, 5580.

TYPHOID DIET No. 5.

This furnishes 5570 calories and is perhaps less bulky.
Milk, 5 oz., 9.00, 11.00 A.M., 1.00 P.M.; 1050 c.c.; calories, 700.

Cream, 3 oz., 7.00, 10.00 P.M.; 630 c.c.; calories, 1260.

Lactose, 15 gm., 1.00 and 4.00 A.M.; 105 gm.; calories, 420.

At 11.00 A.M.:

Eggs (two), calories, 160.

Potato (mashed), 80 gm., calories, 80.

Custard (8 oz.), calories, 500.

Creamed chicken (1 oz.), calories, 50.

Toast (two slices), calories, 150.   Total calories, 950.

At 5.00 P.M.:

Toast (2 slices), calories, 160.

Cereal (2 tablespoonfuls), calories, 290.

Cream (2 oz.), calories, 120.

Lactose (20 gm.), calories, 80.   Total calories, 650.

Use chicken only after convalescence is established.

At 3.00 P.M., lemonade (lactose, 120 gm.).

At 7.00 P.M.:

Egg (one), calories, 80.

Cereal (5 tablespoonfuls), calories, 250.

Cream (2 oz.), calories, 120.

Toast (2 slices), calories, 160.

Butter (20 gm.), calories, 150.

Coffee.

Cream (2 oz.), calories, 120.

Lactose (20 gm.), calories, 90.   Total calories, 960.

Approximate values: Protein, 106 to 115; fats, 212; carbohydrates, 450 to 570.

The larger numbers include chicken and lactose lemonade.

Typhoid Diet without Milk.—Occasionally one undoubtedly meets with a case that cannot tolerate milk in any form, and in such substances Garton[1] had devised a diet leaving milk products entirely out which is about as follows:

6.30 A.M.   Cup of hot coffee, sugar, 2 drams (8 gm.); two slices of zweiback or toast, butter.

8.30 A.M.   One portion of oatmeal or Robinson's prepared barley, according to bowel conditions, with six buttered crackers, saltines.

10.30 A.M.   Six ounces of soup, various kinds (180 c. c.).

12.30 M.   One medium-baked potato, mashed and prepared with butter and salt; two thin slices of buttered toast, hot, and one cup of hot weak tea with 2 drams (8 gm.), of sugar.

2.30 P.M.   Two teaspoonfuls of pudding, bread or tapioca; six saltines.

[1] Mil. Surg., Washington, 1912, xxx, 291.

4.30 P.M.   Two ounces (60 gm.), of rice, farina or cream of wheat mixed with 1 ounce (30 gm.), of butter and 4 drams (16 gm.), of sugar.

6.30 P.M.   Three slices buttered toast.

8.30 P.M.   Six ounces (180 c. c.), of soup.

The feeding periods may be made three hours if preferred by the patient.

Diet in Typhoid Complications.—Intestinal indigestion, as exhibited by diarrhea or tympanites, must be treated etiologically so far as possible, cutting out of the diet anything which apparently disagrees, *e. g.*, high fats may be shown by examination of the stools to produce fatty stools; great fermentation of the stool as tested by Einhorn's saccharometer shows more than the normal production of gas in the tube (5 gm. of a normal stool should produce at most but a small bubble of gas in twelve hours' incubation). This would indicate either a reduction of the carbohydrates or the giving of some diastatic ferment (such as takadiastase) to assist the normal secretions. When the diarrhea or tympanites is slight, or at most very moderate, it is possible to take time to make these more exact observations to arrive at a definite conclusion as to the cause of the disturbance; when, however, the tympanites develops rapidly and assumes menacing proportions, it is necessary to stop all carbohydrate feeding at once. This condition is perhaps best practically combated by the giving of artificially ripened milk in small amounts, diluted or not, and as well, giving some reliable preparation of the Bulgarian bacillus. See page 569 (Bacteriology in Typhoid). This is especially true and accomplishes the desired result in most instances in which the patients have been fed with considerable lactose, but is almost equally efficacious in any form of carbohydrate fermentation. To some extent tympanites is due to lack of intestinal tone, quite as much or more than to actual fermentation, and when patients are properly nourished this is much less apt to be present. The use of broths, egg albumen in fruit juice and peptonized milk also come into consideration.

Intestinal Hemorrhage.—The question always comes up in case of hemorrhage as to whether the patients should continue to be fed or not. If the hemorrhage is severe, so that the patient shows a constitutional reaction to it, by a drop in temperature, increased pulse, or evident anemia, it is safest to suspend all feeding for six to twelve hours, so that the whole canal can be put at rest by morphine and local applications. After this period, however, it is best to begin feeding again, using preferably thoroughly peptonized milk (peptonized one and a half or two hours), so that it may be absorbed high up in the intestine, still giving the lower ileum as much rest as possible. For slight hemorrhages there is no need of suspending feeding liquid nourishment, for the higher the nutrition is kept the better chance there is of there being little hemorrhage.

Perforation.—At the first sign of perforation or its precursor, local peritonitis, all feeding should be at once stopped and the medical man makes way for his surgical brother.

Nausea and Vomiting.—This is an infrequent symptom, but should be treated from the dietetic point of view as laid down in the section on Irritable Stomach, p. 338.

Water.—The feeding of typhoid would be incomplete without special reference to water-drinking. This is a most important matter, and in the presence of a good circulatory system the amount taken should be large, 1500 to 2500 c.c. (1½ or 2½ quarts) per day or more. The removal of certain metabolic by-products by the urine is distinctly favored, and, indeed, a favorable prognosis of a case is often in direct ratio to the urine output.

Paratyphoid Fever.—The dietary regulations set forth for typhoid hold equally for paratyphoid fever.

MALARIAL FEVER.

There are no special indications for diet in this disease other than those which would be useful in any fever. The stomach is often irritable, and vomiting may be present, which may be increased by the quinine; if this is so the feedings indicated for an irritable stomach will be found useful, such as iced fluids in small amounts, Delafield's mixture, buttermilk, or buttermilk and Vichy. The gastric symptoms are rarely severe except at times in the estivo-autumnal type in which case the quinine must be given by hypodermic injection in appropriate solution.

SCARLET FEVER.

The diet in scarlet fever will be more fully discussed in the section on Pediatric Feeding in the Acute Exanthemata, and so far as adult feeding is concerned, much the same rules hold true. The patients should be fed on liquids for the first three weeks, of which milk modified upward, as in the typhoid milk diets, or downward, as in infant feedings, should form the bulk. Indeed, the liquid diets No. 1 and No. 2

as given under Typhoid would be distinctly useful, leaving out eggs in any form at first. After the first three weeks it is still necessary to be careful, by excluding meats and making the bulk of the foods from milk, gruel, cereals, custards, milk toast, etc. Should the kidneys become involved, diets suitable to the particular condition present may be found under the section on Feeding in Renal Diseases.

SMALLPOX.

No special diet is to be recommended for this disease, except that care should be taken during the initial period of fever to give sufficient calories and protein to prevent emaciation and loss of nitrogen, so that during the stage of suppuration the patient may be kept in as strong and vigorous condition as possible. If this rule is carried out convalescence will be shortened. When the fever is high, fluids or semisolids are best, adding soft solids as soon as the patient will take them. The milk, cream, and lactose formulæ recommended for typhoid will be found convenient in making sure the patient gets the full allowance of food, for it is so easy to give a little broth, a little gruel, etc., now and then as the patient wants or will take it, and it will usually be found that the food value of such a diet is away below nutritional requirements. If this hap-hazard plan is followed the patients reach the stage of secondary fever from suppuration in an entirely unnecessarily depleted condition, vastly increasing the risks of this period. During the period of suppuration a return to liquids and semisolids must be made until the patients have strength to take soft solids, which may be given as soon as they will take them. In any event, water should be forced, and as much given at frequent intervals as can be taken, either plain, aërated, or flavored with fruit juices.

CEREBRAL OR CEREBROSPINAL MENINGITIS.

The diet best for these conditions follows the suggestions laid down for any fever, and consists of milk, gruels, lactose, milk and cream mixtures, as in typhoid fever or semisolid feedings, depending on the stage and variety of the disease. Great importance should be given to seeing that the patients take sufficient food to maintain their nutrition to as nearly a normal degree as may be, for, as has been pointed out repeatedly in these pages, the better the nutrition, the better the disease-fighting qualities of the patient and the shorter the convalescence. So long as the patients are conscious or the swallowing reflex remains intact, fluids may be given by a feeding cup or spoon, but when coma becomes marked, or when it is not possible or practical for them to take the necessary food, recourse must be had to feeding by gavage, either through the mouth or nose. (See Gavage.) This should be done at regular intervals, but preferably not oftener than three or possibly four times in twenty-four hours, on account of the possibility of irritating the nose or throat by the passage of the feeding tube.

If the digestion is poor, as it often is in children with these diseases, it may be advisable to predigest the food and give peptonized milk mixtures, and dextrinized gruels, adding other foods cautiously as the digestion improves. At times there is marked vomiting with these cerebral lesions, central in origin. It is wise to continue feedings regularly in spite of the vomiting, but in smaller quantities and at more frequent intervals, even down to half-hourly feedings. One can only determine by trial what the best interval for feeding is or the amount best suited to each case.

If vomiting is increased by feeding it will then be necessary to omit mouth feeding and give what nourishment one can by rectum.

MEASLES.

The dietetic management of measles is for the most part that of any acute infection with fever.

During the early stages nothing but liquid food should be given, together with such soft semifluid food as very soft-boiled egg, gruels, ice-cream, and meat or gelatin jellies giving as nearly the full caloric needs of the individual and as the appetite and digestion will permit. Since the eruption occurs on the mucous surface of the intestines, as well as on the skin, it is necessary to continue the semisolid or very soft character of the food as long as the skin eruption lasts (as the intestinal manifestations presumably remain about the same length of time), for it is quite possible by harsh or rough food to cause a breaking down of some of the areas of intestinal hyperemia, with consequent ulcer formation occurring secondarily. When the eruption has quite faded the diet may be steadily increased, returning to a normal diet early in convalescence.

INFLUENZA (GRIPPE).

The fever is the determining factor in this disease, and the patients may have any simple food that their appetite calls for, following for the most part the suggestions for feeding in fevers in which there are no special dietary indications. Since the manifestations of grippe are so varied, the diet may often be judiciously regulated in view of the particular organs affected, *i. e.*, if the bronchial tree is principally involved the feedings should be regulated as in bronchitis; if the gastro-intestinal form is present, due regard must be had to giving foods which are non-irritating to the stomach and intestine; particularly when there is vomiting, special care is needed. Under these circumstances, after a few hours of absolute gastric rest, one may give small amounts of buttermilk plain or diluted with Vichy.

Delafield's mixture is often well borne when the patients can take nothing else. This consists of equal parts of milk, cream, and Vichy, with cerium oxalate gr. x, soda bicarbonate gr. xx, to each 4 ounces of the mixture. This should be given iced and in dram doses, at first every twenty to thirty minutes, increasing the amount gradually and lengthening the period. Sometimes iced malted milk will be retained or egg white with orange juice and powdered ice. Afterward the patient can take a more liberal diet of soft solids, then rapidly increasing to full diet.

ACUTE ARTICULAR RHEUMATISM.

During the past few years there has been a complete change in the conception of the etiology of this disease, the humoral theory, or, to put it in modern language, the theory of a disturbed body metabolism, as the cause of this disease has been entirely superseded by the proved infectious origin of much of this form of articular inflammation. Much experimental work has been done to prove this latter, and numerous observers have been able, by inoculation of animals with cultures from the throats of rheumatic patients to produce attacks of joint inflammation which closely resemble the conditions found in this disease. The offending organism said to be responsible for this, and obtained from the tonsils, abscesses at the roots of teeth or, in fact, from any focus of pus infection, is a form of streptococcus. Whether there is a distinct strain of this bacterium which causes only rheumatic lesions is exceedingly doubtful, as it is much more likely that it is one of the ordinary groups of streptococci, which, for some as yet unknown reason, has a predilection for the serous membranes of the body, particularly those of the joints and heart. By complement-fixation tests, Hastings claims to have differentiated several different strains of streptococci, all of which are apparently the cause of articular lesions at times. While therefore the humoral theory of this disease has been almost completely given up for a bacterial conception, it is still true that marked metabolic changes accompany the condition, as shown by the excessive acid perspiration and excessive urinary acidity, greater than that which is found in any other disease except possibly in a marked diabetic acidosis. It is not at all unlikely that the metabolic changes which often precede a rheumatic manifestation, may have much to do with the lowered resistance to the streptococci as is the case in rheumatism.

Diet in Acute Articular Rheumatism.—Diet therefore in this disease has a twofold relation, that to the general condition of a bacterial invasion with resulting fever and other usual evidences of infection, and as well, to the metabolic changes which are probably, for the most part, secondary to the infection, or which at least accompany it and may stand in some etiological relationship, if only as a predisposing cause. So far as diet relates merely to the infection, we could stop at the general indications for diet in any fever, but the hyperacid condition of the excretions, notably the sweat and urine, must be taken into account in prescribing a suitable diet, and certain limitations are necessary on this account which would not otherwise be called for. During the first few days of acute fever after a thorough intestinal purge, the diet should consist mainly of milk products, and gruels, such as plain milk; milk, cream and Vichy; junket, Vichy and buttermilk; barley, rice and farina gruels may also be used. Water in large amount is grateful, either plain, as Vichy, and orange or lemonade made with very little sugar. Feedings should be given every two or three hours.

After the first few days of acute illness, and when the appetite begins to improve, additions to the diet may be made of other cereals, stale bread and butter, fruits, especially oranges or scraped or baked apple, baked potato with cream or butter, then green vegetables. Lastly, egg and white-meated fish, such as cod, halibut and bass and chicken. These animal products should not be added until the temperature has been normal for ten days to two weeks, and then in only small amounts. Eggs are an earlier exception, however.

The particular foods which should be avoided during a rheumatic attack, and for some time afterward, are meat soups and meats which, on account of their purine content, tend to produce acid and increase the uric acid in the blood.

Sugar, except in minimal amounts, should be omitted from the diet on account of its tendency to produce acid fermentation in the digestive canal. Tea and coffee are allowable only in great moderation, and well diluted with milk or water. Alcohol should be prohibited in any amount, and is not medically needed. Preserves, cake, and all such foods are to be avoided, as well as some of the hyperacid fruits, such as currants, gooseberries, and certain acid cherries. There is also a strong prejudice against the use of strawberries by rheumatic people not only during an attack but also for a long time afterward. The foundation for this prejudice is not clear, and is certainly not established by scientific analysis but rather from clinical observation. Like some other unexplained clinical data it probably has some sound reason behind it, and until proved innocent, strawberries should be omitted from the rheumatic's dietary.

Subacute Rheumatism.—This stage of a rheumatic infection should be treated dietetically on the same lines as a late stage of the acute process, and the same general rules apply, although here it is rather more necessary to see that the patients take a sufficient quantity of food to make up any loss occasioned by the fever, and a low diet during the most acute stage when the appetite is poor. The same necessity exists for abstinence from the acid-producing foods as in acute rheumatism, notably meat products, except occasionally; sweets and all indigestible foods in general should be avoided.

Chronic Rheumatism (*Chronic Infectious Arthritis*).—This is a disease distinct entirely from gout, although after forty years of age there is often some difficulty in making a differential diagnosis. This is usually facilitated by an estimation of the amount of blood uric acid, easily done by Folin's method. If the disease is not gout as shown by a normal blood uric acid (0.5 to 2 mg. per 100 c.c. of blood) the condition is one of a chronic infection, with often the usual accompaniments of anemia and malnutrition. The diet must be full and almost unrestricted, as the first indications are to nourish the patients satisfactorily and to increase their resistance to the infection. The only restrictions necessary are that meat and sweets should be taken in moderation.

The question of using alcohol in these conditions often comes up, and it may be stated that alcohol is of no direct use except occasionally as an aid to the appetite, and except when needed for this purpose is better left out. Steady users of alcohol are more prone to infections than others, and infections have a stronger hold on even a moderately alcoholic subject than on an abstainer.

In these patients who are subjects of this chronic infection all measures which raise resistance should be employed—fresh air, hydrotherapy, and forced feeding if necessary. In addition, finding the primary focus of infection wherever located, should be done, if possible, with its prompt removal, whether in tonsils, tooth root, pelvic organs, prostate, bone, etc. Often great assistance is rendered by autogenous vaccines in clearing up the persistent symptoms, provided, of course, the focus of infection is found.

Care should be taken not to produce indigestion by overfeeding or giving indigestible foods. Gastro-intestinal catarrh must be avoided by a proper dietary.

TETANUS.

In tetanus it is not so much a question of what food we shall give, but the form in which it is given is most important, and of still greater concern is the method of feeding. In the early stages before the jaws are completely locked, semisolids and liquids may be given by mouth; but even at this stage any disturbance may precipitate a muscular spasm, and great difficulty is often experienced in getting sufficient food into the patients to nourish them. In the later stage, when the jaws are firmly locked, feeding may be done by putting the liquid food in the mouth between the teeth and inside the cheek, allowing it to get into the throat between the teeth or at the back. This is, of course, facilitated if any teeth are missing on one side. If this is not practical, liquids may be given by gavage through a nasal tube cocainizing the nose and pharynx by a nasal spray of a 2 to 4 per cent. solution. This may help to obviate the tetanic spasm so easily brought on by the least external irritation.

If in spite of the cocain the spasms occur, it may be necessary to give a few whiffs of chloroform and then to put down a pint or more of concentrated food such as recommended for suralimentation (see p. 550). This can be done twice a day. Water may be given by mouth in one of these ways, or if reflex spasm is excited a continuous Murphy drip may be used. If the outcome is favorable, feedings can be given by mouth as soon as the jaws are unlocked, with a return to soft solids and normal food as rapidly as the patient's condition warrants it.

YELLOW FEVER.

Since the prophylaxis of yellow fever has been proved so sure and comparatively easy in the United States, only an occasional case imported into a new district is likely to be met with, although the southern countries suffer endemically from this disease.

Most cases present three stages: the first stage of onset with fever, then a stage of remission, which may be permanent, or a third stage may set in of increased severity, which is characterized by the presence of black vomit.

During the first two or three days no food should be given, but water must be supplied in large amounts; if vomiting begins early, so that nothing can be given by mouth, water may be given by rectum or even by hypodermoclysis, although this latter is seldom necessary. Fortunately the rectum and colon are quite tolerant in this disease, and after the onset may be regularly used for rectal feeding and the giving of water, so that although the full food requirements cannot be given in this way, sufficient food can be absorbed to materially help in maintaining nutrition. (See Artificial Nutrition.)

If vomiting is severe it is useless to try to use mouth-feeding in any degree, but during the period of remission the attempt may be made to begin to feed by the mouth with the same foods recommended for feeding in cholera.

If the patients proceed to the third stage with vomiting and diarrhea it is useless to try to give any food by mouth or rectum, but some relief may be obtained by enteroclysis of warm normal saline, and fluid can also be gotten into the circulation by hypodermoclysis or saline venous infusions. It is possible even in this stage that a little iced champagne or crushed ice with diluted brandy may be given by mouth or drop doses of pure carbolic acid in 1 or 1½ ounces of water may be useful in quieting the stomach. In this condition little can be expected from food, and about all one can do is to keep the blood concentration as nearly normal as possible by the use of saline solution by one route or another.

If this third stage is successfully passed and the patient is again able to take nourishment by mouth we can begin with egg albumen in dilute orange juice iced, koumyss or peptonized milk, malted milk, and cold bouillon, gradually returning to a diet of soft solids, and so gradually back to normal feedings.

CHOLERA.

The dietetics of cholera have to do with food in its relation to prevention and its nutritional role during the various stages of the disease.

In every case of cholera the vibrio enters the system by way of the alimentary canal, there being no evidence that it

gains admission in any other way. Since this fact is firmly
established the question of food and water prophylaxis, as in
typhoid fever, assumes paramount importance and whenever there is the least danger of infection all the rules of
prevention must be applied to the food and fluid intake of
all the residents in any threatened district. In order to
accomplish this satisfactorily the following rules should be
observed:

Dietetic Rules in Cholera.—1. No water should be drunk
unless sterilized by boiling; and even water for brushing the
teeth and washing should be sterile.

2. No fluids should be taken unless known to be sterile by
virtue of previous sterilization, full pasteurization or with an
alcohol content of at least 5 per cent., such as wines and
liquors. Beer and ale unless made of sterile water should
not be taken.

3. All vegetables should be thoroughly boiled before using,
nothing raw being taken. Fruits should be eaten only when
cooked.

4. Eating and cooking utensils must be washed only in
boiling water.

5. Ice made of distilled or boiled water alone to be used.

6. The use of acidulated drinks is strongly advocated by
most authorities, as acids are inimicable to the cholera vibrio.
For this purpose lemonade made with the addition of 10 to
15 drops of dilute sulphuric or hydrochloric acids is recommended. Davis recommends the following: Tartaric acid,
15 gm. (½ oz.) in 1000 c.c. (1 quart) of sweetened sterile water
to be drunk freely.

All forms of indigestible foods or foods that are specially
laxative should be omitted from the diet of everyone at a
time of epidemic. After the disease has actually begun in
anyone the diet in the early stage is of great importance, and
should consist of meat jellies, gruels, peptonized milk or
ripened milk, koumyss, zoolak, or buttermilk.

In the middle stage of the disease, practically no food can
be kept down or kept in long enough to do any good, as the
vomiting and purging are extreme. The most that can be
done during this stage is to give cracked ice, with or without
a little champagne or diluted brandy; even these are usually
rejected, and we have to abandon attempts to feed by mouth.
Some writers have advised rectal feeding, but there is little
hope of success, as the peristalsis is so active that nothing
will be retained long enough for absorption. It is, however,
of great assistance in the algid stage to use thorough enteroclysis two or three times a day, inserting the rectal tube

six to eight inches and flushing out the bowel with large amounts of warm saline, using it hot, 105° to 108°.

The usefulness of this is twofold, as it cleanses the bowel and offers an opportunity for the absorption of a fair amount of fluid. The use of the same acid drinks is recommended as long as the stomach will retain them. The most serious problem in these cases is that of supplying sufficient fluid to the tissues, as these patients tend to be desiccated, and many perish from this who, if not so handicapped, would be able to overcome their infection. In order to meet this demand for fluids on the part of the system, water, best in the form of normal saline, must be gotten into the circulation in every way possible, by hypodermoclysis or more rapidly by saline infusion; the latter is more satisfactory, as it is so much more readily available to the dried-out tissues, and as much as 2000 to 3000 c.c. (2 or 3 quarts) may be given at once and repeated when necessary. Sterile saline can also be given intraperitonially. At first the results from the use of this method seemed to promise a great reduction in mortality, as it is so promptly led to clinical improvement; while it does help, the eventual prognosis is not so greatly altered by the procedure as was at first hoped.

Besides normal saline (0.6 per cent. salt solution), Hayem recommends the following intravenous infusion, 1½ or 2 quarts at a time.

Pure sodium chloride, 5 gm. (⅙ ounce).
Pure sodium sulphate, 10 gm. (⅓ ounce).
Water, 1000 c.c. (1 quart).

Since the successful use of human serum (ascitic fluid) by hypodermoclysis (see Artificial Nutrition) has been demonstrated, it would seem that this substance might be successfully employed in cholera, thereby furnishing the body with fluid, some protein, and probably some natural antitoxic substances. So far as is known this method has not been used in cholera, but might well deserve a trial should an opportunity present. When it is evident that improvement has set in, feedings may be begun of one of the liquid foods already referred to, or peptonized milk. If diarrhea still persists, milk preparations, as a rule, are not so well borne, and recourse must be made to farinaceous gruels, at first preferably dextrinized, later mixed with boiled milk or malted milk, meat jellies, clam broth, and oyster soup (served without the oysters) may all be used. Later, getting back to soft farinaceous puddings, then other soft foods, carrying the patient through the convalescence on much the same diet as that used after typhoid fever.

38

PERITONITIS.

Acute Peritonitis.—This is always a surgical condition, and whether an operation is required or not will decide whether any form of diet is indicated.   If operation is needed no food whatever should be given after making the diagnosis; cracked ice may be allowed and water furnished by rectum either as repeated enemata, 4 to 6 ounces, every three or four hours, or a continuous Murphy drip will answer the purpose.

If an operation must be postponed or is contra-indicated for any reason, Ochsner's treatment recommended for acute appendicitis is the best method of procedure (see p. 403). Lavage of the stomach may be performed if vomiting is present, and repeated often enough to keep this under control.

After operation, if there is a more or less general peritonitis, it is best not to give food by mouth for several days, water being supplied as for acute peritonitis, or even given by hypodermoclysis, if in spite of rectal salines the patients seem at all desiccated.   After three or four days if the acute symptoms are subsiding, one can begin to give egg albumen with orange juice and water, whey, broths (without fat), then thin farinaceous gruels, buttermilk either alone or diluted with Vichy, then soft solids, and gradually build up a normal dietary.

Chronic Peritonitis.—If this is tuberculous, or due to a low-grade infection from some one or other of the various bacterial groups, the diet may be full and nourishing, avoiding only indigestible foods or those likely to cause flatulence, such as sweets, potato, uncooked starches, vegetables of the cabbage family, onions, fresh bread, cake, pies, etc.   Any increase of gas is sure to cause discomfort by pulling on adhesions.   It is best to feed rather frequently and in moderate amount; the total caloric value of the food should be high.

Aside from these restrictions the patients may eat what they like, but care should be taken by the physician in charge to see that they get their full quota of food in some form.

CHRONIC INFECTIONS.

The feeding of cases of chronic infections of all sorts is of great importance, for many times the possession of a good stomach and digestion will do more toward saving the day for the patient, who, for example, is the subject of a chronic sepsis, than anything that can be done medicinally.

The chronic tuberculous infections have been discussed under a separate heading, to which the reader is referred, and here we found that it was wise not to overfeed the patient too greatly. On the other hand, in practically all other chronic infections the chief indication is to give as much nourishing food as the patient can possibly digest. Due regard must, of course, be given to the individual digestive capacity, but within that there is no limit. Special attention must be paid to the whims of appetite that are often the index of what will best agree, and as well, all food should be comparatively of slight bulk and concentratedly nourishing, *i. e.*, large amounts of vegetable food and fruits should be avoided, as taking valuable room best reserved for real food. It is also often necessary to feed fairly high quantities of protein, often up to 150 gm. per day or more, care being taken to keep the purine content rather lower than in a normal diet in order that the kidneys in particular shall not be irritated by the excretion of unnecessary amounts of uric acid and other xanthine bases. Often, however, patients do well on less protein.

In cases of any prolonged infection it is especially necessary to pay great attention not alone to the tastes of the patients but to the method of serving the food as well. Food appetizingly served is already half-eaten, to paraphrase a popular saying, and every effort must be made to stimulate a patient's desire for food. Under this latter would come into consideration the use of some form of alcoholic beverage taken with the meal. Depending upon the form of the infection, this is usually allowable, provided the excretory organs are in good condition, and only the lighter forms of drinks are allowed. An occasional glass of light-beer, claret, white wine, seltzer, or even a little whiskey well diluted with Vichy or other carbonated or plain water often adds very greatly to the ease with which food can be taken, and little or nothing extra to the work of the excretory organs.

In order that there shall be no mistake in regard to the quantities of food taken, it is always best to reckon out the patient's needs calorically for their normal height and weight and then to add sufficient calories to cover the extra catabolism occasioned by the fever. Here we can again make use of Coleman's figures as given under Typhoid Fever, as he has shown that in order to keep these patients in nitrogenous equilibrium and body weight it is necessary to give them 40 to 45 calories per kilo, using considerable amounts of carbohydrate as the best sparer of body protein and fat. Of course it is not so necessary to keep to the limited range of food-stuffs that one must in treating an acute condition involving the integrity of the alimentary canal, as in typhoid but the greatest latitude may be granted, even including moderate amounts of meat, in spite of the presence of fever. Watch must be kept of the urine to see that there is no renal irritation or evidence of intestinal putrefaction, for in the presence of either, meat is best left alone. While a large amount of fruit and vegetable food cannot be taken, as already observed, a moderate use of them is not forbidden, and fruit juices are particularly useful in assisting the intake of considerable amounts of water, always a necessity, and also in providing a certain amount of nourishment, as in the case of grape juice, one pint of which contains about 360 calories (von Noorden) taken with meals and diluted with some effervescing water; this latter is of really great assistance.

One word in regard to the intervals of feeding. If a patient has sufficient appetite to take three main meals with an extra bite between meals and at bedtime, this is perhaps the best. As a rule this is not possible when there is considerable fever, in which case one can give a feeding every two hours, and at each alternate feeding, *i. e.*, every four hours, extras are given, such as soft solids, while at the two-hour intervals only a feeding of milk or gruel, etc., is used. Patients who cannot eat advantageously every two hours can be fed every three hours, making in this instance each feeding a soft and liquid feeding together. Each patient must be studied with this in mind in order to get in the greatest amount of food with the minimum of stuffing.

RHEUMATOID ARTHRITIS. ARTHRITIS DEFORMANS.

The etiology of this form of arthritis has been for a long time uncertain, some authorities classing it as a metabolic disease, others as a so-called rheumatic manifestation (infection). The two most prominent theories which traced the trouble to a disturbed metabolism considered it as a form of gout from a faulty purine metabolism, and the other blamed a faulty calcium metabolism for the disease. Accordingly, as one considered it due to either of these disturbances, the diet was modified to meet the demands of gout, *i. e.*, a low purine diet, or was ordered with a low calcium content. Calcium metabolism is a difficult subject, and it has never been clearly shown just what disturbance in the calcium exchange existed in these cases, although a certain amount of retention seemed probable.

On the basis of disturbed calcium metabolism, Bovaird designed the following diet, and in some cases seemed to get a certain amount of improvement; fancied or real.

Low Calcium Diet;
  Bread, 100 gm. (3⅓ oz.).
  Potatoes, 100 gm. (3⅓ oz.).
  Apple, 100 gm. (3⅓ oz.).
  Sugar, 50 gm. (1⅔ oz.).
  Butter, 50 gm. (1⅔ oz.).
  Boiled meat, 250 gm. (8⅓ oz.).
  Fish, 100 gm. (3⅓ oz.).
    Calcium content, 0.315 gm.
    Protein, 80 gm. (2⅔ oz.).
    Carbohydrate, 145 gm. (5 oz.).
    Fat, 100 gm. (3⅓ oz).
    Calories, 2000.

·As modern bacteriological methods have improved, increasing evidence has accumulated in favor of putting this disease among the chronic infections and today among most authorities this view is held.

Why a chronic infection should result in deformed joints in one case and simply enlarged joints in another is not, of course, clear, but both forms, chronic rheumatism and arthritis deformans, have certainly been arrested by the removal of a focus of chronic infection with or without the assistance of autogenous vaccines. It is probable that all these cases fall into this class and that metabolic changes affecting purines, calcium, or what not are secondary to the disturbance caused by the chronic infection.

On this basis (which today seems fairly clearly proved) our dietary regulations have to do again, as in the case of chronic rheumatism, merely with the effects of a chronic infection, such as malnutrition, anemia, etc. On this account the diet should be nourishing and even stimulating, containing a fair proportion of protein, much fat, and a considerable amount of carbohydrate, following largely the patient's appetite, with a due regard to the prevention of indigestion and obesity, both of which complications are rather prone to develop, since the patients are unable to take much exercise, or, in fact, in certain cases, any exercise.

Because of a sedentary life these patients frequently develop a disturbance of their purine metabolism and have gouty manifestations added to their other troubles. It is best therefore not to give the upper limit of protein allowance, and in some cases, besides curtailing the purines, as in gout, the patients are rendered more comfortable by a rather low protein allowance, 50 to 60 gm. per day. Such a reduction is particularly advisable if there is a renal insufficiency, a not uncommon accompaniment of any chronic infection.

Except for the limitations noted, the diet may be practically unrestricted, and those patients who are undernourished will be greatly improved by high calorie feeding, with some attention to muscular exercise by massage, vibration, and active or passive movements. Patients with arthritis deformans who by chance are obese and flabby will be helped by a diet which will remove the excess of fat, allow easier movement of the joints, and by attention to improvement in muscular tone by any one of the foregoing methods, provided the disability is too severe to allow of any form of natural exercise. The best means that Nature provides to fight a chronic infection is a properly nourished body, and the physician's first duty is to put his patient in the best possible condition of nutrition, omitting none of the ways or means that will accomplish this end.

CHAPTER XXXI.

DIET IN RELATION TO SURGICAL OPERATIONS

IT is only comparatively recently that anything like intelligent or painstaking attention has been given to the diet in cases about to be operated upon, and although more or less care has been given in the postoperative period, it has been largely a hit-or-miss attention, and when most needed has received little or inadequate thought. This was notably true in the case of operative procedures upon the digestive tract, where, as one would naturally expect, diet must be of paramount importance. The gravity of this is being realized, and considerable advance has been made in feeding these and other cases with greater exactness and care.

PREOPERATIVE DIET.

Except for abdominal operations it makes little difference how the patients are fed before operation except that the diet should be simple and somewhat lessened in amount the day before. No food whatever should be taken later than twelve to fourteen hours before operation, and the bowels should of course, be previously thoroughly moved.

In contradistinction to this is the care that should be given the diet in a patient about to have an abdominal section. Many cases who seek operation for some chronic trouble, but who are able to be about, reach the hospital or their home, after a busy day more or less tired, possibly somewhat nervous, go to bed, take a laxative and an enema in the morning before operation and wonder (or their surgeon wonders) why there is so much postoperative abdominal distention. The result is readily explained by the fact that the patient is nervously tired, has had lack of dietetic oversight before operation and incomplete intestinal emptying.

General Directions for Cases of Laparotomy.—Whenever possible, patients should go to bed or at least stop their ordinary activities and rest for from thirty-six to forty-eight hours before a major operation; twenty-four hours should be the minimum time. During the one and a half or two days the intestine should be kept fairly well cleared out by catharsis: castor oil, calomel (?), salts or merely cascara, aloes and salines. During the twelve to fourteen hours immediately preceding the operation no food whatever should be taken, but water allowed freely until two or three hours before, after which nothing but mouth washes are permitted. The diet during this preliminary day or two should be of the simplest sort: eggs, broth, purée soups, soft cereals, possibly a little chicken or beef, toast or stale bread and butter, custard, wine jelly (with little sugar), rice pudding. Drinks as weak tea or coffee, water, Vichy. Milk is best not given except as buttermilk to those who like it, and then not over two glasses a day. Koumyss or ripened milk may be used instead, for none of these forms of milk yield the thick curds that raw milk does, and are therefore less disturbing afterward. During the six to eight hours immediately preceding operation, and after the catharsis has begun to be effectual, the patients are given two or three very thorough enemata, with the object of leaving the colon as nearly empty as possible.

In spite of great preoperative care, some cases have a great deal of trouble afterward from gas, and many surgeons feel that the catharsis given, with the idea of clearing the intestine, results principally in irritating it, and while of course removing more or less of the intestinal contents, the food is hurried along without proper digestion, resulting in its fermentation with consequent gas production. These men advocate a light diet for a few days and merely cleansing the lower bowel by high enemata before operation.

Diet Preparatory to Gastric Operations.—When there is to be an operation involving opening the stomach, Finney advocates rendering this organ as nearly sterile as may be by giving only sterile food and drinks for a couple of days before operation, feeling that with a sterile intake the gastric juice will inhibit or kill the few organisms that do get in, so arriving at the antioperative moment with what is practically a sterile stomach; even the feeding utensils are sterile. Antiseptic and sterile mouth washes are used to help to insure the object sought. This can be true only in the presence of a normal or hyperacid gastric contents; with a hypo-acidity or achylia, sterilization of the stomach contents is not a practicability.

All this may result in reducing the danger of infection, but from a practical point of view it is difficult to believe that one can sterilize the buccal cavity and posterior nares. With ordinary care and a short fast before operation, with normal stomach secretion, the stomach is probably as nearly sterile as is necessary.

POSTOPERATIVE DIET.

In the ordinary case of operation, not upon the head or digestive canal and appendages, the postoperative diet may be simply arranged. As soon as the patient recovers from the anesthetic, water may be given in sips, increasing as rapidly as the stomach will tolerate it. In case of continued vomiting it is often a good plan either to wash the stomach out with a stomach-tube or give one or two glasses of water all at once to act in the same way if it is vomited. After a few hours, feedings may be started by giving a little iced milk, koumyss, egg albumen, whey with orange juice, gruel, or broth, increasing to soft diet as rapidly as the patient's appetite demands it.

Postoperative Diet for the Digestive Tube.—In operations about the mouth or throat, such as those for hare-lip, cleft-palate, and tonsillectomy, the diet must be exceedingly bland, only fluids being used, and usually iced food is more grateful than warm. Anything hot, of course, is distinctly uncomfortable or painful.

For cleft-palate operations it is often necessary to train children to take their food from a spoon or dropper before performing the operation, for it is quite impossible for them to nurse from the breast or bottle, or in certain cases it may be even necessary for a time to feed by nasal gavage.

Diet after Tonsillectomy.—At first small bits of cracked ice should be given to suck, and later iced milk is the best food, as it is absolutely non-irritating. Ice-cream is also grateful very early, but salty soups, gruels, or solid food should be postponed until the patient can swallow with comparative comfort. The sensations of the patient are the practical guides in feeding these people, and they may usually have what they like as soon as the throat is sufficiently healed. All rough, hard, scratchy, salt, acid, or peppery food should be given a wide berth.

Postoperative Gastric Diets.—Not enough attention has been given to this subject by surgeons, and taking gastro-enterostomy as a typical gastric operation, we may describe its dietary treatment in detail, other gastric operations being similarly dieted, *i. e.*, gastrostomy, pylorectomy, gastrectomy (partial), or for excision of ulcer or carcinoma.

Diet after Gastro-enterostomy and Other Gastric Operations.—It is only comparatively recently that any particular attention has been paid to the dietary treatment of patients following the operation of gastro-enterostomy, and on the whole it is still sadly neglected, the tendency of many surgeons, if not most, being to feed these patients, postoperatively, very liberally and too soon. It has been the writer's experience to have known of cases, not yet two weeks postoperative given full hospital diet containing, as it does, rather coarse food and even corned beef and cabbage. Why there should be this postoperative dietary lack of care it is difficult to see, except that the results of some cases of gastroenterostomy are so brilliant, despite this failure to give carefully selected food, that those directly responsible for the diets ordered have been prone to think that the chances are equally good for all cases. This, however, is not at all true, and the percentage of cases who are only partially relieved, who have relapses or who are total surgical failures, is still too large to make it anything less than imperative to give a proper diet after this operation. Bearing on this point it is only necessary to quote the following figures to make it evident that the results of operation are not always brilliant. Joslin[1] reports 82 cases of gastro-enterostomy done for gastric or duodenal ulcer, with the following late results: Cured, 47 per cent.; unrelieved, 14 per cent.; relieved, 19 per cent.; died, 20 per cent.

Peck,[2] in 74 cases of duodenal ulcer, found these late results: Cured, 68.9 per cent.; died, 8.1 per cent. The rest improved, unimproved, or untraced. The results of gastric ulcer were a little less favorable.

Records of the Presbyterian Hospital, 31 cases, one to six years postoperative, showed the following results: Cured, 64 per cent.; relieved, 18 per cent.; unrelieved or died, 18 per cent.

Kuttner, in 100 cases, cured 65 per cent.; relieved, 20 per cent.; unrelieved or died, 15 per cent.

Martin and Carrol[3] report the operation unsuccessful in 45 per cent. of cases observed by them.

It is quite true that these results are being constantly improved by better technic and selection of cases, and, indeed, if one could choose operator and case in every instance the resulting cures would probably be over 90 per cent. Since this is not possible, and one has to go by general averages, the necessity of doing everything postoperatively that will tend toward improving the results, is sufficiently evident.

The Diet.—For three days following the operation the patients should receive absolutely no food whatever. After the postoperative vomiting has ceased it is possible to give

[1] Jour. Am. Med. Assn., 1914, lxiii, 1836.
[2] Ibid., August 21, 1915, p. 660.
[3] Ann. Surg., May 15, 1915, p. 557.

small amounts of Celestin Vichy, or ordinary Vichy with the sparkle out of it, 1 or 2 ounces every hour or two. During this period extra water may be furnished the system by the Murphy drip or saline by the rectum may be given, 4 to 6 ounces every three or four hours. For those not afflicted with severe thirst it is even better to withhold water by mouth entirely for one or two days, as in the von Leube gastric ulcer cure. After the preliminary three-day period of starvation the routine of the von Leube or Sippy's alkaline cure may be advantageously begun and carried through, possibly with a little greater rapidity than in the ulcer cure, depending upon the condition of the ulcerated area as determined at the time of operation.

Von Leube Diet.[1]—When feedings are begun the second or third day the patients are given hourly 2 ounces of artificial Vichy, Celestin Vichy or alternating with 2 ounces of milk fully peptonized for two hours. Each day the milk is increased 1 or 2 ounces until 8 ounces are taken every two hours, and the Vichy increased 1 ounce each day until 4 ounces are taken every two hours. In this way fluids are given every hour, either Vichy or the peptonized milk. At the end of a week or ten days there may be added junket, fine cereal, milk toast, and many allow a soft-boiled egg. During the third week creamed fresh fish, such as halibut, or cod, mashed potato, cream of wheat, hominy, spaghetti, purée of vegetables, and creamed soups. Farinaceous desserts, such as farina, tapioca, cornstarch, blanc mange, and custard. The patients will do well to avoid all alcoholic beverages for many months after the operation, but after the second week, tea, cocoa, or a little milk and coffee, if it agrees, may be taken. Everything must be done to avoid increased gastric acidity. and the free use of soda bicarbonate with calcined magnesia one hour after meals, the latter in amounts sufficient to keep the bowels regular, should be given to keep the acidity at the lowest point possible.

It is absolutely essential for the best possible success of the operative results to insist on this routine or some equally conservative diet, for even though there is a new opening, unless the pylorus is occluded, the gastric contents are in part discharged through the pylorus and so pass over a duodenal ulcer; and of course if the ulceration is on the gastric side of the pyloric ring the care in diet is even more self-evidently necessary. Then too, the edges of the new stoma are raw and irritated, and need protection, and great care in the prevention of further irritation which would naturally

[1] As modified by Dr. G. R. Lockwood.

follow the use of injudicious foods. Looking upon the ulceration as still potent for evil, in spite of the advantages derived from a gastro-enterostomy, the necessity for great care in diet cannot be too seriously impressed upon those having the management of such cases.

When gastro-enterostomy is done for a benign stenosis of the pylorus, without ulceration, the need for care in the postoperative diet is still nearly as great on account of the condition of the edges of the new opening as already referred to; and a gastro-jejunal or jejunal ulcer is among the possibilities when unsuitable food is allowed too early or in too large quantities. All cases of gastro-enterostomy should abstain for months from all foods that are mechanically irritating (even after the period of very strict dieting is over), such as seeds, skins of vegetables or fruits, hard or rough foods, also from chemically irritating foods, as condiments, acids, heavy sweets, or those thermally irritating like hot foods or drink.

The Absorption of Food.—The question of the absorption of food after gastro-enterostomy has been of considerable interest, for in the light of the changes affected in the food current it is interesting to know whether these patients absorb their food as well as normal individuals, or whether the changed conditions result in a chronic, although possibly almost imperceptible, loss in food exchanges and consequently in nutrition, with a shortened longevity. This operation has not been done by modern methods long enough to speak with great weight as to longevity, but certainly children who have been operated on by gastro-enterostomy for congenital pyloric stenosis seem to grow and thrive as normal children do, and adults who have had the operation for ulcer or benign stenosis of the pylorus, if clinically cured, apparently are able to maintain normal nutrition, and no instance has come to the writer's notice of a case that has died later on after a clinical cure from any cause that could be due to malnutrition.

In order to test the question from a metabolic stand-point a woman, two years after gastro-enterostomy and clinically cured, with both pylorus and new stoma patent, as proved by x-ray examination, was put on a modified Schmidt diet for a definite period of days and the nitrogen metabolism, fat absorption, and carbohydrate utilization were tested accurately, no deviation from the normal was found.

The following tables are inserted to exemplify the same fact. It will be noted that among the cases in whom the metabolic experiment was made within a few days after the operation, the fat absorption was not as good as it was later on. This is probably the cause of the rather copious stools these cases of gastro-enterostomy have in the weeks immediately after the operation.

ABSORPTION AFTER GASTRO-ENTEROSTOMY.

Subject and conditions.	Time after operation.	Diet.	Fat absorbed per cent	Fat not absorbed per cent.	Nitrogen.	
					Absorbed per cent.	Not absorbed per cent.
1. Non-malignant[1] .	5 months	Mixed	92.3	7.7	91.0	9.0
2. Non-malignant .	7 "	"	92.5	7.5	90.5	9.5
3. Non-malignant .	24 "	"	92.7	7.3	92.1	7.9
4. Non-malignant .	2 "	"	94.7	5.3	92.7	7.3

ABSORPTION AFTER GASTRO-ENTEROSTOMY.[2]

Condition.	Time after operation	Sex and age.	Fat.		Absorbed gm.	Nitrogen.		
			In food, gm.	In feces, gm.		In food, gm.	In urine, gm.	Absorbed gm.
1. Obstructed pylorus .	20 days	F., 40	69.0	8.60	87.5	7.2	7.5	97.1
2. Obstructed pylorus	36 "	F., 52	67.0	17.70	73.7			
3. Non-obstructive hematemesis	11 "	M., 53	118.0	15.90	88.6	14.7	11.5	93.9
4. Obstructive dilatation	18 "	F., 43	122.5	5.25	95.7			
5. Duodenal ulcer . .	14 "	M., 41	210.5	7.00	93.5			
6. Stricture of pylorus .	8 years	M., 68	126.5	...	91.2			

Finney's[3] Diet List following the Operation for Gastro-enterostomy.—*First Day.*—First twelve hours, nothing by mouth, nutrient enemata every four hours alternating with continuous salt solution by Murphy's method.

First Day.—Second twelve hours, water in 4 c.c. (1 dram) doses by mouth every two hours.

Second Day.—Increase water gradually up to 30 c.c. (1 oz.) every two hours.

Third Day.—Water, 30 c.c. (1 oz.) alternating with albumen, 4 c.c. (1 dram); gradually increase quantities of each until

[1] Paterson: Hunterian Lectures, Royal College of Surgeons of England, 1906.
[2] Camerson: British Med. Jour., 1908, i, 144.
[3] Am. Jour. Med. Sc., 1915, cl, No. 4, p. 474.

Eighth Day.—Any liquid, 60 c.c. (2 oz.) every two hours.

Ninth Day.—Any liquid, 90 c.c. (3 oz.) every two hours.

Tenth Day.—Any liquid, 120 c.c. (4 oz.) every two hours. (discontinue rectal feeding).

Eleventh Day.—One soft-boiled egg in addition to any liquid.

Twelfth Day.—Two soft-boiled eggs in addition to any liquid.

Thirteenth Day.—Soft diet.

Fourteenth Day.—Soft diet.

Fifteenth Day.—Very restricted light diet.

Sixteenth Day.—Restricted light diet.

Seventeenth Day.—Restricted light diet.

Eighteenth Day.—Any digestible solid food.

After the eighteenth day the following diet list may be gradually followed, and should be continued for at least four or five months:

Soups, any light soup.

Meats, any easily digested meats, as brains, sweetbreads, beef, mutton, lamb, poultry (best minced and taken either broiled or boiled).

Fish, mainly the white variety, mackerel, bass, as well as oysters (boiled or broiled).

Eggs in any form except fried.

Vegetables, the easily digestible forms, best taken mashed or strained, as asparagus, spinach, peas, beans, potatoes, carrots, farinaceous food; any of the cereals; bread to be taken stale.

Desserts, any of the light puddings.

Fruits, mainly stewed.

Fatty Foods, as cream, butter, and olive oil.

Drinks, as milk, buttermilk, cocoa, carbonated mineral water, and plain water.

The following foods Must be Avoided.—Rich soups, pork, fried foods, veal, stews, hashes, corned meats, twice-cooked meat, potted meat, liver, kidney, duck, goose, sausage, crabs, sardines, lobster, preserved fish, salted or smoked fish, salmon, cauliflower, radishes, celery, cabbage, cucumbers, sweet potatoes, tomatoes, beets, corn, salad, bananas, melons, berries, pineapple, hot bread or cakes, nuts, candies, pies, pastry, preserves, cheese, strong tea or coffee, alcoholic stimulants.

Intestinal Lesions.—The diet for operations performed on the upper intestine follows the same routine as that advised for gastric operations. Those operations performed upon the lower small intestine or colon require less minute detailed care, but the order of first liquids, then soft solids, solids, and mixed foods should be maintained, although the transition from one to another may be more rapid than after operation farther up in the digestive canal.

Diet after Appendectomy.—No food should be given for from forty-eight to seventy-two hours postoperative. Water may be begun as soon as the nausea subsides—small amounts at first and increased as rapidly as the stomach will retain it. The first food should be broth, egg albumen, or Martin's milk,[1] then gruels, cocoa, soft cereals, and gradually back to a full diet.

Diet in Certain Complications, following Abdominal Operations.—Vomiting.—After any abdominal section this symptom may become of paramount importance, taxing the surgeon's skill more than the original operation, for although comparatively little mechanical damage may be done to the wound by vomiting, the interference with nutrition, increase of shock, and desiccation of the tissues may all have exceedingly serious consequences.

If after twenty-four to thirty-six hours the vomiting does not cease, or if it returns and increases on attempts to feed, special measures should be taken for its relief. It is practically useless to persist in feeding if the vomiting continues, so that all fluids or food by mouth should be stopped at once. Any of the measures already recommended (p. 346) to control vomiting may be tried, *e. g.*, dram doses of chloroform water either alone or with 1 drop of 95 per cent. carbolic acid added with 1 ounce of water or the carbolic alone in 1 or 2 ounces of water is often helpful.

Elixir of menthol may be tried. A mustard leaf to the epigastric region, a small hypodermic of morphine, about ⅛ to ¼ grain, sometimes helps. Cracked ice with champagne may be given in small doses. Finally, if nothing else relieves intractable vomiting, the stomach should be washed out at regular intervals, not waiting too long before trying this.

If the vomiting is of the ordinary postoperative type, not due to dilatation of the stomach, although persistent, and none of the procedures, including lavage, give relief, it is best to refrain from using the stomach at all for twelve to twenty-four hours and to feed by rectum as recommended in artificial nutrition (p. 618), giving saline enemata of 4 to 6 ounces (120 to 180 c.c.) between times, with the foot of the bed elevated on shock blocks. At least sufficient fluid can

---

[1] Martin's milk is prepared by making junket, separating the curd and whey, mashing the curd through cheesecloth or in a mortar and adding the whey. Patients can sometimes take this, when they cannot take plain milk.

be given this way to insure the patient's tissues from becoming dried out, and unless the rectum is intolerant it is seldom necessary to furnish water by hypodermoclysis. After a day or two of rectal feeding, another attempt may be made to give food in the form of iced liquids (such as egg albumen, with iced orange juice and water, partially peptonized milk, koumyss, buttermilk, gruels, purée, or clear soups), then to soft solids, such as milk toast, soft cereals, custards, junket, scraped-beef sandwiches, and on to a more normal diet. It is not infrequently found that people will retain some food that they especially crave, although theoretically it may be not at all what one would naturally advise; and again some patients will retain solids or soft solids when they will not retain fluids, and it is always well to try this plan in case of need, using a little dry or buttered toast, zweiback, toasted cracker, or poached egg.

Vomiting from Acute Gastric Dilatation,—If the vomiting is of dark brown or blackish fluid material in large amount, much more than the patient has taken by mouth, frequently repeated, it is probaby due to an acute dilatation of the stomach. The necessary and only relief for this is lavage repeated at first every two to four hours combined with a position of the patient which throws them on the right side, almost on the face; this posture is to relieve the pressure on the duodenum of the gastrohepatic ligament. When the fluid from the stomach is lessened in amount, the lavage can be done less and less frequently, and feedings may be begun which of course should have been stopped as soon as the diagnosis was made. These feedings should consist of some of the usual fluids recommended for irritable stomachs, *e. g.*, egg albumen, peptonized milk, whey, gruels all in small amount, 60 to 120 c.c. (2 to 4 ounces), every two, three or four hours. Even after feedings are begun and all evidence of the gastric dilatation past, for a time the stomach should be washed out every morning. The feedings can be progressively increased in amount and quality as the patient improves, until soft and then full feedings are resumed. During the period of dilatation it may be necessary to furnish the patient with water either by the rectum or by hypodermoclysis.

Prevention of Desiccation of the Tissues.—It not infrequently happens that patients come to operation with the tissues comparatively lacking in water, either due to intractable vomiting or to the fact that water absorption has been interfered with by some stenotic condition of the upper gastro-intestinal tract or excessive diarrhea. Before proceeding to operation this fact should be noted if present and the fluid deficit made up in any way possible by mouth, rectum, or hypodermoclysis, and the operation postponed long enough to overcome this condition.

The same state of affairs may develop after any severe operation in which vomiting is severe and always seriously complicates convalescence. It should not be permitted to escape notice or to continue.

Dietary Measures in Postoperative Intestinal Distention. —This is due to a lack of muscular tone of the intestinal wall sometimes combined with an excessive intestinal fermentation. If the intestinal paresis is severe it is difficult to overcome and forms a very serious complication.

The indications under such circumstances are to omit all feedings, to give water by mouth, small repeated doses of a saline laxative, 4 gm. (1 dram), every hour in water, using Rochelle salts, sulphate of soda, or Epsom salts. A hypodermic of pituitrin often entirely changes the picture and may be repeated every two or three hours for a couple of days, if necessary, or less often as the case may be. Colon irrigations with hot saline or an enema of equal parts of milk and molasses, 120 gm. (4 ounces), may be given, followed by a high enema of soapsuds or plain saline, hypodermics of strychnine sulphate, gr. ¼₀ every three hours, and hot turpentine stupes to the abdomen. There is little chance of influencing the fermentation by drugs, but the giving of cultures of the lactic acid bacillus may be tried if the case is prolonged or subacute.

When peristalsis is again established and the distention under control we may cautiously begin feedings. The particular point which needs attention in the diet from this point on to further convalescence, is, that no easily fermentable food should be given which might in any way increase the amount of intestinal gas. On this account all farinaceous or carbohydrate foods should be omitted from the diet especially all sugars as tending to ferment. The feedings should be at first entirely protein, as egg albumen, bouillon, broth, meat jelly, then fats, as whole egg, clam juice with cream, then as conditions improve we may use some of the partially malted foods, such as malted breakfast food, boiled for two hours in a double boiler, toast or zweiback that is toasted to a hard crisp, which may be eaten with butter, then other cereals, and gradually increase the latitude of the feedings back to a carefully selected mixed diet. . The feedings at first should be given about once in two or three hours in small amounts, increasing gradually to not over 120 c.c. (4 ounces) at a time.

39

This form of diet will usually be well tolerated, will not give rise to increased fermentation, and will be found useful in fermentative conditions of the gastro-intestinal tract aside from the postoperative period.

Diet after Gall-bladder Operations.—When the gall-bladder has been removed at operation the postoperative diet is that of any laparotomy, except that since there may be some temporary disturbance in the flow of bile it is well not to feed fatty foods except in very limited amounts.

When the operation is merely a drainage, and for a time a sinus is left, the diet should be arranged with a view to frequent stimulation of bile production and to making it as fluid as possible. The first object is best accomplished by frequent feedings, since at each feeding the flow of bile is stimulated. The second indication is met by forcing the fluid intake up to 3000 to 4000 c.c. (3 or 4 quarts) of fluid in twenty-four hours. Since most of the bile passes out through the fistula during the early postoperative days it is necessary to sharply restrict all fat in the diet, for bile is essential for the proper emulsification and digestion of fats. The diet should therefore consist of easily digested meats, egg albumen, clear soups, in fact any easily digestible protein. All farinaceous foods are allowed and with the proteins should form the bulk of the diet. Later, soft green vegetables and stewed fruits may be added. As the discharge of bile lessens one may begin to add fats to the diet in the form of thin cream, egg yolk, and crisp bacon.

Diet after Operation for Hemorrhoids.—Since, as a rule, the bowels are confined for about five days after this operation, the matter of diet is not unimportant, for at least the first few evacuations are painful. On this account it is a good plan to give a diet that will leave as little residue as possible even at the expense of complete nutrition not being maintained, so that there will be the least amount of fecal matter to be passed. This can be accomplished by feeding a diet principally protein and fat with the least amount of carbohydrate and no cellulose in the form of vegetables or fruits.

To this end the following articles of diet are advisable. Tea, coffee, water, or a little wine if wanted, or dilute whiskey. Eggs in any simple form, meat without connective tissue, fish, oysters, clear soups, cream, butter, not over three slices of bread per day, fine cereals, such as farina or cream of wheat, jellies, desserts made from gelatin, and water ices. After the fourth day honey and molasses may be allowed in good amounts as laxative and assisting in softening the feces for removal by suitable catharsis when the proper time arrives.

Constipating Diet.—For use after rectal and low intestinal operations. First four days applicable to hemorrhoids and fistula-in-ano cases. In other cases fluids without milk may be continued until the fifth day.

First Day.—Water.

Second day.—Fluids without milk.

Third Day.—Breakfast.—Farina with cream, soft egg, small slice toast, coffee.

Dinner: Clear soup, small piece fish or lean meat, or 4 raw oysters. A slice of bread and butter, gelatine desserts.

Supper; Soft egg on toast, tea.

Fourth Day.—Molasses or honey. (In cases other than hemorrhoids and fistula, do not add until two days before a bowel movement is desired.)

Feeding after Intubation.—Since the introduction and general use of antitoxin in diphtheria, intubation is done less and less often, until now it is rarely necessary compared with conditions before the introduction of the serum. When it is done, however, the question of feeding the child becomes of great importance, and must be carefully carried out. If the food is given in the ordinary way after intubation, a certain amount is quite sure to find its way into the larnyx and cause violent choking. This practically always happens at first; later the child learns to manipulate the food so that it will pass the tube opening. Frequently soft solids cause less trouble than liquids. When choking is a difficulty the child is laid on its back on the nurse's lap, with head hanging backward a short distance over the nurse's thigh; food is then carefully given by spoonfuls and increased as rapidly in amount as it can be taken; usually a few days or even a day of such feeding is all that is necessary, and the child can then learn to swallow without difficulty.

CHAPTER XXXII.

DISEASES OF THE DUCTLESS GLANDS.

In relation to these diseases, diet plays a role of variable value—not so much in a curative or a prophylactic way, so far as the diseases themselves are concerned, as in the symptomatic dietetics in the effects of disease on these glands. Thus in the glycosuria accompanying acromegaly or exophthalmic goiter the diet is arranged largely on the requirements of the individual with respect to this symptom. While this is all true, nevertheless a wrong diet is capable of greatly exaggerating the symptoms of some of the pathological conditions found in these glands, as, for example, the use of a stimulating diet in exophthalmic goiter is distinctly contraindicated. As yet we know too little of the underlying causes of disturbances in the internal secretion of these glands to be able to apply to dietetics here the scientific criteria that are possible in some of the other diseases described in this book, and until the ways are cleared of all obstructions, we must do the best we can in selecting a diet on what is largely clinical experience.

ACROMEGALY.

The causes of diseases of the pituitary gland are by no means clear, and we can only know of their progress by the varying effects upon metabolism. If the whole gland is involved and hyperfunctionates, the increased secretion from the anterior lobe causes the well-known gigantism, that of the posterior, lobe leads to carbohydrate intolerance, with all the clinical manifestations of diabetes, as glycosuria, polydipsia, polyphagia, polyuria, and hyperglycemia.

If the change is degenerative, with loss of function, it leads to an increased carbohydrate tolerance, with consequent increase in body fat often leading to obesity.

In hyperpituitarism of the anterior lobe, feeding the dried gland has been tried, but with little success; the skeletal changes looking toward gigantism usually continue unchecked.

When the hypersecretion affects the posterior lobe we must diet, as in diabetes, since there is diminished carbohydrate tolerance.

If there is hypofunction of the anterior lobe we can give the dried gland by mouth but not with brilliant success. In the diet care must be taken that the carbohydrates are not taken in excess. A full mixed diet is best, combined with pituitary feeding, sometimes supplemented by thyroid extract.

ACUTE THYROIDITIS.

The acute parenchymatous inflammation of the thyroid gland may be secondary to any severe acute infection, either general by the blood route or by local extension from some acute infection of the surrounding tissue. The swelling and tenderness of the gland tell the story, and it is then necessary to feed only the blandest sort of foods. All thyroid stimulants should be omitted, such as meat, soup or any meat products; oatmeal, too, should be forbidden. The acute inflammation is usually of short duration, unless due to an actual pus infection with loss of tissue which must then, of course, be treated surgically.

If the swelling persists and evidence of subacute thyroidism develops or continues, the diet should be as advised for exophthalmic goiter (*q. v.*).

EXOPHTHALMIC GOITER.

The etiology of exophthalmic goiter is still largely a matter of conjecture, but it is probable that in the last analysis we shall find that the cases may be classified as of toxic or neurogenic origin.

When the emphasis is put on the toxic basis we find not a few writers on the subject tracing the trouble to the gastrointestinal canal, so that it is natural to find that here great stress is laid upon the importance of diet. If of neurogenic origin alone, diet will play an important role in the restoration of the organism to a normal basis.

In any event the regulation of the diet certainly has much to do with the intensity of the symptoms, which can usually be diminished or increased by a proper diet or the opposite. Whatever the cause, one fact stands out with great distinctness, namely, that these patients are for the most part poorly nourished and in advanced cases are often emaciated. This is due to the stimulating catabolic effect of the excessive thyroid secretion, proved experimentally by obtaining the same effects on nutrition by the feeding of considerable amounts of dried thyroid substance of the sheep. Falta[1] found that "as there exists an increased exchange in exophthalmic goiter it was believed it could be made up by an

[1] The Ductless Gland Diseases, p. 102.

abundance of albuminous food and he found that the giving of albuminous food increased thyroid function." Rugunger showed "that an almost albumin-free diet, very rich, however, in carbohydrate, can depress the increased exchange to normal." When a large amount of nitrogen-free food is given, with a moderate quantity of protein, there is no fear of a loss of body protein. This reduces the hypersecretion of the thyroid gland and favors keeping intestinal putrefaction at its lowest level. The three chief indications in choosing a diet for these cases of exophthalmic goiter are:

1. To avoid all stimulating foods and drinks.

2. To give a diet which will prevent intestinal putrefaction, so far as possible or at least to keep it at a minimum.

3. To increase the calories in the diet by an abundance of fat and carbohydrate foods, so that the albumin destruction is spared and the patients are made to gain in weight.

Thomson[1] is a strong advocate of the intestinal putrefactive origin of this form of goiter and is very drastic in his elimination of all meat products, and prohibits butcher's meat and oysters, clams and lobsters, and limits the use of eggs to one a day, and advocates one of the fermented-milk preparations, such as buttermilk, artificially ripened milk, or peptonized milk; allows crusty bread, rice, cereals, except oatmeal, and vegetables except peas, tomatoes, beets, turnips, carrots, spinach, beans and asparagus. He also allows cooked fruits except raspberries and strawberries. The vegetables that he especially recommends are potatoes and string beans. Tea and coffee with milk are allowed in small amounts rather grudgingly. Non-oily fish, poultry, quail, and partridge are allowed. In Osler's *Modern Medicine* we find there is no objection to a moderate use of meat in these patients.

Tibbles[2] says that "oatmeal and liver strongly stimulate, animal foods in general moderately stimulate, and a diet of milk, eggs, bread and butter, biscuits, etc., only slightly stimulate the thyroid gland and shows the way to the dietetic treatment of exophthalmic goiter."

The foods that contain considerable quantities of iodin are also to be avoided. (See Table, Part I.)

The milk of thyroidectomized goats has been used and at times to advantage; its efficiency is said to be due to the absence of iodine.

It will be seen from the foregoing quotations that it is no easy matter to choose foods that will keep these various things out of the diet, which for one reason or another are

---

[1] Thomson: Graves's Disease.   [2] Food in Health and Disease, p. 489.

taboo with one or another authority, and still be able to nourish our patients; so that one must keep in mind the three cardinal factors already referred to and construct as nearly in accord with them as possible.

Such a diet might well include foods as follows: fresh-cooked fruits, milk, one or two eggs per day, non-oily fish, as they are lowest in iodine, except codfish; cheese, and fowl occasionally. Potatoes, carrots, endive, kidney beans, pumpkin, celery, onions, corn. Breads, biscuits, macaroni, rice, and all farinaceous foods except oatmeal. Sugars in moderate abundance unless there is an accompanying hyperglycemia or glycosuria, both frequently present in the severe cases. These are all low in iodine, thyroid stimulating content and putrefactive potentiality, and are of high caloric value. Alcohol should be absolutely prohibited.

The final desideratum of furnishing a diet of high caloric value in order to improve nutrition and weight must be observed, as many of these patients have a continuous elevation of temperature and must be overfed, much as we have seen to be essential in typhoid fever, if we wish to preserve or increase body weight, and a high calorie diet is necessary, feeding an extra one-quarter, one-third or even one-half the total calories needed for a normal person of the same weight, made up for the most part of the non-nitrogenous food-stuffs. The lower total quantities of nitrogenous foods are best, keeping the total daily intake down to 70 or 90 gm. protein.

It is necessary, however, according to von Noorden, to avoid too rapid a gain in weight, as this throws too much work upon the heart, and has resulted in his experience, in circulatory collapse, as the strength of the heart does not keep pace with the increased weight. This is seldom a practical danger, as it is usually difficult to get these patients to gain any considerable amount, except in the milder cases.

Diet to Meet Special Indications in Exophthalmic Goiter. —When glycosuria is present it is necessary to reduce the intake of sugars first; if that does not eliminate the glycosuria, then the carbohydrates have to be diminished, and if slight reduction in these does not result in a sugar-free urine, then it will probably be necessary to treat the case as true diabetes. This is fortunately rarely necessary, for, as a usual thing, while there may be a certain amount of hyperglycemia present, particularly in the moderately severe or severe cases, even they often fail to show glycosuria, except occasionally a trace, unless an abnormal amount of carbohydrate is eaten.

Diarrhea.—In the cases that are at all severe this is a very frequent symptom and must be treated intelligently from a dietetic point of view. Naturally it goes without saying that whatever measures of rest or treatment tend to a general improvement of the patient will have a favorable influence on the diarrhea. In spite of this there are cases in whom the diarrhea is an obstinate symptom. These patients have to be treated as one would a case of chronic enteritis, using the diet appropriate for that condition, and it is often a matter of great difficulty to get them straightened out and digesting sufficient food to maintain or increase weight.

A combination of diet, general measures, and astringent medication, if necessary, are usually sufficient unless the case is too severe.

Inanition.—Sufficient has already been said to indicate the needs of these cases. They must be given what amounts to a rest-cure with hyperalimentation principally of the non-nitrogenous foods, with due regard for all the factors already mentioned.

MYXEDEMA OR CRETINISM.

Since the condition of myxedema or cretinism is due to diminished or absent thyroid secretion, we find that clinically all that is necessary is to give these patients thyroid gland (dry extract) in order to bring about a condition normal or approaching it, so that diet plays little part. If, however, one wishes to produce the maximum effect of the artificially fed thyroid it would be well to reverse the diet as recommended for exophthalmic goiter, *i. e.*, give all the thyroid-stimulating foods possible, such as meat and meat products, shell fish, oily fish, and other foods, which we found were of high iodine content. (See Exophthalmic Goiter). There is really little necessity for this, as the thyroid substance and a mixed diet are practically all that are necessary.

ADDISON'S DISEASE.

The loss of normal adrenal secretion in this disease results at first in a general lack of tone of the entire vascular and glandular system, with subsequent loss of flesh and asthenia. Tuberculosis of the adrenals is the usual cause of the disease, and although the accessory glands of the chromaffin system can, to a certain extent, compensate for the hypofunction of the adrenals, this is only true in the earlier stages; later on the dire results of the disease become evident. One must diet symptomatically very largely; if there is gastric disturbance the diets in use for irritable stomach or acute gastritis are of use. If there is diarrhea the diet for intestinal catarrh or chronic diarrhea becomes necessary. If there is merely a depressed digestion, with loss of appetite, one must feed as best one can, giving foods which are simple, very nourishing, and as concentrated as possible. As the thyroid stimulates the adrenals, some help may be obtained by increasing the thyroid secretion by a stimulating diet (such as that containing much meat or meat extract, soups and meat gravies); if this fails, thyroid extract can be given in rather small dosage, 1 or 2 grains, two or three times a day. In order to protect the gastro-intestinal canal from irritation it is essential that the food, besides being simple, concentrated, and nourishing, should be soft and non-irritating, without gristle, skins, seeds, or uncooked cellulose. Mild stimulants to digestion are allowable in small quantities, bitter tonics before meals, a glass of sherry, port, beer, claret, or 1 ounce of whiskey well diluted with Vichy. Alcohol taken in any larger amount is contra-indicated.

CHAPTER XXXIII.

DIET IN MISCELLANEOUS CONDITIONS.

ARTIFICIAL METHODS OF FEEDING.

THE problem of nourishing the body by other means than by mouth feeding has engaged the attention of clinicians and experimental workers for many years. The hope has been constantly entertained that some way could be found by which the entire physiological needs of the body could be met by introducing food by other than the natural route. In pursuance of this hope many methods have been devised to artificially nourish an individual, and the claim has been put forward by one or another investigator that a particular plan has met or almost met the conditions. As laboratory methods have become more exact, and these various ways of artificial feeding have been subjected to more searching analysis, the conclusion is inevitable that so far the most that can be done is to supply from 25 to 35 per cent. of the requirements of nutrition reckoned in necessary heat units, and w th the problem still unsolved as to how to furnish sufficient nitrogen to prevent the undue loss of tissue protein. While this loss can be diminished by feeding peptones or amino-acids and carbohydrates, and possibly a little fat, not enough can be gotten into the system to do more than prevent the excessive nitrogen destruction, and no case has been permanently or completely artificially nourished.

The conditions in which those various ways of feeding are useful are such as prevent the taking of food by the natural route, and include stricture of the upper alimentary canal from whatever cause, peptic ulcer and intractable vomiting, as in the vomiting of pregnancy, etc.

The three methods by which artificial nutrition has been carried out are by rectal feeding, subcutaneous feeding, and intravenous feeding.

Rectal Feeding.—By far the oldest and most serviceable method is that of rectal feeding and although, as already pointed out, it is not sufficient, it at least is of temporary benefit, and has a place of assured usefulness in dietetic therapeutics. As formerly practised, when all sorts of incompletely prepared foods were given by rectum, very little indeed was absorbed, and some years ago the author made metabolism estimations on the absorption of a peptonized milk-and-egg mixture ordinarily used in the large hospitals. It was found that the loss of weight and nitrogen differed little from that seen in starvation, showing that almost nothing was absorbed.[1] This leads naturally to the question as to what the properties of the colon are in regard to normal functions. As an excretory organ, calcium, phosphates, iron, and magnesium are excreted by the large intestine. As a digestive organ, its role is a very minor one; in fact, almost nil, although enzymes from the small intestine do continue their action in the colon, and bacterial action is considerable on carbohydrates, protein, and cellulose. As an absorptive organ it is of very moderate usefulness, although water and salts are well absorbed, amino-acids, monosaccharide sugars, and alcohol to a limited extent, and very much less and more slowly than by the small intestine. Fats are thought by some not to be absorbed at all.[2]

One element in those cases which have been reported successfully nourished for a considerable time by this method is probably that by reverse peristalsis, food has been carried through the ileocecal valve into the small intestine and there absorbed. This is not so improbable as it may at first sight seem, and when one considers how rapidly a bismuth enema is carried from the rectum to the caput coli, often within ten to twenty seconds, as shown by the use of the fluroscope. Therefore given a patent ileocecal valve, food might easily gain access to the small intestine and be there largely absorbed.

Of the food elements introduced in nutrient enemata we must discuss in more detail the fate of protein, carbohydrate, fats, alcohol, salts, and water.

Protein.—The attempt has been made to introduce protein in almost every conceivable form, as egg albumen, chopped meat and pancreas, beef juice, milk, peptone, propeptone, and amino-acids, with the result in general that the nearer the protein molecule approaches its ultimate fate in normal digestion, *i. e.*, as amino-acids, the better is its absorption, so we find peptone better absorbed than albumen, peptone than proteoses, and amino-acids better than peptones.

There are two methods in vogue for determining the absorption of foods introduced into the rectum, one, termed the "washing-out" method, relies upon analysis of what is passed by rectum plus the washings from a high colon irri-

[1] Carter: Arch. Int. Med., April, 1908.
[2] Goodall: Boston Med. and Surg. Jour., clxx, 41.

gation, and comparing the total nitrogen of these two with the nitrogen input. This is, of course, scientifically a very crude method, as there are many opportunities for error. The other, and more accurate method, depends upon *the* estimation of urinary nitrogen, comparing the intake and output. also in some cases calorimetry is used to determine the dynamic action of different food-stuffs. Edsall and Miller[1] found that although 47 per cent. of peptonized milk-and-egg mixture was apparently absorbed, the ethereal sulphates in the urine during the period were so excessively high that the conclusion is inevitable that the apparent absorption was really more due to a disappearance of the protein by putrefaction, so that 47 per cent. is probably an entirely erroneous figure.

Short and Bywaters[2] analyzed various reports of cases fed by the rectum, together with weight charts and urinary findings and concluded that:

1. The daily output of urinary nitrogen from patients given enemata of peptonized milk and eggs (peptonized twenty to thirty minutes) showed that almost no nitrogen was absorbed, and the total nitrogen in the urine was little if any higher than that seen in the urine of fasting men or of patients who received only saline by rectum.

2. Modern physiological opinion holds that proteins are absorbed principally as amino-acids, and the failure of the rectum to absorb ordinary nutrient enemata is largely due to the fact that peptones are usually given instead of amino-acids.

3. Chemically prepared amino-acids or milk pancreatized for twenty-four hours, so that the amino-acids are separated, allows a much better absorption of nitrogen, as shown by the high nitrogen output in the urine.

4. The low output of ammonia nitrogen shows that the high total nitrogen was not due to the absorption of putrefactive bodies when the amino-acids are used.

So far, then, as protein absorption goes there is no doubt but that amino-acids produced chemically from beef, *e. g.*, the preparation called "aminoids," or milk pancreatized for twenty-four hours, *i. e.*, until the casein is brought to amino-acid, is fairly well absorbed, but still not in sufficient amount to prevent a continuous negative nitrogen balance. The Boas and Riegal enemata of milk, egg yolk, wine and arrowroot, or Leube's pancreas, 50 to 100 gm. (1⅔ to 3⅓ oz.). meat, 150 to 300 gm.; fat, 30 to 45 gm. (1 to 1½ oz.); water, 150 c.c. (5 oz.), ground in a mortar and injected into the

[1] Wisconsin Med. Jour., 1903, i, 87.   [2] British Med. Jour., 1913, i, 1361.

rectum, may all be said to be of little value and not worth using in the light of modern investigation, their use is mentioned only to be condemned.

Fats.—There is great difference of opinion regarding the absorbability of fats by the rectum. Friedenwald and Ruhrah believe that fat in emulsion, *e. g.*, egg yolk is absorbed better than is usually believed and recommended the addition of egg yolk to every enema. Short and Bywaters, on the other hand, conclude that very little if any fat is absorbed. Goodall thinks that some fat is taken up by the lymphatics but exceedingly little is absorbed. Taken all together there is little if any experimental evidence that fats are absorbed by the colon except possibly in minimal amounts and too little to be of any nutritive value.[1]

Carbohydrates.—With some of the carbohydrates, notably the monosaccharids, there is every evidence that the colon is able to absorb considerable quantities, and this class forms the backbone of rectal alimentation, provided it is not given in too concentrated a solution, for one of its disadvantages is the fact that it may cause rectal irritation, and one cannot foretell what strength of solution an individual rectum will tolerate. Boyd and Robertson found that ¾ of a 10 to 20 per cent. solution of dextrose was absorbed to a total of 40 to 50 gm. (1½ or 1⅔ oz.) but decided that a total of 30 gm. (1 oz.) was less apt to cause pain and diarrhea. Either pure dextrine glucose or dextrose may be used. Goodall used 500 c.c. (1 pint) of a 3 to 16 per cent. solution of dextrose and after five hours found 42 to 52 gm. (1½ or 1⅔ oz.) was absorbed, with a 10 per cent. solution 157 to 163 gm. (5 or 5½ oz.) was absorbed and with a 15 per cent. solution as much as 144 to 193 gm. was taken up, and he contends that the amount of sugar destroyed by bacterial action varies from 0.5 to 1 per cent. Many observers, however, find that the weaker solutions up to 5 per cent. are better tolerated, causing less rectal irritation. This latter may in part be due to the fermentation of the sugar which can be prevented by adding 1 part of thymol to 4000 parts of the solution. When lactose was substituted for the dextrose it was found that the ammonia nitrogen in the urine rose rapidly, showing that it was not well absorbed. This did not happen when dextrose was used. The addition of absolute alcohol to the rectal feeding increases its food value, but care must be taken not to use strong solutions, as they promptly produce rectal

---

[1] There is apparently good reason to believe that animal fats of low melting-point such as cod-liver oil are absorbed by the skin and form one possible method of artificial nutrition, especially in infants, if the oil is well rubbed into the skin of axillæ and groins where the glandular and lymphatic supply is rich.

irritation. The following combination of dextrose, alcohol and saline represents a serviceable feeding, supplying 555 calories and will be absorbed approximately in eight hours.

Dextrose, 50 gm. (1⅔ oz.).
Absolute alcohol, 50 gm. (1⅔ oz.).
Normal saline solution, 1000 c.c. (1 qt.).

The same authority found that if large enemata with the same proportions of dextrose and alcohol were used absorption was not so complete, and this was also true of enemata of the same size but of higher concentration. When this can be tolerated by the rectum it is especially useful in: (1) Simple exhaustion. (2) In certain septic conditions, especially good for the heart muscle. (3) As an antidote to chloroform and phosphorus poisoning or anything that causes fatty liver, as the fatty changes may often be prevented by giving glycogen-forming material. (4) In diabetic acidosis and acetonemia. (5) After abdominal operations, particularly in undernourished or desiccated individuals.

This enema may be alternated with milk pancreatized for twenty-four hours, or the dextrose and alcohol be added in 2 to 5 per cent. strength as follows:

Dextrose, 20 to 50 gm. (1⅔ oz.) 80 to 205 calories.
Alcohol, 20 to 50 gm. (1⅔ oz.), 140 to 350 calories.
Pancreatized milk, or commercial amino-acids, 1000 c.c. (1 qt.), 200 calories.
Salt, 9 gm.

This solution may be given in 250 c.c. (8 oz.) dose every four hours, and represents about 420 to 755 calories (1000 c.c. of peptonized milk, has merely the caloric value of the protein for rectal feeding; the fat and lactose are probably little utilized).

Hutchinson[1] recommends a solution of unboiled starch as unirritating and well absorbed, but does not present data which are convincing.

Precautions in Rectal Feeding.—There are certain precautions which must be observed if one expects to have success in rectal feeding, otherwise they will certainly not be successful:

1. The rectum must be kept very clean by a good irrigation of saline once a day.

2. The food must be sterilized, the peptonized milk in particular must be brought to a boil after peptonization is complete.

3. When the rectum becomes irritated by using solutions which are too strong the strength must be reduced and the rectum given a rest of a few hours after a saline cleansing.

[1] Food and Dietetics, p. 519.

4. All enemata should be given with the foot of the bed raised on shock-blocks and the patient should remain in this position for at least an hour after it.

5. It may be necessary to add 5 to 10 drops of deodorized tincture of opium if the rectal irritability cannot be otherwise controlled.

It is often advantageous to give the dextrose solution by the Murphy drip, which is done by putting the solution at 105° F. in an irrigator and keeping this warm by means of cloths wrapped about the apparatus, or by placing a lighted electric bulb in the fluid to keep up its temperature. The fluid flow is then regulated by a stop-cock or merely by pinching the rubber tube by an artery clamp so that the fluid will drip from 60 to 90 drops per minute. This can often be continued for hours, depending on the rectal toleration.

Subcutaneous Feeding.—This division of artificial nutrition has engaged the efforts of many experimenters, but as yet the goal seems as far off as ever, for although it is possible to supply a certain amount of protein and carbohydrate and fat by the hypodermic route, the quantities are too small to be at all sufficient for nutritional requirements. This method is far less distinctly valuable than the rectal routine of feeding, but when for any reason it is impossible to use the rectum, it may be used to some, but, taken altogether, slight advantage.

Protein.—Protein in many forms has been used, as egg albumen, peptone, alkali albuminate, and propeptones, but all these forms cause irritation, abscess and a breaking down of tissue besides setting up a renal irritation.[1] Experimentally it was possible in dogs by giving small repeated and increasing doses of skimmed milk peptonized one and a half hours to supply protein, so that the nitrogenous balance showed only a loss of 0.3 to 0.5 gm. per day, but for ordinary use milk peptone when injected hypodermically must be considered dangerous on account of its toxicity, and should not be used.[2] More promising was the use of blood serum or ascetic fluid given hypodermically,[3] and in this way a certain amount of nitrogen can be supplied to the system which is made use of. Blood serum contains about 1 per cent. nitrogen and ascetic fluid, 0.17 to 1 per cent., so it can be seen that in order to supply sufficient protein to maintain nitrogenous equilibrium even in Chittenden's low estimate of 0.12 gm. nitrogen per kilo daily, it would take for a man

[1] Gautier: Diet and Dietetics, p. 529.
[2] Carter: Arch. Int. Med., April, 1908.
[3] Carter: Am. Jour. Med. Sc., August, 1911.

of 70 kilos from 840 c.c. to 4200 c.c. of fluid depending upon whether blood serum or ascetic fluid were used, entirely too large an amount for practical daily use. A certain amount may be used, up to 300 or 400 c.c. daily, probably without detriment to the organism, and although this has not been used in such large amounts in man, larger amounts proportionally have been injected in dogs without seeming detriment, and nitrogen can be given to them in this way to a certain and often large extent which is absorbed, metabolized and excreted; nevertheless, during the test periods there was always a negative N balance of from 0.04 to 4.35 gm. nitrogen for a two- or three-day period, the starvation balance for two days being 3.83 gm. nitrogen.

If serum or ascetic fluid is aseptically drawn it can be used without sterilization, but if there is any doubt it should be heated to 55° C., which causes it to become opalescent but not coagulated.[1]

Salter[2] injected 100 to 120 c.c. (3⅓ to 4 oz.) of horse serum heated to 65° C. without albuminous coagulation, and noted that the nitrogen excretion in the urine was increased.

Fats.—Comparatively little accurate experimental work has been done with the hypodermic injection of fats from an exact metabolic point of view, but it has been found that sterilized olive oil can be injected in amounts of 30 to 40 c.c. (1 or 1⅓ oz.) daily, preferably 10 c.c. in three or four places, and that it is absorbed and metabolized is evidenced by the diminution in the excretion of nitrogen. In this way Hutchinson believed he could supply 500 calories. There is no doubt but that oil so injected is utilized, but the absorption is very slow, and its usefulness as a means of artificial nutrition is not at all clear. Subcutaneous injections of egg yolk with one-third its weight of normal saline, and strained through cheesecloth, have been given, increasing from 1 to 10 c.c. given in the buttocks; although tried in children, its use has not been checked by careful observation, and is not to be recommended.

Carbohydrate.—The one form of carbohydrate which has been successfully used by the hypodermic route is dextrose. Voit,[3] in 1896, used a 10 per cent. solution and found it could be injected under the skin without glycosuria, although it was too painful and caused too much infiltration of the tissue to be useful. Kausch[4] began with a 2 per cent. solu-

---

[1] Reinach: Berl. klin. Wchnschr. March 20, 1899.
[2] Guy's Hosp. Rep., 1896, liii, 241.
[3] München. med. Wchnschr., August 4, 1896.
[4] Deutsch. med. Wchnschr., 1911, No. 1, 8.

tion of dextrose, using up to 1000 c.c.; if he used a stronger solution, 8 to 10 per cent., it was promptly excreted in the urine, but without renal irritation.   He also observed that the poorer the patient's general nutrition was the better the sugar was borne.   Gautier found that 60 to 80 gm. (2 or 2⅔ oz.) of glucose in 1000 c.c. (1 qt.) of water with 5 or 6 gm. salt added was well absorbed when given by subcutaneous injection, but even this is not sufficient to furnish more than a fraction of the normal requirements.

Intravenous Feeding.—This has been tried with various foods, principally milk and sugar solutions.   The method is of slight if any practical usefulness, although if it is necessary for quick action, Goodall advises giving an isotonic dextrose solution (5.4 per cent.) in Ringer-Loche solution intravenously.   The following is the formula recommended, especially for children.

Dextrose, 55 gm. (1⅓ oz.).
Potassium chloride, 0.2 gm. (3 grains).
Calcium chloride, 0.2 gm. (3 grains).
Sodium carbonate, 0.1 gm. (1½ grains).
Aq. destil. q. s. ad., 1000 c.c. (1 qt.).

Kausch recommends the following solution for intravenous use when necessary:

Dextrose, 50 gm. (1⅔ oz.).
Sodium chloride, 9 gm. (⅓ oz.).
Adrenalin chloride (1 to 1000 sol.), 10 gtt.
Aq. destil. q. s. ad. 1000 c.c. (1 qt.).
Filter and boil and give intravenously twice daily.

One cardinal rule in giving dextrose solutions either subcutaneously or intravenously is that they must be given very slowly, as otherwise they are excreted by the kidneys with inadequate absorption.   Woodyatt and Wilde[1] in some experiments on animals and later with human application, determined that a man of 70 kilos (154 pounds) at rest may receive intravenously and utilize completely 63 gm. glucose per hour without showing glycosuria.   This is equivalent to 252 calories per hour or 6048 per day.   The normal tolerance limit for glucose expressed as velocity is established, as these authors say, at close to 0.85 gm. of glucose per kilo (2.2 pounds) of body weight hourly.   This solution is given by a specially constructed apparatus by which the rate of the solution's flow can be accurately regulated.

The giving of food solutions intraperitoneally has been tried but should not be used under any circumstances, as too little is gained and an added shock is put upon the system.

[1] Jour. Am. Med. Assn., December 11, 1915.

40

To critically summarize these various methods of artificial nutrition, it may be said that the rectal route is the only one that is so far at all clinically satisfactory and that by this means roughly one-third the caloric requirements may be given in the form of dextrose solution with a certain amount of protein in the form of amino-acids, and, of course, water and salts in entirely sufficient amount if the rectum is tolerant. If for any reason the rectum is not usable, a fair amount of nitrogen can be given by the hypodermic injection of serum or ascetic fluid and from 20 to 40 gm. of dextrose as a 2 to 4 per cent. solution and possibly 30 to 40 gm. of fat as olive oil. Intravenously proteins and fat are not available, but a certain amount of dextrose can be given up to 55 gm. (?) in a 5 per cent. solution in Ringer-Loche fluid, although in either the subcutaneous or intravenous injection of dextrose a certain amount is apt to be lost through the kidneys unless given very slowly.

DIET IN PREGNANCY AND ITS COMPLICATIONS.

Many and varied have been the dietetic rules laid down for this condition, almost entirely founded on clinical experience, or supposed experience, and in turn almost every form of food has been under the partial ban of exclusion.

During the earlier months of pregnancy the appetite and ordinary metabolism need only be considered in choosing a diet, except when marked nausea exists. In the later months Cragin recommends giving meat not more than three times a week, and, since much depends upon the regularity of the bowel movements, some attention must be given to anticonstipation elements in the diet; fruit, fresh, stewed or dried, and green vegetables, all in considerable amounts are very serviceable. In spite of such a diet most patients require, as pregnancy advances, some additional laxative substance or drug.

Nausea and Vomiting of Pregnancy.—Some women are bothered by morning nausea or vomiting more or less during the first three or four months of pregnancy, in fact a certain amount of this is the rule, but after the fourth month the sensation generally disappears and the appetite, which has usually been poor or capricious during this period, returns to normal and may continue up to the end of the pregnancy. At times the nausea and vomiting are so extreme as to menace life and are presumably of toxic origin accompanying an acute yellow atrophy of the liver as postmorten examination in these fatal cases usually shows. There have been many theories advanced to explain the mild morning vomiting of pregnancy and the pernicious form but to quote an Editorial in the Journ. Am. Med. Assn., June 7, 1919, the theories advanced in explanation of these phenomena are unsatisfactory because most of them are at best only part of the possibilities presented by this particular type of nausea and vomiting. There are various factors which point to some metabolic factor in the origin of both the mild and pernicious form of vomiting. The ketonuria also present is an added indication of a metabolic upset. The symptoms appear most often in the morning after a twelve hour period of starvation.

The diet for the mild grades of discomfort should be of simple, easily digested food, avoiding fats, rich sauces, salt or smoked meat (unless the appetite craves these, when they may be given in small amounts), heavy sweets, etc. Food should be taken often and in small amounts; and it may be of assistance to have the patient take a couple of crackers on waking or a small cup of fairly strong tea, then resting awhile before breakfast.

Lynch[1] lay stress in the early and mild cases of vomiting in pregnancy in the habit factor as needing care in treatment. He advises putting the patients to bed and stopping all food and drink by mouth for twenty-four hours. Colonic irrigation are given daily and bromids 40 to 60 gr. (4 to 5 gm.) given by rectum every four hours. A solution of glucose and soda is given by rectum 8 to 10 oz. (240 to 300 c.c.) given several times daily. The first time the patient is fed she should be told to control her vomiting if possible, that the vomiting habit is easy to form but hard to break. The first meal should be dry as possible. Those cases with gastric hyperacidity respond best to a diet of protein, limited fats and carbohydrates. A diet of meat with toasted bread and butter, and a small amount of milk or cream is especially recommended by Lynch. The rectal glucose solution and soda controls the acidosis and this symptom is usually observed when the supply of actually utilized carbohydrates is low, *e. g.*, when sugars fail to be oxidized as in diabetes mellitus.

A shortage of physiologically available carbohydrates, usually expressed in the glycogen supply of the tissues, often leads to the infiltration of the liver with fats, an indication of carbohydrate starvation in the body, as fat is not deposited in the liver while carbohydrates are still available.

Duncan and Harding[2] have argued that pregnancy and a short period of hunger (over night) might account for the

[1] Jour. Am. Med. Assn., August 16, 1919, p. 492.
[2] Canada Med. Assn. Jour., 1918, viii, 1057.

periodicity of the morning sickness due to a temporary relative lack of glycogen in the liver leading to a fatty infiltration.

Applying this idea chemically they have endeavored to correct this assumed deficiency of carbohydrate supply in cases of varying severity of nausea and vomiting, by giving glucose, lactose, mainly the latter and have supplemented this by a diet high in carbohydrates.

They give very gratifying reports in seventy cases treated on this principle which is certainly worth an extended trial. Carson[1] says that percussion of the 5th dorsal spine causes a pyloric opening reflex which results in the almost immediate emptying of the stomach; a useful procedure (if a fact) in nourishing these and other cases of severe vomiting.

In the most severe form of vomiting of pregnancy very little success is experienced in nourishing the patients, all the methods recommended for an irritable stomach may be tried, colon irrigations, etc., but in the really severe cases emptying the uterus is the procedure that becomes necessary. Just the time at which this latter procedure is indicated is a matter of nice judgment and, of course, should never be decided upon singly, but only after full consultation. Until an operation is deemed necessary everything to quiet the stomach that offers any reasonable hope of success should be tried, *e. g.*, lavage, cocaine or menthol mixtures, cracked ice, sinapisms, drop doses of 95 per cent. carbolic acid in 1 or 2 ounces of water, followed by a trial of iced fluids jellies, and koumyss, or some dry solid like toast.

Alcohol is best let alone, as a habit is more easily established in pregnant women and on account of its well-known and harmful influence on the fetus.

Nephritis.—Close watch must be kept of the pregnant woman's urinary output and should albumin appear, a few days of an absolute milk diet will be necessary. If the albumin clears up then a return to soft diet may be made, principally a lactofarinaceous diet; as improvement continues vegetables and fruit may be added, but animal protein, except milk and eggs, is better left out of the menu for a considerable time after the urine becomes normal.

Should grave symptoms of uremia develop all the methods ordinarily employed to combat this condition should be used, *e. g.*, milk diet, hot packs, colon irrigation, saline infusions, veratrum viride, and phlebotomy if necessary, emptying the uterus if no other measures seem to suffice. If there is edema with the uremic manifestations, the diet should be one of the salt-poor diets (see p. 453).

[1] Med. Rec., 1917, xcii, 897.

In any event the diet as recommended for acute nephritis is indicated. If the outcome is favorable, without the necessity of terminating labor, the diet during the remainder of the pregnancy must be regulated with the utmost care, largely as advised in chronic nephritis.

Mild Autointoxication.—The symptoms of this condition are not outspoken, but consist of a little headache, a general feeling of lassitude, lack of ambition and possibly vague digestive disturbances. These are often the precursors of more serious trouble and should not be ignored; with such a condition to treat, a thorough emptying of the bowel is necessary, followed daily by a colon irrigation of hot saline. The diet should be reduced in quantity and meat and meat soups excluded until after the symptoms clear up. Massage and passive movement or active exercise as walking or light dumbbell exercise will help in a return to normal conditions. Such symptoms can for the most part be obviated if the patients will take care not to overeat and to take regular and systematic exercise throughout their pregnancy. Regular walking and abdominal exercises such as raising the legs while lying prone or coming up to a sitting posture from the prone position, help to furnish exercise, strengthen the abdominal muscles, aid in preventing constipation, and give much better "pushing" power at the time of greatest need.

Contracted Pelvis or with an Oversized Fetus.—Various dietary regulations have been tried with a view to influencing the size of the child in order that it may pass a small pelvic outlet without difficulty, and of these the best known is Prochwnick's diet, of which the main principles are, reducing the carbohydrates and fluids during the last two or three months of pregnancy in the hope that the growth of the fetus may be kept back (retarding the ossification of the bones). De Lee[1] thinks the diet useless, but there are others who believe it accomplishes its purpose, although it should only be undertaken under medical supervision. It is probably an extremely useless procedure.

Prochwnick's Diet:[2]

Breakfast. Small cup of coffee, 100 c.c. (3 oz.); bread, 30 gm. (1 oz.); a very little butter.

Dinner: Meat, fish or one egg with a little sauce; vegetables cooked with butter or cream; lettuce; small piece of cheese.

Supper: The same as at dinner, with bread, 30 gm. (1 oz.); butter and a little milk.

[1] De Lee: Principles and Practice of Obstetrics, p. 729.
[2] Centralbl. f. Gynecol., 1889, 33.

Forbidden: Soup, pastries, sugar, beer, and potatoes. Water up to 1 pint a day or a light wine, 300 to 400 c.c. (10 to 14 oz.) is the only fluid allowed.

Puerperium.—During the first eighteen hours postpartum the mother should have liquids sufficient to quench the thirst, a cup of tea, water, Vichy, or broth. After this, coffee, milk, toast, soft cereals, milk toast, and so back to normal diet. After the bowels have been moved on the second day the amount of food can be steadily increased, always giving plenty of water and small midmorning and afternoon feedings.

Foods Best Avoided.—Acid fruits, such as grapefruit, lemonade, sour oranges, strawberries, plums, tomatoes, and onions all may cause colic in the infant. Peas, potatoes, tunips, and beans so often give rise to flatulence that they are best left out of the diet until the mother is able to exercise and be about.[1]

The following is the postpartum diet recommended by Edgar:

Diet List after Normal Confinement.

First two days:

Liquids: Milk, hot or cold; beef tea, weak tea; beef broth or chicken broth; beef juice; egg shake; clam broth; simple soups and cocoa.

Solids: Thin bread and butter; saltine or soda crackers; milk toast; dry or buttered toast; dropped or soft-boiled eggs; any breakfast cereal thoroughly cooked.

After first two days:

Liquids: As above with addition of coffee.

Solids: Any breakfast cereal; scrambled, soft-boiled, or dropped eggs; broiled white fish; lamb chop; beef-steak; roast lamb; broiled, baked, or creamed chicken; baked, mashed or stewed potatoes; macaroni; celery; lettuce; fruits; fresh vegetables, such as peas, asparagus, and string beans in season and in moderation; boiled or baked custard, curds and whey; wine jelly; simple puddings, such as rice, tapioca.

Avoid: Nursing mothers should avoid whatever previously disagreed with them and usually also pork, veal, corned beef, cabbage, turnips, cucumbers, corn, beans (canned and dried), vinegar, strawberries, and melons unless thoroughly ripe.

Sample Breakfasts:

(1) Any breakfast cereal; soft egg; tea. (2) Orange; cereal and cream; scrambled egg; tea or cocoa. (3)

Edgar: The Practice of Obstetrics, p. 673.

Cereal; broiled white fish; bread and butter; tea, coffee, or cocoa. (4) Lamb chop; stewed potatoes; toast; tea, coffee, or cocoa. (5) Orange; scrambled or dropped egg; minced chicken; graham bread; coffee.

Sample Dinners:
(1) Broiled or roast chicken; sweet potato; baked cup custard. (2) Roast lamb; mashed potato; macaroni; wine jelly. (3) Roast beef; celery; mashed potato; rice pudding. (4) Simple soup; chicken; stewed potatoes; baked cup custard. (5) Raw oysters with any of the above.

Sample Suppers:
(1) Creamed chicken on toast; milk or cocoa. (2) Oyster stew; bread and butter; cocoa. (3) Minced chicken on toast; baked apple and cream; tea. (4) Dropped eggs on toast; graham bread and butter; cocoa or tea. (5) Raw oysters with any of the above.

SPRUE.

Since the acquisition by the United States of the tropical islands of Porto Rico and the Manila group, and with the return of missionaries from the East, cases of sprue are increasingly seen and the need for a proper dietary is correspondingly necessary. Most of the cases seen are past the acute stage on arrival here, and the feeding problem is not so urgent as at the onset; relapses occur, however, in this climate, and it is then necessary to return to such diets as are best for the acute condition. Manson,[1] whose experience with tropical diseases makes his advice of paramount importance, insists on the absolute necessity of the milk diet in the early stages and during a relapse, and says "failure to realize this or to attempt half-way measures is responsible for most of the serious consequences of this disease."

The milk cure as recommended by Manson is as follows: For the first twenty-four hours 60 ounces of milk are allowed; the milk should not be drunk but sipped with a spoon in very small amounts. After the first day the quantity of milk should be increased at the rate of $\frac{1}{2}$ pint a day or every other day until 100 ounces are taken in twenty-four hours. This amount should be continued for ten days, and then if everything is satisfactory the amount may be gradually increase up to 6 or 7 pints. The length of time this should be kept up is as Manson says "for six weeks, dating from the time the stools become solid and the mouth free from irrita-

[1] Tropical Diseases, New York, 1908.

tion." No other food or drink whatever should be permitted. After this a raw egg, artificially malted cereals, well-boiled arrow-root, stale bread, or zweiback and butter. Later chicken broth and a little fruit. Still later fish, and chicken. Cases that cannot take plain milk may be given it peptonized or as koumyss, etc. The fruit treatment in connection with milk has also found much favor in certain quarters and the taking of bananas and apples has been found useful. Strawberries seem to be especially helpful, and Manson begins by giving one or two berries with each milk feeding, increasing the amount until 2 or 3 pounds are taken daily. Preserved fruits, especially peaches and pears, are allowed in case strawberries are not to be had. In the light of our present knowledge the usefulness of the strawberries may well be due to its contained water soluble B (vitamines).

Occasionally a patient is found who cannot take milk in any form or in whom the milk treatment fails; these cases often do well on meat juice, and after a day or two, scraped meat, later the thoroughly toasted bread or biscuits, and a gradual advance as already described. During the early stages of treatment a certain amount of nourishment can be introduced by means of nutritive enemata. (See Section on Rectal Feeding.) As the patients get on a more mixed diet it will often be seen that the stools are distinctly fatty and an examination for the normal ferments shows markedly deficient trypsin and amylase with or without a high total free fat above the normal (25 per cent. in feces). The stools may seem digested, but the assimilation is poor and the body weight remains fixed low or decreasing.

These evidences of impaired pancreatic digestion are quite regularly present in practically all the cases at some stage of the disease, and much benefit is derived by giving commercially prepared ferments, as diastase and dried pancreatic extracts (in salol or keratin-coated capsules). When the gastric digestion is impaired, as shown by the results of a test-meal analysis, dilute hydrochloric acid and pepsin are helpful.

As little or nothing is known of the etiology of this disease the dietary routine is, of course, purely an empirical one and has been built up entirely on clinical experience. The determination of gastric or pancreatic loss of function to a greater or less degree is a matter of routine examination, and taking advantage of the findings often results in the increased absorption of food, with consequent gain in weight.

DENTAL CARIES.

It is common knowledge that dental caries is on the increase, and although it is also true that more attention is given to the teeth than formerly, and some of the bad effects of the caries are minimized, the original statement holds true. Durand[1] calls attention anew to the influence of diet on the development and health of the teeth, quoting various authorities, and comparing the dental caries of the present-day children with evidences of the same trouble in the examination of prehistoric skulls. An examination of 10,500 English and Scotch school children, showed dental caries in 86 per cent.;[2] among 19,725 children in northern Germany, 95 per cent.; and in the United States the record was little better. Among ancient British and Anglo-Saxon skulls decay was found in only 15 per cent.; of Anglo-Saxon, 2.9 per cent.; British of stone age, 21.8 per cent.; bronze age, 32 per cent.[3]

A good many different factors have been blamed for this condition, prominent among which are the softness of the foods given, requiring little chewing, the extreme temperatures at which foods are fed, varying from ice-cream to hot coffee and the tremendous per capita increase in the consumption of sugar throughout the civilized world. Bearing on this last point Seagrave, for the Seattle Department of Public Health, examined the teeth of 2000 children from two to seven years of age who had been fed for the first six months of life on either breast milk, cow's milk mixtures or sweetened condensed milk, with the following results:

Food.	Number examined	Number showing caries	Percentage of caries
Breast milk	829	366	42.6
Cow's milk mixture . . .	232	102	42.9
Sweetened condensed milk .	61	41	72.1

Durand's figures bearing on the same conditions are as follows:

Breast milk	418	118	28.2
Cow's milk mixtures . . .	102	30	29.4
Sweetened condensed milk .	32	17	53.1
Sweetened condensed milk (private cases)	104	77	74.0

Durand says "the significance of these statistics is that a poorly balanced diet, high in carbohydrate (particularly sugar—Ed.) and low in fat, protein, and mineral constituents fed during the period in which the teeth are developing and

[1] Jour. Am. Med. Assn., 1916, lxvii, 8, p. 564.
[2] Rose, in British Dental Association Report, quoted by Smale.
[3] Mummery: Tr. Odont. Soc., ii, 215.

calcifying in the jaws, seems to have rendered them doubly susceptible to decay after they erupted."

From this it is evident that the proper feeding for children does not include condensed milk, except for very short periods of time to combat, for instance an intestinal indigestion, nor sweets in generous amount at any time.

The diet should be breast milk or properly modified cow's milk, giving vegetables, fruits, and meat as early as possible, these latter may often be given as early as the sixth month. It is also advisable to give a child foods that require chewing, as "strips of tough meat, bacon rind, bones, tough crusts, hard bread, and later apple, celery, lettuce, etc." Durand emphasizes the fact that the last article of food eaten should not be some sweet carbohydrate which will leave a decaying residue, but an acid fruit which produces a highly alkaline saliva with a high percentage cf ptyalin. In a practical test by Wallace[1] 14 children were fed on these principles and at the ages from five to seven years there was not the slightest evidence of caries.

DIET IN CANCER.

In the absence of definite knowledge of the etiology of cancer any method of dietetic treatment must necessarily be empirical and although many methods of diet have been tried to combat the disease, it must be said that in human cancer the progress and results have been exceedingly meagre and hardly encouraging.

In 1880 Beneke[2] found cancer cells rich in cholesterine and observation had shown that cancer was more frequent in carnivora than in herbivora and more frequent among people who were great meat eaters. On this basis Beneke's diet was designed with little nitrogenous food. Kessler[3] designed a diet low in sulphur on the basis of this knowledge that the sulphur metabolism is disturbed in cancer, giving only sulphur free foods or with a minimum content.

For nitrogenous foods he allows:

Fish: Halibut, salmon, white fish, cod, mackeral herring, shad, black fish, Spanish mackeral and porgy.

No meat of ox or blood (rich in sulphur).

Buttermilk is also bad and egg yolk, not white.

Vegetables allowed are: truffles, rhubarb, beets, chicory, pumpkin, lettuce, beans, peas, romain salad, chestnuts.

Cereals: Wheat, oatmeal, rice, corn bread, barley, buckwheat, poppy seed, graham bread.

[1] Dental Record, London, 1912 p 56.
[2] Deutsch Arch. fur Klin Med., xv, 1880.
[3] New York Med. Jour., Nov. 30, 1917.

Fruits; Almonds, olives, plums, oranges, huckleberries,
strawberries.
Casein and butter, as they are almost sulphur free.
Sample menu of Kessler's diet:
Breakfast: Tea or coffee with sugar and cream.
(No milk on account of lactalbumin which is high in
sulphur).
Fresh or cooked fruit.
One of the cereals allowed.
Dinner: Soup of fruit, cereals, or vegetables (not meat).
Beans, peas, lentils.
Meat, two ounces at most.
Potato dumplings, carrots, beets or other edible roots.
Boiled or preserved fruits, rice and salad.
Casein is added to the food to bring up the protein to normal or is given as medicine 1 to 3 drams (4 to 12 gm.) every
three hours.
Supper: Fruit with rice, potato and butter, salads.
Centanni[1] says the idea of dietetic treatment of malignant
disease is not new, but hitherto the experiments have been
made with a diet which starved all the cells. The consequence was that the normal cells were too weak to contend
with the cancer cells and the malignant disease was merely
whipped up by the modified diet. Centanni, on the other
hand, sought to modify the diet in such a way that it amply
sufficed for the nourishment of all the cells, cancer cells included, but the substances in the diet which promote growth
were all carefully excluded, and others added which tend to
inhibit growth. Modern research has demonstrated a number
of food substances which promote growth—he calls them "blastins" and he emphasizes that cancer cells do not differ essentially from normal cells except in their "tumultuous multiplication." By depriving them of those elements in the food
the fundamental office of which is to sustain the multiplicative function, auxetics, Wuchsstoffe or blastins, and for
which the cancer cells display exceptional avidity, the tumor
cells languish and die. Among the facts which testify to
the correctness of this assumption are Haaland's experiences
—confirmed by others—to the effect that gestation prevents
successful grafting of tumors and checks the growth of those
already implanted. The physiologic growth of the fetus
victoriously combats the pathologic growth of the cancer.
In Centanni's research he experimented with ninety-three
series of from four to ten mice each. On ordinary food, 100
per cent. of the tumor grafts "took" and some grew to be

[1] Reforma Med., 1918, xxxiv, No. 32.

larger than the body of the mouse to start with. Given the restricted diet ten days beforehand, none of the grafts "took" or only feebly grew. On this diet, tumors already established, up to 2 or 2.5 cm. in diameter, became arrested and were finally reabsorbed without leaving a trace. Large tumors softened and decayed to a friable mass. The most striking results were obtained when the main mass of the tumor was resected and the remainder became reabsorbed as the animals were kept on the blastin-free diet. The growth promoting substances are certain vitamines, certain internal secretions, and certain chemical substances. In his experimental diet he took particular pains to exclude the anti-scurvy vitamine and nuclein and phosphorus compounds, and denatured the food by heating to 125 or 130 C. The outlook for application of the principle to man seems hopeful as human beings are particularly sensitive to lack of vitamines, while the size of the cancer in proportion to the whole body is immeasurably smaller than in the experiments related. On the other hand, the results will take much longer to become manifest. The method is harmless, as any disturbances from a dietetic deficiency would be recognized early and could be promptly remedied. Experienced medical supervision would be indispensable.

DIET RECOMMENDED FOR SPEAKERS AND SINGERS

These people, as a rule, should eat a mixed diet, obeying the rules of moderation and hygiene as should others. It is best for the voice not to take food for a few hours before it is to be used, so that people who sing or expect to make a speech in the evening have the habit of eating a light meal at about 5 P.M., and nothing then until after the performance, when they again take something to eat. All sorts of dietary fads have arisen among professional singers and actors of taking some one special form of food before using the voice and find no harm, but there is little evidence that these special foods have a specific effect or lack of it. Their chief usefulness lies in the fact that it is usually confined to one article of diet in small amount so that no particular effect follows its use.

When the voice is husky, sucking a lemon with a small lump of sugar imbedded in it helps some people, others find dram doses of whiskey and glycerin or whiskey, glycerin and lemon juice of value. The value, however, of many of these things is more fancied than real.

DIET ADAPTED TO THE USE OF BRAIN WORKERS.

The requirements of food for brain workers do not differ materially from those of other people leading a sedentary life, for, contrary to the general opinion, brain work does not require as much food as muscular work of a corresponding degree of intensity. It is necessary for these people to take more food than those who are absolutely quiet without any occupation, but the difference is slight. On the other hand, while the quantity may be only that of the person at ordinary activity there is the greatest necessity for care in the selection of the kind of food to be eaten. It is necessary to avoid indigestible foods of all kinds, as these people are prone to indigestion, and on account of their lack of exercise have not the vitality for digestion that their more active brothers have. The food should therefore be simple with the avoidance of heavy meats, such as pork, veal, corned or salt meat or fish, pies, pastry, heavy sweets as preserves, rich sauces and salads, devilled crabs, etc.

Fish was formerly thought to be of special value in the diet of brain workers on account of its large percentage of phosphorus, the brain also requiring a larger amount of phosphorus than the rest of the body, as shown by its chemical analysis. The theory has been completely disproved, and fish is only so much protein so far as feeding goes.

Brain workers should take alcohol only in the greatest moderation, or better none at all, as without exercise the injurious effects of alcohol are greatly exaggerated.

DIET FOR ATHLETES.

Much has been written on the subject of diet in connection with feats of muscular strength, more particularly for athletes, and one may get a variety of opinions for the asking. Much of the subject is founded on the personal experience and observations of trainers, and although a good deal of scientific work has been done in America, particularly, and forms a basis for many of the rules, the greater part is based on clinical observation. It has been a rule that those engaged in severe muscular effort should eat a larger proportion of protein food than should those who live an ordinary life or who take a moderate amount of exercise.

The experiments of Chittenden have shown that a man may thrive on about one-third the ordinary allowance of protein and yet be capable of a large, though perhaps not excessive, amount of muscular work. While this is an established fact it is a question that needs longer experience to prove that the same rule holds true for those engaged in severe work, and it is probable that rather more than this minimum protein allowance is the optimum for athletes, although protein destruction does not go on at a much higher rate in athletes. The mere fact that excessive effort has always been accompanied by a very large protein intake does not necessarily mean that this is the best regimen, for above all, the excretory organs should not be given an extra amount of unnecessary work by the ingestion of an excessive diet, particularly of the proteins.

Carbohydrates and fats spare the protein combustion and should constitute a considerable excess proportion of the athlete's diet, and the fact that the effort is to be excessive and of short duration calls for a different proportion of the food elements compared with that needed for sustained muscular work. Thus, in short, running dashes, feats of strength which are quickly over, there is need of a greater proportion of carbohydrates (sugars) for although the specific dynamic action of protein is greater the heat derived from this is not available for work.[1] When a sustained muscular effort is to be made fats are of great importance as well. An interesting illustration of the latter is seen in the diet of the Western cowboys, who find that if they have a long piece of hard work ahead of them, with little chance to eat a proper meal until night, they can accomplish this most easily if their meal before starting contains a large percentage of fat. This is because the combustion of fat is much slower than that of either protein or carbohydrate, and its availability as food reaches its maximum a much longer time after its ingestion.

Three meals a day are better for all athletes than repeated small meals, and the diet should be a generally mixed one.

The association of gradually increasing work and increasing diet is an important one, and the food required by a man in training, to a certain extent, should keep pace with his muscular development; in other words, training consists in a gradual increase of effort and diet should be increased accordingly, *i. e.*, the largest diet should not be allowed in the early days of training. The end of training should also be marked by a decreased diet, not always a simple matter, for it is easy to acquire the habit of large eating, and its continuance after the necessity for it is past. This disproportion is said to be the cause of much of "farmer's indigestion," a continuance of a large dietary during the winter when there is comparatively little muscular effort required in the running of the farm.

[1] Paul E. Howe.

When it comes to actual figures to express the needs of the body for severe muscular work, we can, of course, only deal with averages, keeping in mind the underlying principles of diet already referred to.

The following figures are presented so that there may be compared some diets actually in use with standards expressive of the body's requirement during severe muscular exercise.

Rowing	Protein	Fat	Carbohydrate	Calories
Average of six crews	155 gm. (5 oz.)	177 gm. (6 oz.)	440 gm. (14½ oz.)	4085
Football average of two teams	225 gm. (7½ oz.)	354 gm. (12 oz.)	633 gm. (21 oz.)	6812
Standard(Voit) hard muscular work	145 gm. (5 oz.)	100 gm. (3½ oz.)	450 gm. (15 oz.)	3370
Hard muscular work (Playfair)[1]	185 gm. (6 oz.)	71 gm. (2⅓ oz.)	568 gm. (19 oz.)	3750

From this comparison it will be seen that the diet actually used by the crews differs little from the Voit standard, whereas the football teams consumed a very much greater proportion of all three food elements. This is comparable to the difference in the length of time consumed in the contests—a rowing race of four miles lasting usually from thirteen to fifteen minutes; a football game, an hour, with one short intermission—the caloric needs also of the latter being apparently about 50 per cent. greater. These dietaries are of course founded on experience perhaps rather than on actual food requirements.

Sugar.—Much has been written on the usefulness of considerable amounts of sugar for athletes but definite conclusions based on accurate experimentation are lacking. There is no doubt but that sugar forms a readily usable form of carbohydrate, with high caloric value, and may, in moderation, form part of an athlete's diet; but that one should take excessive amounts of it for this purpose is not in all probability a wise thing, as it may easily result in a disturbed digestion, both gastric and intestinal, accompanied by fermentation.

The diet for athletes, as already stated, should be a mixed one, consisting of meats, fish, eggs, milk, cereals, stale bread, roll, or toast, occasionally baked potato, macaroni, rice or other farinaceous articles, a moderate allowance of sugar, fats of all sorts, especially butter, cream, and fat meat. Green vegetables, ripe fruits, fresh or stewed. Water taken

[1] Bulletin 21, U. S. Dept. Agriculture.

largely between meals or an hour before and after exercise (but never iced). Some trainers allow weak tea and coffee, but it is probably that those in training are better off without either. The same rule applying to all alcoholic beverages, although an occasional glass of mild beer may have a tonic effect when the appetite is uncertain.

Foods to Avoid.—Soups, except an occasional purée. Tough, indigestible meats, as veal, pork, salted meats or fish, except occasionally a bit of bacon. Gravies, rich entrées, spiced food, hot breads and cakes or rich cake (cookies and a little dry, simple cake are allowable). Candy and pies. Wine, beer, ale, spirits, tea and coffee.

Dietary Rules for Athletes.

1. Eat slowly and masticate all food thoroughly.

2. Do not exercise violently for at least an hour to an hour and a half after meals, better two or three hours.

3. Do not eat immediately after exercise, allow at least thirty to forty-five minutes for actual rest.

4. Do not wash food down with any fluids, a moderate amount of fluid with meals is permissible, but should be drunk between mouthfuls or at the end of the meal.

5. Water in any desired amount may be taken during the day, the bulk of it is best taken between meals or at least a half-hour before eating.

6. Do not eat an excess of any kind of food with the idea that the more food one takes the stronger one will be, the opposite is much nearer the truth.

7. Remember that milk is a food and should never be used merely to quench one's thirst.

8. Avoid tea and coffee and alcoholic beverages.

THE FEEDING OF UNCONSCIOUS PATIENTS.

In many if not most unconscious patients the swallowing reflex is preserved, so that food is automatically sent down the esophagus as soon as it reaches the posterior pharyngeal wall. In such cases it is possible to feed a certain amount by the spoon or slipping a small catheter into the side of the cheek on the dependent side and pouring liquid food into the funnel very slowly. If only a quantity equal to a normal swallow is given at a time, this does very well; faster feeding or the giving of greater amounts will cause laryngeal irritation and choking.

If this method is not easily accomplished the simplest way is to feed by gavage through the nose or mouth, which ever proves easier. This is done as follows:

A small-sized, smooth-rubber catheter is lubricated with vaseline or some lubricating jelly and passed through the nose down the throat beyond the laryngeal opening or through the mouth to the same point. A glass funnel is then attached to the distal end, and the liquid food, warmed, is poured slowly down. When the feeding is finished, in removing the tube close the lumen by bending or squeezing it between the thumb and forefinger. This will prevent the few remaining drops from getting into the larynx.

The food best adapted to this use are some of the milk, cream, and lactose mixtures recommended for typhoid fever patients (p. 575), to which raw eggs, beaten up, may be added, or thin cereal or the food formula given under suralimentation, may be tried. The intervals of feeding should be as long as possible, preferably not oftener than three times in the twenty-four hours The caloric needs of the individual must be considered in arranging for the exact quantity to be used in the twenty-four hours.

FOOD POISONING.

The importance of poisoning by food is impressed by practical experience upon everyone at some time in their lives, and he is fortunate who is not rendered helpless or worse by such an experience. At one time or another almost every article of food belonging to anyone of the classes of food constituents has been blamed for causing symptoms of poisoning, many of them, legitimately, others in error. Individual susceptibility plays a great part in the precipitation of symptoms, and in a given instance, where a number of persons are poisoned at the same time after eating approximately the same amount of the tainted food, some are made much more ill than others, while at the same time some are entirely unaffected. This is particularly well seen in the hypersusceptibility of certain persons to a particular protein showing an anaphylactic reaction when another is untouched by the same condition.

Food Poisons May be Divided into:
1. Endogenous (to the food).
2. Exogenous.

1. In endogenous poisonous foods the poison is an inherent quality of the food, as muscarine in mushrooms. The blood of some eels is poisonous from preformed physiological products. Some mollusks and fish are believed to be poisonous at certain phases of their sexual life. Certain fish are highly poisonous even when fresh, probably from leucomains and

41

basic alkaloidal substances elaborated by the cell metabolism.[1]

2. Exogenous poisonous foods are the more common and may be divided into (*a*) poisonous compounds, such as the metals, arsenic, tin, antimony, lead, zinc, and copper; (*b*) animal parasites such as trichinæ, etc.; (*c*) the most frequent form is due to bacteria and fungi. Food infection is thus the most frequent form of food poisoning and can affect every sort of food imaginable.

Milk as one of the chief articles of diet is particularly subject to contamination; it is an ideal culture medium for certain bacteria, giving rise to all sorts of gastro-intestinal inflammatory conditions in infants, besides acting as a carrier in typhoid, streptococcus sore throat, scarlet fever, and cholera. Milk poison as such or galactotoxismus is analogous to meat or fish intoxication. Tryotoxicon also produced in milk, cheese, and ice-cream (discovered by Vaughan in 1885), is probably not the product of one organism but of several.

Meat Poisoning.—Three kinds:[2]

1. Due to eating meat from diseased animals. This is usually associated with the Bacillus enteritides or paratyphi.

2. Due to eating putrefied meat, usually associated with Bacillus proteus and Bacillus coli.

3. Due to "sausage poison" produced by the anaërobic Bacillus botulinus.

The first kind is often from freshly killed meat, the other two when the meat has been kept awhile. The first two kinds of poisoning are of the gastro-enteric type and the third gives symptoms referable to the central nervous system.

Fish Poisoning.—1. Poisoning in which the poison exists in the living animal.

2. Those in which the poison develops subsequently.

Certain fish or parts, *e. g.*, roe or ovarian tissue, are sometimes poisonous, giving rise to choleraic symptoms, paralyses, convulsions, and often death. This poison is present in the "fugu" roe, also the roe of barbs (German fish) when eaten in May is poisonous, and, according to Kobert, the liver and bile of a number of fish are poisonous. Some mussels and snails are poisonous. Oysters convey typhoid when fattened in polluted beds. Shell fish usually give rise to poisoning by either anaphylaxis or direct bacterial poisoning, which may show itself in three forms:

[1] Ref. Handbook Med. Sc., 1914, 3d edition, iv, 420.
[2] Bolderon: Food Poisoning, p. 15.

1. Gastro-enteric type with nausea, vomiting and diarrhea.

2. Exanthemic type showing skin eruptions, erythematous, vesicular or urticarial.

3. A type of poisoning much like botulism and affecting the central nervous system.[1]

Vegetable Poisoning.—Potato poisoning was at first thought to be due to solanin, but the quantity of solanin even in two pounds of potatoes is too small to cause symptoms, and it is more probable that potato poisoning is due to bacterial decomposition of potatoes by proteus bacilli, as observed by Dieudonne.[2] The poisoning from potatoes is more apt to occur when the potatoes are cooked one day and kept in large pots or containers until the next day, before being eaten, and in warm weather the decomposition can take place very rapidly. Most of the outbreaks of potato poisoning have taken place in July and August, and usually when new potaoes are used.

Poisoning by Canned Goods.—Meats, fish, and vegetables which, if not absolutely sterilized when canned, undergo putrefaction with the evolution of gas, which can be known by inspecting the can, for under such circumstances the top of the can is convex or bulging, and when it is opened a foul odor and gas escape.

Canned salmon has a particularly bad reputation among fish. Numerous outbreaks have been reported after eating canned vegetables. String beans have been often at fault; but no matter which vegetable is to blame there is no question but that all these outbreaks of poisoning can be traced to a bacterial origin of one or another kind.

In the vegetable poisoning we have moulds as a factor, which is not true of meat or other animal products, such as fish, roe, eggs, and milk, which are strictly bacterial in origin; thus, for example, we find ergot of rye the cause of ergotism.

It would be possible to go on indefinitely multiplying examples of poisoning by almost every form of food which had become infected, but enough has been said to point to the importance of the subject to persons in health, and to those already suffering from disease an additional burden of intoxication, from such a cause, may easily prove fatal.

What, then, has this subject to do with dietetics? Everything from the point of view of prophylaxis, very little when the mischief has already been done. There are, however, certain dietetic and culinary precautions which should be observed, most of which are so self-evident as hardly to need mention.

[1] Ibid., p. 915.   [2] Deutsch. Militär Ztschr., 1904.

Dietary Precautions.—1. Only fresh food should be bought from a reliable dealer, unless the buyer is able to decide for himself just what is fresh.

2. Meat that tastes "queer," oysters that are spoiled, and meat that is bitter, strong, or rancid should be ejected from the mouth, no matter in whose society. It can be artistically done.

3. Cooking thoroughly, broiling, roasting, or boiling kills most of the bacteria, but is usually ineffectual in removing the products of decomposition or in making them ineffective. Ordinary boiling does not kill all kinds of bacteria; most are readily killed but some resist prolonged boiling. Bacillus botulinus is easily decomposed by heat, while Bacillus paratyphi produces a poison which cannot be eliminated even by boiling a long time.[1]

4. Not less than a 15 per cent. solution of salt should be used as brine for salting, and smoking food must be done very thoroughly, or in either case the bacteria will not be destroyed.

5. Fish if frozen fresh, will keep almost indefinitely without loss of essential good qualities, palatability, or change in sanitary characteristics.[2] But if the fish are frozen after being infected when they are thawed for cooking the poisonous effects will be seen as readily as if they had not been frozen.

6. Food should be eaten as soon as convenient after cooking, and should not be kept for long intervals. If necessary to keep food over, particularly in hot weather, it should be cooked again just before eating.

7. Canned goods should never be used if the can is seen to have a convex top, as this is always due to imperfect sterilization, with resulting fermentation and putrefaction, the bulging being caused by the gas under pressure. These cans are called "swells" or "blow" cans.

8. All canned food should be thoroughly cooked through before serving, to kill any possible organisms, and if the entire canful is not used at one meal it should be kept in stone or enamel ware on ice and not in the can.

9. Meat and potatoes after being cooked together should not be kept over night as a ptomain (?) is developed that is exceedingly apt to cause a severe diarrhoea particularly if the food is not kept on ice.

If by chance it becomes necessary to prescribe a diet for a patient who is suffering from food-poisoning one should fol-

[1] Munchen. med. Wchnschr., 1902, xlix, 1817.
[2] Biochem. Bull. Col. University, New York, October, 1913, p. 54.

low the rules laid down for the diet of the concomitant condition which it causes, *e. g.*, diet for acute gastritis, gastro-enteritis, or enterocolitis, according to which part of the intestinal canal is affected. It is needless to say that if any food is remaining in the stomach or intestine, patients must have gastric lavage, quick and effectual catharsis, and high colonic irrigations.

SPECIAL DIETARY CURES.

As long as food is necessary to man, just so long will there be dietary fads, and greater or less stress will be put upon the omission or taking of one or another class of food-stuff, largely according to the effect upon the individual originating the special form of dietary. While this is so, there develops, as a result of these various diets, valuable suggestions which may be applied with equal benefit to other forms of more normal dietaries. Thus, many of Fletcher's ideas are excellent and useful for anyone to apply—so, too, the emphasis placed upon the taking of more vegetable foods, fruits, nuts, etc., is valuable— but few people are willing to abide by a hard-and-fast method of eating, and rightly, as the individual equation is always important and must be considered. There are, of course, many more forms of dietary cure than the few mentioned in the text, but it hardly seems worth while going into the subject more extensively.

The Vegetarian Diet.—Vegetarianism, as a propaganda, has been so befogged by prejudice, ignorance, and inaccuracy that it has never received support from any considerable proportion of the inhabitants of the temperate zone, and lack of opportunity has, of course, shut out from its use those who live in excessively cold climates. Many of the inhabitants of the tropics, on the other hand, voluntarily have assumed a modification of this diet, largely as a matter of expediency, and because they found that a flesh diet was not one that gave them the best physical results. Thompson calls attention to historical and anthropological facts, such as the structure of the teeth in prehistoric skulls, the character and length of the digestive canal, organs and secretions to prove that man has always been omnivorous, and that he is intended to be, is evidenced by the presence of free hydrochloric acid and pepsin in the gastric secretion, which are of no particular use in the digestion of vegetable protein. Of the diets of aboriginal people, some were largely vegetarians, some largely meat-eaters, depending on the seasons and the opportunities for obtaining principally one or the other form of food, but all have been mixed feeders when possible. Some famous men have been vegetarians, but one suspects that they would have been famous anyhow regardless of their diet, and Hall[1] says that history fails to show that a people on a vegetable diet ever rose very high in the scale of civilization, most of the world's work being done by people in the temperate zone, where a mixed diet is the rule. Those who advocate a vegetarian diet do so on these grounds:

1. Physiological, in that vegetarianism tends to prolong life, make it healthier, and produces a better temperament.

2. Economical, in that it is less costly to the individual and the state.

3. Moral, in that humanity forbids the slaughter of animals for food.[2]

In support of the physiological grounds for a vegetable diet, Newman[3] holds that:

1. The rich who eat meat largely are the ones subject to gout, arteriosclerosis. etc.

2. That vegetarians recover more quickly from wounds.

3. That they are less liable to epidemic diseases.

4. That cases of extreme longevity are usually found among those that live exclusively on a vegetarian diet.

These claims, of course, are categorically contradicted by the advocates of a mixed diet.

While it is true that nitrogenous equilibrium can be maintained when the protein of peas, beans, and some leaf proteins is substituted for that of meat and milk, it is necessarily done at the expense of a dietary excessive in amount, for although the protein of vegetable origin is assimilable it is not nearly so much so as that of animal origin. McCollum has also shown by animal experiments that the protein derived from seeds of plants alone is incapable of supporting life but that the protein of the leaves of plants must be added in order to maintain the equilibrium. Vegetable protein is so intimately associated with the cellulose and starch, it is metabolized with difficulty, as much as 17 per cent. being lost.[4] The extreme of this is perhaps best seen in mushrooms where the percentage of protein is very high, so accounting for its popularity as a food, whereas, chemical analysis of the stools shows that practically none of its contained protein is assimilated.

The greater bulk of this diet has certain disadvantages:

1. In that the stomach and bowels are somewhat distended, as seen in cattle with their large bellies, also noted

---

[1] Nutrition and Dietetics, p. 46.
[2] Rutgers: Ztschr. of Biol., 1888, xxiv, 351.　　　[3] Essays on Diet, p. 87.
[4] Thompson: Dietetics, p. 33.

among certain cases of the Irish, where a similar condition known as "potato belly" is well-known. This tends to the enfeeblement of the digestive organs and diarrhea. The average stool of the meat-eater is 120 gm.; that of a vegetarian 333 gm.[1]

2. So much muscular effort is necessary to digest the food that it necessitates a large amount of blood and nervous energy.

3. The great amount of water is a disadvantage and causes softness from retained water, and probably accounts for the low resistance to disease often seen in vegetarians.

In comparing the protein of meat and vegetables we find.[2]

100 parts of lean beef contain 89 parts of protein.
100 parts of fat beef contain 51 parts of protein.
100 parts of pea flour contain 27 parts of protein.
100 parts of wheat contain 16 parts of protein.
100 parts of rice contain 7 parts of protein.

This illustrates that vegetable protein to be sufficient must be eaten in large amount. When it comes to a consideration of the vitality of vegetarians we meet with opposing views, those recommending mixed feeding feeling sure that vitality is much higher than under a vegetarian regimen. The Japanese, on the other hand, although largely vegetarians, have great vitality but small stature; but, as a matter of fact, few of them are exclusively vegetarians, for, as a people, they eat much fish and consume milk and eggs.

There are three classes of so-called vegetarians.

1. Those who eat nothing but cereals and vegetables.

2. Those who together with vegetable and farinaceous foods, also consume animal protein in the form of eggs and milk.

3. Fruitarians living exclusively on fruits, nuts and cereals. There are comparatively few strict vegetarians of the first and third classes and when one hears of people being vegetarians, it will almost always be found that at least milk and eggs are included in their diet.

Metabolism of Vegetarians.—Recently an effort has been made to advocate a vegetarian regimen on a strictly scientific basis[3] and the "measure of the basal gaseous metabolism, which may be considered as the carbon-dioxide production and oxygen consumption during complete muscular repose, and at least twelve hours after the last meal, gives an admir-

[1] Voit: Ztschr. f. Biol., 1889, xxv, 232.
[2] Hutchinson: Food and Dietetics, 3d edition, p. 173.
[3] Buttner: A Fleshless Diet, F. A. Stokes & Co., 1910.

able index of the metabolic activity."[1] Benedict and Roth[2] have followed this out on persons who have been vegetarians for years, and found that heat production per twenty-four hours as computed from the gaseous exchange showed that the vegetarians produced 25.5 calories per kilo and the non-vegetarians of like height and weight, 26.4 calories; also, there was too little difference between the respiratory quotients to be taken as evidence of a larger glycogen storage in vegetarians as compared with non-vegetarians.

The evidence thus shows there is no advantage in a strictly vegetarian diet, and although it is possible to live and thrive fairly well on such a diet, its disadvantages are too great to make it probable that, except for short periods and possibly in the tropics, it will ever become a universal diet. The anthropological history of the world shows that in the earliest times men often lived largely on meat; when civilization brought class distinctions the poorer classes ate less meat, the richer classes more meat, increasingly so. Of late there has been a distinct reaction in the meat-eating of the wealthier classes, and one sees less meat and more vegetable food consumed than formerly. Civilized people become more sedentary in their habits as they progress upward in the scale of civilization, and find they need less of the stimulating qualities of animal protein; and, because, also, on account of their sedentary habits, people find that the ingestion of considerable quantities of animal protein, with the consequent increase in intestinal putrefaction, gives rise to symptoms of toxemia, which have assumed a very definite place in the pathology of disease.

Vegetarian Diets.—When it is necessary or advisable to make use of the vegetarian regimen plus the usual addition of milk and eggs for additional and less bulky protein we find an endless variety of menus which one may choose from, of which, the following are a few samples:[3]

Meat substitutes:

Cheese souffle, corn and cheese, Welsh rarebit, baked cracker and cheese. Cheese rolls. Nut and cheese roast. Cheese and vegetable roll. Fried bread with cheese. Cheese ramequins. Cheese croquettes. Cheese fingers, etc. Macaroni and cheese. Rice and cheese. Rice, peas, beans and lentils.

Macaroni and kidney beans. Chestnuts with hard sauce. Chestnut purée and mushroom. Boiled, creamed and broiled scalloped eggs and milk.

---

[1] Jour. Am. Med. Assn., lxiv, 17, 1425.
[2] Proc. Nat. Acad. Sc., 1915, i, 100.
[3] Gillmore: Meatless Cookery.

Sample Breakfast Menus:

Oranges; boiled rice; hashed browned potatoes; whole wheat gems; cocoa.

Fruit; hominy; baked bananas; potato cakes; toasted white bread; cereal, coffee.

Grapes; shredded wheat biscuit; fried tomatoes, corn cake; chocolate, etc.

Luncheons:

Asparagus on toast; stewed tomatoes; cottage cheese; prune fluff; spinach on toast; lettuce sandwiches; apple sauce; banana salad; rice soup; potato croquettes; tomato sandwiches; Malaga grapes.

Dinner:

Cream of vegetable soup; macaroni au gratin; mashed sweet potatoes; spinach; fruit salad; ginger pudding.

Cream of potato soup; fried bananas; lima beans; mashed turnips; apple and celery salad; tapioca pudding.

Tomato soup; new potatoes; cheese fritters; tomatoes; lettuce salad; ice-cream.

Fletcherism.—In the past, numberless propaganda of specialized diet, methods of eating, water-drinking, and the thousand and one fads which sweep the community have all been brought forward and urged with the industry of the religious zealot. In many of them there is a certain amount of common sense, and some patients are unquestionably helped, but many of the methods quickly fall into disrepute when they are found not to be beneficial to all alike.

The system of dietetics, or possibly the philosophy of dietetics, crystallized by Horace Fletcher, has stood more scientific investigation, with better results than almost any of them, and now has the enthusiastic support of many eminent men of science.

"Fletcherism," as it is called, was formerly put down as a new fad with the most salient feature of excessive mastication as the keynote, but Fletcher tells us[1] that this is not a true characterization of his method by any means, although he does recommend thorough mastication, which to rapid eaters certainly seems excessive. This method of eating was arrived at by personal experimentation after Fletcher had been rejected by a life insurance company as a bad risk, and the results in his case were surely successful, as he has repeatedly been able to undergo physical effort with less wear and tear than most of his younger contemporaries. The five principles upon which Fletcherism is founded are:

[1] Horace Fletcher: "Fletcherism:" What It Is.

"1. Wait for a true, earned appetite.

"2. Select from the food available that which appeals most to the appetite and in the order called for by appetite.

"3. Get all the good taste there is in food out of it in the mouth, and swallow only when it practically 'swallows itself.'

"4. Enjoy the good taste for all it is worth and do not allow any depressing or diverting thought to intrude upon the ceremony.

"5. Wait; take and enjoy as much as possible what appetite approves; Nature will do the rest."[1]

A great point is made of mouth digestion with fine comminution of the food, giving the ptyalin a chance to act upon the starch and convert it as far as possible toward the ultimate maltose before swallowing it. The action of ptyalin is arrested by the acid in the gastric secretion and is only completed later in the intestine by pancreatic amylase. The discovery was made that if food is properly prepared for swallowing, it is difficult to keep from swallowing it, as the pharyngeal reflex is so strong. The same rule applies to liquids as to solids, and it is not so much a matter of what one eats, if one is hungry for it, as how one eats.

Fletcher disposes of the common criticism that his method will upset the meal schedule of the best-regulated family by saying that a week's trial will determine how many meals a person should eat as a rule, two or three according to the amount of appetite, and the meals should be taken at a regular meal hour.

If when a meal is due there is no appetite, wait until the next, and if appetite calls for food before it is due, this is usually easily quieted by a drink of water. After a time the new habits become second nature and the regulation of the meal hour presents no difficulty, as habit determines the new schedule, whether it be for one or more meals a day.

The following method of attaining physiological economy in nutrition has been formulated by Fletcher and is included now in the Instructions to the Medical Department of the United States Army under the following heading:

METHOD OF ATTAINING ECONOMIC ASSIMILATION OF NUTRIMENT AND IMMUNITY FROM DISEASE, MUSCULAR SORENESS AND FATIGUE.

1. Feed only when a distinct appetite has been earned.

2. Masticate all solid food until it is completely liquefied and excites in an irresistible manner the swallowing reflex or swallowing impulse.

[1] Ibid., p. 8.

3. Attention to the act and appreciation of the taste are necessary, meantime, to excite the flow of gastric juice into the stomach to meet the food, as demonstrated by Pawlow.

4. Strict attention to these two particulars will fulfill the requirements of Nature relative to the preparation of the food for digestion and assimilation; and this being faithfully done, the automatic processes of digestion and assimilation will proceed most profitably and will result in discarding very little digestion-ash (feces) to encumber the intestines or to compel excessive draft upon the bodily energy for excretion.

5. The assurance of healthy economy is observed in the small amount of excreta and its peculiar inoffensive character, showing escape from putrid bacterial decomposition such as brings indol and skatol offensively into evidence.

6. When digestion and assimilation have been normally economic, the digestion-ash (feces) may be formed into little balls ranging in size from a pea to a so-called Queen olive, according to the food taken, and should be quite dry, having only the odor of moist clay or of a hot biscuit. This inoffensive character remains indefinitely until the ash completely dries, or disintegrates like rotten stone or wood.

7. The weight of the digestive-ash may range (moist) from 10 grams to not more than 40 to 50 grams a day, according to the food; the latter estimate being based on a vegetarian diet, and may not call for excretion for several days; smallness indicating best condition. Foods differ so materially that the amount and character of the excreta cannot be accurately specified. Some foods and conditions demand two evacuations daily. Thorough and faithful Fletcherizing settles the question satisfactorily.

8. Fruits may hasten peristalsis; but not if they are treated in the mouth as sapid liquids rather than as solids, and are insalivated, sipped, tasted, into absorption in the same way wine-tasters test and take wine, and tea-tasters test tea. The latter spit out the tea after tasting, as otherwise it vitiates their taste and ruins them for their discriminating profession.

9. Milk, soups, wines, beer and all sapid liquids or semi-solids should be treated in this manner for the best assimilation and digestion as well as for the best gustatory results.

10. This would seem to entail a great deal of care and bother, and lead to a waste of time.

11. Such, however, is not the case. To give attention in the beginning does require strict attention and persistent care to overcome life-long habits of nervous haste; but if the attack is earnest, habits of careful mouth treatment and

appetite discrimination soon become fixed and cause deliberation in taking food unconsciously to the feeder.

12. Food of a protein value of 5 to 7 grams of nitrogen and 1500 to 2500 calories of fuel value paying strict attention to the appetite for selection and carefully treated in the mouth, has been found to be the quantity best suited to economy and efficiency of both mind and body in sedentary pursuits and ordinary business activity; and also, such habit of economy has given practical immunity from the common diseases for a period extending over more than fifteen years, whereas the same subject was formerly liable to periodical illness. Similar economy and immunity have shown themselves consistently in the cases of many test subjects covering periods of ten years, and applies equally to both sexes, all ages and other idiosyncratic conditions.

13. The time necessary for satisfying complete body needs and appetite daily, when the habit of attention, appreciation and deliberation have been installed, is less than half an hour, no matter how divided as to number of rations. This necessitates industry of mastication, to be sure, and will not admit of waste of much time between mouthfuls.

14. Ten to fifteen minutes will completely satisfy a ravenous appetite if all conditions of ingestion and preparation are favorable.

15. Both quantitative and qualitative supply of saliva are important factors; but attention to these fundamental requirements of right eating soon regulates the supply of all of the digesive juices, and in connection with the care recommended above, ensures economy of nutrition and probably immunity from disease.

The results claimed by Fletcher for his method include attaining the optimum weight for the individual, freedom from muscular soreness after exercise, absence of fatigue and feeling tired, freedom from colds and the ordinary infections with a continuous feeling of well-being.

The results in certain cases at least are all Fletcher claims for them.

Fruit Cures.—The use of fruits in disease is twofold, first as part of an invalid's general diet, and secondly as a specific cure for disease.

On the score of the first it may be said that in most diseases, whether accompanied by fever or not, fruit in some form is almost always allowable unless there are digestive contra-indications and even in these cases fruit juices can usually be used. As a part of the diet it counts little for its food value and is ordinarily left out of account on that score, but its refreshing qualities, vegetable acids and laxative effect, make fruit of great value in disease. If the fruit is ripe and easily digested it may be taken raw, but if otherwise is best cooked. About the only fruits that are not good for sick people are raw pineapples, very seedy fruit, or dried fruits. Naturally some people have an idiosyncrasy for certain fruits, and we find one patient cannot take bananas, another is made ill by strawberries and so on, but outside of such contra-indications, fruits may be taken freely, either whole or as fruit juices alone or mixed with water and sugar.

When we come to examine the claims of the various fruit cures it is at once seen that whatever claims are made, the fact must be at once recognized that an exclusive fruit diet is an insufficient diet and that it is not a feasible way to nourish people, although a certain amount of food may be furnished the system in this form. In the case of people who greatly overeat and are in consequence overweight and plethoric, a fruit cure does good by virtue of its low food value and its laxative effect, both of great assistance in such conditions.

Grape Cure.—In this form of fruit cure popular abroad and in California among a few people, grapes are eaten in addition to other food, beginning with a moderate amount and gradually increasing. In this manner two pounds of grapes are given at first as follows: One-half pound on waking— one-half pound at 11 A.M. another at 5 P.M.—still another at bedtime. This may be increased to three or four or even five pounds per day in some cases. As the diet is of low protein content it is of use in renal insufficiency or in gout, on account of the "roughage;" it is helpful in constipation and again in obesity, if little other food is taken it results in reduction on account of its low caloric value.

CHAPTER XXXIV.

FOOD PROTECTION. ACCESSORY FOODS. BEVERAGES

FLIES, FOOD AND ILLNESS.

THE relation between flies and sickness is too well-known to need much more than passing notice in a book on dietetics were it not for the fact that food, the third link in the chain, is all important, for by this vehicle, when infected by fly-carried bacteria, no end of damage may be done. That the house should be screened from flies, and particularly the kitchen, all food should be screened and all flies killed if they do gain admittance, goes almost without saying. In addition to this they should be attacked in their breeding place, the manure piles of the country being the chief spots. This latter can be fairly effectively done if every day the fresh manure is well wetted down with a solution of from one-fourth to one pound of copper sulphate to the gallon of water, the stronger solutions killing 67 per cent., the weaker 57 per cent. of the maggots. Even better than this is the use of borax, 1½ pounds (dry) to 8 bushels of manure will kill 98 to 99 per cent. of the maggots. Calcined colemanite, 2 pounds to 8 bushels, showed the same high percentage of larvicidal action. In addition the use of these latter substances have no ill effect on the manure for its future usefulness as a fertilizer.[1]

BEVERAGES FOR THE SICK.

Flaxseed Tea:[2]

2 tablespoonfuls of flaxseed, 1½ tablespoonfuls of cream of tartar, 1 quart of boiling water, syrup and slices of lemon.

Wash flaxseed, add water (boiling) and cream of tartar, and allow to simmer until liquid is reduced a half. Strain, cool, add a little syrup, and serve with cut lemon.

Orange-albumen Water:[3]

White of 1 egg, 2 tablespoonfuls crushed ice, ⅓ cup orange juice, syrup.

Beat the egg white, add orange juice, and syrup if needed. Strain over crushed ice.

[1] Plowman: Fighting the Fly Peril, p. 116.
[2] Farmer: Food Cookery for the Sick, p. 72.   [3] Ibid.

Wine Whey:[1]

¼ cup of milk, 3 tablespoonfuls sherry.

Scald milk, add the wine, and let stand five minutes. Strain through cheesecloth (double) and serve.

Egg lemonade:[2]

1 egg, 1 tablespoonful sugar, 2 tablespoonfuls lemon juice, ¼ cup cold water, 2 tablespoonfuls sherry, 2 tablespoonfuls crushed ice.

Beat eggs lightly, add water, sugar, lemon juice and wine. Strain over crushed ice. Not necessary to use the wine.

Artificial Buttermilk or Ripened Milk:

1000 c.c. (1 quart) fresh milk (fat-free for certain cases). Sterilize at 212° F. for twenty minutes. Cool to blood heat, 98° F., and pour into sterile bottles. Add proper amount of lactic acid bacillus culture (tablets or liquid). Stand for twenty-four hours at 95° F. Thoroughly beat with egg beater and put on ice.

Irish Moss Jelly:[3]

⅛ cup Irish moss, lemon juice to taste, 1 cup water, syrup.

Soak moss in cold water to cover, drain and pick over. Put in double boiler with one and one-half cups of cold water, cook for forty-five minutes and strain.

Peptonized Milk[4] (cold process):

1 tube Fairchild's peptonizing powder (or any good preparation), ½ cup cold water, 1 pint milk.

Dissolve powder in a little of the water, add the rest of the water, then the milk, shake and put on ice.

Fully Peptonized Milk:

Same as cold process, but put in clean bottle and stand in water at 115° F. for two hours, shaking occasionally and keeping temperature of water at 115°. When finished it should appear thin and have a slightly greenish-yellow tint. It should then be scalded and put on ice. If only partial peptonization is wanted, the process can be stopped at the end of ten, twenty or thirty minutes.

Koumyss:[5]

1 quart milk, ¼ yeast cake, 1½ tablespoonfuls of sugar, 1 tablespoonful lukewarm water.

Heat milk to 75° F., add sugar and yeast cake dissolved in the warm water. Pour into sterilized beer bottles to within one and one-half inches of the top. Cool and shake. Put the bottles inverted where they can remain

---

[1] Farmer: Food Cookery for the Sick, p. 72. [2] Ibid.
[3] Ibid. [4] Ibid. [5] Ibid.

at about 70° F., for ten hours, then put on ice and keep for forty-eight hours, shaking occasionally.

Egg Nogg:[1]

1½ tablespoonful sherry or 1 tablespoonful of brandy or rum, ¾ tablespoonful of sugar, few grains of salt, ⅔ cup cold milk.

Beat egg slightly, add sugar, salt, and liquor, then gradually add milk. Strain and serve.

Cocoa Shells:[2]

⅓ cup cocoa shells, 2 cups boiling water.

Boil the shells and water two hours, keep adding water as it boils away. Strain and serve with equal parts of hot milk, sugar to taste.

Albumen Water:[3]

White of 1 egg, ½ cup cold water.

Stir egg with silver spoon or fork, this sets albumen free, add water. Strain and serve. If necessary, it may be flavored with fruit juices.

Cereal Gruels[4] general directions:

Use a double boiler. Keep correct proportions of receipts. Cook at boiling temperature, 212° F. Serve daintily.

Arrow-root Gruel:[5]

2 teaspoonfuls arrow-root, 2 tablespoonfuls cold water, 1 cup boiling water, salt q. s., sugar, lemon juice, brandy or wine if required.

Mix arrow-root and cold water to smooth paste, add to boiling water or milk. Cook in double boiler two hours. Salt, strain and serve. 205 calories.

Barley Gruel:[6]

1 tablespoonful barley flour, 2 tablespoonfuls cold milk, 1 cup scalded milk, salt.

Blend the barley with cold milk and stir into scalding hot milk. Cook in double boiler twenty minutes. Season with salt, add sugar if desired. Strain. 248 calories.

Flour Gruel:[7]

¾ cup scalded milk, ½ tablespoonful flour, ¼ cup cold milk, speck of salt.

Scald milk. Mix flour with cold milk to smooth mixture, stir in scalding hot milk. Cook in double boiler one-half hour, or on back of stove in saucepan. 212 calories.

[1] Farmer: Food Cookery for the Sick, p. 72.　　　[2] Ibid.
[3] Ibid.　　　[4] Pattee: Diet in Disease, 1916, p. 236.
[5] Ibid.　　　[6] Ibid.　　　[7] Ibid.

Farina Gruel:[1]

½ tablespoonful farina, ¼ cup cold water, ½ cup boiling water, ½ cup scalded milk, salt.

Mix farina with cold water, add to the boiling water, and boil thirty minutes. Add scalding hot milk, salt q. s. A little sugar may be added, or an egg may be beaten and poured into it. 102 calories.

ARTIFICIAL FOODS.

The use of artificial foods is much more prevalent abroad than in America, and although they have a distinct field of usefulness, they are not so generally useful as one might think. One of their chief advantages is to reinforce natural foods when one wishes to give concentrated food of small bulk.

Plasmon.—Plasmon is made from milk protein; it is a tasteless powder of white color, soluble in warm (but not hot) water, and is about 70 per cent. protein.

Nutrose.—Nutrose is also a casein preparation, but combined with soda, making it easily soluble in water, represents about 90 per cent. protein.

Somatose.—Somatose is made of meat digested, chiefly to albumoses, and is highly nutritious.

Beef Meal.—Beef meal is prepared by digesting meat artificially and is of high nutritive value—77 per cent. protein, 13 per cent. fat. It may be added to milk, soups, or milk preparations.

Peptones.—Panopeptones, Witte's peptones. Armour's or Carnick's, vary from 1.5 per cent. to 10 per cent. nitrogen, and although concentrated foods, they are not practical for any but temporary use; large amounts upset the stomach or produce diarrhea.

Roberat.—Roberat is manufactured from the protein of wheat, corn, and rice. It is a purin-free food, or practically so, and may be used in gouty conditions, being added to other foods.

Aleuronat.—Aleuronat is a ███████ flour, 80 to 90 per cent. protein, with 7 per cent. carbohydrate. This is used principally in making diabetic "near" bread, or is mixed with wheat flour in definite proportions, according to the carbohydrate tolerance.

Tropon.—Tropon is a protein food made from fish and vegetables. This is sold separately or mixed with malt or chocolate, and since it is practically tasteless, it can be mixed with almost any food to reinforce it.

[1] Pattee: Diet in Disease, 1916, p. 236.

OLIVE OIL AND ITS DIETARY USAGE.

Olive oil expressed from the ripe olive, either foreign or domestic (California), is largely used in medicine; in fact it is the basis of many of the oily medicinal preparations, and enters very considerably into the treatment of various diseases, principally of the digestive tract. As a general thing, when any part of the digestive canal is affected by lesions leading to stenosis in any degree, olive oil is a favorite remedy.

Stenosis of the Esophagus.—Here olive oil is given in considerable quantities up to 4 ounces several times a day. always before food is taken. In this way the tube is lubricated and soothed and the passage of suitable liquid or semiliquid food is facilitated. It also has a high caloric value as a food, and 4 ounces of it represents about 1000 calories; as much as this is not usually taken at one time, but may be.

Pyloric Stenosis.—In pyloric stenosis either from a juxtapyloric ulcer or from an old cicatrix, it does good in the same way, but in addition, like all oils, it has a marked effect in checking the flow of free hydrochloric acid. So in hyperchlorhydria from whatever cause, olive oil is often useful for this latter reason. Its usefulness in ulcer is often great, particularly when this is associated with pylorospasm, and especially in such cases its control of gastric hyperacidity is marked.

Gastric Dilatation.—In gastric dilatation dependent on narrowing at the pylorus, some relief is often obtained if the narrowing is due to spasm; when there is a definite stricture from cicatricial tissue the most it can do is to allow the maximum dilatation, in view of the actual narrowing, by the relief of irritation.

Cholelithiasis.—For many years olive oil given on an empty stomach was a popular remedy for gall-stones, large numbers of which were said to have been passed by this method. On investigation the large numbers of so-called "gall-stones" have proved to be nothing more nor less than inspissated olive oil mixed with a little bile and intestinal contents. The oil is frequently passed in faceted small masses which on appearance seem to be gall-stones, but on further examination prove to be only the oil in this form. As a matter of fact, however, the pylorospasm often excited by cholelithiasis is relieved, so that the patient connects this relief with the passage of these false "gall-stones" and thinks himself cured. Olive oil also increases the flow of bile, and so does good in any condition of bile stasis.

Gastric Hyperacidity.—The symptoms associated with gastric hyperacidity are frequently relieved by taking olive oil on an empty stomach prior to meals. This is due to the fact that oils and fats depress the flow of gastric juice, so actually reducing the acidity and consequently to some extent at least, the frequently associated pylorospasm. Ulcer of the stomach, so often a cause of gastric hyperacidity, is favorably influenced by a course of olive oil treatment, the oil being given before meals, beginning with 4 c.c. (1 dram) and increasing up to 15 c.c. (½ ounce) or even 30 c.c. (1 ounce). Some patients who cannot take oil before meals may take it directly afterward, when it also does good, but probably not to so great a degree.

As a matter of fact it is to be regretted that all people cannot take olive oil, for many patients who might otherwise benefit from its use are unable to do so on account of a marked gastric disturbance, causing principally eructations and a disagreeable after-taste. In these persons peanut oil may be better tolerated and be just as effectual. In the same way an emulsion of sweet almonds may be equally efficient and is prepared as follows, according to Cohnheim:

Blanch a dessertspoonful of sweet almonds and remove the skins, both being accomplished by boiling water. After being dried they are ground to powder and the powder added to a cup of boiling water. This is well rubbed with a spoon and strained through cheesecloth. About 200 c.c. of this emulsion may be made from the dessertspoonful of almonds. This should be slightly sweetened and taken before meals as one would olive oil.

CHAPTER XXXV.

TABLE OF FOOD VALUES, WEIGHTS AND MEASURES

AVERAGE CHEMICAL COMPOSITION OF AMERICAN FOODS.[1]

Food material.	Water. Per cent.	Protein. Per cent.	Fat. Per cent.	Carbohy-drates. Per cent.	Calories per 100 gm.{
ANIMAL FOOD.					
A. Beef.					
Fresh:					
Chuck, including shoulder .	65.0	19.2	15.4	. . .	222
Loin	61.3	19.0	19.1	. . .	255
Sirloin butt, as purchased .	62.5	19.7	17.7	. . .	246
Porterhouse steak . . .	60.0	21.9	20.4	. . .	280
Ribs	57.0	17.8	24.6	. . .	302
Round	67.8	20.9	18.6	. . .	184
Beef Organs:					
Brain	80.6	8.8	9.3	. . .	122
Kidney	76.7	16.6	4.8	0.4	115
Beef liver	71.2	20.4	4.5	1.7	133
Sweetbreads, as purchased .	70.9	16.8	12.1	. . .	181
Tongue	70.8	18.9	9.2	. . .	163
Cooked:					
Roast, as purchased . .	48.2	22.3	28.6	. . .	357
Round steak, fat removed, as purchased . . .	63.0	27.6	7.7	. . .	185
Loin steak:					
Tenderloin, broiled . .	54.8	23.5	20.4	. . .	287
Canned:					
Boiled beef, as purchased .	51.8	25.5	22.5	. . .	314
Corned beef	51.8	26.3	18.7	. . .	282
Roast beef, as purchased .	58.9	25.9	14.8	. . .	243
B. Veal.					
Fresh:					
Breast	68.2	20.3	11.0	. . .	185
Leg	71.7	20.7	6.7	. . .	146
Loin	69.5	19.9	10.0	. . .	174
Rib	69.8	20.2	9.4	. . .	170
Shoulder and flank, medium fat	65.2	19.7	14.4	. . .	215
Kidney, as purchased .	75.8	16.9	6.4	. . .	129
C. Lamb.					
Fresh:					
Breast or chuck		19.1	23.6	. . .	298
Leg, hind	58.6	18.6	22.6	. . .	287
Shoulder	51.8	18.1	29.7	. . .	351
Forequarter	55.1	18.3	25.8	. . .	315
Hindquarter	60.9	19.6	19.1	. . .	258
Cooked:					
Chops, broiled . . .	47.6	21.7	29.9	. . .	367
Leg, roast	67.1	19.7	12.7	. . .	198

[1] From Atwater and Bryant (Abstract, United States Department of Agriculture, Bulletin No. 28, 1906.

Food material.	Water. Per cent.	Protein. Per cent.	Fat. Per cent	Carbohy-drates. Per cent.	Calories per 100 gm
ANIMAL FOOD.					
D. MUTTON.					
Fresh:					
Chuck, lean	64.7	17.8	16.3	...	225
Leg, hind	63.2	18.7	17.5	...	239
Shoulder	60.2	17.5	21.8	...	274
Forequarter	52.9	15.6	30.9	...	352
Cooked:					
Mutton, leg, roast . . .	50.9	25.0	22.6	...	313
E. PORK.					
Fresh:					
Ham	50.1	15.7	33.4	...	375
Pickled, salted, and smoked:					
Ham, smoked, boiled, as purchased	51.3	20.2	22.4	...	291
fried, as purchased . .	36.6	22.2	33.2	...	400
Bacon, smoked	20.2	10.5	64.8	...	646
F. SAUSAGE.					
(As purchased.)					
Bologna	55.2	18.2	19.7	...	258
Frankfurt	57.2	19.6	18.6	1.1	258
Pork	39.8	13.0	44.2	1.1	468
Sausage meat . . .	46.2	17.4	32.5	...	374
G. POULTRY.					
Fresh:					
Chicken, broiler . . .	69.7	20.7	8.3	...	196
young, dark meat . .	70.1	20.8	8.2	...	187
light meat . . .	70.3	21.9	7.4	...	184
Duck, breast	73.9	22.3	2.3	...	151
Guinea-hen meat, not includ-ing giblets	68.9	23.4	6.5	...	191
Pheasant meat, not includ-ing giblets	70.0	24.7	4.6	...	180
Pigeon meat, not including giblets	63.2	22.9	12.1	...	243
Quail meat, not including giblets	66.3	25.4	7.0	...	208
Squab meat, not including giblets	56.6	18.5	23.8	...	324
Turkey, dark meat . . .	57.0	21.4	20.6	...	316
cooked	53.7	39.2	4.3	...	265
light meat	63.9	25.7	9.4	...	235
cooked	58.5	34.6	4.9	...	240
Preserved Poultry Meat:					
Potted turkey . . .	56.0	17.2	22.0	...	306
chicken	56.1	19.4	20.3	...	306
Canned chicken soup .	87.1	2.9	3.3	5.1	66
gumbo soup . .	91.0	2.4	0.2	4.8	35
boned chicken . .	57.6	27.7	12.8	...	274
H. FISH.					
Fresh:					
Cod, whole	82.6	16.5	0.4	1.2	103
Bass, black, whole . . .	76.7	20.6	1.7	1.2	103
sea, whole	79.3	19.8	0.5	1.4	86
striped, whole . . .	77.7	18.6	2.8	1.2	102
Blackfish, whole	70.1	18.7	1.2	1.1	80

Food material.	Water. Per cent.	Protein. Per cent.	Fat. Per cent.	Carbohy-drates. Per cent.	Calories per 100 gm.
ANIMAL FOOD.					
H. FISH.—*Continued.*					
Fresh:					
Bluefish, entrails removed .	78.5	19.4	1.2	1.3	90
Butterfish, whole . . .	70.0	18.0	11.0	1.2	176
Eels, salt water	71.6	18.6	9.1	1.0	161
Haddock, entrails removed	81.7	17.2	0.3	1.2	74
Halibut, steak or sections .	75.4	18.6	5.2	1.0	125
Herring, whole . . .	72.5	19.5	7.1	1.5	146
Mackerel, whole . . .	73.4	18.7	7.1	1.2	142
Perch, white, whole . . .	75.7	19.3	4.0	1.2	117
as purchased . . .	28.4	7.3	1.5	0.4	44
yellow, whole . . .	79.3	18.7	0.8	1.2	84
Pickerel, pike, whole . .	79.8	18.7	0.5	1.1	81
Pike, gray, whole . .	80.8	17.9	0.8	1.1	80
Pompano, whole . . .	72.8	18.8	7.5	1.0	147
Pogy (scup), whole . . .	75.0	18.6	5.1	1.4	123
Salmon, whole . . .	64.6	22.0	12.8	1.4	209
Shad, whole	70.6	18.8	9.5	1.3	165
roe, as purchased . .	71.2	20.9	3.8	1.5	133
Smelt, whole	79.2	17.6	1.8	1.7	89
Spanish mackerel, whole .	68.1	21.5	9.4	1.5	175
Trout, brook, whole . .	77.8	19.2	2.1	1.2	98
Preserved and canned:					
Cod, salt	53.5	25.4	0.3	...	90
Herring, smoked . . .	34.6	36.9	15.8	...	299
Mackerel, salt, dressed .	43.4	17.3	26.4	...	316
Salmon, canned . . .	63.5	21.8	12.1	...	201
Sardines, canned . .	52.3	23.0	19.7	...	278
Shellfish, etc., Fresh:					
Clams, round, removed from shell, as purchased .	80.8	10.6	1.1	5.2	75
Oysters, solids, as purchased	88.3	6.0	1.3	3.3	51
Scallops, as purchased . .	80.3	14.8	0.1	3.4	76
I. EGGS.					
Hens', uncooked . . .	73.7	13.4	10.5	...	159
boiled	73.2	13.2	12.0	...	169
whites	86.2	12.3	0.2	...	55
yolks	49.5	15.7	33.3	...	376
Egg, boiled, 1 egg (50 gm.)	36.6	6.6	6.0	...	169
		Total, 1 egg	...		83
J. DAIRY PRODUCTS, ETC.					
(As purchased.)					
Butter	11.0	1.0	85.0	...	795
Buttermilk	91.0	3.0	0.5	4.8	36
Cheese, American, pale	31.6	28.8	35.9	0.3	453
red	28.6	29.6	38.3	...	477
California flat . . .	34.0	24.3	33.4	4.5	429
Cheddar	27.4	27.7	36.8	4.1	473
Cheshire	37.1	26.9	30.7	0.9	399
Cottage	72.0	20.9	1.0	4.3	112
Dutch	35.2	37.1	17.7	...	316
Full cream	34.2	25.9	33.7	2.4	430
Limburger	42.1	23.0	29.4	0.4	369
Neufchatel	50.0	18.7	27.4	1.5	337
Roquefort	29.3	22.6	29.5	1.8	375
Swiss	31.4	27.6	24.9	1.3	443
Cream	74.0	2.5	18.5	4.5	201
Koumyss	89.3	2.8	2.1	5.4	53

Food material	Water. Per cent.	Protein. Per cent.	Fat. Per cent.	Carbohydrates. Per cent.	Calories per 100 gm.
ANIMAL FOOD.					
J. **DAIRY PRODUCTS, ETC.—**					
Continued.					
Milk, condensed, sweetened	26.9	8.8	8.3	54.1	335
unsweetened (evaporated cream)	68.2	9.6	9.3	11.2	172
skimmed	90.5	3.4	0.3	5.1	37
whole	87.0	3.3	4.0	5.0	72
whey	93.0	1.0	0.3	5.0	28
K. MISCELLANEOUS.					
(As purchased.)					
Beef-juice	93.0	4.9	0.6	...	25
Calf's-foot jelly	77.6	4.3	....	17.4	89
Oleomargarine	9.5	1.2	83.0	...	777
VEGETABLE FOOD.					
A. FLOUR, MEALS, ETC.					
Barley meal and flour	11.9	10.5	2.2	72.8	362
Buckwheat flour	13.6	6.4	1.2	77.9	357
Cornmeal, granular	12.5	9.2	1.9	75.4	365
Corn Preparations:					
Cerealine	10.3	9.6	1.1	78.3	370
Hominy	11.8	8.3	0.6	79.0	364
cooked	79.3	2.2	0.2	17.8	84
Oatmeal	7.3	16.1	7.2	67.5	410
boiled	84.5	2.8	0.5	11.5	63
gruel	91.6	1.2	0.4	6.3	34
water	96.0	0.7	0.1	2.9	15
Rolled oats	7.7	16.7	7.3	66.2	408
Rice	12.3	8.0	0.3	79.0	359
boiled	72.5	2.8	0.1	24.4	112
flaked	9.5	7.9	0.4	81.9	371
flour	8.5	8.6	6.1	68.0	370
Rye flour	12.9	6.8	0.9	78.7	359
meal	11.4	13.6	2.0	71.5	367
Wheat, entire	11.4	13.8	1.9	71.9	369
gluten	12.0	14.2	1.8	71.1	367
Graham	11.3	13.3	2.2	71.4	368
Prepared (self-raising)	10.8	10.2	1.2	73.0	353
Wheat Preparations:					
Cracked and crushed	10.1	11.1	1.7	75.5	371
Farina	10.9	11.0	1.4	76.3	371
Flaked	8.7	13.4	1.4	74.3	373
Gems	10.4	10.5	2.0	76.0	374
Glutens	8.9	13.6	1.7	74.6	378
Macaroni	10.3	13.4	0.9	74.1	367
cooked	78.4	3.0	1.5	15.8	91
Noodles	10.7	11.7	1.0	75.6	367
Shredded	8.1	10.5	1.4	77.9	375
Spaghetti	10.6	12.1	0.4	76.3	366
Vermicelli	11.0	10.9	2.0	72.0	358
B. BREAD, CRACKERS, PASTRY, ETC. (As purchased.)					
Bread:					
Brown	43.6	5.4	1.8	47.1	231
Corn (johnny cake)	38.9	7.9	4.7	46.3	266
Rye	35.7	9.0	0.6	53.2	260
Wheat:					
Buns	29.0	6.3	6.5	57.3	321
Cinnamon	23.6	9.4	7.2	59.1	347
Currant	27.5	6.7	7.6	57.6	334

Food material.	Water. Per cent.	Protein. Per cent.	Fat. Per cent.	Carbohydrates. Per cent.	Calories per 100 gm.
VEGETABLE FOOD.					
B. Bread, Crackers, Pastry, etc.—*Continued.*					
Bread, Wheat: Hot cross	36.7	7.9	4.8	49.7	281
Graham	35.7	8.9	1.8	52.1	267
Biscuit, home-made	32.9	8.7	2.6	55.3	287
soda	22.9	9.3	13.7	52.6	381
Rolls, French	32.0	8.5	2.5	55.7	287
Vienna	31.7	8.5	2.2	56.5	287
White, biscuit	35.2	8.0	1.4	54.3	269
home-made	35.0	9.1	1.6	53.3	270
all analyses	35.3	9.2	1.3	53.1	268
Whole wheat	38.4	9.7	0.9	49.7	251
Zwieback	5.8	9.8	9.9	73.5	434
Crackers:					
Soda	5.9	9.8	9.1	73.1	424
Boston (split)	7.5	11.0	8.5	71.1	416
Egg	5.8	12.6	14.0	66.6	454
Graham	5.4	10.0	9.4	73.8	429
Oatmeal	6.3	11.8	11.1	69.0	434
Oyster	4.8	11.3	10.5	70.5	433
Pretzels	9.6	9.7	3.9	72.8	375
Saltines	5.6	10.6	12.7	68.5	442
Water	6.4	11.7	5.0	75.7	405
All analyses	6.8	10.7	8.8	71.9	420
Cake:					
Bakers'	31.4	6.3	4.6	59.9	302
Chocolate layer	20.5	6.2	8.1	64.1	364
Drop	16.6	7.6	14.7	60.3	316
Frosted	18.2	5.9	9.0	64.8	374
Fruit	17.3	5.9	10.9	64.1	388
Gingerbread	18.8	5.8	9.0	63.5	368
Sponge	15.3	6.3	10.7	65.9	396
Cookies, Cakes, etc.:					
Molasses cookies	6.2	7.2	8.7	75.7	421
Sugar cookies	8.3	7.0	10.2	73.2	423
Ginger snaps	6.3	6.5	8.6	76.0	418
Lady fingers	15.0	8.8	5.0	70.6	371
Macaroons	12.3	6.5	15.2	65.2	435
Doughnuts	18.3	6.7	21.0	53.1	441
Pie:					
Apple	42.5	3.1	9.8	42.8	280
Cream	32.0	4.4	11.4	51.2	334
Custard	62.4	4.2	6.3	26.1	183
Lemon	47.4	3.6	10.1	37.4	262
Mince	41.3	5.8	12.3	38.1	294
Squash	64.2	4.4	8.4	21.7	185
Puddings:					
Rice custard	59.4	4.0	4.6	31.4	182
Indian meal	60.7	5.5	4.8	27.5	180
Tapioca	64.5	3.3	3.2	28.2	159
Tapioca with apple	70.1	0.3	0.1	29.3	122
Ice-cream	66.9	5.2	10.1	17.7	189

Food material.	Water. Per cent	Protein. Per cent.	Fat. Per cent.	Carbohy- drates. Per cent.	Calories per 100 gm.
VEGETABLE FOOD.					
C. SUGARS, STARCHES, ETC.					
(As Purchased.)					
Candy	....	....	....	96.0	391
Honey	18.2	0.4	....	81.2	335
Molasses, cane	25.1	2.4	....	69.3	284
Starch, tapioca	11.4	0.4	0.1	88.0	364
Sugar, coffee or brown	....	....	....	95.0	389
granulated	....	....	....	100.0	410
maple	....	....	....	82.8	339
powdered	....	....	....	100.0	410
D. VEGETABLES.					
Artichokes, as purchased	79.5	2.6	0.2	16.7	80
Asparagus, cooked, as pur-chased	91.1	2.1	3.3	2.2	48
Beans, butter, green	58.9	9.4	0.6	29.1	163
String beans, cooked	95.3	0.8	1.1	1.9	21
fresh, as purchased	83.0	2.1	0.3	6.9	40
Beets, cooked	88.6	2.3	0.1	7.4	41
Cabbage	91.5	1.6	0.3	5.6	32
Carrots, fresh	88.2	1.1	0.4	9.3	46
Cauliflower, as purchased	92.3	1.8	6.5	4.7	31
Celery	94.5	1.1	0.1	3.3	19
Corn, green	75.4	3.1	1.1	19.7	104
Cucumbers	95.4	0.8	0.2	3.1	18
Eggplant	92.9	1.2	0.3	5.1	29
Greens, beet, cooked, as pur-chased	89.5	2.2	3.4	3.2	54
Lentils, dried, as purchased	8.4	25.7	1.0	59.2	357
Lettuce	94.7	1.2	0.3	2.9	20
Mushrooms, as purchased	88.1	3.5	0.4	6.8	46
Okra	90.2	1.6	0.2	7.4	39
Onions, fresh	87.6	1.6	0.3	9.9	49
prepared, as purchased	91.2	1.2	1.8	4.9	42
Parsnips	83.0	1.6	0.5	13.5	66
Peas, dried, as purchased	9.5	24.6	1.0	62.0	365
green	74.6	7.0	0.5	16.9	102
cooked, as purchased	73.8	6.7	3.4	14.6	119
Potatoes, raw or fresh cooked	78.3	2.2	0.1	18.4	85
boiled, as purchased	75.5	2.5	0.1	20.9	97
cooked chips, as purchased	2.2	6.8	39.8	46.7	589
mashed and creamed, as purchased	75.1	2.6	3.0	17.8	111
sweet, raw or fresh	69.0	1.8	0.7	27.4	126
cooked and prepared, as purchased	51.9	3.0	2.1	42.1	204
Pumpkins	93.1	1.0	0.1	5.2	26
Radishes	91.8	1.3	0.1	5.8	30
Rhubarb	94.4	0.6	0.7	3.6	23
Sauerkraut, as purchased	88.8	1.7	0.5	3.8	28
Spinach, fresh, as purchased	92.3	2.1	0.3	3.2	24
cooked, as purchased	89.8	2.1	4.1	2.6	57
Squash	88.3	1.4	0.5	9.0	47
Tomatoes, fresh, as purchased	94.3	0.9	0.4	3.9	23
Turnips	89.6	1.3	0.2	8.1	41

Food material.	Water. Per cent.	Protein. Per cent.	Fat. Per cent.	Carbohydrates. Per cent.	Calories per 100 gm.
VEGETABLE FOOD.					
D. Vegetables.—*Continued.*					
Canned as Purchased.					
Asparagus	94.4	1.5	0.1	2.8	19
Beans, baked	68.9	6.9	2.5	19.6	132
string	93.7	1.1	0.1	3.8	21
lima	79.5	4.0	0.3	14.6	79
red kidney . . .	72.7	7.0	0.2	18.5	106
Brussels sprouts . . .	93.7	1.5	0.1	3.4	21
Corn, green	76.1	2.8	1.2	19.0	103
Okra	94.4	0.7	0.1	3.6	19
Peas, green	85.3	3.6	0.2	9.8	56
Pumpkins	91.6	0.8	0.2	6.7	33
Squash	87.6	0.9	0.5	10.5	52
Succotash	75.9	3.6	1.0	18.6	103
Tomatoes	94.0	1.2	0.2	4.0	23
F. Fruits, Berries.					
Apples:					
Edible portion . . .	84.6	0.4	0.5	14.2	64
As purchased (refuse, 25.0)	63.3	0.3	0.3	10.8	49
Apricots	85.0	1.1	. . .	13.4	59
Bananas:					
Edible portion . . .	75.3	1.3	0 6	22.0	101
As purchased (refuse, 35.0)	48.9	0.8	0.4	14.3	66
Blackberries, as purchased .	86.3	1.3	1.0	10.9	15
Cherries, as purchased .	76.8	0.9	0.8	15.9	76
Cranberries, as purchased .	88.9	0.4	0.6	9.9	47
Currants, as purchased .	85.0	1.5	. . . .	12.8	58
Figs, fresh, as purchased .	79.1	1.5	. . . .	18.8	84
Grapes, as purchased . .	58.0	1.0	1.2	14.4	74
Huckleberries	81.9	0.6	0.6	16.6	76
Lemons:					
Edible portion . . .	89.3	1.0	0.7	8.5	45
As purchased (refuse, 30.0)	62.5	0.7	0.5	5.9	32
Muskmelons:					
Edible portion . . .	89.5	0.6	. . . .	9.3	41
As purchased (refuse, 50.0)	44.8	0.3	. . . .	4.6	20
Nectarines	82.9	0.6	. . . .	15.9	67
Oranges:					
Edible portion . . .	86.9	0.8	0.2	11.6	53
As purchased (refuse, 27.0)	63.4	0.6	0.1	8.5	37
Peaches:					
Edible portion . . .	69.4	0.7	0.1	9.4	42
As purchased (refuse, 18.0)	73.3	0.5	0.1	7.7	34
Pears:					
Edible portion . . .	64.4	0.6	0.5	14.1	65
As purchased (refuse, 10.0)	76.0	0.5	0.4	12.7	57
Pineapple	89.3	0.4	0.3	9.7	44
Prunes	79.6	0.9	. . . .	18.9	81
Raspberries, as purchased .	85.8	1.0	. . . .	12.6	56
Strawberries	90.4	1.0	0.6	7.4	40
Watermelons:					
Edible portion . . .	92.4	0.4	0.2	6.7	31
As purchased (refuse, 59.4)	37.5	0.2	0.1	2.7	13
Dried.					
Apples, as purchased . .	28.1	1.6	2.2	66.1	298
Apricots, as purchased .	29.4	4.7	1.0	62.5	284
Citron, as purchased . .	19.0	0.5	1.5	78.1	336

Food material.	Water. Per cent.	Protein. Per cent.	Fat. Per cent.	Carbohy-drates. Per cent.	Calories per 100 gm.

VEGETABLE FOOD.
F. FRUITS, BERRIES, ETC.—
Continued.

Food material.	Water. Per cent.	Protein. Per cent.	Fat. Per cent.	Carbohy-drates. Per cent.	Calories per 100 gm.
Currants, as purchased . .	17.2	2.4	1.7	74.2	330
Dates	15.4	2.1	2.8	78.4	336
Figs, as purchased . . .	18.8	4.3	0.3	74.2	325
Pears	16.5	2.8	5.4	72.9	360
Prunes	22.3	2.1	....	73.3	309
Raisins	14.6	2.6	3.3	76.1	354

Canned and Jellies.
Preserves, etc., as purchased:

Food material.	Water.	Protein.	Fat.	Carbohy-drates.	Calories
Apples, crab	42.4	0.3	2.4	54.4	247
sauce	61.1	0.2	0.8	37.2	161
Apricots	81.4	0.9	....	17.3	75
Blackberries	40.0	0.8	2.1	56.4	254
Blueberries	85.6	0.6	0.6	12.8	61
Cherries	77.2	1.1	0.1	21.1	91
Figs, stewed	56.5	1.2	0.3	40.9	173
Marmalade (orange peel) .	14.5	0.6	0.1	84.5	349
Peaches	88.1	0.7	0.1	10.8	49
Pears	81.1	0.3	0.3	18.0	78
Strawberries, stewed .	74.8	0.7	....	24.0	101
Prune sauce	76.6	0.5	0.1	22.3	95

G. NUTS.

Food material.	Water.	Protein.	Fat.	Carbohy-drates.	Calories
Almonds	4.8	21.0	54.9	17.3	668
Beechnut	4.0	21.9	57.4	13.2	678
Brazil nuts (Bertholletia ex-celsa), edible portion . .	5.3	17.0	66.8	7.0	720
Butternuts: Juglans cinerea . . .	4.4	27.9	61.2	3.5	698
Chestnuts:					
Edible portion . . .	45.0	6.2	5.4	42.1	246
As purchased (refuse, 16.0)	37.8	5.2	4.5	35.4	208
Cocoanuts	14.1	5.7	50.6	27.9	608
Cocoanut, prepared, as pur-chased	3.5	6.3	57.4	31.5	689
Filberts	3.7	15.6	65.3	13.0	725
Hickory nuts	3.7	15.4	67.4	11.4	737
Lichi nuts	17.9	2.9	0.2	77.5	332
Peanuts:					
Edible portion . . .	9.2	25.8	38.6	24.4	564
As purchased (refuse, 24.5)	6.9	19.5	29.1	18.5	427
Peanut butter, as purchased .	2.1	29.3	46.5	17.1	623
Walnuts, California . .	2.5	18.4	64.4	13.0	728

H. MISCELLANEOUS.

Food material.	Water.	Protein.	Fat.	Carbohy-drates.	Calories
Chocolate	5.9	12.9	48.7	30.3	631
Cocoa	4.6	21.6	28.9	37.7	511

UNCLASSIFIED FOOD MATERIALS.
ANIMAL AND VEGETABLE.
A. SOUPS.
Home-made (as purchased).

Food material.	Water.	Protein.	Fat.	Carbohy-drates.	Calories
Beef	92.9	4.4	0.4	1.1	26
Bean	84.3	3.2	1.4	9.4	65
Chicken	84.3	10.5	0.8	2.4	61
Chowder, clam . . .	88.7	1.8	0.8	6.7	43
Meat stew	84.5	4.6	4.3	5.5	81

Food materia .	Water. Per cent.	Protein. Per cent.	Fat. Per cent.	Carbohy-drates. Per cent.	Calories per 100 gm.
UNCLASSIFIED FOOD MATERIAL.					
A. SOUPS.—*Continued.*					
Canned (as purchased).					
Asparagus, cream of	87.4	2.5	3.2	5.5	63
Bouillon	96.6	2.2	0.1	0.2	11
Celery, cream of	88.6	2.1	2.8	5.0	55
Chicken	93.8	3.6	0.1	1.5	22
gumbo	89.2	3.8	0.9	4.7	43
Consommé	96.0	2.5	....	0.4	12
Corn, cream of	86.8	2.5	1.9	7.8	59
Julienne	95.9	2.7	....	0.5	13
Mock turtle	89.8	5.2	0.9	2.8	41
Mulligatawny	89.3	3.7	0.1	5.7	40
Oxtail	88.8	4.0	1.3	4.3	46
Pea	86.9	3.6	0.7	7.6	52
cream of green	87.7	2.6	2.7	5.7	60
Tomato	90.0	1.8	1 1	5.6	41
Turtle, green	86.6	6.1	1.9	3.9	58
Vegetable	95.7	2.9	....	0.5	14
B. MISCELLANEOUS.					
Hash	80.3	6.0	1.9	9.4	80
Mincemeat, commercial	27.7	6.7	1.4	60.2	288
home-made	54.4	4.8	6.7	32.1	214
Salad, ham	69.4	15.4	7.6	5.6	157
Sandwich, egg	41.4	9.6	12.7	34.5	299
chicken	48.5	12.3	5.4	32.1	232

TABLE OF MEASURES AND WEIGHTS.

4 saltspoonfuls	=	1 teaspoonful
3 teaspoonfuls	=	1 tablespoonful
4 tablespoonfuls	=	¼ cup or ½ gill
16 tablespoonfuls (dry)	=	1 cup
16 tablespoonfuls (wet)	=	1 cup
2 gills	=	1 cup (8 oz. or 250 c.c.)
2 cups	=	1 pint (16 oz. or 500 c.c.)
2 pints	=	1 quart (32 oz. or 1000 c.c.)
4 quarts	=	1 gallon (128 oz. or 4000 c.c.)
2 tablespoonfuls butter	=	1 ounce (30 gm.)
4 tablespoonfuls flour	=	1 ounce (30 gm.)
2 tablespoonfuls granul'd sugar	=	1 ounce (30 gm.)
2 tablespoonfuls liquid	=	1 ounce (30 c.c.)
5 tablespoonfuls liquid	=	1 wineglassful

APOTHECARIES' MEASURES.

60 minims (M)	=	1 fluidram (4 c.c.)
8 fluidrams	=	1 fluidounce (30 c.c.)
16 fluidounces	=	1 pint (500 c.c.)
2 pints	=	1 quart (1000 c.c.)
4 quarts	=	1 gallon (4000 c.c.)

APOTHECARIES' WEIGHTS.

20 grains	=	1 scruple (1⅓ gm.)
3 scruples	=.	1 dram (4 gm.)
8 drams (480 grains)	=	1 ounce (30 gm.)
12 ounces	=	1 pound (360 gm.)

APPROXIMATE MEASURES.

1 teaspoonful	= about	1 fluidram (4 c.c.)
1 dessertspoonful	=	2 fluidrams (8 c.c.)
1 tablespoonful	=	4 fluidrams (15 c.c.)
1 wineglassful	=	2 ounces (60 c.c.)

RELATIVE VALUE OF METRIC AND APOTHECARIES' MEASURE.

Cubic centimeters.	Fluid-ounces.	Cubic centimeters.	Fluid-ounces.	Cubic centimeters.	Fluid-drams.	Cubic centimeters.	Minims.
1000 =	33.81	400 =	13.53	25 =	6.76	4.00 =	64.80
900 =	30.43	300 =	10.14	10 =	2.71	3.00 =	48.60
800 =	27.05	200 =	6.76	9 =	2.43	2.00 =	32.40
700 =	23.67	100 =	3.38	8 =	2.16	1.00 =	16.23
600 =	20.29	75 =	2.53	7 =	1.89	0.50 =	8.11
500 =	16.90	50 =	1.69	6 =	1.62	0.25 =	4.06
473 =	16.00	30 =	1.01	5 =	1.35	0.06 =	1.00

RELATIVE VALUE OF APOTHECARIES' AND METRIC MEASURE.

Minims.	Cubic centimeters.	Minims.	Cubic centimeters.	Fluid-ounces.	Cubic centimeters.	Fluid-ounces.	Cubic centimeters.
1 =	0.06	30 =	1.90	1 =	30.00	21 =	621.00
2 =	0.12	35 =	2.16	2 =	59.20	22 =	650.00
3 =	0.18	40 =	2.50	3 =	89.00	23 =	680.00
4 =	0.24	45 =	2.80	4 =	118.40	24 =	710.00
5 =	0.30	50 =	3.08	5 =	148.00	25 =	740.00
6 =	0.36	55 =	3.40	6 =	178.00	26 =	769.00
7 =	0.42			7 =	207.00	27 =	798.07
8 =	0.50	Fluid-drams		8 =	236.00	28 =	828.80
9 =	0.55			9 =	266.00	30 =	887.25
10 =	0.60	1 =	3.75	10 =	295.70	31 =	917.00
11 =	0.68	1¼ =	4.65	12 =	355.00	32 =	946.00
12 =	0.74	1½ =	5.60	13 =	385.00	48 =	1419.00
13 =	0.80	1¾ =	6.51	14 =	414.00	56 =	1655.00
14 =	0.85	2 =	7.50	15 =	444.00	64 =	1892.00
15 =	0.92	3 =	11.25	16 =	473.11	72 =	2128.00
16 =	1.00	4 =	15.00	17 =	503.00	80 =	2365.00
17 =	1.05	5 =	18.50	18 =	532.00	96 =	2839.00
18 =	1.12	6 =	22.50	19 =	591.50	112 =	3312.00
19 =	1.17	7 =	26.00			128 =	3785.00
20 =	1.25						
25 =	1.54						

RELATIVE VALUE OF METRIC AND AVOIRDUPOIS WEIGHT.

Grams.	Ounces.	Grains.	Grams.	Ounces.	Grains.
28.35 =	1		125.0 =	4 +	179
29.00 =	1 +	10	150.0 =	5 +	127
30.00 =	1 +	25	200.0 =	7 +	24
32.00 =	1 +	56	250.0 =	8 +	358
33.00 =	1 +	72	300.0 =	10 +	255
34.00 =	1 +	87	350.0 =	12 +	152
35.00 =	1 +	103	400.0 =	14 +	48
36.00 =	1 +	118	500.0 =	17 +	279
37.00 =	1 +	133	550.0 =	19 +	175
38.00 =	1 +	149	600.0 =	21 +	72
39.00 =	1 +	164	650.0 =	22 +	405
40.00 =	1 +	180	700.0 =	24 +	303
50.00 =	1 +	334	750.0 =	26 +	198
60.00 =	2 +	50	800.0 =	28 +	96
70.00 =	2 +	205	850.0 =	29 +	429
80.00 =	2 +	300	900.0 =	31 +	326
85.00 =	3		950.0 =	33 +	222
100.00 =	3 +	230	1000.0 =	35 +	120

RELATIVE VALUE OF AVOIRDUPOIS AND METRIC WEIGHT.

Avoirdu- pois ounces.		Grams.		Avoirdu- pois pounds.		Grams.
⅛	=	1.772		1.0	=	453.60
⅜	=	3.544		2.0	=	907.18
¼	=	7.088		2.2	=	1000.00
½	=	14.175		3.0	=	1360.78
1	=	28.35		4.0	=	1814.37
2	=	56.70		5.0	=	2267.55
3	=	85.05		6.0	=	2721.55
4	=	113.40		7.0	=	3175.14
5	=	141.75		8.0	=	3628.74
6	=	170.10		9.0	=	4082.33
7	=	198.45		10.0	=	4535.92
8	=	226.80				
9	=	255.15				
10	=	283.50				
11	=	311.84				
12	=	340.20				
13	=	368.54				
14	=	396.90				
15	=	425.25				
Avoir. pounds.						

RELATIVE VALUE OF APOTHECARIES' AND METRIC WEIGHT.

Grains.		Grams.		Grains.		Grams.		Drams.		Grams.
1.0	=	0.0625		24	=	1.55		1	=	3.90
2.0	=	0.1300		25	=	1.62		2	=	7.80
3.0	=	0.1950		26	=	1.70		3	=	11.65
4.0	=	0.2600		27	=	1.75		4	=	15.50
5.0	=	0.3240		28	=	1.82		5	=	19.40
6.0	=	0.4000		30	=	1.95		6	=	23.30
7.0	=	0.4600		32	=	2.10		7	=	27.20
8.0	=	0.5200		33	=	2.16		Ounces.		
9.0	=	0.6000		34	=	2.20		1	=	31.10
10.0	=	0.6500		35	=	2.25		2	=	62.20
11.0	=	0.7150		36	=	2.30		3	=	93.30
12.0	=	0.7800		38	=	2.47		4	=	124.40
14.0	=	0.9070		39	=	2.55		5	=	155.50
15.0	=	0.9720		40	=	2.73		6	=	186.60
15.5	=	1.0000		44	=	2.86		7	=	217.70
16.0	=	1.0400		48	=	3.00		8	=	248.80
18.0	=	1.1600		50	=	3.25		9	=	280.00
20.0	=	1.3000		52	=	3.40		10	=	311.00
21.0	=	1.3600		56	=	3.65		48	=	1492.80
22.0	=	1.4250		58	=	3.75		100	=	3110.40

RELATIVE VALUE OF METRIC AND APOTHECARIES' WEIGHT.

Grams.		Grains.		Grams.		Grains.
1	=	15.43		9	=	138.90
2	=	30.86		10	=	154.32
3	=	46.30		100	=	1543.23
4	=	61.73		125	=	1929.04
5	=	77.16		150	=	2374.85
6	=	92.60		175	=	2700.65
7	=	98.02		1000	=	15432.35
8	=	123.46				

Table of 100 calory portion giving actual amount of protein, fat, and carbohydrate and the percentage of calories in protein, fat, and carbohydrate in each portion.

Name of food.	Portion containing 100 calories roughly described.	Weight of 100 calories.		Actual amount of protein, fat, and carbohydrate in each portion on of 100 calories.			Percentage of calories in protein, fat, and carbohydrate, in 100 calory portion.		
		Grams.	Oz.	Protein.	Fat.	Carbohydrate.	Protein.	Fat.	Carbohydrate.
COOKED MEATS.									
Beef, round, boiled (fat)	Small serving	36.0	1.3	9.1	7.1		40.0	60.0	
Beef, round, boiled (lean)	Large serving	62.0	2.2	17.1	4.7		90.0	10.0	
Beef, round, boiled (medium)	Small serving	44.0	1.6	11.2	8.8		60.0	40.0	
Beef, fifth right rib, roasted	Small serving	32.0	1.2	7.1	9.1		25.0	75.0	
Beef, ribs boiled	Small serving	30.0	1.1	5.2	10.4		27.0	73.0	
Beef, ribs boiled	Very small serving	25.0	0.87	5.3	7.3		21.0	79.0	
Calf's foot jelly, as purchased	......	112.0	4.0	4.8	...	19.0	19.0	...	81.0
Chicken, as purchased, canned	One thin slice	27.0	0.96	7.4	3.4		23.0	77.0	
Lamb chops, boiled, edible portion, average	One small chop	27.0	0.96	5.8	8.0		24.0	76.0	
Lamb, leg, roast	Ordinary serving	50.0	1.8	9.8	6.3		40.0	60.0	
Mutton, leg, boiled	Large serving	34.0	1.2	8.5	7.6		35.0	65.0	
Pork, ham, boiled (fat)	Small serving	20.5	0.73	4.1	4.5		14.0	86.0	
Pork, ham, roasted (fat)	Small serving	27.0	0.96	4.4	10.8		19.0	81.0	
Turkey, as purchased, canned	Small serving	28.0	0.99	3.7	8.4		23.0	77.0	
Veal, leg, boiled	Large serving	67.5	2.4	13.9	4.5		73.0	27.0	
UNCOOKED MEATS.									
Beef, loin, edible portion, average (lean)	Ordinary serving	50.0	1.8	9.5	9.6		40.0	60.0	
Beef, loin, porterhouse steak, edible portion, average	Small steak	36.0	1.3	7.9	7.3		32.0	68.0	
Beef, loin, sirloin steak, edible portion, average	Small steak	40.0	1.4	7.5	7.4		31.0	69.0	
Beef, ribs, lean, edible portion, average	Ordinary serving	52.0	1.8	9.2	13.7		42.0	58.0	
Beef, round, lean, edible portion, average	Ordinary serving	52.0	1.8	13.2	10.7		54.0	46.0	
Beef, tongue, edible portion, average	Ordinary serving	63.0	2.2	11.7	5.7		47.0	53.0	
Beef, juice	......	62.0	2.2	19.6	2.4		78.0	22.0	
Chicken (broilers) edible portion, average	Large serving	90.0	3.2	18.6	7.4		79.0	21.0	
Clams, round, in shell, edible portion, average	Twelve to sixteen	395.0	14.0	22.2	2.3	10.9	56.0	8.0	36.0
Cod, whole, edible portion	Two servings	210.0	7.4	15.0	0.5		95.0	5.0	
Goose (young), edible portion, average	Half serving	25.0	0.88	5.5	13.7		16.0	84.0	
Halibut steaks or section, edible portion, average	Ordinary serving	138.0	4.9	15.0	4.1		61.0	39.0	
Liver (veal), as purchased, average	Two small servings	81.0	2.8	15.0	4.2		61.0	39.0	
Lobsters, whole, edible portion, average	Two servings	79.0	2.8	19.1	2.1	4.6	78.0	20.0	2.0
Mackerel (Spanish), whole, edible portion, average	Ordinary serving	117.0	4.1	12.2	5.3		50.0	50.0	
Mutton leg, hind, lean, edible portion, average	Ordinary serving	57.0	2.0	9.3	8.7		41.0	59.0	
Oysters, in shell, edible portion, average	One dozen	193.0	6.8	11.5	2.5	6.3	49.0	22.0	29.0
Pork, loin chops, edible portion, average	Very small serving	50.0	1.8	4.5	9.1		18.0	82.0	
Pork, ham, smoked, lean, edible portion, average	Small serving	27.0	0.97	4.5	7.7		18.0	82.0	

[1] Reproduced by special permission of Prof. Irving Fisher, Jour. Am. Med. Assn., 1907, xlviii, 1320.

Table of 100 calory portion giving actual amount of protein, fat, and carbohydrate and the percentage of calories in protein, fat, and carbohydrate in each portion.

Name of food.	Portion containing 100 calories roughly described	Weight of 100 calories — Grams.	Oz.	Actual amount of protein, fat, and carbohydrate in each portion of 100 calories — Protein.	Fat.	Carbohydrate.	Percentage of calories in protein, fat, and carbohydrate in 100 calory portion — Protein.	Fat.	Carbohydrate.
Pork, bacon, smoked, medium fat, edible portion, average	Small serving	36.0	1.3	5.9	13.9	....	29.0	71.0	....
Salmon (California) anterior section, edible portion, average	Small serving	15.0	0.53	1.5	9.7	....	6.0	94.0	....
Shad, whole, edible portion, average	Ordinary serving	42.0	1.5	9.1	5.0	....	30.0	70.0	....
Trout, brook, whole, edible portion, average	Two small servings	60.0	2.1	11.2	5.7	0.7	46.0	54.0	....
Turkey, edible portion, average	Two small servings	100.0	3.6	19.2	2.1	1.2	80.0	20.0	....
	Two small servings	33.0	1.2	7.5	3.1	....	29.0	71.0	....
VEGETABLES.									
Artichokes, as purchased, average, canned	....	430.0	15.0	11.1	0.86	71.8	14.0	....	86.0
Asparagus, as purchased, average, canned	....	540.0	19.0	4.3	6.7	4.5	33.0	5.0	62.0
Beans, baked, canned	Small side dish	75.0	2.66	5.2	1.9	14.7	21.0	18.0	61.0
Beans, lima, canned	Large side dish	126.0	4.44	5.4	0.4	18.4	21.0	4.0	75.0
Beans, string, cooked	Five servings	480.0	16.66	3.8	5.3	9.1	15.0	48.0	37.0
Beets, edible portion, cooked	Three servings	245.0	8.7	5.6	0.2	18.3	2.0	23.0	75.0
Beans, string, cooked	Five servings	480.0	16.66	3.8	5.3	9.1	15.0	48.0	37.0
Beets, edible portion, cooked	Three servings	245.0	8.7	5.6	0.2	18.3	2.0	23.0	75.0
Cabbage, edible portion, cooked	....	310.0	11.0	4.9	0.9	17.3	20.0	8.0	72.0
Carrots, edible portion, average, cooked	....	215.0	7.6	1.8	0.65	15.3	10.0	8.0	82.0
Cauliflower, as purchased, average	....	312.0	11.0	5.6	1.5	14.6	23.0	15.0	62.0
Celery, edible portion, average	....	540.0	19.0	6.0	0.5	17.8	24.0	5.0	71.0
Corn, sweet, cooked	One side dish	99.0	3.5	2.8	1.2	19.0	13.0	10.0	77.0
Cucumbers, edible portion, average	....	565.0	20.0	4.5	1.1	17.5	18.0	10.0	72.0
Egg plant, edible portion, average	....	350.0	12.0	4.2	1.0	17.8	17.0	10.0	73.0
Lentils, cooked	....	89.0	3.15	22.9	0.9	52.6	27.0	1.0	72.0
Lettuce, edible portion, average	....	505.0	18.0	6.0	1.5	14.6	25.0	14.0	61.0
Mushrooms, as purchased, average	....	215.0	7.6	7.5	0.8	14.6	31.0	8.0	61.0
Onions, fresh, edible portion, average	....	200.0	7.1	3.2	0.8	19.8	13.0	5.0	82.0
Onions, cooked	....	240.0	8.4	2.9	4.3	11.7	12.0	40.0	48.0
Parsnips, edible portion, average	Two large servings	152.0	5.3	2.4	0.7	20.5	10.0	7.0	83.0
Peas, green, cooked	One and a half serving	85.0	3.0	5.7	2.9	12.4	23.0	27.0	50.0
Potatoes, baked	One serving	86.0	3.05	1.7	0.08	15.8	11.0	1.0	88.0
Potatoes, boiled	One good sized	102.0	3.62	2.5	0.1	21.3	11.0	1.0	88.0
Potatoes, mashed (creamed)	One large sized	89.0	3.14	2.3	2.6	15.8	10.0	25.0	65.0
Potatoes, chips	One serving	17.0	0.6	1.1	6.7	8.0	4.0	63.0	33.0
Potatoes, sweet, cooked	One-half serving	49.0	1.7	1.4	1.0	20.6	6.0	9.0	85.0
Pumpkins, edible portion, average	Half of average potato	380.0	12.0	3.8	0.38	19.8	15.0	4.0	81.0
Radishes, as purchased	....	480.0	17.0	6.2	0.48	27.4	18.0	3.0	79.0
Rhubarb, edible portion, average	....	430.0	15.0	2.5	3.0	15.5	10.0	27.0	63.0

Food	Serving	Wt.							
Spinach, cooked, as purchased	Two ordinary servings	174.0	6.1	3.6	7.4	4.5	15.0	66.0	19.0
Squash, edible portion, average		210.0	7.4	2.9	1.0	19.0	12.0	10.0	78.0
Succotash, canned, as purchased, average	......	100.0	3.5	3.6	1.7	18.6	15.0	9.0	76.0
Tomatoes, fresh, as purchased, average	Ordinary serving	430.0	15.0	3.9	0.86	16.7	21.0	16.0	69.0
Tomatoes, canned	Four av. tomatoes	431.0	15.2	5.1	0.5	17.2	....	7.0	72.0
Turnips, edible portion, average	Two large servings	246.0	8.7	3.1	....	20.0	13.0	4.0	83.0
DAIRY PRODUCTS.									
Butter, as purchased	Ordinary pat or ball	12.5	0.44	0.1	10.6	....	0.5	99.5	54.0
Buttermilk, as purchased	One and a half glasses	275.0	9.7	8.2	1.3	13.2	34.0	12.0	2.0
Cheese, American, pale, as purchased	One and a half cubic inches	22.0	0.77	6.3	7.8	0.06	25.0	73.0	16.0
Cheese, cottage, as purchased	Four cubic inches	89.0	3.12	18.6	0.8	3.8	76.0	8.0	2.0
Cheese, full cream, as purchased	One and a half cubic inches	23.0	0.82	5.9	7.7	0.55	25.0	73.0	2.0
Cheese, Neufchatel, as purchased	One and a half cubic inches	29.5	1.05	5.6	8.2	0.45	22.0	76.0	1.0
Cheese, Swiss, as purchased	One and a half cubic inches	23.0	0.8	6.3	5.7	0.3	25.0	74.0	2.0
Cheese, pineapple, as purchased	One and a half cubic inches	20.0	0.72	7.4	3.5	....	25.0	73.0	9.0
Cream	One-quarter ordinary glass	49.0	1.7	1.2	9.0	2.2	5.0	86.0	42.0
Koumyss		188.0	6.7	5.2	3.9	10.0	21.0	37.0	67.0
Milk, condensed, sweetened, as purchased	......	30.0	1.06	2.6	2.4	16.2	10.0	23.0	....
Milk, condensed, unsweetened (evaporated cream) as purchased		59.0	2.05	5.7	7.6	....	24.0	....	....
Milk, skimmed, as purchased	One and a half glasses	255.0	9.4	8.6	0.78	....	37.0	....	....
Milk, whole, as purchased	Small glass	140.0	4.9	4.7	5.6	....	19.0	....	....
Whey, as purchased	Two glasses	360.0	13.0	3.6	1.0	....	15.0	....	....
FRUITS (DRIED).									
Apples, as purchased, average	......	34.0	1.2	0.54	0.74	32.4	24.0	50.0	26.0
Apricots, as purchased, average	......	35.0	1.24	1.6	3.0	21.47	37.0	7.0	56.0
Dates, edible portion, average	Three large	28.0	0.99	0.58	0.78	21.9	19.0	52.0	29.0
Figs, edible portion, average	One large	31.0	1.1	1.3	....	23.0	15.0	10.0	75.0
Prunes, edible portion, average	Three large	32.0	1.14	0.7	....	23.4	....	....	....
Raisins, as purchased	......	31.0	1.1	0.8	1.0	23.6	....	....	....
FRUITS (FRESH OR COOKED).									
Apples, as purchased	Two apples	206.0	7.3	0.6	0.6	22.0	3.0	7.0	90.0
Apples, sauce	Ordinary serving	111.0	3.9	0.2	0.8	41.3	7.0	3.0	90.0
Apricots, edible portion, average	......	168.0	5.92	1.84	....	22.5	2.0	7.0	91.0
Apricots, cooked	Large serving	131.0	4.61	1.1	....	22.6	5.0	....	95.0
Bananas, yellow, edible portion, average	One large	100.0	3.5	1.3	0.6	22.0	3.0	....	97.0
Blackberries, as purchased, average	......	170.0	5.9	2.2	1.7	18.5	3.0	9.0	88.0

FISHER'S TABLE OF ONE HUNDRED CALORY PORTIONS.—Continued.

Table of 100 calory portion giving actual amount of protein, fat, and carbohydrate and the percentage of calories in protein, fat, and carbohydrate in each portion.

Name of food.	Portion containing 100 calories roughly described	Weight of 100 calories.		Actual amount of protein, fat, and carbohydrate in each portion of 100 calories.			Percentage of calories in protein, fat, and carbohydrate in 100 calory portion.		
		Grams.	Oz.	Protein.	Fat.	Carbohydrate.	Protein.	Fat.	Carbohydrate
Blueberries, canned, as purchased		165.0	5.8	1.0	1.0	21.0	4.0	9.0	87.0
Blueberries		128.0	4.6	0.76	0.76	20.7	3.0	8.0	89.0
Cantaloupes	Half ordinary serving	243.0	8.6	0.72	...	11.0	6.0	...	94.0
Cherries, edible portion, average		124.0	4.4	1.1	0.9	19.7	5.0	10.0	85.0
Cranberries, as purchased, average		210.0	7.5	0.8	1.2	20.7	3.0	12.0	85.0
Grapes, as purchased, average		136.0	4.8	1.3	1.6	19.5	5.0	15.0	80.0
Grapefruit		215.0	7.57	1.7	0.4	12.9	7.0	4.0	89.0
Grape juice	Small glass	120.0	4.2	...	...	72.0	...	...	100.0
Lemons, edible portion		215.0	7.57	2.1	1.5	12.2	9.0	14.0	77.0
Nectarines		147.0	5.18	0.8	...	23.5	4.0	...	96.0
Olives, ripe	About seven olives	37.0	1.31	0.5	7.7	1.2	2.0	91.0	7.0
Oranges, as purchased, average	One very large	270.0	9.4	1.3	0.2	18.7	6.0	3.0	91.0
Oranges, juice	Large glass	188.0	6.62	...	...	37.0	...	...	100.0
Peaches, as purchased, average	Three ordinary	290.0	10.0	1.4	0.3	22.3	7.0	2.0	91.0
Peaches, juice	Ordinary glass	136.0	4.8	...	...	18.0	...	...	100.0
Pears	One large pear	173.0	5.4	1.0	0.8	44.3	4.0	7.0	89.0
Pineapples, edible portion, average		226.0	8.0	0.9	0.6	22.0	4.0	6.0	90.0
Raspberries, black		146.0	5.18	2.4	1.4	18.0	10.0	14.0	76.0
Raspberries, red		178.0	6.29	2.6	...	22.4	8.0	...	92.0
Strawberries, as purchased, average	Two servings	260.0	9.1	1.5	1.5	19.2	10.0	15.0	75.0
Watermelon, as purchased, average	Two servings	760.0	27.0	1.5	0.7	22.0	6.0	6.0	88.0
CAKES, PASTRY, PUDDING AND DESSERTS.									
Cake, chocolate layer, as purchased	Half ordinary square piece	28.0	0.98	1.7	2.2	12.7	7.0	22.0	71.0
Cake, gingerbread, as purchased	Half ordinary square piece	27.0	0.96	1.5	2.4	18.0	6.0	23.0	71.0
Cake, sponge, as purchased	Small piece	25.0	0.89	1.5	2.7	16.5	7.0	25.0	68.0
Custard, milk	Ordinary cup	122.0	4.29	5.1	7.7	32.0	26.0	56.0	18.0
Custard, tapioca	Two-thirds ordinary	69.5	2.45	2.3	2.1	18.4	9.0	12.0	79.0
Doughnuts, as purchased	Half a doughnut	23.0	0.8	1.7	4.8	12.2	6.0	45.0	49.0
Lady fingers, as purchased		27.0	0.95	2.3	1.3	19.0	10.0	12.0	78.0
Macaroons, as purchased		23.0	0.82	1.4	3.4	15.0	6.0	33.0	61.0

Food	Measure								
Pie, apple, as purchased	One-third ordinary piece	38.0	1.3	1.1	3.7	16.3	5.0	32.0	63.0
Pie, cream, as purchased	One-fourth ordinary piece	30.0	1.1	1.3	3.4	15.3	5.0	32.0	63.0
Pie, custard, as purchased	One-third ordinary piece	55.0	1.9	2.3	3.4	14.3	9.0	32.0	59.0
Pie, lemon, as purchased	One-third ordinary piece	38.0	1.35	1.3	3.8	14.2	6.0	36.0	58.0
Pie, mince, as purchased	One-fourth ordinary piece	35.0	1.2	2.0	4.3	13.3	8.0	38.0	54.0
Pie, squash, as purchased	One-third ordinary piece	55.0	1.9	2.4	4.6	12.0	10.0	42.0	48.0
Pudding, apple sago	Half ordinary serving	88.0	3.02	2.0	0.8	23.7	6.0	3.0	91.0
Pudding, brown betty	Very small serving	56.6	2.0				7.0	12.0	81.0
Pudding, cream rice	Half ordinary serving	75.0	2.65	3.0	3.4	23.5	8.0	13.0	79.0
Pudding, Indian meal	Small serving	56.6	2.0	3.0	2.6	15.4	12.0	25.0	63.0
Pudding, apple tapioca		79.0	2.8	0.2	0.07	23.0	1.0	1.0	98.0
Tapioca, cooked	Ordinary serving	108.0	3.85	3.5	3.4	30.4	1.0	1.0	98.0

SWEETS AND PICKLES.

Food	Measure								
Honey, as purchased	Four teaspoonfuls	30.0	1.05	0.1		24.3	1.0		99.0
Marmalade (orange peel)		28.3	1.0	0.2	0.02	24.0	0.5	2.5	97.0
Molasses, cane		35.0	1.2	0.8		24.0	0.5		99.0
Olives, green, edible portion	Seven olives	32.0	1.1	0.2	6.0	2.5	1.0	84.0	15.0
Olives, ripe, edible portion	Seven olives	38.0	1.3	0.2	6.0	2.5	2.0	91.0	7.0
Sugar, granulated	Three teaspoonfuls or one and a half lumps	24.0	0.86			24.0			100.0
Sugar, maple	Four teaspoonfuls	29.0	1.03			35.0			100.0
Syrup, maple	Four teaspoonfuls	35.0	1.2			35.0			100.0

NUTS.

Food	Measure								
Almonds, edible portion, average	About eight	15.0	0.53	3.1	8.2	2.6	13.0	77.0	10.0
Beechnuts		14.8	0.52	3.3	8.5	1.9	13.0	79.0	8.0
Brazil nuts, edible portion	Three ordinary size	14.0	0.49	2.3	9.3	1.0	10.0	86.0	4.0
Butternuts		14.0	0.5	3.9	8.5	0.5	16.0	82.0	2.0
Cocoanuts		16.0	0.57	0.9	8.0	4.4	4.0	77.0	19.0
Chestnuts, fresh, edible portion, average	Ten nuts	40.0	1.4	2.4	2.1	17.0	10.0	20.0	70.0
Filberts, edible portion, average		14.0	0.48	2.1	9.1	1.8	9.0	84.0	7.0
Hickory nuts		13.0	0.47	2.0	8.7	1.5	9.0	85.0	6.0
Peanuts, edible portion, average	Thirteen double	18.0	0.62	4.6	8.0	4.4	20.0	63.0	17.0
Pecans, polished, edible portion	About eight	13.0	0.46	1.8	12.0	2.5	6.0	87.0	7.0
Walnuts, California, edible portion	About six	14.0	0.48	2.5	9.1	1.8	10.0	83.0	7.0

Table of 100 calory portion giving actual amount of protein, fat and carbohydrate and the percentage of calories in protein, fat, and carbohydrate in each portion.

Name of food.	Portion containing 100 calories roughly described.	Weight of 100 calories. Grams.	Oz.	Actual amount of protein, fat, and carbohydrate in each portion of 100 calories. Protein.	Fat.	Carbohydrate.	Percentage of calories in protein, fat, and carbohydrate in 100 calory portion. Protein.	Fat.	Carbohydrate.
CEREALS.									
Bread, brown, as purchased, average	Ordinary thick slice	43.0	1.5	2.3	0.77	20.2	9.0	7.0	84.0
Bread, corn (johnny cake), as purchased, average	Small square	38.0	1.3	3.0	1.7	17.5	12.0	16.0	72.0
Bread, white, home-made, as purchased	Ordinary thick slice	38.0	1.3	3.4	0.6	20.2	13.0	6.0	81.0
Cornmeal, granular, average	......	27.0	0.96	2.5	0.5	20.3	10.0	5.0	85.0
Crackers, graham, as purchased	Two crackers	23.0	0.82	2.3	2.1	16.8	9.0	20.0	71.0
Crackers, oatmeal, as purchased	Two crackers	23.0	0.81	2.7	2.5	15.8	11.0	24.0	65.0
Hominy, cooked	Large serving	120.0	4.2	2.6	0.2	21.3	11.0	2.0	87.0
Macaroni, average, cooked	Ordinary serving	110.0	3.85	3.3	1.6	17.3	14.0	15.0	71.0
Oatmeal, average, boiled	One and a half serving	159.0	5.6	4.4	0.8	18.2	18.0	7.0	75.0
Rice, uncooked	......	28.0	0.98	2.2	0.8	22.0	9.0	1.0	90.0
Rice, boiled, average	Ordinary serving dish	87.0	3.1	2.4	0.8	21.2	10.0	1.0	89.0
Rice, flakes	Ordinary cereal dish	27.0	0.94	2.9	0.77	19.7	8.0	1.0	91.0
Rolls, Vienna, as purchased, average	One large roll	35.0	1.2	2.9	0.77	19.7	12.0	7.0	81.0
Shredded wheat	One biscuit	27.0	0.94	3.5	0.4	22.5	13.0	4.5	82.5
Spaghetti, average	......	28.0	0.97	3.4	0.11	21.3	12.0	1.0	87.0
Wheat flour, entire wheat, average	......	27.0	0.96	2.6	0.24	13.5	15.0	5.0	80.0
Wheat flour, graham, average	......	27.0	0.96	2.4	0.48	14.0	15.0	5.0	80.0
Wheat flour, patent roller process, family and straight grade spring wheat, average	......	27.0	0.97	2.9	0.3	20.2	12.0	3.0	85.0
Zweiback	Size of thick slice of bread	23.0	0.81	2.2	2.3	16.9	9.0	21.0	70.0
MISCELLANEOUS.									
Eggs, hen's, boiled	One large egg	58.0	2.1	7.9	7.2	.....	32.0	68.0	.....
Eggs, hen's, whites		181.0	6.4	22.0	.....	.....	100.0	.....	.....
Eggs, hen's, yolks	Two yolks	27.0	0.94	4.2	9.0	.....	17.0	83.0	.....
Soup, beef, as purchased, average	Very large plate	380.0	13.0	16.7	1.5	.....	69.0	14.0	17.0
Soup, bean, as purchased, average		150.0	5.4	4.8	2.1	14.0	20.0	20.0	60.0
Soup, cream of celery, as purchased, average	Two plates	180.0	6.3	3.7	5.0	9.0	16.0	47.0	37.0
Consomme, as purchased		830.0	29.0	20.7	.....	3.3	85.0	.....	15.0
Clam chowder, as purchased	Two plates	230.0	8.25	4.1	1.8	15.4	17.0	18.0	65.0

TABLE SHOWING THE NUTRITIVE VALUE OF THE FOOD MATERIALS CALCULATED FOR THE QUANTITIES COMMONLY REQUIRED IN COOKING SMALL PORTIONS.[1]

Food material (uncooked).	Measure.	Weight.		Protein. Gms	Fat. Gms.	Carbo-hydrates Gms.	Fuel value. Calories.
		Oz.	Gms.				
A							
Almonds shelled	1 cup	5⅔	160.0	33.6	87.8	27.7	1035.0
Apples, fresh	1 medium	5+	150.0	0.5	0.5	16.0	70.0
Apples, dried	1 cup	3	85.0	1.4	1.8	56.2	247.0
Apricots, dried	1 cup	5	142.0	6.6	1.4	88.5	354.0
Arrowroot	1 tbsp.	½	14+	....	....	13.8	55.0
Asparagus	1 bunch	44 (2¾ lbs.)	1247.0	22.4	2.4	41.0	276.0
B							
Bacon	1 serving	⅝	18.0	1.6	10.4	....	100.0
Bacon	1 lb.	16	454.0	43.0	269.4	....	2597.0
Bananas	1 medium	3½	100.0	0.8	0.4	14.0	64.0
Barley, pearl	1 tbsp	1	27.0	2.2	0.3	19.8	90.0
Barley, crushed	1 tbsp.	½	14+	1.1	0.1	11.3	51.0
Barley, flour	1 tbsp.	½+	16.0	1.3	0.2	12.5	57.0
Barley, flour	1 cup	8	227.0	19.0	2.5	174.3	796.0
Bass (edible portion)	1 serving	3½	100.0	18.6	2.8	....	100.0
Bass (edible portion)	1 lb.	16	454.0	84.3	12.6	....	452.0
Bean flour	1 tbsp.	3/10	8.0	1.8	0.1	4.8	28.0
Bean flour	1 cup	4⅜	125.0	29.3	2.3	77.5	448.0
Beans string	1 serving	4	113.0	2.4	0.3	5.8	44.0
Beef broth	1 serving	3½	100.0	1.8	1.02	....	16.5
Beef broth	1 quart	32	907.0	16.5	9.3	....	149.0
Beef juice	1 serving	3½	100.0	4.9	0.6	....	25.0
Beef marrow	1 tbsp.	½	14 1	0.31	13.1	....	120.0
Beef marrow	1 lb.	16	454.0	9.92	420.8	....	3828.0
Beefsteak, porterhouse	1 serving	3½	100.0	19.1	18.0	....	238.0
Beefsteak, porterhouse	1 lb.	16	454.0	86.6	81.2	....	1077.0
Beefsteak, rump	1 serving	3½	100.0	21.0	13.7	....	207.0
Beefsteak, rump	1 lb.	16	454.0	94.8	62.1	....	938.0
Beefsteak, sirloin	1 serving	3½	100.0	16.5	16.1	....	211.0
Beefsteak, sirloin	1 lb	16	454.0	74.8	73.0	....	957.0
Beefsteak, top of round	1 serving	3½	100.0	19.5	7.3	....	144.0
Beefsteak, top of round	1 lb.	16	454.0	88.45	33.1	....	652.0
Blue fish, edible portion	1 serving	3½	100.0	19.4	1.2	....	88.0
Blue fish, edible portion	1 lb.	16	454.0	87.8	5.44	....	401.0
Brandy	1 tbsp.	½	14+	....	....	....	42.0
Bran	1 cup	2½	71.0	7.8	1.5	43.4	218.0
Brazil nuts, shelled	1 lb.	16	454.0	76.94	302.88	31.68	3048.0
Brazil nuts, shelled	1 nut	¼	....	1.2	4.74	0.05	47.6
Brazil nuts shelled	1 tbsp. chopped	¼	....	3.6	14.22	0.15	142.8
Bread, white	1 slice	1	28.4	2.6	0.3	15.0	73.0
Bread, white	1 loaf	12	340.0	31.6	4.1	179.3	881.0
Bread crumbs (dry)	1 cup	4⅜	136.0	12.6	1.6	71.7	352.0
Bread, Boston brown	1 small slice	1	28.4	1.5	0.5	13.3	64.0
Bread, gum gluten	1 slice	1	28.4	8.4	0.3	8.5	70.3
Bread, gum gluten	1 loaf	13	386.5	114.0	4.0	116.3	957.2
Butter	1 tbsp.	½	14+	0.1	12.1	....	109.0
Butter	1 cup	8	227.0	2.2	193.0	....	1744.0
C							
Carrots	1 small	2	57.0	0.5	....	4.2	20.0
Cauliflower	1 serving	4	113.0	2.0	0.6	5.2	35.0
Celery	1 serving	2	57.0	....	....	1.4	6.0
Cheese, American	1 tbsp.	½	15.0	4.0	5.0	....	62.0

[1] A. F. Pattee: Practical Dietetics, p. 64, 10th edition. Reproduced by special permission. The weights assigned to the various measurements in this table have been determined carefully, but are the results of a limited number of experiments, and hence must be regarded as only approximate. The food values are given with sufficient accuracy to be within the limits of error of computations made on average analysis of food-stuffs.

Food material (uncooked).	Measure.	Weight.		Protein. Gms.	Fat. Gms.	Carbo-hydrates Gms.	Fuel value. Calories.
		Oz.	Gms.				
Cheese, American (fresh grated)	2 tbsp.	1	28.4	8.0	10.0	....	124.0
Cheese, cottage	1 serving	1	28.0	5.9	0.28	1.2	31.0
Cheese, creamed	2 tbsp. (1½ cu. inch)	8	23.0	6.1	8.1	0.5	100.0
Chicken, edible portion	1 serving	3½	100.0	21.4	2.5	....	108.0
Chicken	1 lb.	16	454.0	97.5	11.3	....	492.0
Chocolate, unsweetened	1 square	1	28.4	3.65	13.8	8.59	173.0
Chocolate, unsweetened	1 lb.	16	454.0	58.5	220.9	137.4	2772.0
Clams, edible portion	1 serving	3½	100.0	8.6	1.0	2.0	51.0
Clam bouillon	1 serving	3½	100.0	0.2	....	0.2	2.0
Clam bouillon	1 quart	32	906.0	2.0	0.8	1.6	23.0
Claret (10 per cent. alcohol)	1 tbsp.	½	14.0	....	....	....	10.0
Cocoa	1 tbsp.	¼	7+	1.5	2.0	2.5	35.0
Cod, fresh (edible portion)	1 serving	3½	100.0	16.5	0.4	....	70.0
Cod, fresh	1 lb.	16	454.0	74.8	1.8	....	315.0
Cod fish, salt, boneless	1 serving	2	57.0	15.7	0.2	....	64.0
Cod fish, salt, boneless	1 lb.	16	454.0	125.6	1.4	....	515.0
Condensed milk	1 teaspoon	0.388	11.0	0.88	1.057	6.07	37.31
Condensed milk	......	1	28.35	2.27	2.72	15.66	96.2
Condensed milk	1 can	16	450.0	36.33	43.79	250.6	1541.8
Consomme	1 serving	3½	100.0	2.5	....	0.4	12.0
Consomme	1 quart	32	906.0	10.0	....	1.6	46.0
Corn	1 cup	10	28.4	7.9	3.4	53.9	278.0
Cornmeal	1 tbsp.	⅓	10.0	0.8	0.2	7.1	33.0
Cornmeal	1 cup	5	142.0	13.0	2.6	106.8	504.0
Cornstarch	1 tbsp.	⅓	10.0	....	....	9.5	38.0
Cornstarch	1 cup	5½	156.0	....	....	148.2	592.0
Cracker crumbs	1 cup	5+	151.0	16.5	9.0	110.2	588.0
Crackers, water	1 large	⅓	10.0	1.2	0.5	7.6	40.0
Cream, thin (18%)	1 tbsp.	½	14.0	0.4	2.8	0.7	29.0
Cream, thin (18%)	1 cup	8	227.0	5.6	41.9	10.2	440.0
Cream, thick (40%)	1 tbsp.	½	14.0	0.3	6.0	0.5	57.0
Cream, thick (40%)	1 cup	8	227.0	4.99	90.7	6.8	864.0
Cucumbers, fresh (edible portion)	......	1	28.4	23.0	0.06	0.89	5.0
Currants, fresh	1 cup	5	142.0	2.12	....	18.0	81.0
Currants, dried	1 cup	8	227.0	5.44	3.84	84.0	728.0
D							
Dates	1 cup, with stones	8	227.0	4.0	5.6	160.8	710.0
Dry peptonoids, soluble	1 tbsp.	2	159.0	6.0	....	8.0	57.0
E							
Eggs, whole average size (without shell)	1	1½	45.0	5.4	4.2	....	60.0
Eggs, white	1	8/16	25.0	3.3	....	....	13.0
Eggs, yolk	1	½	13.0	2.1	4.5	....	48.0
F							
Farina	1 tbsp.	⅓	10.0	1.0	0.1	7.2	34.0
Farina	1 cup	6	170.0	18.7	2.3	129.8	616.0
Figs	1 fig	1	28.4	1.3	0.1	22.2	95.0
Figs	½ lb.	8	227.0	9.7	0.7	168.2	718.0
Filberts, shelled	1 lb.	16	454.0	70.72	296.16	58.88	3184.0
Filberts, shelled	1 doz.	¾	....	3.3	13.89	2.76	150.0
Filberts, shelled	1 tbsp. (chopped)	½	....	2.21	9.26	1.84	100.0
Flour, barley	1 tbsp.	½+	16.0	1.3	0.2	12.5	57.0
Flour, barley	1 cup	8	227.0	19.0	2.5	174.3	796.0
Flour, gum gluten	1 tbsp.	⅓	8.0	3.46	0.12	3.48	29.0
Flour, gum gluten	1 cup	5	142.0	60.0	2.3	63.0	512.7
Flour, Graham	1 tbsp.	⅓	8.0	1.3	0.2	6.8	34.0
Flour, Graham	1 cup	5	142.0	18.8	3.2	101.2	509.0
Flour, rice	1 tbsp.	½	16.0	1.4	0.04	10.2	58.0
Flour, rice	1 cup	8½	241.0	18.9	0.7	187.8	870.0
Flour, rye	1 tbsp.	⅓	8.0	0.5	0.07	6.3	28.0
Flour, rye	1 cup	5	142.0	9.6	1.3	111.5	496.0
Flour, wheat (roller process)	1 tbsp.	⅓	8.0	0.9	0.08	6.0	28.0
Flour, wheat (roller process)	1 cup	5	142.0	15.9	1.4	106.2	500.0
Fowl (edible portion)	1 serving	3½	100.0	19.3	16.3	....	224.0
Fowl (edible portion)	1 lb.	16	454.0	87.5	73.9	....	1015.0

Food material (uncooked).	Measure.	Weight.		Protein. Gms.	Fat. Gms.	Carbo-hydrates Gms.	Fuel value. Calories.
		Oz.	Gms.				
G							
Gelatin, granulated .	1 tbsp.	3/10	8.5	7.8	....	....	31.0
Gelatin, granulated .	1 box	1 1/5	34.0	31.1	....	....	125.0
Gelatin, shredded .	½ box	3/5	17.0	15.6	....	....	62.0
Gum gluten flour . .	1 tbsp.	⅓	8.0	3.46	0.12	3.48	29.0
Gum gluten flour . .	1 cup	5	142.0	60.0	2.3	63.0	512.7
Gum gluten flour . .	1 lb.	16	450.0	191.0	7.3	200.0	1629.7
Gum gluten bread .	1 slice	1	28.4	8.4	0.3	8.5	70.3
Gum gluten bread .	1 loaf	13	386.5	114.0	4.0	116.3	957.2
Gum gluten biscuit .	1 biscuit	¼	7.0	2.94	0.13	3.15	25.5
Gum gluten noodles .	1 cup	3½	100.0	45.0	4.2	32.5	350.0
Greens	1 serving	4	113.0	2.3	0.3	3.6	27.0
Grapes, Malaga . .	1 doz.	2	57.0	0.74	0.9	10.88	55.0
Grapes, Malaga . .	1 lb.	16	454.0	4.5	5.4	65.3	328.0
Grape juice . . .	1 tbsp.	½	14.0	....	....	3.8	15.0
Grape juice . . .	1 cup	8	227.0	....	....	60.0	240.0
H							
Haddock, edible portion	1 serving	3½	100.0	17.2	0.3	....	72.0
Haddock, edible portion	1 lb.	16	454.0	77.9	1.36	....	324.0
Halibut, edible portion	1 serving	3½	100.0	18.6	5.2	....	121.0
Halibut, edible portion	1 lb.	16	454.0	84.3	23.5	....	549.0
Ham, fresh, lean . .	1 serving	3½	100.0	24.8	14.2	....	227.0
Ham, fresh, lean . .	1 lb..	16	454.0	112.6	64.4	....	1029.0
Hickory nuts, shelled	1 lb.	16	454.0	69.76	305.6	51.68	3234.0
Hickory nuts, shelled	¼ cup (chopped)	1½	....	6.54	28.5	4.83	303.0
Hickory nuts, shelled	1 tbsp. (chopped)	½	....	2.18	9.5	1.61	101.0
Hominy	1 tbsp.	½	14.0	1.2	0.1	11.2	50.0
Hominy	1 cup	8	227.0	18.9	1.4	179.2	805.0
Honey	1 tbsp.	1	28.35	0.13	....	23.0	92.0
Ice Cream (homemade)	1 qt						1400.0
Jell-O	1 box	3½	100.0	11.2	....	86.4	395.0
Jell-O	1 serving	⅝	16.0	1.9	....	14.4	66.0
K							
Koumyss	1 qt.	34⅜	975.0	2.2	2.1	1.5	328.0
L							
Lamb chops . . .	1 serving	3½	100.0	18.7	28.3	....	329.0
Lamb chops . . .	1 lb.	16	454.0	84.8	128.3	....	1494.0
Lard	1 tbsp.	½	14.0	....	14.0	....	127.0
Lard	1 lb.	16	454.0	....	484.0	....	4083.0
Lemon juice (1 lemon)	3 tbsp.	1½	42.0	....	....	4.2	17.0
Lentil flour . . .	1 tbsp.	3/10	9.0	2.3	0.9	5.3	31.0
Lentil flour . . .	1 cup	5	144.0	37.0	1.4	85.0	500.0
Lettuce	1 head	8	227.0	2.3	.0 5	5.7	36.0
Liquid peptonoids .	1 tbsp.	½	15.0	0.8	....	2.1	28.0
Lobster, edible portion	1 serving	3½	100.0	18.1	1.1	0.5	84.0
Lobster, edible portion	1 lb.	16	454.0	82.08	4.96	2.24	382.0
M							
Macaroni	1 cup	3¾	108.0	14.7	1.0	81.1	392.0
Mackerel, fresh (edible portion)	1 serving	3½	100.0	18.7	7.1	....	139.0
Mackerel, fresh (edible portion)	1 lb.	16	454.0	84.8	32.16	....	629.0
Mackerel, salted . .	1 serving	3½	100.0	16.3	17.4	....	222.0
Mackerel, salted . .	1 lb.	16	454.0	73.9	78.9	....	1007.0
Malted milk, Horlick's	1 tbsp.	½	14.0	2.3	1.2	9.5	59.0
Milk, whole . . .	1 tbsp.	7/10	20.0	0.06	0.8	1.0	14.0
Milk, whole . . .	1 cup	8⅝	244.0	8.0	9.3	12.2	169.0

Food material (uncooked).	Measure.	Weight.		Protein. Gms.	Fat. Gms.	Carbohydrates Gms.	Fuel value. Calories
		Oz.	Gms.				
Milk, whole . . .	1 quart	34⅜	975.0	32.2	39.0	48.8	675.0
Milk, skimmed . .	1 tbsp.	7/10	20.0	0.7	0.06	1.0	7.0
Milk, skimmed . .	1 cup	8⅝	244.0	8.3	0.7	12.5	89.0
Milk, skimmed . .	1 quart	34⅜	975.0	33.1	2.9	49.7	358.0
Molasses	1 tbsp.	⅞	27.0	0.6	....	18.7	77.0
Molasses	1 cup	11	317.0	7.6	....	219.7	909.0
Mutton chops . . .	1 serving	3½	100.0	16.0	33.1	....	362.0
Mutton chops . . .	1 lb.	16	454.0	72.5	150.1	....	1640.0
N							
Noodles, gluten . .	1 cup	3½	100.0	45.0	4.2	32.5	434.0
O							
Oatmeal, granulated .	1 tbsp.	½	14.0	1.8	0.9	9,9	55.0
Oatmeal, granulated .	1 cup	8	227.0	28.8	14.7	158.2	880.0
Oats, rolled . . .	1 tbsp.	⅙	5.0	0.7	0.3	2.7	16.0
Oats, rolled . . .	1 cup	2½	71.0	11.8	5.2	46.9	282.0
Olive oil, Nicelle . .	1 tbsp.	½	15.0	....	15.0	....	135.0
Olives	2 or 3	½	14.0	0.1	2.8	1.2	31.0
Onion	1 serving	4	113.0	1.8	0.3	11.2	56.0
Orange	1 medium	5	142.0	1.2	0.3	17.4	77.0
Orange juice . . .	1 tbsp.	½	14.0	....	....	1.6	6.0
Orange juice . . .	1 cup	8	227.0	....	....	25.6	104.0
Oysters	2	1	28.4	1.7	0.3	1.0	14.0
Oysters	1 cup (solid)	6	170.0	10.5	2.0	6.3	84.0
P							
Panopepton . . .	1 tbsp.	½	15.0	1.0	....	2.5	30.0
Peaches, fresh . . .	1 medium	4	113.0	0.8	0.1	11.3	50.0
Peaches, dried . .	1 cup	3	85.0	1.4	1.8	56.2	247.0
Peach juice . . .	1 tbsp.	½	14.0	....	....	1.1	5.0
Peach juice . . .	1 cup	8	227.0	....	....	17.6	80.0
Peanuts, shelled . .	1 cup	5	142.0	36.55	54.7	34.55	777.0
Peanut butter . .	1 tbsp.	9/16	16.0	4.8	7.7	2.8	100.0
Peas, green . . .	1 serving	4	113.0	7.7	0.5	19.6	114.0
Peas, canned . . .	1 cup	6½	184.0	6.6	0.4	18.0	100.0
Pea flour	1 cup	5	144.0	36.9	1.5	93.0	533.0
Pea flour	1 tbsp.	5/16	9.0	2.3	1.0	5.8	33.0
Pecans, shelled . .	1 cup	5½	156.0	15.0	110.0	23.8	1145.0
Pineapple, fresh (edible portion)	......	8	227.0	0.9	0.7	22.0	98.0
Pineapple, canned .	1 slice	3	85.0	0.4	0.6	31.0	130.5
Pineapple, canned .	1 cup	8	227.0	0.9	1.6	82.6	348.0
Pineapple, canned .	1 can	24	680.0	2.6	4.8	247.0	1044.0
Port wine (10 per cent. alcohol)	1 tbsp.	½	14.0	....	....	....	10.0
Potatoes, white . .	1 medium	3½	100.0	2.2	0.1	18.4	83.0
Potatoes, sweet . .	1 medium	3½	100.0	1.8	0.7	27.4	123.0
Prunes	1 cup	5	142.0	2.5	....	88.1	363.0
Prunes	3 prunes	1	28.4	0.5	....	17.6	72.0
Q							
Quail	1 serving	3½	100.0	21.8	8.0	....	159.0
R							
Raisins	1 doz.		9.0	0.2	0.3	6.5	29.0
Raisins	1 cup	4⅓	113.0	2.6	3.4	77.6	352.0
Raspberries, fresh, black (edible portion)	1 cup	5	142.0	2.4	1.4	17.8	94.0
Raspberry juice . .	1 cup	8	227.0	....	....	22.6	90.0
Rhubarb	......	1	28.4	0.2	0.2	1.0	6.0
Rhubarb	......	16	454.0	2.7	3.2	16.3	105.0
Rice	1 tbsp.	½	15.0	1.1	0.04	11.2	50.0
Rice	1 cup	8½	240.0	18.1	0.7	179.1	795.0
Rum	1 tbsp.	½	14.0	....	....	....	38.0

Food material (uncooked).	Measure.	Weight. Oz.	Weight. Gms.	Protein. Gms.	Fat. Gms.	Carbo-hydrates Gms.	Fuel value. Calories.
S							
Salmon, edible portion	1 serving	3½	100.0	22.0	12.8	....	203.0
Salmon, edible portion	1 lb.	16	454.0	99.6	57.9	....	922.0
Saltines	1 wafer	⅛	3.0	0.4	0.5	2.4	15.0
Sardines, canned . .	1 serving	3½	100.0	23.0	19.7	....	269.0
Sardines, canned . .	1 can	16	454.0	104.3	89.2	....	1221.0
Shad (edible portion)	1 serving	3½	100.0	18.8	9.5	....	161.0
Shad (edible portion)	1 lb.	16	454.0	85.1	43.0	....	729.0
Shad roe	1 serving	3½	100.0	20.9	3.8	26.0	128.0
Sherry	1 tbsp.	½	14.0	....	....	....	13.0
Spinach	1 serving	4	⅓	2.3	0.3	3.6	27.0
Squabs	1 serving	3½	100.0	16.3	36.2	....	391.0
Squash	1 serving	3½	100.0	1.4	0.5	9.0	46.0
Strawberries (ed. port.)	1 serving	4	113.0	1.0	0.7	7.9	42.0
Strawberrier (ed. port.)	1 cup	6	170.0	1.5	1.0	11.9	63.0
Strawberry juice . .	1 cup	8	227.0	....	....	11.4	45.0
Suet	1 tbsp.	½	14.0	0.66	11.59	....	107.0
Suet	1 lb.	16	454.0	21.28	371.0	....	3425.0
Sugar, granulated .	1 tbsp.	½+	15.0	....	....	15.0	60.0
Sugar, granulated .	1 cup	7½	210.0	....	....	210.0	840.0
Sugar, loaf . . .	1 lump	¼	7.6	....	....	7.6	30.0
Sugar, loaf . . .	1 cup	6½	184.0	....	....	184.0	736.0
Sugar, powdered . .	1 tbsp.	½	12.0	....	....	12.0	48.0
Sugar, powdered . .	1 cup	6½	184.0	....	....	184.0	736.0
Sugar of milk . . .	......	....	1.0	....	....	100 0%	4.1
Sugar of milk . . .	1 teaspoon (av. size)	0.164	5.0	....	....	100.0%	20.5
Sugar of milk . . .	1 tbsp.	0.564	16.0	....	....	100.0%	65.6
Sweetbreads . . .	1 serving	3½	100.0	16.8	12.1	....	176.0
Sweetbreads . . .	1 lb.	16	454.0	76.2	54.8	....	798.0
Sweetbreads . . .	1 pair (med. size)	8	227.0	38.1	27.4	....	399.0
T							
Tapioca, pearled . .	1 tbsp.	½	14.0	0.03	....	12.3	49.0
Tapioca, pearled . .	1 cup	6½	184.0	0.4	....	159.5	640.0
Tapioca, minute . .	1 tbsp.	½	14.0	0.03	....	12.2	49.0
Tomatoes	1 tbsp.	½+	15.0	0.2	0.03	0.6	4.0
Tomatoes	1 cup	8	227.0	2.7	0.5	9.0	51.0
Tomatoes	1 medium (whole tomato)	5	142.0	0.5	0.3	3.0	16.0
Trout (edible portion)	1 serving	3½	100.0	17.8	10.3	....	164.0
Trout (edible portion)	1 lb.	16	454.0	80.6	46.7	....	743.0
Turnip	1 serving	3½	100.0	1.3	0.2	8.1	39.0
Turkey (edible portion)	1 serving	3½	100.0	21.1	22.9	....	290.5
Turkey (edible portion)	1 lb.	16	454.0	95.7	103.9	....	1317.0
W							
Walnuts, English . .	1 cup	5½	156.0	25.8	98.8	25.1	1093.0
Walnuts, English . .	1 meat	....	1.0	0.17	0.63	0.16	7.0
Whey	1 glass	6½	184.0	1.8	0.5	9.3	50.0
Whitefish (ed. port.) .	1 serving	3½	100.0	22.9	6.5	....	150.0
Whitefish (ed. port.) .	1 lb.	16	454.0	103.8	29:4	....	681.0

INDEX

A

Lightning Source UK Ltd.
Milton Keynes UK

176755UK00002B/51/P